THE ANCESTRAL DIET REVOLUTION

HOW VEGETABLE OILS AND PROCESSED
FOODS DESTROY OUR HEALTH –
AND HOW TO RECOVER!

*Prevent, Treat, and Often Reverse Most Chronic Diseases,
Including Overweight, Obesity, Heart Disease, Cancers, Metabolic Syndrome,
Diabetes, Alzheimer's, Macular Degeneration, Autoimmune Disease, Anxiety,
Depression, and Much, Much More, With Natural, Ancestral Diets*

CHRIS KNOBBE, MD
& SUZANNE ALEXANDER, M.Ed.

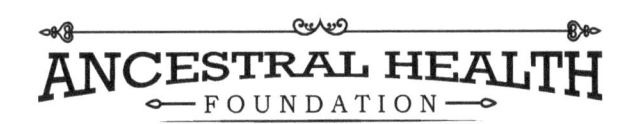

ANCESTRAL HEALTH
FOUNDATION

Copyright © 2023 by Chris A. Knobbe, Ancestral Health Foundation

Cover Design by: Ana Secivanovic

Book Formatting by: Jennifer Woodhead and Ana Secivanovic

Graphs and Tables (not otherwise attributed) by: Chris Knobbe, MD, Syed Murad Ali Jaffery, ACCA, MA, and Marija Stojanoska, MSc

ISBN: 978-1-7340717-4-0

Published by Ancestral Health Foundation
Boulder, Colorado
First eBook and Print Editions, 2023

All rights reserved. In accordance with the U.S. Copyright Act of 1976, this work in its entirety is protected by United States International Copyright law. Any attempt to duplicate all or any part of this work, by re-creating, scanning, uploading, electronic sharing, or otherwise without the express written consent of the authors constitutes unlawful piracy, copyright infringement, and theft of intellectual property.

Any attempt to summarize this work, in any manner beyond one or two brief paragraphs with appropriate citation, may be considered to infringe upon U.S. and international copyright and intellectual property rights, is unlawful, and may be subject to legal action to the full extent of the law. For any review or quote beyond one or two paragraphs, please contact the authors. Thank you for your support of the authors' legal and intellectual property rights.

This book contains certain opinions from the authors. It is intended to provide general nutritional advice deemed to be beneficial for the prevention and treatment of many chronic diseases. This book is made available to the public with the understanding that the authors are not engaged in delivering personalized or individual medical, health, or treatment advice. The authors and publisher specifically disclaim all responsibility for any liability, loss, or risk – personal or otherwise – by the use and application of any of the contents of this book.

DEDICATION

Dedicated to the pioneering work and memory of Weston A. Price, without whom this research and book may have ever even begun. One day when we meet in Heaven, I'll finally be able to thank you. I only hope that my life's work will meet with your approval.

In memory of my sister, Jan, whose life and love still inspire me each day.

To you, Suzie, what an honor and privilege to ever even know a person so selfless as you. Your life, love, commitment, and integrity inspire me each day. Thank you for working tirelessly and endlessly, day in and day out, with your only reward being the benefit of others whose lives we touch.

And most of all, for my daughter, Kyla, who could never know how much I love her. Your life, love, joy, and spirit have brought more meaning to my life than anything else ever could.

– C.K.

In loving memory of my father, Dr. William Alexander, and brother, Glyn: Your extraordinary love lives on in my heart.

To my mother, Roxane: I'm so in awe of how you handle the loss of your vision from AMD and never allow adversity to weaken your faith and trust in God. I love you so much!

To Chris: I can't thank you enough for giving me this incredible opportunity to work so closely with you to bring this book to fruition. It has been a tremendous honor to learn from you and to watch you at work, always giving every ounce of your being to your research, seeking the truth, and dedicating your life to healing others.

For you, my beautiful daughters, Alexandra, Roxana, and precious granddaughter, Claire: My most treasured blessings from God. You are the light of my life. I'll love you forever!

PSALM 118:28-29

– S.A.

PRAISE FOR
THE ANCESTRAL DIET REVOLUTION

"Dr. Chris Knobbe has done it again! If Chris hasn't convinced you yet, *The Ancestral Diet Revolution* will show you that the number one action you can take to be healthy and slim is to avoid all industrial seed oils! Then, embrace the foods of your ancestors and enjoy your journey to perfect health!"

> Sally Fallon Morell, President
> The Weston A. Price Foundation
> Author of the book, *Nourishing Traditions*

"Chris Knobbe has produced evidence linking omega-6 seed oils as a driver of overweight, coronary heart disease, cancers, type 2 diabetes, and many chronic diseases. I support this book."

> Loren Cordain, PhD
> Founder of the term "Paleo Diet"
> Author of *The Paleo Diet*, *The Paleo Answer*, and *The Real Paleo Diet Cookbook*

"Dr. Knobbe's book, *The Ancestral Diet Revolution*, presents a vast body of research, both published and original, which culminates in profound conclusions: We can prevent and reverse overweight, obesity, and most all chronic diseases, simply by avoiding processed foods and, primarily, by the avoidance of industrial seed oils. This book is not only revolutionary, methodical, and scientific, but the new and originally produced supportive evidence is absolutely stunning."

> Dr. Aseem Malhotra
> Consultant Cardiologist, United Kingdom, NHS
> Author of the book, *A Statin Free Life*
> World Renowned Public Health Advocate

"Seed oils are perhaps the single greatest driver of illness and disease today, and they are pervasive in our food supply. In this book, Chris has done a fantastic job of breaking down the history of their intrusion into our food, the science of why they are harmful, and how you can massively improve your health by avoiding them. If you care about your health, read this book and share with those you care about."

> Paul Saladino, MD
> AKA "Carnivore MD"
> Author of the book, *The Carnivore Code*
> Host of the Podcast: "Fundamental Health with Paul Saladino, MD"

"Chris Knobbe has written a masterpiece of work with his latest book, *The Ancestral Diet Revolution*. Regardless of your food preferences, an in-depth review of basic scientific principles supports the removal of toxic, nutrient-deficient, inflammatory, pro-oxidative seed oils from your diet. Perhaps surprisingly, the reader will come to understand why chronic diseases like type 2 diabetes, obesity, cancer, heart disease, Alzheimer's, macular degeneration, and many others are increasing despite evidence of declining sugar and carbohydrate use over the past 2 decades. A convincing argument for eating whole foods while eliminating seed oils seems plausible and strongly supported by the evidence. I would strongly recommend this book to all healthcare professionals, dieticians, nutrition coaches, or anyone interested in improving their health and well-being."

> J.R. Cripps MD FRCSC (Emeritus)
> Nutrition Network Practitioner
> Assistant Professor of Surgery
> Northern Ontario School of Medicine (NOSM), retired

"The Ancestral Diet Revolution is a must-read for anyone interested in optimizing health and preventing or reversing chronic disease. The book provides a comprehensive review of the science as well as the evolutionary wisdom that should guide your dietary choices. Dr. Knobbe and Ms. Alexander provide the blueprint that you need to achieve your best health results."

> Philip Ovadia MD
> Cardiothoracic Surgeon
> Metabolic Health Specialist
> Author of the book, *Stay Off My Operating Table*

"There are many books about nutrition, but very few books like **The Ancestral Diet Revolution.** Blending what is known of the ancestral diet of our ancestors for eons, modern nutrition research, along with a strong dose of common sense, is the perfect recipe for nutrition guidance that will improve your overall health and set you up for a long and happy health-span!"

> Ken D. Berry, MD, Family Practitioner
> Host: KenDBerryMD YouTube Channel
> Author of the book, *Lies My Doctor Told Me: Medical Myths That Can Harm Your Health*

"Dr. Chris Knobbe leaves no stone unturned in his blistering exposé of ALL the hidden dangers of the most alarming food toxin hidden in plain sight – vegetable oils."

> Professor Aaron P. Blaisdell, PhD
> Director, UCLA Comparative Cognition Lab
> UCLA Brain Research Institute / UCLA Evolutionary Medicine Program
> Co-Founder, Ancestral Health Society
> Editor-in-Chief, Journal of Evolution and Health

"Seed oils. Bad stuff.

"Our food is fried in them… at restaurants, at takeout's, at home. Most packaged consumables are soaked with them. Cheap. Not essential. Not healthy. Guzzled down by the bucket load.

"We've been encouraged by our health system to ingest seed oils for over 40 years. Saturated fat has been discouraged, with no strong evidence. And to our detriment.

"Unlike natural saturated fat, industrially-produced seed oils are a metabolic disrupter, driving insulin resistance and chronic disease… a worldwide epidemic of chronic disease. And blindness.

"Chris Knobbe's timely and important book sheds a powerful light on the far-reaching harms of this insidious and ubiquitous fat.

"Avoid seed oils. Avoid ultra-processed substances. Butter is better. Most things are better."

> Dr. James Muecke, AM
> Eye Surgeon and Blindness Prevention Pioneer
> Australian of the Year - 2020
> Co-Founder Sight for All

"Ophthalmologist Dr. Chris Knobbe has written a book full of convincing evidence that it is the seed oils in the modern diet rather than sugar that constitute the major cause of chronic disease. This well-illustrated and fully referenced book challenges traditional beliefs and should be read by anyone interested in the link between nutrition and chronic disease. Fascinating reading!"

    Professor Peter Brukner, OAM, D Sc, MBBS, FACSP
    Sport and Exercise Medicine Physician
    Professor of Sports Medicine, La Trobe University, Melbourne, Australia
    Chair, *SugarByHalf* & *Defeat Diabetes*

"*The Ancestral Diet Revolution* is an incredibly well-researched book that makes a compelling case that the dramatic increase in the consumption of industrially processed vegetable and seed oils - often promoted to the public as "healthy" - has been a major contributor to a simultaneous rise in a wide variety of devastating chronic diseases. As a nutritional epidemiologist, I have been frustrated by the many flawed studies and deep financial conflicts of interest that have led to mistakes in dietary policy that have harmed our health.

"*The Ancestral Diet Revolution* is not only thoroughly supported by an extraordinary amount of citations from the medical literature, it is a thoroughly engaging read that vividly describes the history of dietary intake patterns from traditional cultures to today, through illustrative photographs and documentation of the increases in diet-related chronic disease that have occurred when excessive amounts of seed oils have entered the diet. Scientific mechanisms underlying the harms of industrially processed vegetable and seed oils are presented.

"Importantly, *The Ancestral Diet Revolution* also offers practical dietary solutions that will undoubtedly help reverse the rising tide of chronic disease that is occurring worldwide. I highly recommend that healthcare professionals and the general public alike read this eye-opening book."

    Chris D'Adamo, Ph.D.
    University of Maryland School of Medicine
    Director, Center for Integrative Medicine
    Assistant Professor, Department of Family and Community Medicine
    Department of Epidemiology and Public Health

"A compelling, articulate, scientific and common sense argument of the proximate cause of modern diseases. The toxicity of 'vegetable oils' is explained in granular detail from historical, population-based data as well as animal studies. It is a must-read for anyone who wants to be healthy and free of obesity, diabetes, dementia, heart disease, and cancer."

>   Nadir Ali, MD
>   Low Carbohydrate Interventional Cardiologist
>   Founder: Low Carb Houston

"Anyone seeking insight into nutrition and health is hit by an instant deluge of information overload. Each week brings a mountain of publications along with a plethora of websites, blogs, podcasts, and videos. Contradictions abound: vegan or carnivore; plant-based or animal-based (with or without paradoxes); low-carb or low-fat; low-protein or high-protein? Having battled through the macros, then, should we time-restrict our eating and analyze our gut microbiome, or give up and focus on the specifics of mTOR, DNA methylation and telomere length?

"When opposing beliefs are held with religious fervor, rational debate fails. Add to this the massive financial drivers directing Big Food and Big Pharma, along with the ravenous needs of university funding and a self-perpetuating medical publication industry, and impartial guidance becomes a Holy Grail.

"Through a meticulous examination of the medical history of our last 200 years, along with comparative epidemiology and dietary change across the globe, Dr. Knobbe constructs a cogent and compelling argument for defects in basic nutrition as a primary cause of the devastating diseases of modern civilization.

"The tenets of ancestral health are well-recognized, and the potential toxicity of seed oils has been acknowledged for some years, but through a data-driven approach and a scrupulous analysis of the correlation between diet and our most common diseases, Dr. Knobbe focuses the spotlight on a single, identifiable and modifiable aetiology. With an understanding of the cellular effects of seed oils and the broader ramifications of their many potentially pathological actions, the jigsaw falls into place. The resulting picture is alarming, the facts are stark, and without change, the prospect of robust health in the developed world looks bleak.

"This book provides an excellent and well-referenced argument in support of a massive dietary change for billions. Anticipating the necessary paradigm shift in the thinking of governments and global health agencies appears hopelessly optimistic, but by presenting a unifying concept to the different sides of the nutritional health debate, Dr. Knobbe may at least unite and focus what has been a disparate group. Until then, I strongly advise you to consider Dr. Knobbe's arguments carefully, take the necessary steps to improve your own health, and share this critically important message."

> Andrew J. Luff, MA, FRCS, FRCOphth
> Founding Ophthalmologist, Sapphire Eyecare
> Vitreoretinal Surgeon
> Professor, University of Chichester, United Kingdom

"Dr. Chris Knobbe has done a tremendous job in making the argument that hyper-processed foods and one of their most common ingredients, the industrial seed oils, have played a unique and fundamental role in the undeniable public health crisis. With over 1300 scientific references and tremendous attention to the historical record, Dr. Knobbe makes a very powerful argument that perhaps these new additions to our diets are not something we were designed to eat and are clearly harming us. Beautifully illustrated and full of graphical information, this book belongs in the personal library of anyone that cares about their health!"

> Shawn Baker, MD
> Orthopedic Surgeon and World-Class Athlete
> Modern-Day Founder of the Carnivore Diet
> Author of the best-selling book, *The Carnivore Diet*

"The book is well written, engaging, and perfected with illustrations synchronized with text on the same pages – what a pleasure and growth as we read it. It has this original insight of what has been causing this complex of epidemics of chronic diseases and even cancers.

"After more than a decade of researching the evidence of ancestral nutrition and tracking the contemporary changes from creation and introduction of industrialized food in our diet, this book is written with the very profound knowledge of this subject.

"Very impressive, it cites within the text more than 1,300 relevant references of scientific papers, documents, and current publications of worldwide organizations and government reports that give a solid base for harvesting data of production and consumption of foods by the people of the country

– nothing is left off table. It allows the reader to go after these references at will. It is carefully and generously written for the best and easy understanding for the reader.

"In contrast to the short duration of epidemiological studies that are based on asking someone to recall what and how much one has eaten in the last year and making extrapolations assuming that one kept that diet for many years to infer causality on disease or health, the writers' approach was based on long term epidemiologic data of different groups of people contrasting their ancestral health and diet with those after dietary changes were introduced over generations – This is solid epidemiologic evidence not seen yet!

"I am thankful to the authors for this true wake-up call based on facts interrelated with logic and science. I have already implemented this teaching in my daily choices and life."

>Julio Lutterbach, MD
>Pediatric Cardiologist and Clinical Instructor
>University of Colorado School of Medicine, Cardiology
>Children's Hospital Colorado

"The *Ancestral Diet Revolution* is a modern-day masterpiece and a must-read for every medical student that rotates through my clinic...and for every patient too! This book makes a strong case that it won't be the research labs in the ivory towers producing the next great pharmaceutical that will turn around this modern epidemic of chronic diseases, but rather, looking back at the eating habits of our healthy ancestors!

"Dr. Knobbe combines a fascinating journey back in history with modern-day science to make a very strong case for modern processed foods, and seed oils in particular, being the driving force behind the chronic inflammation-based modern disease epidemic. I predict that societies and medical professionals of today who embrace the truth found in *The Ancestral Diet Revolution* will reap the reward of health, and those who continue on with the modern-day, processed food diet will continue to trudge along in the quagmire of seemingly 'unpreventable' chronic disease."

>Ben Edwards, MD
>Family Practice Physician
>Veritas Medical Founder and Medical Director
>Host of "You're the Cure!" Radio Show

"I love new ideas, and this is a provocative one supported by strong epidemiology — it is definitely a hypothesis worth testing!"

>Richard Johnson, MD
>Professor of Medicine, Internal Medicine and Nephrology
>University of Colorado School of Medicine
>Author of *"Nature Wants Us To Be Fat"*

"Dr. Knobbe has spent many years researching why chronic diseases have exploded in the U.S. and modern societies. Through Dr. Knobbe's extensive research and passion to help others, he takes the reader on an edge-of-your-seat journey. This amazing life-changing book highlights why the main culprit of chronic disease is not high saturated fat intake or even sugar, but rather, it is seed oils.

"The Ancestral Diet Revolution has over 1000 references highlighting many cultures, revealing how cancer, cardiovascular disease, and even blindness from macular degeneration can be traced to the introduction of seed oils. Wow, congratulations and a big thank you, Dr. Knobbe, for an incredible life-changing wake-up call and an enlightening reading experience!"

>Dr. Kerry Gelb, Optometric Physician
>Radio Host and Podcast Host
>Documentary writer and host (*Open Your Eyes* film and podcast)

"Dr. Knobbe gives us a priceless compendium of the research that the food and drug industries all want us to ignore. This life-changing science should make the medical news, and the fact that it doesn't speaks volumes. The sheer weight of damning evidence against seed oils will blow you away."

>Cate Shanahan, MD
>Medical Director, ABC Metabolic Health Center
>LA Lakers PRO Nutrition Creator
>NY Times Bestselling Author of *Deep Nutrition* and *The FATBURN Fix*

"It is a scientific and practical struggle to make sense of the roles of macronutrient proportions, sugars, refined carbs, and various proteins and fats in our health and well-being. Same regarding plant-based versus animal-based nutrients. How can we come to understand what's causing the modern plague of chronic, non-communicable diseases? What's the role of dietary inputs? In the middle of this conundrum, the Diet Wars confuse more than edify. By going into the historical record, pulling together critical bits from research, and forcing us to clearly view the evidence, Chris Knobbe has given us a gift of profound insight into the mechanisms of modern chronic diseases.

"Is there a nutritional component that consistently tracks with the onset and increases of chronic non-infectious diseases? The answer is yes. It's the commercial seed oils (and other sources) that have loaded our modern diet with excess Omega-6 fatty acids (and the especially destructive linoleic acid). Many pieces of the puzzle now fit together. We can now see that high-carb vs. low-carb or plant vs. animal is not the core issue. What emerges instead is the dominant role played by linoleic acid in provoking obesity and disease.

"There are many good books, but few truly warrant the label "game changer." This book by Chris Knobbe is one of the few. Those who read with curiosity and an open mind will find an entirely new way of understanding many of the disease processes haunting our modern lives. As a researcher and clinician, I am so thankful that Chris delivered this heroic piece of work."

>Gary V. Koyen, Ph.D.
>Founder & CEO of Cruxpoint Health Breakthrough, Inc.

WHY ARE WE DYING?

"While it is accepted that the only certainties in life are death and taxes, there's a growing interest in the causes of and solutions to premature death. In millennia past, average life expectancy was much shorter due mainly to deaths in childbirth, infections, starvation and being killed in tribal warfare. None of these things apply today so why is the developed world getting fatter and sicker by the day? In westernized, industrialized countries, healthy life expectancy (health span) has been going backward for decades. In recent years life expectancy (lifespan) itself first plateaued and then began to decline, despite our ever-growing investment in health systems.

"What are the root causes of today's biggest killers – namely type 2 diabetes, heart disease, cancer, and dementia? Why has heart disease, a disease virtually unknown 100+ years ago, doubled, redoubled, quadrupled, and doubled again until it became the single largest killer, killing one in three of us? The answer has to be lifestyle related, and many of us have fingered sugar and processed carbs as the suspect.

"Dr. Knobbe argues differently. He would have us believe that it's the ascendancy of seed (aka vegetable) oils in the human diet that is the prime offender. In his tour-de-force new book, he presents a comprehensive analysis of the worldwide epidemiological evidence in support of his arguments.

"Ultra-processed foods, laden with seed oils, are not only toxic in themselves but are short on the essential nutrients (vitamins, minerals, animal protein, and natural fats) that we humans need to survive and thrive. It's not (he argues) about the calories, nor can it be primarily our sugar consumption, because the obesity epidemic continues apace despite REDUCTIONS in both carbohydrates and sugars in various populations in recent decades. However, the one constant is the inexorable rise of vegetable oils in the human diet.

"If you want to live long and die well, as I do, this book is a thought-provoking 'must-read!'"

    Graham Phillips, B Pharm, Dipp Comm Pharm, FRPharmS
    AKA "The Pharmacist Who Gave Up Drugs"
    London, England

"The Ancestral Diet Revolution is a must-read for anyone looking to escape from the modern industrial food system. Authors Chris Knobbe and Suzanne Alexander illustrate the dangers of vegetable oils and processed food and explain how an ancestral dietary approach is the key to regaining human health."

    Dr. Bill Schindler, PhD
    Co-Star of the National Geographic Channel series, "The Great Human Race"
    Author of the book, *Eat Like a Human: Nourishing Foods and Ancient Ways of Cooking to Revolutionize Your Health*

"Many of us are aware of problems when processed food is consumed. However, most people have not yet learned of the harmful effects of vegetable oils. Our family rid our pantry of them in 2014, never to return! We have not missed them as there are good alternatives.

"This is a beautifully written book, well researched, laid out, and easily readable. Do your health a favour and read it!"

>Dr. Rod Tayler FANZCA, Anesthesiologist
>Founder of Low Carb Down Under
>Albert Park, Victoria, Australia

"This is an excellent book. Dr. Knobbe makes a very compelling case for the recent and persistent rise in chronic diseases being directly related to the hard shift away from our ancestral human diet to one of highly processed foods and seed oils, something that I strongly agree with. He lays out hard evidence from decades' worth of peer-reviewed literature, along with historical records and anthropological data, with over 1,300 separate references in total. This is a thoroughly well-thought-out and researched book, which reads like a novel but could, and probably should, be used in university-level nutritional science courses. If you want to understand the root cause of most modern diseases and learn how you can prevent or even reverse them, this book is a must-read."

>Anthony Chaffee, MD
>Neurosurgical Resident
>Host of "The Plant Free MD" Podcast

"I received my Ph.D. in Mechanical Engineering from the University of Illinois and planned on becoming a University Professor. However, from the time of high-school through graduate school, a series of progressively daunting health challenges affected me, including amenorrhea (no period for 12 years), autoimmunity, gut issues, polycystic ovarian syndrome (PCOS), insomnia, iron overload, and orthorexia, all of which haunted me and threatened my overall well-being. All of this occurred while I ate an omega-6 heavy diet, over-exercised, remained lean and committed to a rigorous college athletic program. Similar health challenges affected my younger sister, Sarah. During this time of self-discovery, I became progressively more passionate about nutrition and regenerative agriculture. So instead of becoming a university professor, I decided to become a first-generation regenerative farmer, and my sister Sarah and I initiated Angel Acres Farm. Dr. Chris Knobbe's work on the dangers of seed oils and high omega-6 diets strongly influenced my own diet, but he also inspired me to produce chicken eggs with low omega-6 linoleic acid (LA) levels.

"We are now proud to say that, while following low omega-6 ancestral diets ourselves, we're not only recovering our own health, but we're providing healthy low omega-6 LA eggs, milk, and meats, for hundreds of families across the country.

"I cannot recommend Dr. Knobbe's book, *The Ancestral Diet Revolution*, enough. It is a paradigm-shifting book with critically important concepts on ancestral diets and health supported by thousands of scientific studies. If you care about maintaining or recovering your own health, learning why it is vital that our diets are low in linoleic acid, or are in need of evidence to share with family and friends why they should be eating more ancestrally, this book is a must-read! You will walk away with a very clear understanding of how we should be eating and how inverted the current food pyramid is!"

> Ashley Armstrong, PhD, MS, BS, Mechanical Engineering
> Proprietor, Angel Acres Farm, Marcellus, Michigan
> Host: "Rooted in Resilience" Podcast

"An eye-opening book that brings to light a key element of our health care crisis. Dr. Knobbe is bold to take on this sensitive subject and bring out to the masses critical information that can have a profound and lasting impact on everyone's health."

> Mariela Glandt, MD
> Endocrinologist
> Founder: OwnaHealth and Metabolix NGO, Tel Aviv, Israel

"The evidence Chris has brought against seed oils in this book, The Ancestral Diet Revolution, in regard to overweight, obesity, coronary heart disease, cancer, diabetes, metabolic syndrome, Alzheimer's disease, and more, rises to the level of causative inference. As a biochemical engineer, I'm all about finding root causes. Look no further. This is the answer!"

> Ivor Cummins, BE (Chem), CEng MIEI PMP (Biochemical Engineering)
> Co-Author of the book, *Eat Rich Live Long* (with "Denver's Diet Doctor," Jeff Gerber, MD)
> Host of "The Fat Emperor" Podcast, Dublin, Ireland

"Out of the box thinking. Brilliant. This historical treasure trove of seminal information on the history of seed oils and their nefarious impact on our overall modern health, including cardiac, neurologic, cancer, endocrine, and retinal disease, is necessary reading for all physicians and retina docs aspiring to better patient care. Dr. Chris Knobbe's book, *The Ancestral Diet Revolution*, is a truly masterful anthology about the deleterious impact of processed foods, and this critical historical read documents a profiteering industry that touted and marketed 'seed oils' as vegetable oils to 'benefit' children. The modern physician needs to understand that our patients want "wellness."

"We retinal physicians have been browbeaten to follow Western 'evidence-based' medicine such as age-related eye disease (AREDS2) guidelines as the only way forward to slow degenerative disease, such as age-related macular degeneration (AMD). We need to be open to other contributing dietary and environmental impacts upon disease. Globalization has taught us to consider differences in the incidence of disease and to weigh the western diet as a greater contributor to ill health. Time to iterate and embrace 'rethinking.'"

> Robin D. Ross MD, MPH, CPH
> Clinical Assistant Professor, University of Arizona College of Medicine Phoenix
> Director, Global Retina Institute; Scottsdale, Arizona, USA

"It is no wonder that Dr. Chris Knobbe, an ophthalmologist, has seen the past, present, and future of the health of the world and its root causes. The rise of these modern chronic diseases, such as cancer, heart disease, macular degeneration, and diabetes, were rare until the foods and lifestyle of the Western world infiltrated the developing countries. The real nourishing foods, minds, and hearts of previous centuries are seen as too simple and oftentimes as distasteful or, ironically, as harmful, while the current lifestyle is unquestionably adopted and accelerated to every person throughout the world. This viral mass production is the true pandemic to which we must awaken our minds and seek to find the real essence of life in nature, in foods, in movement, and with our community and the world around us. Open your eyes to that which harms, although ever so slowly, as not to be noticed, until the boiling point of disease is upon you. The cause is attributed to age, genetics or bad luck, while the culprits of the Western lifestyle live on freely, propagating to our future generations. Dr. Knobbe's book is eye-opening. May you see and live full of health."

> Dr. Kevin Ham, MD, B.Sc Biochemistry

CONTENTS

PRAISE FOR THE ANCESTRAL DIET REVOLUTION

INTRODUCTION ... 13

CHAPTER 1:
LEARN FROM THE PAST TO HEAL IN THE PRESENT ... 19

Why Only Ancestral Diets Are Low in Omega-6 Linoleic Acid – or "LA" ... 20
The Science and Legacy of Weston A. Price ... 23
Native, Ancestral, Traditional, and Westernized Diets – A Brief Explanation ... 27
Food Processing in History ... 27
Added Sugars – Nutrient-Deficient Food ... 27
Seed Oils ('Vegetable Oils') – In 1865, They Were Not Considered Food! ... 28
Refined Wheat Flour and Other Refined Grains ... 38
Artificially Produced Trans-Fats ... 39
Processed Foods: Added Sugars, Refined Flours, Seed Oils, and Trans Fats ... 43
Sugar and Processed Carbohydrates Often Proposed as the Main Dietary Problem ... 43
Seed Oils Imposed Upon Processed Carbohydrates: A Deadly Combination ... 43
More Early 20th Century Research – E.V. McCollum – Seed Oils Cannot Sustain Life ... 47
Why Does Allopathic Conventional Medicine Recommend Seed Oils? ... 50
Chapter 1: Summary ... 52

CHAPTER 2:
PROCESSED FOODS AND SEED OIL DANGERS ... 55

The Emergence of Coronary Heart Disease and Markedly Increasing Cancer ... 56
An Early Word on Dietary Management of Disease Conditions ... 58
Processed Foods Vs. Natural Animal and Plant Foods – and Chronic Disease Outcomes ... 58
Westernized Chronic Diseases Are Rare or Virtually Absent in Hunter-Gatherers and Populations Consuming Native, Traditional Diets ... 62
Coronary Heart Disease Is a 20th Century Phenomenon ... 66

Birth of the Diet-Heart Hypothesis … 75

Smoking and CHD: Must Understand to Get the Whole Picture … 81

"Highly Unsaturated Fatty Acids" or HUFA, Increase CHD, and Come From LA … 82

The Much Ballyhooed Omega-6 to Omega-3 Ratio: Can We Fix it With More Omega-3s? … 83

Mid to Late 20th Century: Coronary Heart Disease Emerges in Africa … 87

The Maasai Tribe: Highest Saturated Animal Fat Consumption in the World, But Virtually No Heart Disease … 89

The Traditional Tokelauans – 50% Saturated Fat Diet, Yet No Coronary Heart Disease! … 93

The Tokelauans Devastating Health Transition – Driven by Processed Foods, Sugars, and Seed Oils … 96

Cancer is Another 20th Century Plague – Markedly Increasing in Parallel to Seed Oils … 100

Cancer Escalation in China – Along with Obesity, CHD, Diabetes, & Other Chronic Diseases – In Proportion to Seed Oils … 103

Rodent Studies Show Seed Oils Induce Far Higher Cancer Rates – With a Threshold Effect … 106

Chapter 2: Summary … **110**

CHAPTER 3:
MORE ON PROCESSED FOODS AND SEED OIL DANGERS … 113

Epidemics of Obesity, Diabetes, Metabolic Syndrome, Alzheimer's Disease, Autoimmune Diseases, Macular Degeneration, and More – All Aligned with Seed Oil Consumption … 114

Obesity Is Largely a Result of the Introduction of Seed Oils … 114

Body Mass Index (BMI) Increasing Since the 19th Century in All Age Groups! … 115

Seed Oil Consumption and Obesity in the World, Developed and Developing Countries, the U.S. and Vietnam – Circa Year 2000 … 124

Type 2 Diabetes Is a Disease Almost Entirely of Seed Oil Consumption – Escalating Even While Sugar Decreases! … 125

Metabolic Syndrome – Another Chronic Disease Driven by Seed Oils … 133

Alzheimer's Disease and Dementia – Parallel Rise with Seed Oils … 137

Autoimmune Diseases – Once Medical Rarities – Have Exploded in the 20th and 21st Centuries … 139

More than 100 Autoimmune Diseases Skyrocketing in Incidence and Prevalence … 140

Multiple Sclerosis (MS) Rises in Parallel to Seed Oils. … 140

Inflammatory Bowel Disease: Ulcerative Colitis and Crohn's Disease … 142

Autoimmune Diseases Skyrocket Globally in Correlation to Seed Oils … 143

Major Cause of Blindness – Age-Related Macular Degeneration – Is Yet Another Seed Oil Catastrophe … 145

Are Rare Diseases Becoming More Common Due to Processed Foods and Seed Oil Consumption? … 149

But Doesn't Low Life Expectancy in the 19th and Early 20th Centuries Account for Low
Chronic Disease Prevalence During that Era? 150

Can We Blame "Bad Genes" for Increasing Chronic Disease? 153

Chapter 3: Summary **156**

CHAPTER 4:
HOW AND WHY LINOLEIC ACID MAY BE HARMING YOU 159

Essential Fatty Acids: Omega-6 LA and Omega-3 ALA: Must Have, But in Small Amounts! 160

Paracelsus Paraphrased: 'The Dose Makes the Poison' 163

Why Seed Oils Are Far More Devastating than Sugar or Processed Carbs 165

Seed Oils Are Rich in Omega-6 LA, Which Accumulates in Our Body Fat 166

Omega-6 LA is Stored in Our Body Fat with a Half-Life of Nearly 2 Years! 169

New Zealand Māori – Once Brilliantly Healthy, With the Lowest Adipose LA% Ever Documented
– Now Suffer Devastating Health Effects of Seed Oils 170

LA% in Body Fat (Adipose) Increasing Over Time – Globally – In Parallel with Increasing
Seed Oil Consumption and Obesity 175

Sweden – LA Rises from 4% to 7% in Body Fat, With Parallel Rise in Obesity 177

U.K. – Like the U.S., Obesity & Chronic Disease Rising with Seed Oils, While Sugar Consumption Falls! 179

Australia and Australian Aboriginals: Populations With Rising Seed Oils, Obesity
and Chronic Disease – While Both Sugars and Carbs Fall 181

Papua New Guineans of Tukisenta: Extreme "High Carb" But Healthy! 186

High-PUFA Diets: Why They're Dangerous and Saturated Fats Are Healthy 190

How is Omega-6 LA Excess Driving Coronary Heart Disease? 190

It's Not Native LDL, But Rather, Oxidized LDL that is the Primary Driver of CHD 191

Why High-Fat Diets Have Often Been 'Proven' Dangerous 195

The Greenland Inuit or 'Eskimos' – Carnivores but Healthy and Heart Disease Free on Their Ancestral Diet 196

Diet and Disease in the Inuit: Obesity, Diabetes, and CHD Emerge with Seed Oil and Margarine Consumption 202

High Levels of Long-Chain Omega-3 Fats – Less Heart Attacks but More Strokes? 205

The Traditional Inuit Diet is Now Westernized – A Look Back at LA% in the Traditional Diet 207

Is Israel a 'Paradox'? The Quintessential Nation following the AHA's 'Heart Healthy Diet' Replete with
Vegetable Oils – But is it Working? 208

Chapter 4: Summary **213**

CHAPTER 5:
WHAT THE DEEPER SCIENCE SAYS — 217

Why Your LA Must Be Low! — 218
Simplified Molecular Biology of How and Why Excess LA Drives Obesity and Chronic Disease — 219
Seed Oils and High LA Diets Are Highly Pro-Oxidative — 219
Seed Oils Are Pro-Inflammatory — 226
Toxicity from Seed Oils: OxLAMs & ALEs Add Even More Harm — 226
HNE, the Classic and Most Toxic ALE, Increases with Cooking of Vegetable Oils — 231
Malondialdehyde (MDA): Another Destructive ALE from Seed Oils — 234
Acrolein, the Major Toxicant in Cigarette Smoke: Higher in Vegetable Oils! — 235
Carboxyethylpyrrole (CEP) – More Fallout from Seed Oil Excesses — 237
Omega-6 LA Excess, Mitochondrial Dysfunction, Overweight and Chronic Disease — 238
In a Low LA Diet, Oxidation is Low and Mitochondria Work Like a Marvel of Engineering — 238
In an Omega-6 LA Rich Diet, Oxidation is High and Mitochondria Begin to Fail — 239
Seed Oils Displace Animal Fats and Vitamins A, D, and K2: the Coup de Grâce of Seed Oil Devastation — 242
Vitamin A Deficiency: A Rampant Condition — 243
We Now Face a Pandemic of Vitamin D Deficiency, Despite Supplements — 247
Sunlight, Melatonin Production, and Mitochondrial Health: Beyond Vitamin D — 250
Vitamin K2 – The Final Fat-Soluble Vitamin to Complete the "Healthy Trio" — 252
Sugars Vs. Seed Oils: Why ALEs from Seed Oils Are Far Worse than AGEs from Sugars — 255
Animal Studies – Seed Oils Rapidly Induce Obesity, Diabetes, Fatty Liver, Insulin Resistance, and Heart Failure — 259
Another Study Indicates that High Omega-6 LA Diets Induce Obesity and Disease in Rodents — 260
More Animal Studies Prove Severe Weight Gain, Metabolic Disaster, and Heart Failure with Seed Oils — 263
Carnosine to the Rescue – the Sacrificial Sink for AGEs and ALEs — 264
Chapter 5: Summary — 266

CHAPTER 6:
THE MOST COMPELLING EVIDENCE OF ALL — 269

Seed Oils Are Devastating the Health of Japanese, Including Okinawans — 270
Increasing Global Chronic Disease Parallels the Rise in Vegetable Oil Consumption Historically — 278
Obesity and Chronic Disease Escalate Exponentially Worldwide, While Carbs Are Stable, Sugars Rise 5%, and 'Vegetable Oils' Approximately Double: 1975-2014 — 281
Healthy Populations: What Do They Not Consume? — 285

Healthy Babies and Children: Raising Them Ancestrally	286
Veganism and Vegetarianism: What Can We Learn? Advice and Cautions	290
Healthy Populations: Macronutrient Ratios Do Not Matter!	293
Omega-6 LA in Healthy Versus Chronic Disease-Riddled Populations	295
Why Do Low Carb Diets Work (When they do)?	295
Why Are Seed Oils Still in the Food Supply?	297
Have We Established Causality? Can We Convict Seed Oils for Obesity & Chronic Disease?	297
Chapter 6: Summary	**302**

CHAPTER 7:
THE ANCESTRAL DIET PROTOCOL 305

Processed Foods – Must Avoid!	306
High PUFA Seed ('Vegetable') Oils to Avoid	308
Fruit Oils – Coconut, Palm, Palm Kernel, Olive, and Avocado Oils – Far Safer	308
Nuts and Seeds Are Immense Sources of Omega-6 LA: Proceed with Caution!	311
Linoleic Acid (LA) in Ancestrally Raised Vs CAFO-Raised, Corn & Soy-Fed Animals	313
Ancestrally-Fed Vs Corn- and Soy-Fed Beef – The Main Problem with CAFO Beef	313
Ancestrally Fed Versus Corn- and Soy-Fed Chicken	314
Ancestrally Fed Versus Corn- and Soy-Fed Pork	315
LA Concentration in Beef Burgers Versus Plant-Based 'Burgers'	316
Ancestral Versus Other Varieties of Eggs	316
Wild-Caught Versus Farm-Raised Corn- and Soy-Fed Fish	317
The Benefits of a Low LA Ancestral Diet	320
Chapter 7: Summary	**321**

CHAPTER 8:
EAT ANCESTRALLY AND MOVE 325

Eliminate Processed Foods – It's Worth Repeating	326
Fractals of Health: Take the Next Big Steps	326
More Optimal Health: Consume Pasture-Raised Animals and Wild-Caught Fish	328
Most Optimal Health: Add Offal, Cod Liver Oil, Fish Eggs, and Other Nutrient-Rich Sources of Vitamins and Minerals	329

Final Dietary Tweaks: Based on Nutrient Testing	331
Exercise and Fitness: Final Critical Components of Health	331
Options for Farm Fresh Produce and Ancestrally Fed Meats	332
Our 10 Major Rules to Take Charge of Your Health Destiny	333
Chapter 8: Summary	**336**
EPILOGUE	339
WHERE TO FIND US	341
FOUNDATIONAL WEBSITES	341
A FEW OF OUR FAVORITE QUOTES	342
ENDNOTES	344
ABOUT THE AUTHORS	399

NUTRITION AND MEDICAL DISCLAIMER

This book is for general informational purposes only and does not provide individualized specific medical advice. The contents of this book should not be used to self-diagnose any condition, nor is it intended to be a substitute for a medical exam, diagnosis, treatment, prescription, recommendation, or cure. It does not create a doctor-patient relationship between the authors and yourself, or any reader.

Use of the contents of this book is at the reader's discretion. Please do not rely on this information as a substitute for professional medical advice, diagnosis, or treatment. If you have concerns or questions regarding your health, please consult a medical professional. The authors' statements within this book have not been evaluated or approved by the Food and Drug Administration. In fact, in this book, much of the evidence and conclusions submitted for your consideration do indeed conflict with the current and long-standing dogma and dietary advice of allopathic medicine.

You are personally and ultimately responsible for all decisions pertaining to your own health. Each individual has unique dietary needs and, perhaps, restrictions. By choosing to read this book, you hereby assume all responsibility for any use of its contents.

The authors and publishers are not responsible for any adverse reactions, effects, or consequences resulting from the use of dietary advice provided herein. We suggest that you not change your health regimen or diet without consulting your own personal physician.

INTRODUCTION

"Let's be clear: the work of science has nothing whatever to do with consensus. Consensus is the business of politics. Science, on the contrary, requires only one investigator who happens to be right, which means that he or she has results that are verifiable by reference to the real world. In science consensus is irrelevant. What is relevant is reproducible results.
The greatest scientists in history are great precisely because they broke with the consensus."

— MICHAEL CRICHTON, MD

INTRODUCTION

At the end of the American Civil War in 1865, the health of people all around the world stood in stark contrast to that of today. Chronic diseases were practically unheard of. Being overweight was exceedingly uncommon, and with only about 1% of all Americans qualifying as obese, that condition bordered on rarity.

Except for a few scholarly physicians, almost no one in the world had ever heard of a heart attack, and published reports of cases numbered fewer than ten. Cancer was attributable as the cause of death in only about 0.5% of cases, which might well be considered sporadic.

Diabetes was an extreme medical rarity, affecting fewer than three people per 100,000 (0.0028%), an unfathomable number by today's standards. Alzheimer's disease, dementia (of the non-syphilitic type), and age-related macular degeneration (a leading cause of blindness today) were all unknown. Autoimmune diseases, such as lupus, multiple sclerosis, and type 1 diabetes, all appear to have been unusual and possibly rare.

In short, being overweight and suffering from chronic diseases – the conditions and diseases that plague us today – were practically unknown. But why?

The most parsimonious explanation is that *the world had virtually no processed foods*, but more importantly, *the world had almost no vegetable oils*.

In fact, if you had mentioned the term "vegetable oils" to anyone in the world before 1865, they probably would have looked at you in bewilderment. The term hadn't even been coined. In that era, most of the world had not seen or consumed edible oil, and if they had, it was most likely olive oil (although there were trifling amounts of sesame and peanut oils in Asia and insignificant amounts of coconut, palm, and palm kernel oils, mostly in Africa and some tropical regions).

Just after the American Civil War, cottonseed oil was introduced into the American food supply, but it was a hard sell since Americans knew of cottonseed oil only as machine oil or lamp oil. Not to be deterred, manufacturers resorted to adulterating olive oil with cottonseed oil or mixing it with lard or butter to create "oleomargarine." Curiously, the same general practices persist today.

By the end of the nineteenth and beginning of the twentieth century, cottonseed oil manufacturers were generating handsome returns. The allure of profits led other industrialists to introduce soybean oil into the food supply in 1909. Then in 1911, Proctor & Gamble introduced Crisco, a semisolid chemical concoction derived from cottonseed oil, which would begin to compete with the traditional cooking fats – lard, butter, and beef tallow.

Over the next few decades, Industrial Revolution opportunists followed in their predecessors' "pioneering" footsteps, eventually producing the oils of corn, canola, rapeseed, grapeseed, sunflower, safflower, rice bran, and a few others. The Edible Oil Industry was born.

Over the next century, this industry succeeded in almost completely replacing added animal fats in the diet with so-called 'vegetable oils,' a euphemism with early twentieth-century roots, given that none of the oils are derived from vegetables. Pork lard became a relic of historical interest, beef tallow utilization and consumption fell into disfavor, and butter consumption dwindled to record lows.

The so-called 'heart-healthy' vegetable oils reigned as king. Early twentieth-century claims touting Proctor & Gamble's "new cooking fat," Crisco, as a "discovery" that would "affect every family in America" proved eerily prescient. By 1950, edible cooking oils, margarines, and Crisco, all unknown just eighty-five years previously, were poised to eventually almost completely replace animal fats for the added fats in the diet.

By 1961, with coronary heart disease reaching unprecedented levels and evidence that vegetable oils reduced blood cholesterol, American physiologist Ancel Keys introduced the "diet-heart hypothesis," an enigmatic theory which held that saturated fats elevated cholesterol, and cholesterol caused heart disease.

The American Heart Association, in affiliation with Keys, bolstered the theory with widespread advice for Americans to avoid saturated fats and embrace vegetable oils. Within a few decades, Keys and the American Heart Association had the support of Harvard, Mayo Clinic, Tufts University, Cleveland Clinic, and other prestigious institutions.

Curiously, however, investigative science journalists, researchers, and scientists collectively uncovered critically relevant, but hidden facts. The bulk of these chronic diseases, including the two big killers – coronary heart disease and cancer – were once either rare or unusual, as reviewed earlier.

The question thus became, what induced this onslaught of chronic disease? It couldn't possibly have been saturated fat, which had been consumed in large amounts in many diets since time immemorial.

Over the past eleven years, our combined research and investigations have proven one irrefutable fact:

Wherever vegetable oils are introduced into populations, a massive trail of destruction follows.

This includes increases in coronary heart disease (CHD), cancers, metabolic syndrome, type 2 diabetes, dementia, Alzheimer's disease, age-related macular degeneration (AMD), autoimmune diseases, and many other chronic disease conditions, many of which are proven to have increased at least thousands-of-fold, and perhaps infinitely.

And while obesity was found in only about 1% of Americans in the nineteenth century, as of 2018, obesity had risen to 42.5%, with another 31% being overweight, bringing the combined total of overweight and obese Americans to 74%. Worse yet, obesity in America is projected to reach 49% – essentially half of all Americans – by the year 2030.

As of 2015, a full 88% of Americans could not meet just five criteria of metabolic health, including healthy levels of blood glucose, triglycerides, HDL, blood pressure, and waist circumference, without associated medications. Just three years later, in 2018, it was shown that 93% of Americans failed to meet optimal cardiometabolic health based on an assessment of body fat, blood glucose, blood lipids, blood pressure, and clinical cardiovascular disease.

So you may be wondering, what are ancestral diets, how do they fundamentally differ from westernized diets, and where do vegetable oils fit into all of this? Ancestral diets are essentially the diets of our ancestors. They do not contain processed foods. And processed foods are based primarily upon the presence of refined (added) sugars, refined flours, vegetable oils, and trans fats.

For the sake of brevity, ancestral diets do not contain seed oils since the latter are products primarily born out of the Industrial Revolution. Consumption of vegetable oils in modernized, processed food-laden diets, induces "high LA diets," whereas the absence of vegetable oils is generally consistent with "low LA diets." And what is "LA," you ask?

LA is an abbreviation for linoleic acid, an essential fat of the omega-6 variety abundant in vegetable oils. In fact, LA accounts for only about 2% of the total fats in ancestrally raised animal sources, whereas most vegetable oils tend to range between 10% and 70% LA. Consumption of these high omega-6 LA-containing vegetable oils on any regular basis induces the accumulation of omega-6 LA within our body fat and cellular membranes.

And why does this matter? The omega-6 fat linoleic acid (LA), especially after accumulating in bodily tissues, drives a physiologic environment that is pro-oxidative, pro-inflammatory, toxic, and nutrient-deficient. This sets the stage for undesirable weight gain, metabolic chaos, and numerous chronic diseases.

In 1865, when vegetable oils did not exist in the United States, omega-6 LA accounted for only about 1/100th of the average American diet, but by 2008, LA accounted for an extraordinary 1/8th of the diet. And since 2008, vegetable oil consumption has continued to rise!

Vegetable oils represent the single-greatest change to the diet of mankind in all of history. If we look back to the year 1900, 99% of the added fats in the human diet were animal fats – mostly lard, butter, and beef tallow. But by 2005, 86% of added fats were vegetable oils. And with that came a massive consumption of omega-6 LA and a whole host of chronic diseases, most of which were completely unknown in the mid-nineteenth century before the introduction of 'vegetable oils.'

In this book, we will argue that vegetable oils are biological poisons, and just like any toxin, the more one consumes, the greater the harm. Their historical introduction and gradual increase proved to be a sophisticated means to insert a pernicious poison into a population, utilizing a slow, insidious displacement of animal fats, all the while advertising the oils and their derivatives as 'healthy.'

It is indisputable that conventional medicine fails to connect all these dots. Why? Because physicians educated in allopathic medical schools are not taught to consider the root cause of disease. Their teachings espouse the theory that chronic diseases result primarily from aging, "bad genes," and lifestyle choices, the latter of which are mostly related to smoking, excess alcohol consumption, or lack of exercise.

However, it is evident that if we cannot define the root cause of a condition or disease, we generally can neither prevent it nor properly treat it. Thus, a profoundly deep investigation and exposé is in order.

The public has grown weary of the floundering of modern medicine and nutritional theories. An article in *The Atlantic* recently began, "Much of what medical researchers conclude in their studies is misleading, exaggerated, or flat-out wrong." A recent study published in the *British Medical Journal* indicates that only 18% of clinical recommendations in medicine today are evidence-based.

This book, on the other hand, is a treatise in which we will show an overwhelming abundance of scientific evidence that enables us to derive causal inference with respect to vegetable oils and chronic disease. In other words, this evidence, we believe, will lead to accepted scientific theory that will one day be considered a fundamental law of nature, no different from any mathematical theorem or law of physics.

The scientific evidence presented herein includes that from numerous populations observed over many decades (even up to a century or more), correlative analyses, strength of the evidence, dose-response effects, experimental studies in animals, biological plausibility, and ultimately, a formal analysis of causality using the Bradford Hill criteria.

INTRODUCTION

Almost no statistics will be offered to draw these conclusions. They're rarely needed. In fact, we believe in the old adage, "If you need statistics to prove your point, you probably don't have one."

In light of that, we will show increases in obesity, coronary heart disease, cancers, diabetes, Alzheimer's disease, and many other diseases, often on the order of many-fold over shorter periods of time and up to many thousandfolds over long periods of time, all in correlation to markedly rising vegetable oils, leaving little room for speculation.

It will become obvious that while consumption of vegetable oils has increased infinitely on a global scale over the past 155 years, in parallel, so have chronic diseases. The evidence is incontrovertible.

Once we have a deep, fundamental understanding of the cause, treating the problem becomes simple, fundamental, and relatively easy. There's no more guesswork. No calorie counting, no futile exercise regimens designed for weight loss (they don't work), no low-fat or low-carb dieting. Just simple, straightforward ancestral dietary plans, eating the foods we want and desire, but with the ingredients from nature, instead of factories.

In this book, we'll provide simple strategies to implement an ancestral diet – the diet of our ancestors – which will not only prevent overweight or chronic disease but will also treat these conditions if they currently exist.

Sure, it will take vigilance and due diligence on your part if you wish to implement and stick with an ancestral diet, but rest assured, the benefits will rapidly accumulate.

Excess weight will almost effortlessly plunge. More importantly, the risks of heart attacks and heart disease, cancers, strokes, dementia, Alzheimer's disease, macular degeneration, and many other diseases will rapidly abate. Thousands and thousands of testimonials cannot be wrong.

By the time you've finished reading this, you can immediately begin to implement your own ancestral diet! It's simple. Start now by getting most all vegetable oils out of your diet. Then implement the additional strategies we've outlined.

It is our suggestion that you read every sentence in this book. The deity is in the details, and critically important foundational principles are scattered throughout these chapters. If you follow the formulas revealed within these pages, it is likely you will live a long, healthy life, free of disease, and full of abundance, joy, and peace of mind. Don't wait. Begin today!

It is truly an honor and pleasure to present this book to you. We thank you for buying it. Please share this book and your enthusiasm for its contents with your family, friends, and colleagues. You may save their lives as well as your own.

Let's begin…

CHAPTER 1

Three Aboriginal Australians on Bathurst Island in 1939. In 1929, 75% of Bathurst islanders supported themselves on local fauna and flora.

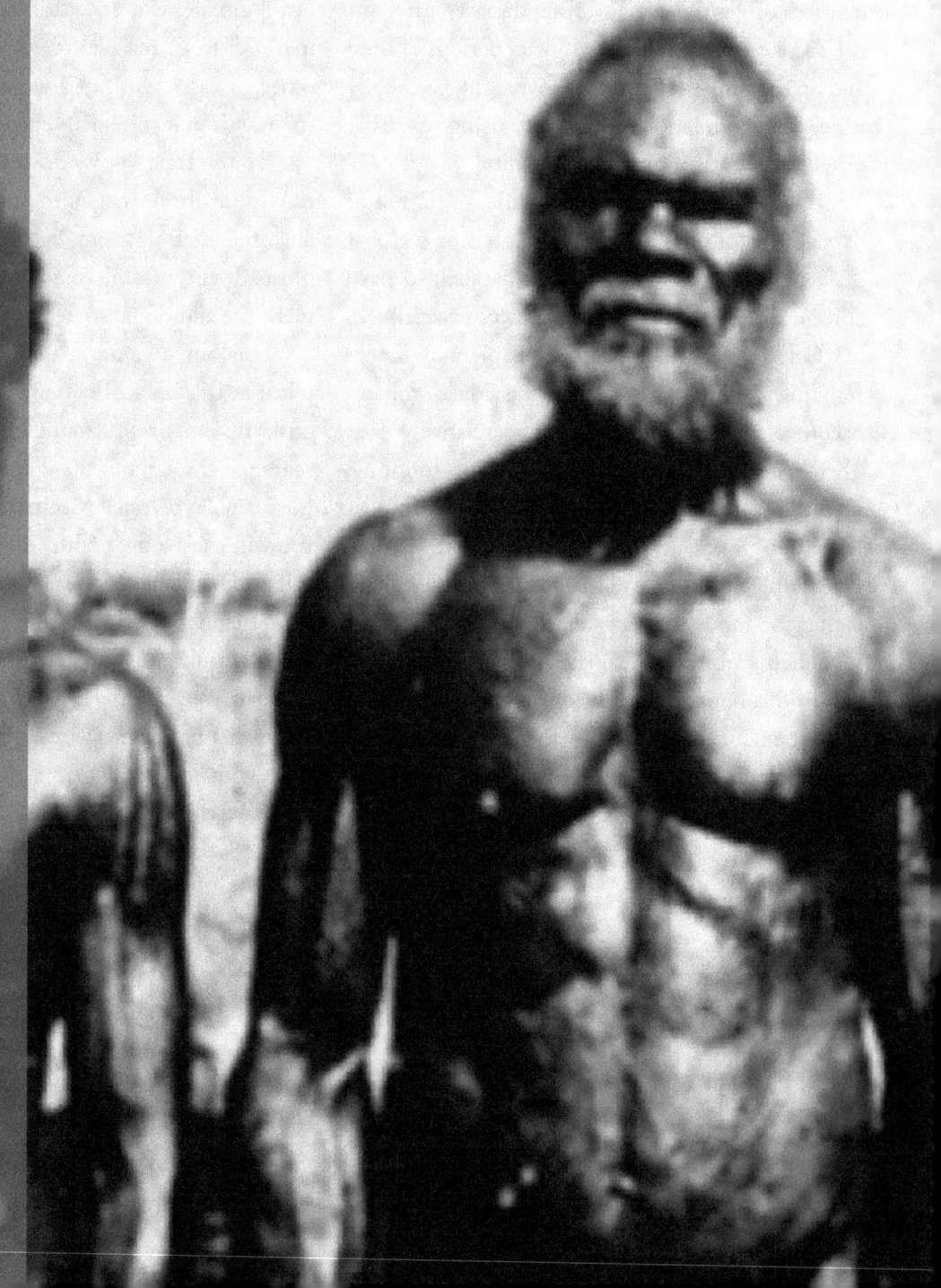

CHAPTER 1

LEARN FROM THE PAST TO HEAL IN THE PRESENT

"It is easier to fool people than to convince them they've been fooled."

— MARK TWAIN (APOCRYPHAL)

CHAPTER 1

Have we all been fooled? Have we been fooled for more than 60 years, duped into a belief system that the so-called 'vegetable oils' are healthy, when a mountain of evidence 'proves' they're not?

Could the 'vegetable oils,' which we'll generally call seed oils – since they're mostly from seeds and never from vegetables – be the primary and proximate cause of overweight, obesity, coronary heart disease (CHD), hypertension (high blood pressure), strokes, cancers, type 2 diabetes, metabolic syndrome, Alzheimer's disease, dementia, autoimmune diseases, age-related macular degeneration (AMD), and so much more, all while the "diet dictocrats" such as the American Heart Association,[461] Harvard School of Public Health,[462] Tufts University Department of Nutrition,[463] Mayo Clinic Department of Nutrition,[464] and many other academics, all tell us they're 'healthy,' 'heart-healthy,' 'lower the bad cholesterol,' and should be substituted for 'unhealthy animal fats'?

Taking it a step further, might the dietary advice, which purports that 'sugar is the villain' in obesity, diabetes, metabolic syndrome, and so much more, also be misaligned with the truth? And could it also be true that low carbohydrate ('low carb') diets might also be missing the primary problem, even when they work? Could it be that low sugar and low carbohydrate diets work, not primarily because they're eliminating sugar and 'carbs,' but because they're simultaneously eliminating a stealth fat that lurks within processed foods and most carbohydrate-rich foods everywhere? And might this elusive omega-6 fat, which is rather hidden in seed oils, be exacting its toll slowly, progressively, chronically, and insidiously, destroying our normal and healthy metabolism, all while its reputation is protected under the guise of being 'heart healthy'?

This is the hypothesis that we will present and defend in this book – the hypothesis that seed oils per se are the greatest threat to our health – driving overweight, heart disease, cancers, diabetes, metabolic syndrome and most other chronic diseases as well. In fact, we will boldly state that the history, correlations, deep science, metabolic pathways, and practically every shred of evidence related to overweight and chronic disease, will support this hypothesis.

WHY ONLY ANCESTRAL DIETS ARE LOW IN OMEGA-6 LINOLEIC ACID – OR "LA"

"LA" as used in this book, refers to a fat – or technically a fatty acid -- that we believe to be the primary contributor to virtually all chronic diseases. In fact, most doctors are not even aware of it, and precious few are aware of how pernicious it is when consumption is high.

What is it? *Linoleic acid, or LA.*

Linoleic acid, or LA, is an essential omega-6 fatty acid (or more simply fat), which is present in exceedingly small amounts in nearly all natural fat sources.[1] However, it is present in exponentially greater amounts in 'vegetable oils,'[1] which we'll generally refer to as seed oils, since they're primarily from seeds and never derived from vegetables.

Over the last 155 years, LA in the human diet has increased from about 2 to 3 grams a day up to 20 to 40 grams per person per day in many westernized diets.[2] In fact, our calculations confirm that, in the U.S. in the year 1865, before seed oils were available, LA consumption was about 2.2 grams/person/day (generally abbreviated g/day) in the American diet.[3]

However, with the advent of seed oil invention, production, and consumption, which began in the year 1866 in the U.S., LA consumption rose from approximately 2.2 g/day in 1865, to 4.84 g/day in 1909, to 18 g/day in 1999, and finally to 29 g/day by 2008.[4,5,6] Ergo, as a percentage of the diet, omega-6 LA consumption was almost exactly 1% of total dietary calories in 1865, about 2% in 1909, 7% in 1999, and 11.8% by 2008. Yet, seed oil consumption continues to climb, even since 2008, pushing omega-6 LA consumption even higher than the last cited figures.[4,3]

These are astonishing figures, that is, that today, the single omega-6 fat (fatty acid), linoleic acid (LA), which made up approximately 1/100th of the American diet just 157 years ago (1865), now makes up an average of 1/8th of our diet (as of 2008) and possibly more. And while considered an essential fat,[7] when consumed in excessive amounts, which we believe over 99% of westernized people do, LA (an omega-6 polyunsaturated fatty acid or PUFA) acts as a metabolic poison.[8,9,10,11]

LA is the primary omega-6 fat in seed oils, accounting for approximately 90% of the omega-6 composition of such oils.[12] We postulate and submit that, seed oils, which are the major dietary components of omega-6 LA in diets worldwide, are the single greatest driver of overweight and chronic diseases. Such chronic diseases include coronary heart disease, hypertension, strokes, cancers, type 2 diabetes, Alzheimer's disease, age-related macular degeneration (AMD), Alzheimer's disease, dementia, overweight, obesity, and virtually every chronic disease known to man. The "lynchpin" of all of these diseases is this omega-6 fat, linoleic acid, or LA and its associated derivative components.

LA exists in every processed and unprocessed food which contains even the slightest amount of fat.[13] However, LA is exceedingly high in westernized, processed food-laden diets,[14] all of which are loaded with seed oil content, and all of which are collectively associated with overweight and chronic disease.[15]

It is important to realize that many foods considered natural and unprocessed really aren't. Some classic examples are animals and fish that are fed *grains* rather than foods naturally consumed in the wild, and as a result are loaded with exceedingly high levels of LA.[16] For example, in 1981, the amount of LA found in pork from ancestrally raised pigs that consumed leaves, roots, coconut fruit, insects and small animals on the island of Tokelau, was only 2.0%.[17]

Contrast that to concentrated animal feeding operations (CAFOs) in the U.S. where pigs are fed genetically modified corn and soy, which raises typical grocery store pork LA up to 20.0% and higher.[18] This is also true for the new artificial or synthetic meats that have large levels of LA. In one comparative analysis, the median level of LA in meat-based beef burgers was 2.65% of the total fat, whereas the plant-based burgers median level was 15.66%, which is 5.9 times greater.[19] However, compare those levels to the average 51% LA in soybean oil, which is the most commonly consumed edible oil in the U.S.[20]

So called 'vegetable oils,' which we may also refer to as seed oils, edible oils, or high PUFA (polyunsaturated fatty acid) oils, have risen from nearly zero consumption globally in the year 1865, to now occupy almost one third of all calories in the U.S., nearly one-fourth of all calories in 12 westernized countries, and about one-seventh of all calories in 64 countries.[124] These countries collectively include the most populous countries in the world.[124]

CHAPTER 1

In parallel with ever-increasing seed oil consumption, chronic diseases have risen from being unusual, rare, or unknown, to being so commonplace that even young children recognize their names. And why is this so? Because today, most of these disease conditions that were unknown just about 120 years ago in the year 1900, are now the leading causes of disease, suffering, and death (review in Chapters 1 through 5). Naysayers of this hypothesis will assert that the rising seed oil and omega-6 LA consumption are not necessarily the cause of the epidemics of overweight, obesity, and chronic disease. 'Correlation is not causation' they will assert. But when does correlation rise to the level of causation? When have we met all (or enough) of the criteria laid out by Sir Austin Bradford Hill to establish causality?[21][22]

There are many questions in Nutrition and Medicine that demand answers. We're all aware that saturated fats have been vilified since about 1960, but is there any validity to this whatsoever? Has saturated fat increased in correlation to the epidemics of obesity, heart disease, cancers, and more? Or have seed oils, with their high omega-6 fat? And if LA, which is currently derived mostly from seed oils, is accumulating in our bodies, what are the consequences of that and what are the biological mechanisms of disease?

How could these seemingly harmless euphemistically named 'vegetable oils' exact so much destruction? Are they even from vegetables – any of them? Furthermore, is sugar the villain it has been made out to be? Or is it, at least in part, receiving the blame for the devastation that seed oils have caused, since the two generally "run together"? Are low carbohydrate diets a requirement to lose excess weight and be healthy? Or are carbohydrates innocent and catching unfair blame as well? Can we turn the rising tide on this epidemic of overweight and chronic disease? Is there a single collective solution to the entire problem?

Throughout this book, we will answer every one of these questions, and not only support the evidence with scientifically published data, but we will make sense of exactly how and why seed oils could drive so much disease, suffering, and death. Our major goal is to cover this topic in enough detail to drive home the message, while being as brief as possible. That said, the subject matter, in our view, demands substantial review and evidence to formally cover the topic. This is not just "another diet book" geared at weight loss. Everyone must consume some type of diet and, like it or not, that diet will dictate not just one's weight and body habitus but, far more importantly, one's health, or lack thereof. One's chosen diet may very well dictate the difference between a life filled with agony and cut decades short, or a long life filled with vitality, energy, and youthfulness.

So while application of the knowledge gained by reading this book will indeed help you to lose undesirable weight (if needed), far more importantly, it will help to prevent and treat most any chronic disease condition or conditions you might already suffer from. We want you to not only have more years of life, but more "life in your years," more time spent in good health, more time with children and grandchildren, and more of everything in life that you desire.

With this brief introduction, we hope you will join us in a journey of evaluating diets in history around the world, which unveils the true and underlying causes of overweight and chronic disease.

We'll begin this journey with a pertinent history of nutrition, which reveals that seed oils are

relatively new to man, they're man-made, they're extraordinarily high in omega-6 LA, and when populations begin to consume them to any significant degree, a trail of destruction follows.

Such physical destruction includes marked increases in overweight, obesity, coronary heart disease, hypertension, metabolic disease, type 2 diabetes, cancers of almost every type, autoimmune disease, Alzheimer's disease, dementia, age-related macular degeneration (AMD), dental cavities, dental malocclusion (misalignment), birth defects, and many, many more chronic diseases, all of which escalate exponentially as seed oil consumption increases.

THE SCIENCE AND LEGACY OF WESTON A. PRICE

It has been said that, "Without reference to the past the present is incomprehensible and the future unpredictable."[1166] In light of this, throughout this book, we will go to great lengths to delve into the history of nutrition, with painstaking efforts to connect the emergence of chronic disease to modernized, processed foods. As will become evident, most chronic diseases – the same diseases that are household name today – were once unknown. The question is why? Weston A. Price was one of the pioneering researchers largely responsible for developing fundamental concepts in nutrition that would begin to provide answers to that question.

Between the years of approximately 1932 and 1939, Weston A. Price completed an epic body of pioneering anthropological nutrition research, which could never again be replicated, but which established marked evidence that modernized, man-made, processed foods reliably induce an epidemic of chronic degenerative disease. Price produced numerous scientific papers on the subject,[23] [24] [25] [26] [27] which finally culminated in a textbook entitled, *Nutrition and Physical Degeneration,* published in 1939 with a second edition in 1945.[28]

Price, who was both a scientist and a dentist, observed by the 1920s and early 1930s, that dental decay and physical degenerative disease in the U.S. was already so rampant that he couldn't establish what he referred to as "suitable controls" or "standards of excellence." By these terms, Price referred to the degree to which man's mind and body might develop and maintain itself under the best of circumstances, that is, with proper nutrition. With a firm understanding of the body of nutrition science for that era, Price left the U.S. to evaluate the health of native, traditional-living populations all around the world, in order to establish the effects of native, traditional diets as compared to the effects of "modernized foods."

Price sought out "primitive racial stocks," which were genetically homogeneous groups, all of whom not only lived within the same geographic latitude, longitude, and climate, but whose only differences were the foods they consumed. The traditional living people, who generally resided where they could not be reached by any roads or ports, had virtually no access to westernized, processed foods – the foods Price called the "displacing foods" – whereas their nearby genetic cohorts, which could generally be reached by roads or ports, had ample access to such "modernized" (processed) foods.

Thus, in one shear stroke of genius, Price eliminated genetics, climate, and geographic locale as factors of influence in physical degenerative disease. Over a period of about seven years, Price evaluated many populations and tens of thousands of people, on a case-by-case basis, on five continents, in fourteen nations, and in hundreds of tribes and village,

CHAPTER 1

Weston A. Price, DDS

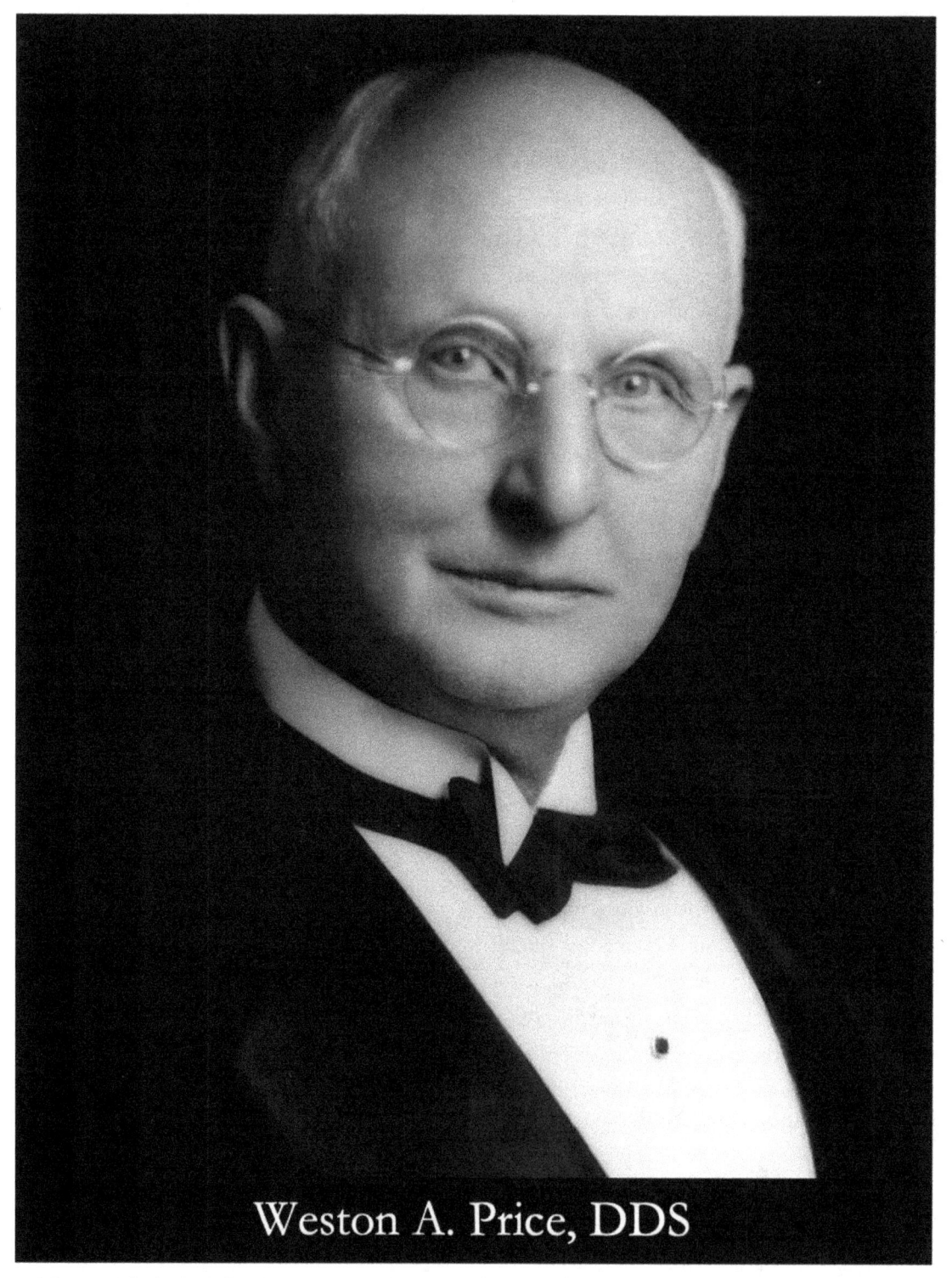

Weston A. Price, DDS. Image courtesy of Price-Pottenger Nutrition Foundation.
© Price-Pottenger Nutrition Foundation, Inc. All rights reserved.

as such populations transitioned from native, traditional diets to westernized diets. Given that entire diets cannot be controlled in people for more than perhaps a few weeks or months, evaluating people in what Price referred to as "Nature's laboratory" was again, a stroke of genius.

Diet, as it turned out, was indeed the key factor in either health or disease. Individuals and entire populations that continued to consume their native, traditional diets, remained in brilliant health, with naturally straight, beautiful, and healthy teeth, which were generally more than 99% free of dental caries (cavities). Furthermore, they maintained great immunity to birth defects, degenerative conditions, and chronic diseases (see images below).

On the other hand, those who consumed westernized, man-made, processed foods, which Price referred to as the "displacing foods of modern commerce," succumbed to many varied chronic, degenerative disease conditions. In essence, the more that any population substituted the "displacing foods" for traditional foods, the greater the development of physical degeneration, which generally began with dental caries (cavities), narrowed and malformed dental arches in children, with consequent misaligned (crooked) teeth, and dental decay in adults.

This was followed by the development of degenerative disease conditions, including arthritis, cancers, and loss of immunity to infectious dis-

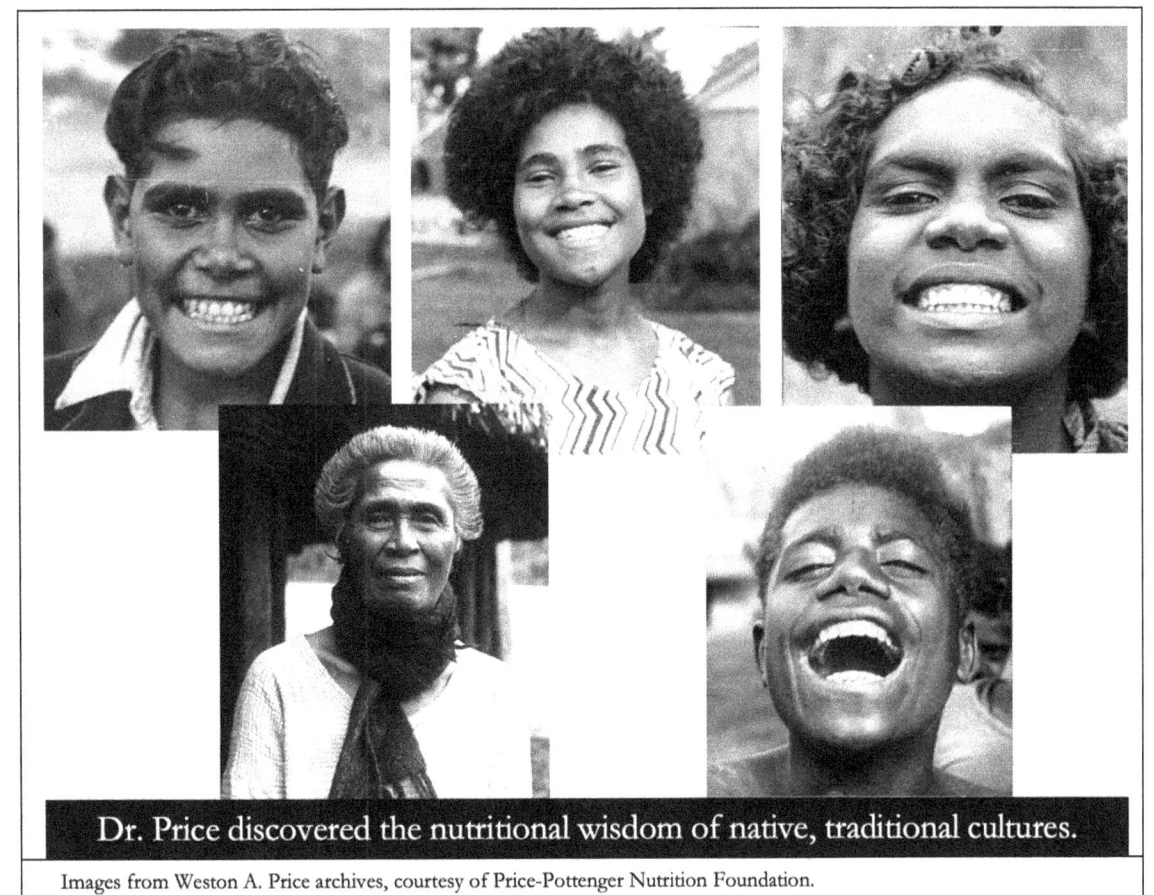

Dr. Price discovered the nutritional wisdom of native, traditional cultures.

Images from Weston A. Price archives, courtesy of Price-Pottenger Nutrition Foundation.
© Price-Pottenger Nutrition Foundation, Inc. All rights reserved.

eases such as tuberculosis. Those consuming the "displacing foods" developed numerous other maladies, including birth defects such as cleft palate and clubfoot, but also conditions that we generally think of as "psychological," such as depression and suicidal ideation. Children raised on such foods developed permanent and irreversible physical and mental handicaps (see images below) and Price even suggested that such "modernized foods" were associated with moral decay at a societal level.[28]

Price observed that the westernized diets, sometimes referred to by native, traditional living people as the "foods of the white man," contained increasing amounts of nutrient-deficient foods. According to Price, the nutrient-deficient foods included white sugar, refined white wheat flour, white rice, syrups, jams, confectionary, canned goods, and "vegetable fats," the term he used for vegetable oils.[29] He referred to these foods as the "displacing foods of modern commerce" to designate that such foods displaced the nutrient-dense foods of traditional living cultures.

Price sent back thousands of food samples from people living on native, traditional diets, and analyzed their nutrient-density against those of the American foods of his day, which was the 1930s. The native, traditional populations' foods, on average, contained ten times more fat-soluble vitamins, that is, vitamins A, D, and K2 primarily, four times more water soluble vitamins, which is all the B vitamins and C,[30] and 1.5 to 60 times more minerals, than did the American diets of the 1930s.[31] Thus,

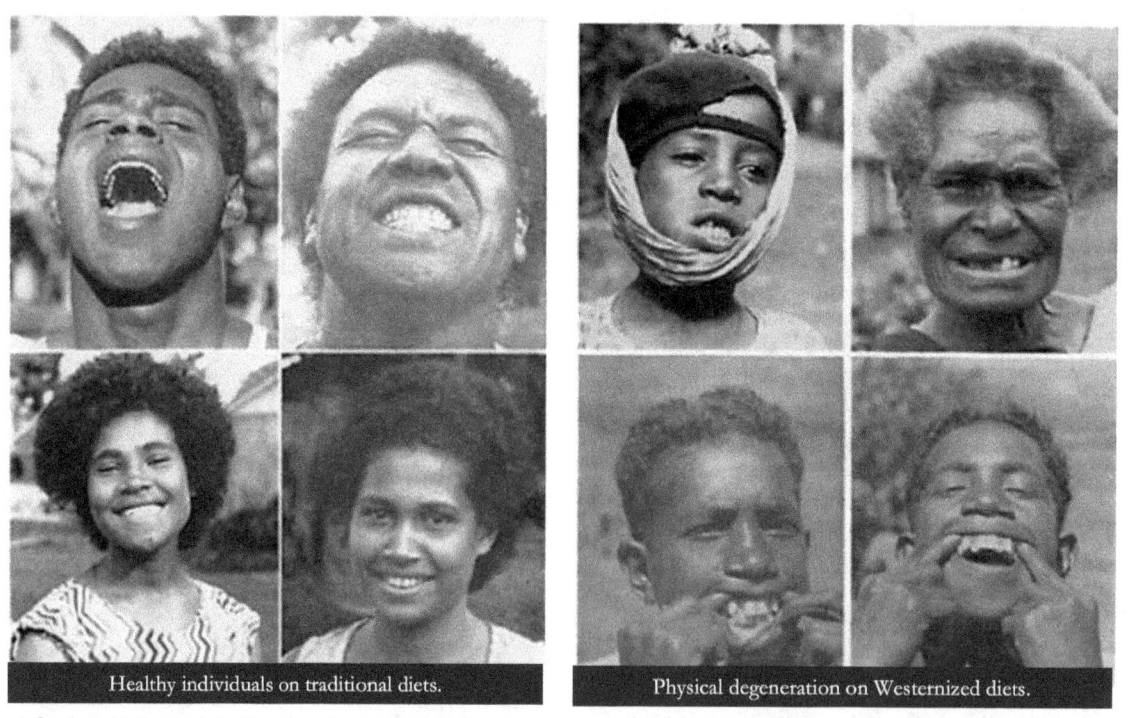

Healthy individuals on traditional diets.   Physical degeneration on Westernized diets.

Left 4 photos: Healthy individuals with healthy teeth on five continents while consuming native, traditional diets. These people generally had neither toothbrush nor floss.
Right 4 photos: Dental misalignment, cavities, abscesses, loss of teeth and physical degeneration on Westernized diets.
Images from Weston A. Price archives, courtesy of Price-Pottenger Nutrition Foundation. © Price-Pottenger Nutrition Foundation, Inc. All rights reserved.

Price established that nutrient-density was a key and critical component of healthy diets, and successful diets all around the globe avoided the same thing, i.e., the "displacing foods of modern commerce."

Price's work, which brought causal inference in the link between processed food, dental disease, and chronic disease, has been ignored by orthodox, allopathic medicine as well as medical schools, dental schools, and allied health professions, with nary a single reference to his works in recent decades. However, the Price-Pottenger Nutrition Foundation, with roots going back to 1952, and the Weston A. Price Foundation, founded in 1999, have both sought to evangelize Price's work. Many today, including myself, still consider Weston A. Price the "Father of Nutrition."

NATIVE, ANCESTRAL, TRADITIONAL, AND WESTERNIZED DIETS – A BRIEF EXPLANATION

We may use the terms "native," "ancestral" or "traditional diets" interchangeably, all of which indicate diets derived from locally produced foods as well as the foods of a given population's ancestors. We will use these three terms generally to indicate most any diet worldwide before 1866, when seed oils, artificially produced trans fats, and refined grains in the form of white flours generally didn't exist (for perhaps 99+% of the world), and when refined (and added) sugars were minimal on a global scale.

The term "westernized diet" as used in most scientific papers, however, generally indicates diets that are "rich in saturated fat, total fat, sugar, and salt," and our definition of this term will differ almost entirely. In our view, the term "westernization" encompasses diets that contain and are often replete with seed oils, refined flours, sugars, and trans fats. However, we will not include an abundance of fat, saturated fat, or salt as indicators of "westernization."

FOOD PROCESSING IN HISTORY

History reveals that until the year 1866, perhaps 99.75% of the world's population had little or no ultra-processed foods, with the exception of added sugars, which were only available in small quantities up until that time.[4]

The current NOVA classification affirms that the addition of "salt, sugar, oils or fats, or other food substances to the original food" defines the food as processed, along with a number of other processes (e.g., heat, pressure, sterilization, pasteurization, freezing, and canning) which all share in common an ultimate goal of extending shelf life while also minimizing production costs.[32]

The term "processed food," therefore, for the purposes of this book, will be defined essentially as those foods containing added sugars, refined flours (mostly wheat flour), 'vegetable' (seed) oils, and artificially produced trans fats. As can be seen, this definition is a more succinct version of Weston A. Price's definition. These foodstuffs, with the exception of added sugars, had little to no existence in any markets on a global scale until the late 19th century.[33] [34]

ADDED SUGARS – NUTRIENT-DEFICIENT FOOD

Whereas added sugars in the diet have been available for centuries, the remaining processed foods have all entered the food supply since 1866, essentially. Up until the late 19th and early 20th centuries, sugar was consumed only in small quantities on a global scale, in part, because it was difficult to produce and therefore, prohibitively expensive.[35]

Researchers Stephan Guyenet and Jeremy Landen, at the University of Washington, found that the average U.S. sugar consumption was 6.3 pounds per person per year in in 1822, which rose to a high of 107.7 pounds per person per year by 1999.[36] This is an increase of over 17-fold during this period of time (1822- 1999), and represents an average consumption of 32 teaspoons per person per day at its greatest.

More modernized cultivation and production methods have made sugar vastly more available and less expensive, which is a hallmark feature of all such processed foods today. Thus, increasing consumption of processed food via displacement of more naturally and organically produced foods has become the norm.

SEED OILS ('VEGETABLE OILS') – IN 1865, THEY WERE NOT CONSIDERED FOOD!

Beginning in 1866, seed oils – again, historically referred to as 'vegetable oils' – entered the food supply in very small quantities and for the vast majority of the world, for the first time in human history.[37] The first of these seed oils to enter the food supply in the U.S. and for nearly the entire world was cottonseed oil.[37]

Certainly, there were a very few isolated instances of edible oils (peanut,[38] sesame[39]) or tropical oils (olive,[40] coconut,[41] palm and palm kernel[42]) having been produced in relatively small quantities in a few cultures throughout the ages, but for perhaps 99.7% of the world's population, seed oils had never been consumed as food, until after the American Civil War ending in 1865.

Certainly, there is no evidence prior to 1865 for any significant production of seed oils via high-pressure, high-heat seed presses combined with petroleum-derived hexane solvent baths, chemical alkalinization, bleaching, and deodorization, which is the process used for most seed oils since the early 20th century.[43] [44] [45]

As mentioned, the bulk of such highly processed and polyunsaturated oils, which are derived primarily from seeds and not from vegetables, began with cottonseed oil production in the mid-1860s. Americans weren't so keen on consuming cottonseed oil as food, however, as they had previously known cottonseed oil only as lamp oil and machine oil.[37] This made the sale of cottonseed oil as 'food' a tough sell. Not to be deterred, cottonseed oil manufacturers found other opportunities, one of which was to adulterate olive oil with cottonseed oil.

This became obvious by the year 1880, when the French, who were well aware of how olive oil should taste, made a formal complaint to U.S. authorities that cottonseed oil was being sold in France under the name of olive oil.[37] In fact, some 73,782 barrels of the adulterated olive oil had been shipped to Europe in 1879. As such, cottonseed oil began to compete with olive oil, under its own name, but perhaps even more greatly as an adulterant.

Author D.A. Tompkins, in his 1902 textbook, *Cotton Seed Oil, History and Commercial Features*, wrote, "The first [cottonseed] mill was built in Natchez, Miss., in 1834... [but the oil wasn't consumed as food]. Immediately after the Civil war of 1860-65, several mills were built, some of which succeeded, and some failed [some oils entered the human food supply]... By 1880, the business of crushing cottonseed had developed into a distinct and entirely legitimate business, but the process employed, and everything pertaining to the industry was held in great secrecy... The oil was found

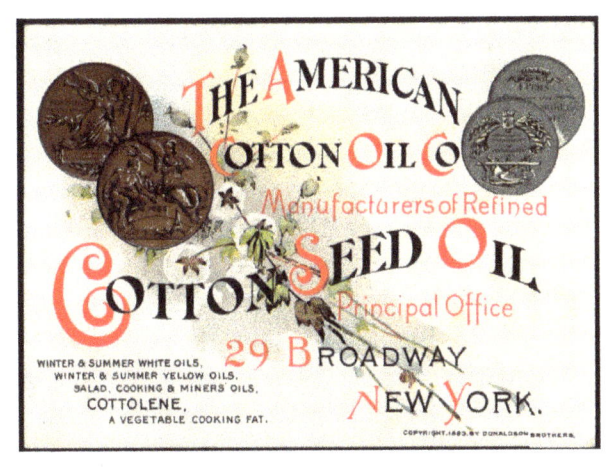

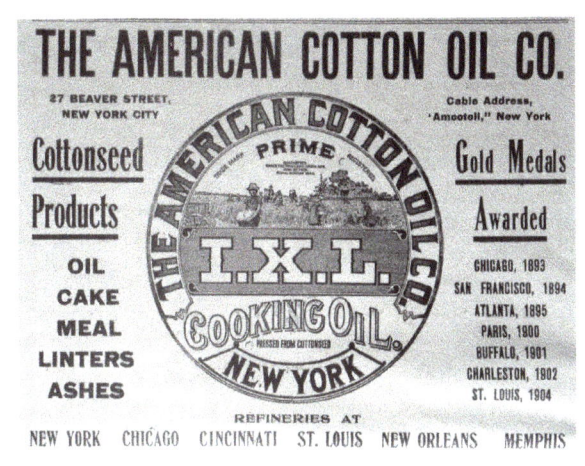

Left: Advertisement for the American Cotton Oil Company, 1893. Right: Advertisement for the American Cotton Oil Company, 1911. Images in the Public Domain.

to be about the same as olive oil, and the cake and meal was largely exported and used in England, and on the Continent, for stock [cattle] food. What was purchased in America was principally used as a fertilizer. The oil was used principally as a substitute for, or an adulterant of, olive oil, and readily sold in the crude state, at from 50 to 60 cents per gallon."[46]

The other opportunity cottonseed oil manufacturers sought was perhaps less underhanded, and involved the mixing of cottonseed oil with beef fat, producing one of the first ever "shortenings." This new product was sold under the brand name "Cottolene." On page 30, notice the image of the trademark application by N.K. Fairbank & Company, registered October 11, 1887, which secured "Cottolene" as a brand to be recognized in the U.S.[47] This set the stage for oils and margarines or shortenings to supplant and replace lard, butter, and beef tallow as nearly the only non-animal-based cooking fats available worldwide. By the end of the 19th century, cottonseed oil began to be manufactured and sold as an artificial butter and was also compounded with lard as an adulterant and sold to unsuspecting customers.[37]

In 1897, Robert Ganz and Company, proprietors of cottonseed oil manufacturing, published a book under the title, *The Manufacture of Cottonseed Oil and Allied Products*, which served in part as a manual for other proprietors to begin, operate, and make profitable their own cottonseed oil mill.

Ganz wrote, "Ten or twelve years ago [about 1885-1887] in cotton-growing districts, where an abundantly reproductive soil furnished lavish supplies of seed at low prices, the prospect of reaping a golden harvest by transforming the crude material [cottonseed] into the manufactured products of oil and cake was of the most alluring character. It was recognized that the oil commanded a high figure, while the cake [the left-over crushed seed remnants, sold for cattle feed] could be readily disposed of on a permanently active market – conditions which are remarkable by reason of their absence in current times… Mills sprung up as if by magic, and the whirr of machinery was heard for the first time in many of the distant cotton-growing districts. The opinion was wide-spread that he who used the most seed, and therefore made the most oil and cake, made the most money."[48]

Ganz' book provided a complete listing of all known cottonseed oil mills operating in 1897, both foreign and domestic, and he specifically

CHAPTER 1

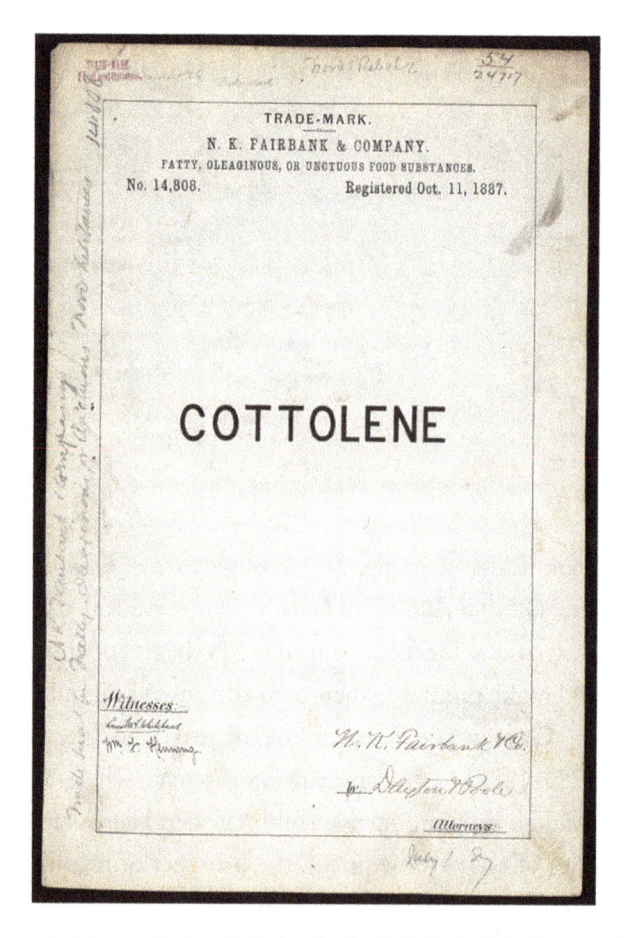

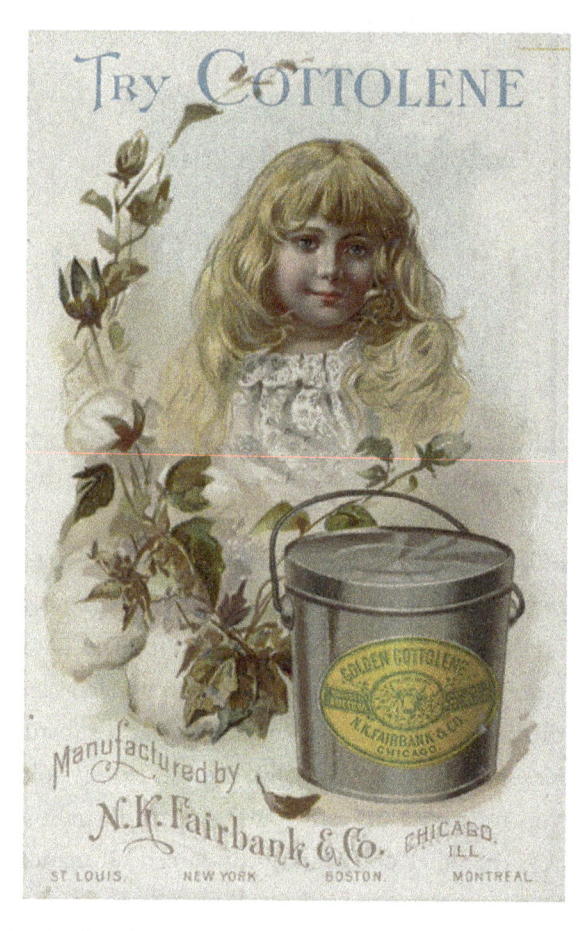

Left Image: Trademark Registration by N.K. Fairbank & Company for Cottolene brand Fatty, Oleaginous, or Unctuous Food Substance. Registered Oct 11, 1887. Image courtesy of the U.S. Library of Congress, photo in the Public Domain. Right Image: Cottolene Advertisement, courtesy of Alan and Shirley Brocker Sliker Collection, MSS 314, Special Collections, Michigan State University Libraries.

listed some 268 cottonseed oil mills in the U.S., 21 mills in England, but none in any other country at that time with the exception of a single oil mill in all of Asia, which was operated in Shanghai.[49] As we'll see, this has vast implications for health, and repeatedly what we have observed is that the United States and the United Kingdom were the epicenters of the emergence of chronic diseases, including coronary heart disease, vastly increasing rates of cancer, obesity, diabetes, etc., while the Asian countries, who were among the last to adopt production and consumption of such seed oils, enjoyed far greater health until the late 20th century (all to be reviewed in this chapter and chapters two through five). Most of Africa has been the last to adopt seed oils as food.

On the topic of cottonseed oil use, an issue of *Popular Science* from that turn-of-the 20th-century era summed up cottonseed (and cottonseed oil) with the single phrase, "What was garbage in 1860 [cottonseed] was fertilizer in 1870, cattle feed in 1880, and table food and many things else in 1890."[50]

Cottonseed oil, the first available seed oil in the U.S., was followed next by soybean oil production

30

in 1909, which was eventually followed by the production of numerous other so-called 'vegetable oils' or "edible oils," including corn, canola, rapeseed, grapeseed, sunflower, safflower, rice bran, and a few others of diminutive consumption.[45]

Thus, an entire industry for a 'food' that had

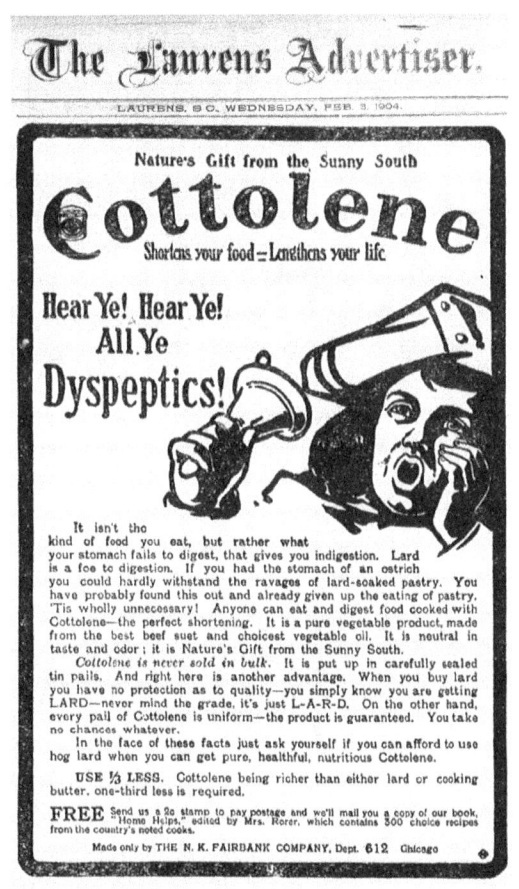

Image courtesy of the U.S. Library of Congress, in the public domain. The Laurens Advertiser (newspaper). Feb 3, 1904.

never previously existed, i.e., the Edible Oil Industry, was born.[45] Such industry sought to replace traditional animal fats (e.g., lard, butter, and beef tallow) and, in some cases, the tropical oils (e.g. coconut) and fruit oils (e.g., olive oil), with oils that required intensive mechanical and chemical production, but which could also be produced on large scales inexpensively and for great profit.[50] Such oils could readily be sold for far less than butter, lard, or beef tallow, for far greater profit. In the year 1918, the *Business Digest and Investment Weekly* referred to vegetable oil production as a "new organization of trade" affirming that "The lower grades of [vegetable] oil have been utilized in industry to a great extent for years, but never before have vegetable oils been used so freely as foodstuffs."[51]

Our published previous work, with data derived collectively from the U.S. Census Bureau, USDA Economic Research Service (ERS), and the Food and Agriculture Organization of the United Nations (FAO), shows on page 32, Figure 1.1, that the U.S. total vegetable oil consumption rose from almost precisely zero grams per person per day in 1865, to 1.62 g/day in 1900, to 19.0 g/day in 1960, to 80g/day by 2010.[4] A review of the literature yields no evidence that seed oils (excluding sesame oil, consumed in small amounts in Asia) existed to any substantial degree in any populations globally through the year 1865.

Therefore, seed oil consumption has risen infinitely on a global scale, since the year 1865. In the year 1900, seed oil consumption averaged 1.62 g/day in the U.S., which rose to 80g/day by 2010. In this 110-year period alone, seed oil consumption thus rose approximately 49.4-fold. Furthermore, the edible oil consumption in the year 1900 was just as likely to have been olive oil as cottonseed oil, the latter of which was the only other highly polyunsaturated fatty acid (PUFA) oil available at that time.[4]

On a calorie basis, in 2010, 80g of seed oils consumed per day amounts to 720 calories, or approximately 32% of U.S. caloric consumption.[4] *Thus, nearly one-third of U.S. population's diets were supplanted and replaced with seed oils during this 145-year period (1865-2010).* Furthermore, seed

CHAPTER 1

FIG. 1.1

Total Vegetable Oil Consumption – USA

From 0 to 80 g/day in 145 Years (2010)

80 g Oil = 720 Calories
32% of U.S. Caloric Intake

99% of Added Fats from Animal Fat

100% of Added Fats from Animal Fat

86% of Added Fats from Vegetable Oils (2005)

U.S. Dietary Guidelines "Low Fat"

Y-axis: Grams Per Capita Per Day (0–90)
X-axis: 1860–2020

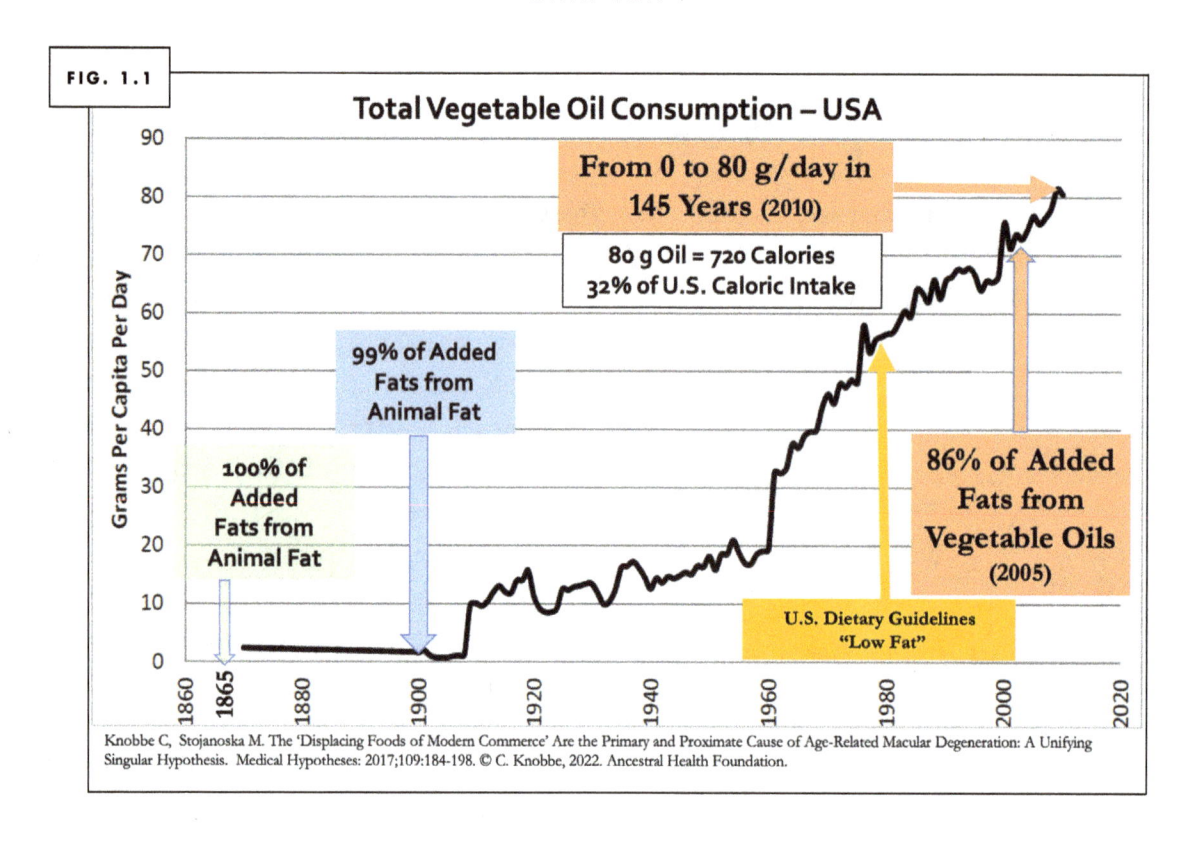

Knobbe C, Stojanoska M. The 'Displacing Foods of Modern Commerce' Are the Primary and Proximate Cause of Age-Related Macular Degeneration: A Unifying Singular Hypothesis. Medical Hypotheses: 2017;109:184-198. © C. Knobbe, 2022. Ancestral Health Foundation.

FIG. 1.2

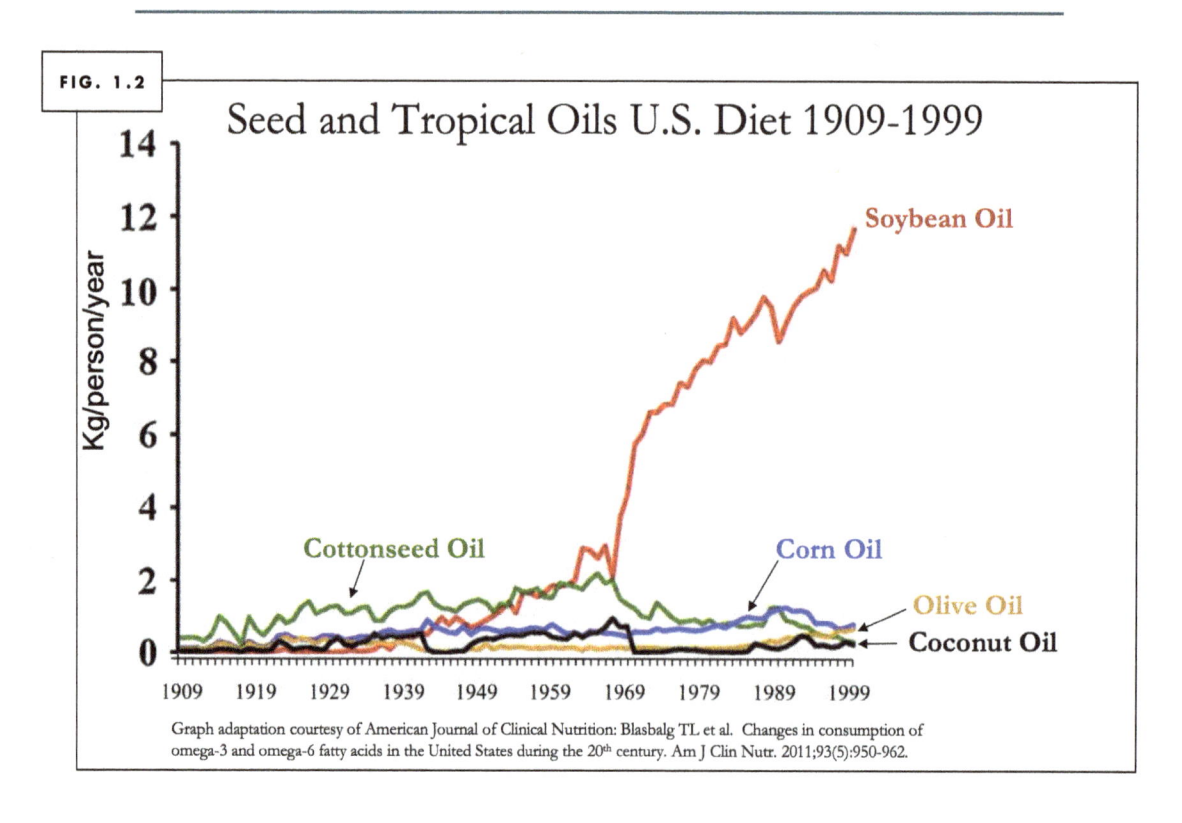

Seed and Tropical Oils U.S. Diet 1909-1999

Y-axis: Kg/person/year (0–14)
X-axis: 1909–1999

- Soybean Oil
- Cottonseed Oil
- Corn Oil
- Olive Oil
- Coconut Oil

Graph adaptation courtesy of American Journal of Clinical Nutrition: Blasbalg TL et al. Changes in consumption of omega-3 and omega-6 fatty acids in the United States during the 20th century. Am J Clin Nutr. 2011;93(5):950-962.

FIG. 1.3

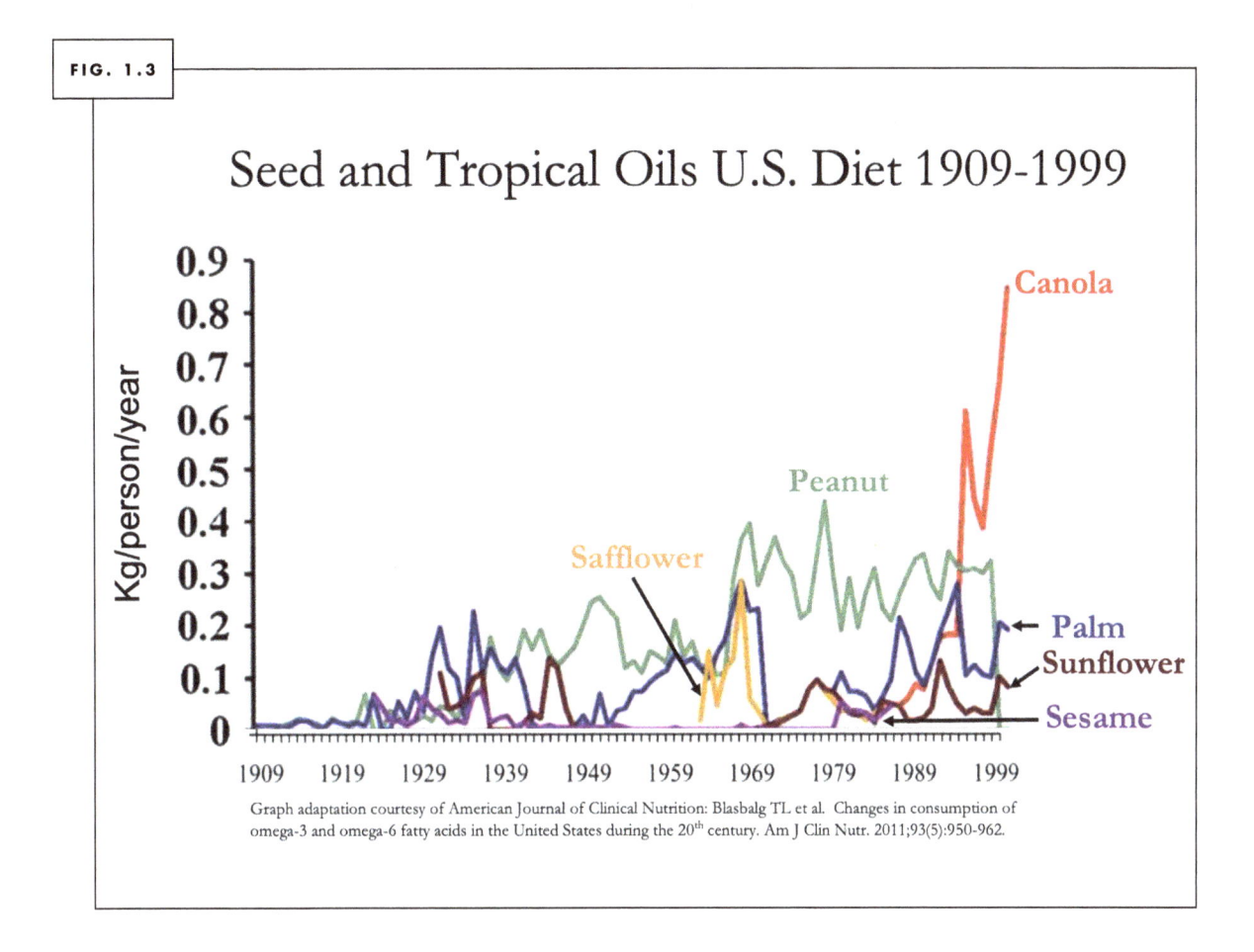

Seed and Tropical Oils U.S. Diet 1909-1999

Graph adaptation courtesy of American Journal of Clinical Nutrition: Blasbalg TL et al. Changes in consumption of omega-3 and omega-6 fatty acids in the United States during the 20th century. Am J Clin Nutr. 2011;93(5):950-962.

oil consumption continues to rise both in the U.S. and globally (to be reviewed). ***This, we believe, is the single greatest change to the diet in all of history (see Figures 1.2, 1.3, and 1.4).***

The USDA Economic Research Service (ERS) also supports these findings, confirming that total PUFA (omega-6 and omega-3 fats) alone elevated from 13g/day in 1909 to 45 g/day in 2008 (see the graph on page 35, "U.S. PUFA Consumption, 1909 – 2005", 2006 – 2008 data not shown).[52] Total PUFA, of course, does not account for all of the calories in oils consumed, as the remainder of the fatty acids (fats) in such oils include not only the polyunsaturated fats, but also the monounsaturated and saturated fats.

Only 0.5% of total caloric energy consumed as LA

FIG. 1.4

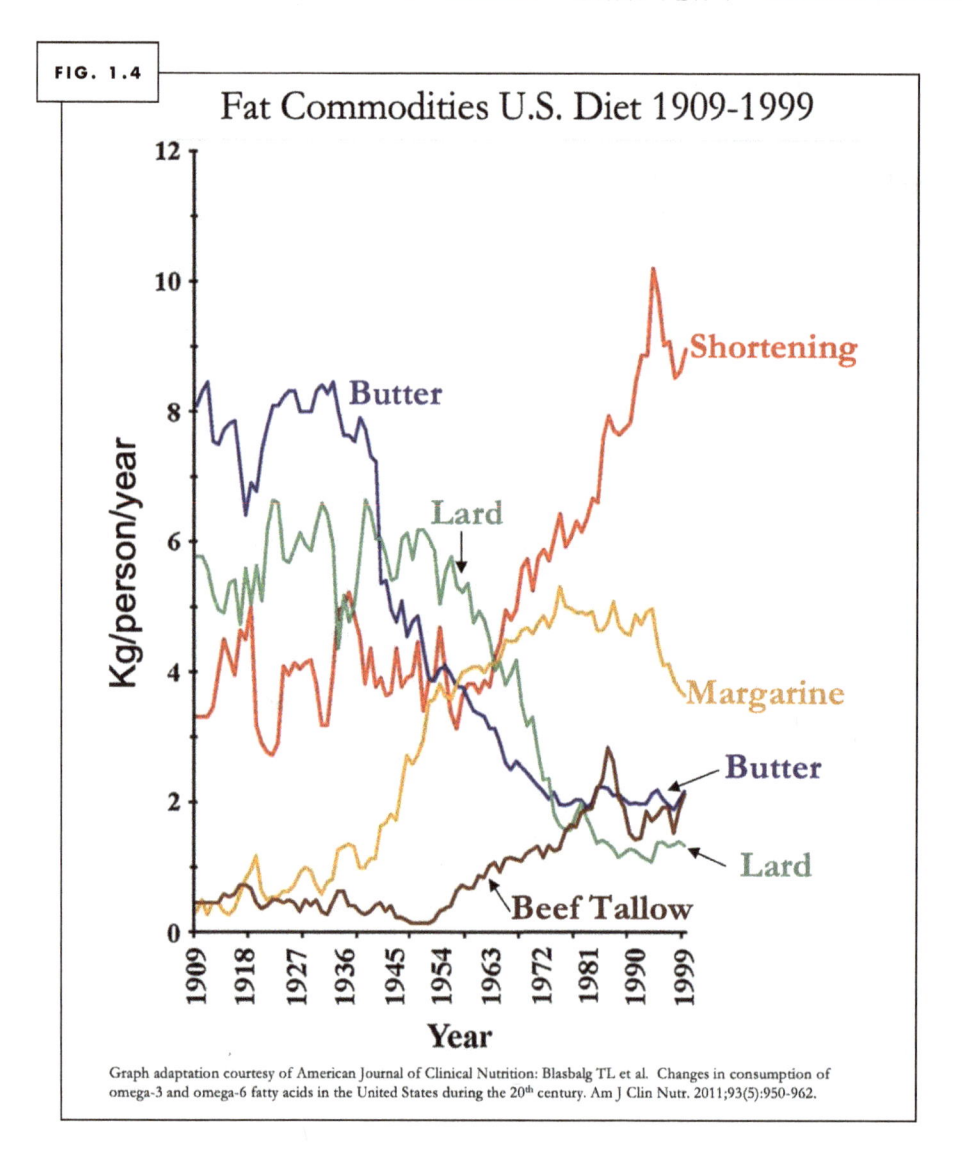

Fat Commodities U.S. Diet 1909-1999

Graph adaptation courtesy of American Journal of Clinical Nutrition: Blasbalg TL et al. Changes in consumption of omega-3 and omega-6 fatty acids in the United States during the 20th century. Am J Clin Nutr. 2011;93(5):950-962.

is considered essential.[53] [54] Linoleic acid (LA) is also by far the most abundant of the dietary PUFAs and has been shown to account for approximately 90% of omega-6 PUFA consumption.[55]

In land-locked regions, LA consumption historically, prior to the introduction of seed oils, would have been based primarily on pasture-raised animal consumption, such as beef, chicken, pig, and lamb, generally with very small amounts present in most natural and unprocessed plant foods. Researchers John Speth and Katherine Spielmann analyzed numerous grass-fed ungulates, including beef, bison, deer, antelope, elk, caribou, moose, Dall sheep, and Bighorn sheep, and found that they only averaged 2.3% LA in their adipose tissue, providing the typical hunter-gatherer with an estimated 0.35% of total calories as LA, for those surviving substantially on such animals.[56]

Other studies have confirmed such findings in 100% grass-fed animals; for example, in one study the LA content of the total fatty acids (total fat) in beef was only 2.01%.[57] This strongly suggests that the total amount of LA in the diet that is essential is even less than 0.5% and may be even less than the

U.S. PUFA Consumption, 1909-2005

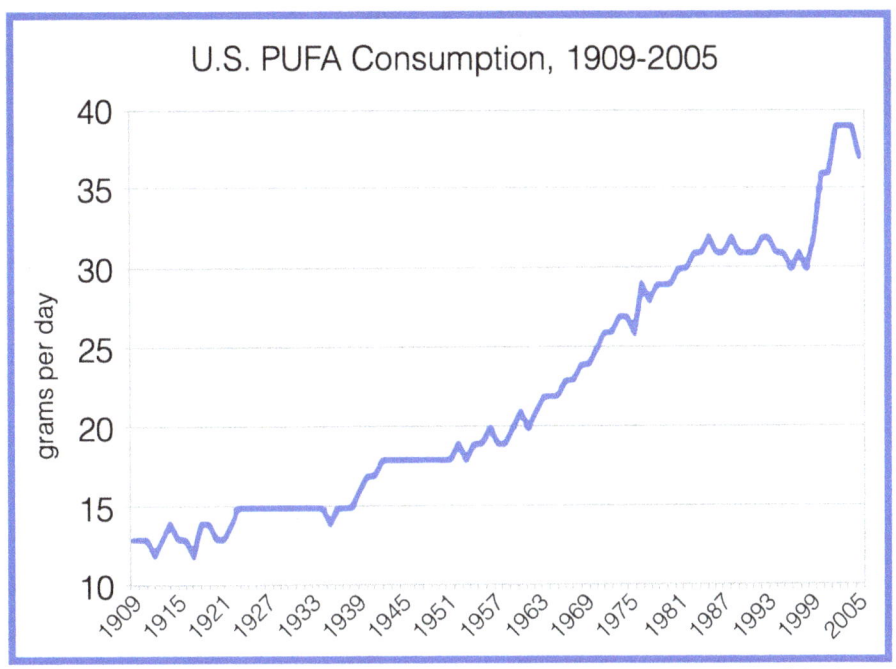

Total Polyunsaturated Fatty Acid (PUFA) Consumption, 1909-2005. USDA Economic Research Service.

0.35% that typical hunter-gatherers would consume.

Using grass-fed animal fat data as a basis, we have been able to model expected LA consumption in American diets in the year 1865 (i.e., before seed oil introduction) and have calculated that only approximately 2.2 g of LA would have been consumed per day.[3] This estimation is based on 40% of calories having been consumed from animal fats, such as beef, chicken, pork, lamb, butter, eggs, and milk, with approximately 2.5% of animal fat calories as LA, with total calorie consumption assumed to be the same as Americans of 1971 (NHANES 1971). Caloric consumption in 1971 averaged 1955 calories/day (specifically kcal/day, however, we'll use "cal/day" from here on).[58]

Thus, LA consumption in 1865 was approximately 1.0% of total energy consumed. Tanya Blasbalg and colleagues at the NIH confirmed that in 1909, 2.23% of energy in the U.S. was consumed as LA, which followed the introduction (and low-level consumption) of cottonseed and soybean oils,[59] and this translates to 4.84 g/day of LA. In 1999, the NHANES 1999-2000 data showed an average of 2250 total cal/day consumed[58] and Blasbalg and colleagues data showed that 7.21% of energy consumed was LA,[59] which translates to 18.0 g/day of LA. Stephan Guyenet, PhD, showed that average LA consumption in 2008 in the U.S. was 29 g/day, which is 11.8% of energy.[60]

Thus, LA consumption in the U.S. rose from about 2.2 g/day or 1.0% of consumed energy in 1865, to 4.84 g/day or 2.23% of energy in 1909, to 18.0 g/day or 7.21% of energy in 1999, and to 29g/day or 11.8% of energy by 2008. This is a 13-fold increase based on mass and nearly a 12-fold increase based on percentage, over a period of 143 years.

If one refers back to the previous graphs in this chapter, including "Total Vegetable Oil Consumption – USA," "U.S. PUFA Consumption 1909-2005," and "Omega-6 Linoleic Acid (LA)%

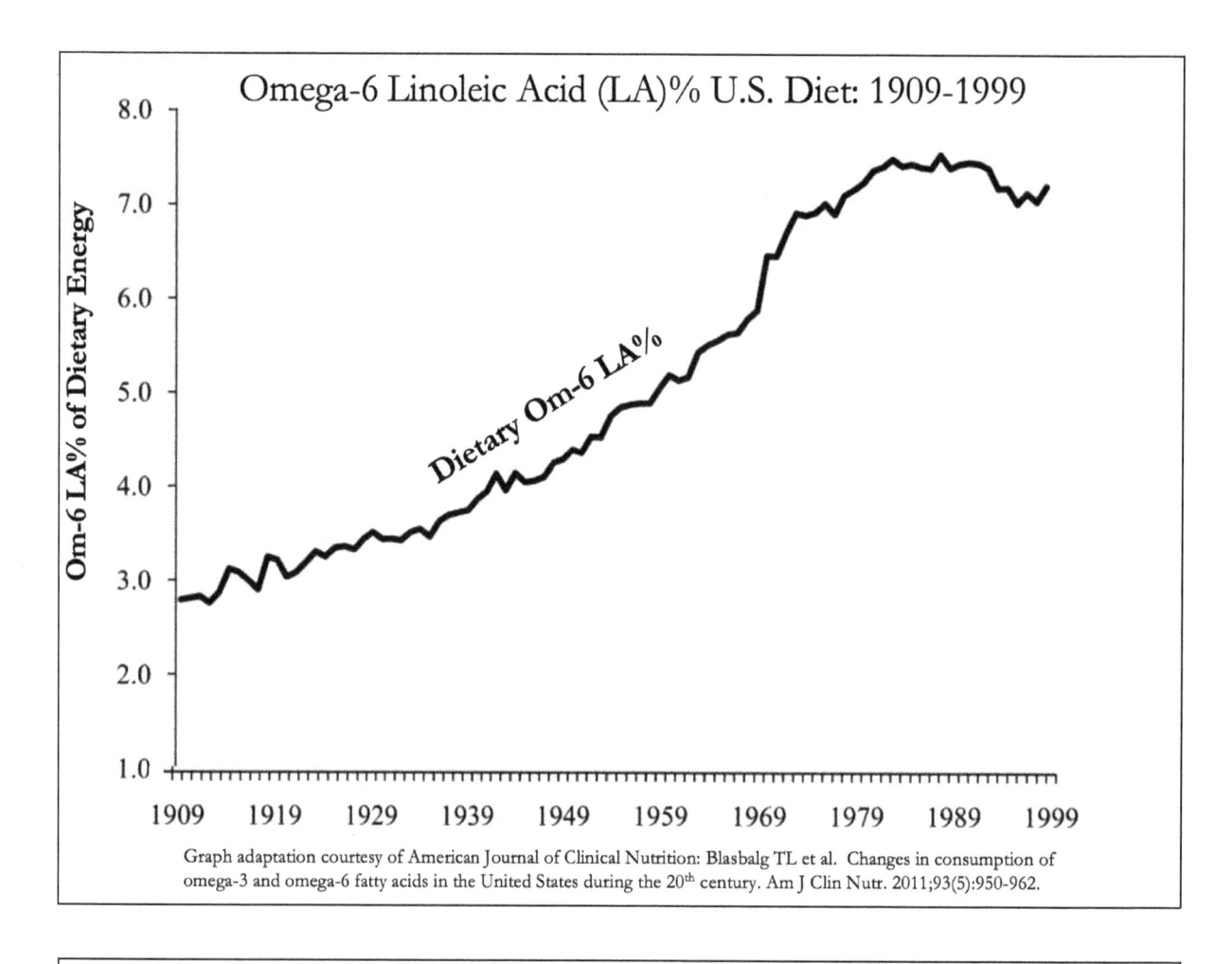

CHAPTER 1

Omega-6 Linoleic Acid (LA)% U.S. Diet: 1909-1999

Dietary Om-6 LA%

Graph adaptation courtesy of American Journal of Clinical Nutrition: Blasbalg TL et al. Changes in consumption of omega-3 and omega-6 fatty acids in the United States during the 20th century. Am J Clin Nutr. 2011;93(5):950-962.

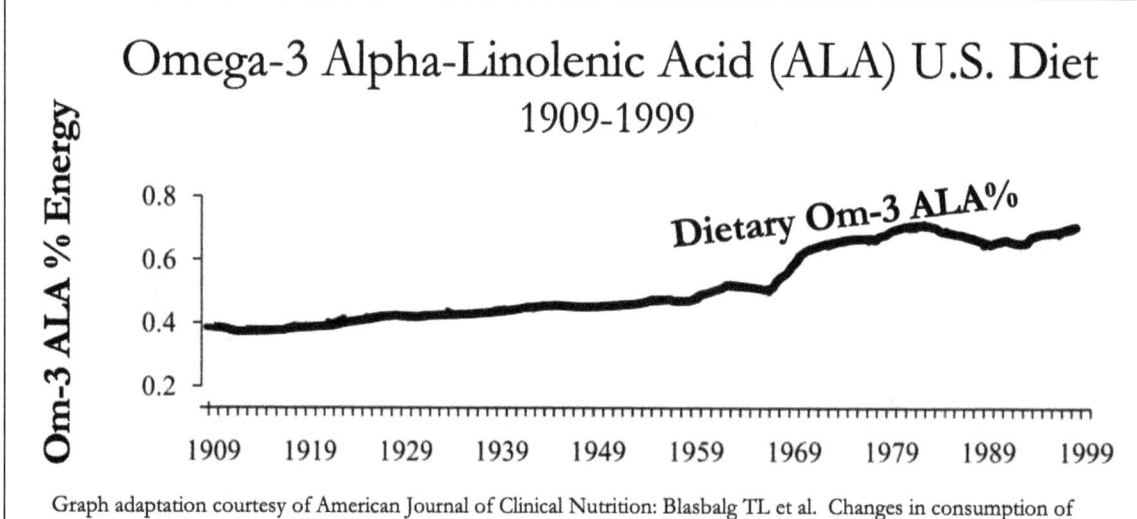

Omega-3 Alpha-Linolenic Acid (ALA) U.S. Diet 1909-1999

Dietary Om-3 ALA%

Graph adaptation courtesy of American Journal of Clinical Nutrition: Blasbalg TL et al. Changes in consumption of omega-3 and omega-6 fatty acids in the United States during the 20th century. Am J Clin Nutr. 2011;93(5):950-962.

U.S. Diet: 1909-1999," it becomes obvious that it is seed oil consumption that drives high omega-6 LA consumption. It is indeed the most important factor, albeit not the only factor (high LA in animals inappropriately fed corn, soy, and seed oils is an additional factor, see Chapter Six).

During this same interval, 1909 to 1999, dietary omega-3 alpha-linolenic acid (ALA) consumption elevated 85%, from 0.39% of energy consumed (calories) to 0.72% of energy.[5] That is, omega-3 ALA nearly doubled in the 20th century, during the same time that obesity, coronary heart disease (CHD), cancers, diabetes, Alzheimer's disease, age-related macular degeneration (AMD), and most every other chronic disease has increased exponentially, yet there's been a pervasive belief that omega-3 supplementation is beneficial.[61]

Of course, omega-3 ALA in the diet competes with the enzymes that convert LA to longer chain mediators of inflammation, which may well be beneficial in those consuming levels of LA that are too high,[61] but nevertheless, a lack of omega-3 fats is surely not the inherent primary problem.

These recent levels of seed oil (and thus, LA) consumption are the exact recipe for obesity, diabetes, and metabolic disaster, unquestionably.[62,63,64,65] Furthermore, seed oil consumption continues an unmitigated global ascent in consumption,[66] while obesity, heart disease, and chronic disease all escalate continually, and globally.[66]

John Kearney, PhD, professor of biological sciences at the Dublin Institute of Technology, in an extensive review of the global food transition over the past 60 years (since about 1960), confirmed, "The consumption of vegetable oils has significantly increased in all regions of the world (threefold in developing countries and twofold in industrial countries). These increases in developing countries are most marked in China, Brazil, and India…"[66]

Kearney's data for the doubling and tripling of seed oil consumption for developed and developing countries, respectively, is for the years 1963 to 2003, specifically. Seed oil consumption has continued to escalate markedly since 2003, as we will present subsequently. Kearney continued, "While animal fats were consumed at slightly higher levels than vegetable oils back in the early 1960s [globally] (most notably in Oceania and Europe), reverse trends have seen a marked decline in the consumption of animal fats in parallel with the rise in vegetable oil consumption."[66]

As reviewed by Professor Kearney, we're witnessing a global processed food transition and the most marked change in that period has been seed oil consumption. Furthermore, as Kearney reviewed, seed oils are replacing animal fats, with a "marked decline" in animal fat consumption. This is a double disaster.

If we examine omega-6 LA consumption as a fraction of the diet, in the U.S., LA accounted for approximately 1/100th of total calories in 1865 and that number elevated to more than 1/8th of total calories by 2008. Once again, this appears to be the single greatest change to the diet in all of history.

If we also use the greater number of 0.5% of energy as LA as being essential, we observe that we consumed twice that amount in 1865, about four times that amount in 1909 and, by 2008, LA consumption was 23.6-fold greater than necessary. This is virtually impossible to accomplish without either seed oils or extraordinary amounts of nuts and seeds in the diet, which would be a rarity. The LA levels consumed in the U.S. in 1865 were certainly extremely healthy, at 1.0% of energy consumed.

However, even in 1909, when LA consumed

was at 2.23% of energy, this may be bordering on excess, as diets above approximately 2% of energy as LA are not generally ancestral (to be reviewed subsequently). Of course, by 1909 Americans were consuming both cottonseed oil and soybean oil, in very small quantities, which were not available until after the Industrial Revolution, when edible oil manufacturing began.

Production of the high PUFA seed oils generally requires intense heat and pressure, seed oil presses, a petroleum-derived hexane solvent bath, and finally, chemical alkalinization, bleaching, and deodorization, often with process temperatures exceeding 480 to 500 °F (249 – 260 °C).[67][68][69][70] These are the reasons that these oils not only have been referred to by many as "factory fats" but also because they're saddled with the toxic advanced lipid oxidation end products (ALEs), which will be reviewed subsequently.

If it weren't for the deodorization step, these oils would actually reek of rancidity, which means they would actually stink.[71] But again, seed oil refining chemists and engineers developed processes in the early 20th century to produce such oils in vast quantities and in such a manner that they're virtually odorless and tasteless. This has allowed manufacturers to easily incorporate these dirt-cheap oils into foods without us actually knowing.

With regard to the omega-6 LA content, some will argue that increasing consumption of an essential nutrient in the diet is not harmful, however, this is not true. We must respect the fact that *every single necessity for life, including water, oxygen, salt, vitamins, and virtually every chemical known, is toxic at high levels.*[72] As Paracelsus' dictum clearly states, *"The dose makes the poison."*[72]

Throughout this book, you will see again and again that LA in high doses leaves a massive trail of destruction. At high levels it is metabolic poison. In fact, at high levels of consumption, it exerts its deleterious effects through pro-oxidative, pro-inflammatory, toxic, and nutrient deficient pathways, which all converge to synergistically exact destruction on the consumer.[3]

REFINED WHEAT FLOUR AND OTHER REFINED GRAINS

To make health matters even worse, in the 1880s, the first ever large-scale operations of refined wheat flour began as a result of the introduction of roller-mill technology, which was introduced almost simultaneously in the U.S., U.K., and Hungary.[73] This was a new technology which could shear away the bran and germ of wheat, to produce refined white wheat flour. Such refined white flours are devoid of naturally occurring nutrients due to the fact that the bran and the germ of wheat contain the omega-3 and omega-6 oils, B-vitamins, and most of the minerals.[74][75] So while white flour was considered desirable and often preferred for baking, its consumption leads markedly to loss of water-soluble B vitamins and minerals, which are especially important for those whose diets depended largely on wheat. However, as processed foods – including sugars and seed oils – further supplant whole, unprocessed foods, nutrient-deficiencies of vitamins and minerals continue to stack up.

The USDA Economic Research Service (ERS) confirmed that, "From a low starting point in the 1600s, consumption of wheat flour rose to about 225 pounds per capita in 1880, and then fell to about 110 pounds a century later."[76] By 2011, wheat consumption averaged 132.5 pounds per capita per year.[76] Today, wheat accounts for about 20% of the world's diet.[77]

As of 2005, Loren Cordain, PhD and colleagues, found that 85.3% of cereal grains, which would be mostly wheat, were consumed in the U.S. as "highly processed refined grains."[78] Furthermore, the USDA ERS confirms that, as of 2010, grains accounted for 518 cal/day or about 23.4% of calories, the bulk of which is wheat.[79][80] The Whole Grains Council found that during the 2013-2016 time interval, 84% of grains are refined, leaving only 16% of grains consumed by Americans as whole grains.[81] Thus, refined wheat alone – a nutrient-deficient food – currently contributes an estimated 15 to 20% of the diet of the average American.

ARTIFICIALLY PRODUCED TRANS-FATS

There is a pervasive belief system that artificially produced trans-fats are no longer in the food supply, but this belief is patently and verifiably false, for numerous reasons, which will be reviewed.

In 1911, Proctor & Gamble introduced the first ever artificially produced trans-fats on a massive scale, under the brand name Crisco,[82] and this product was specifically produced and marketed to supplant and replace the more expensive butter and pork lard (rendered pork fat). Crisco and other trans-fats are produced by bubbling hydrogen gas through edible oils (originally, cottonseed oil) under high temperature and pressure in the presence of nickel or other metal catalysts.[83][84]

The resulting product is a semi-solid that is white, malleable, has a relatively low melting point, and a resemblance that is similar to lard. Crisco was marketed as a more economical alternative to butter and lard, and Proctor & Gamble's marketing campaign touted that the product was "easily digestible," a "rich, wholesome cream of

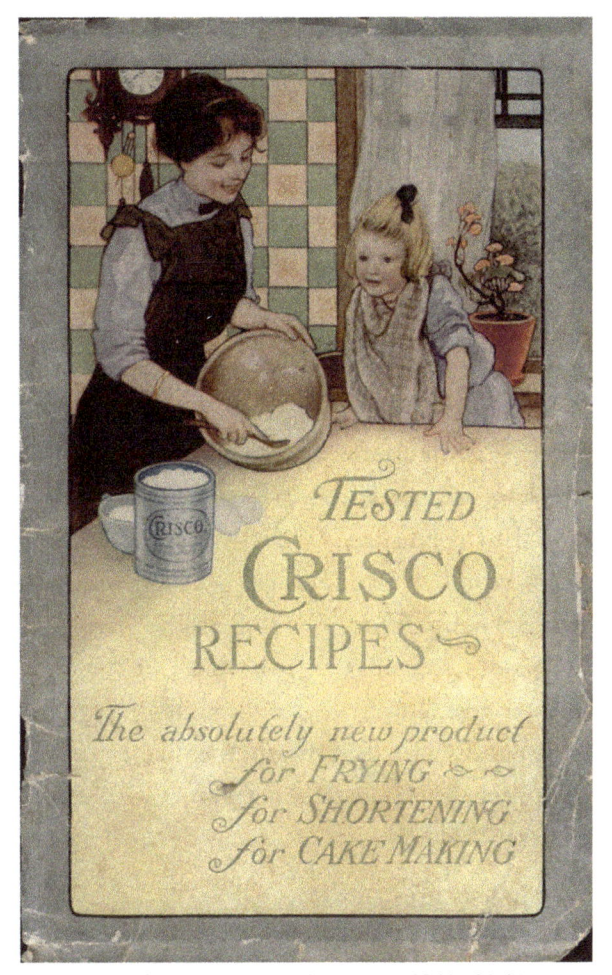

Crisco Cookbook Cover. Sliker Collection, MSS 314, Michigan State University Libraries. Image in Public Domain.

nutritious food oils in sanitary tins," "the ideal fat," "a scientific discovery which will affect every kitchen in America," and even purported that Crisco would enhance the character of children who consumed it.[82][85][86]

A mass marketing campaign was enormously successful and many populations around the world embraced the notion that Crisco was indeed "the healthier alternative to butter and lard" just as Proctor & Gamble's campaign touted. In a review article published in The Atlantic, authors wrote, "The unprecedented product rollout resulted in the sales of 2.6 million pounds of Crisco in 1912 and

60 million pounds just four years later."[123] Proctor & Gamble's (P & G) marketing was not only evasive, but created euphemisms, repeatedly.

According to Smithsonian Magazine, "Crisco [according to P & G] was made from '100% shortening,' it's marketing materials asserted, and 'Crisco is Crisco, and nothing else.' Sometimes they gestured towards the plant kingdom: Crisco, they asserted, was 'strictly vegetable,' 'purely vegetable' or 'absolutely all vegetable.' At their most specific, advertisements claimed that Crisco was made from 'vegetable oil,' a relatively new phrase that Crisco helped to popularize."[87] Thus was born the term 'vegetable oil,' which, of course, is a euphemism for what are almost exclusively seed oils.

Indeed, seed oils ('vegetable oils') are the starting point for industrially produced trans-fats[88] and in recent decades these nearly wax-like molecules have been proven to have vastly negative health effects, including cardiovascular disease, cancer, diabetes,[89][90] potential fetal and infant developmental defects, and neurologic damage.[88] On the other hand, the naturally occurring trans-fats, vaccenic acid (VA) and conjugated linoleic acid (CLA), which are produced in the gut of ruminant animals (e.g., beef and bison), are different from a chemical standpoint and entirely different when it comes to our health. CLA and VA are found in the meats and milk of ruminants and, in fact, have been discovered to produce numerous health benefits.[91]

CLA, for example, has been shown to prevent obesity, cancer, diabetes, hypertension (high blood pressure), and even metabolic syndrome (which is a combination of hypertension, abnormal lipids, insulin resistance, elevated blood sugars, and visceral obesity).[92][93]

German born biochemist, Fred Kummerow, PhD, professor of comparative biosciences, who had been researching trans-fats since the 1950s, published the first papers suggesting causative links between trans-fats and metabolic disturbance in 1957[94] as well as a possible link between polyunsaturated oils (e.g. corn) and heart disease.[95]

With regard to CHD, in 1957, Kummerow clearly did not support the consumption of seed oils in place of natural animal fats, stating, "It may be desirable to lower consumption of foods high in calories, such as French-fried potatoes, potato chips, and party snacks, if these items are consumed at the expense of high protein-containing foods, such as milk, eggs, and meat... high protein foods such as milk, meat, and eggs should serve as the foundation of our diet, even though these food items also contain animal fats. Adding fruits and vegetables will help to supply vitamins and make this diet complete in all essentials."[95]

Clearly, Kummerow denigrated the food items high in polyunsaturated seed oils (French-fries, potato chips, and party snacks), while defending and exonerating the natural fats of milk, eggs, and meat as foods causative of heart disease.

More than five decades later, in 2009, at the age of 94, Kummerow filed a petition with the U.S. Food and Drug Administration (FDA) seeking to ban artificial trans-fats from the U.S. food supply.[96] This came after decades of published research on the negative health effects of trans-fats and numerous attempts by Kummerow to get manufacturers to discontinue their use of trans-fats in foods, which summarily failed.

Some four years later, in 2013, the FDA had still not responded to Kummerow's petition, prompting him to file a lawsuit against the FDA and the U.S. Department of Health and Human Services.

This legal action sought to compel the FDA to take steps to ban artificially produced trans-fats from the U.S. food supply. Kummerow's petition boldly stated, "Artificial trans-fat is a poisonous and deleterious substance, and the FDA has acknowledged the danger."[97]

Three months after Kummerow's lawsuit was filed, artificially produced trans-fats were removed from the U.S. FDA's "Generally Regarded As Safe" (GRAS) status with a preliminary statement in 2013, which was followed by a finalized determination and announcement on June 16, 2015.[98] In the FDA's initial determination, food manufacturers were allowed three years to remove industrially produced trans-fats from processed foods.[98] Then, on May 21, 2018, the FDA extended the compliance deadline for food products "manufactured before June 18, 2018," referencing "that, due to shelf lives ranging from 3 to 24 months, a variety of products… will be in distribution…"[99] The new deadline was set as January 1, 2020, with such foods containing industrially produced trans-fats being "subject to enforcement action by FDA." Under the 2018 ruling, the latest compliance date to remove trans-fats, for specific food items under petitioned use, was January 1, 2021.

However, near the end of the year in 2021, our independent review of processed foods continues to show that numerous items still contain "hydrogenated oil," and it is known that industrially produced trans-fats are present in these products as well.[100] Manufacturers use of hydrogenated oils instead of partially hydrogenated oils is allowed by the FDA since the hydrogenated oils are theoretically fully saturated oils but, as reviewed, such is not the case and trans-fats are still present even in "fully hydrogenated oils."[100]

Furthermore, we still find some foods on the store shelves containing "partially hydrogenated oils," which is an absolute confirmation that even more than eight years following the FDA's announcement that trans-fats were to be removed from GRAS status, some food manufacturers continue to show blatant disregard for the ruling and have failed to remove these dangerous products from their foods. To our knowledge, none have faced legal actions, penalties, or sanctions imposed by the FDA.

As of late 2021 and beyond, perhaps the most important consideration to our health with regard to trans-fats, is that seed oils themselves have been proven in many studies to contain these dangerous components. These studies have been conducted over a period of more than 45 years with clear and repeated evidence that "High temperature treatment can cause the formation of trans-fat in oils through oxidation process [oxidative processes]."[101]

This has further been linked to the high-temperatures utilized in the deodorization process of seed oil production, which is the final step in seed oil manufacturing.[102][103] This procedure and other heat treatments of seed oils have repeatedly produced what researchers have called "isomerization of omega-6 linoleic acid (LA) and omega-3 alpha linolenic acid (ALA)," which is organic chemistry lingo to describe trans-fat production.[107][104][105][106]

The first study to confirm the presence of industrially produced trans-fats in seed oils, to our knowledge, was conducted by R.G. Ackman and colleagues in 1974; the group discovered the presence of "linolenic acid artifacts" which were produced as a result of the high-temperature deodorization procedure required of many seed oils.[107] These so-called "artifacts" were confirmed in their analyses to be industrially produced trans-fats. In 1992, French researchers examined eight different salad oils and five food samples containing either rapeseed or soybean oils and found that the total industrially produced trans-fats accounted for up to 3% of the fatty acids (fats).[108]

In that study, the primary omega-3 fatty acid, linolenic acid (18:w3) was shown to produce about 13-14 times more trans-fats by volume present as compared to omega-6 linoleic acid (LA, 18:2). In 1993, fifteen samples of commercial edible soybean and rapeseed oils from Belgium, Great Britain, and Germany were analyzed for trans-fatty acid content and only one of the thirteen samples contained trace amounts of trans-fats, while the others contained between 1.0% and 3.3% trans-fats.[109]

A study completed at the University of Florida in 1994 found that soybean and canola oils purchased in the U.S. contained industrially produced trans-fats ranging from 0.56% to 4.2%.[110] These authors clearly stated, "Consumers will obtain isomerized essential fatty acids [trans-fats] from vegetable oils currently marketed in the U.S."[110] In another study of vegetable oils originating from Belgium, published in 1996, 19 different edible oils were evaluated, finding that trans-fats accounted for anywhere from 0.0% to 4.6% of the total fats, with a mean of 1.1%.[111] Soybean oil was up to 2.1%, peanut oil up to 1.2%, corn oil up to 4.6%, and sunflower oil up to 1.8%; olive oil was the only sample that had non-detectable levels of trans-fats. In studies completed in China in 2010 and 2011, a total of 93 samples of seed oils were analyzed for trans-fats, finding trans-fatty acid content to average 1.15% in soybean oils, 1.37% in rapeseed oils, 1.41% in sunflower oils, and 2.01% for corn oils.[112]

From what appears to be the largest study of trans-fats in seed oils to date, these authors clearly stated, "Trans fatty acid is widely present in edible oils at low levels."[112] In yet another paper published in the Journal of the American Oil Chemists Society (AOCS), in 2013, researchers confirmed that canola oils contained between 1.21% and 1.73% trans-fats as a percentage of total fat, with corn oil ranging from 0.36% to 0.99%, grapeseed oil 0.44%, peanut oil 0.39%, safflower oil 0.13% to 0.67%, sunflower oil 0.13% to 0.78%, "vegetable oil" 0.74% to 2.18%, and olive oil a negligible 0.03% to 0.04%.[113]

Thus, in numerous studies conducted over a period of more than 45 years on at least three continents, seed oils have repeatedly been shown to harbor substantial levels of trans-fats. The U.S. FDA has not directly addressed this. And as previously stated, without seed oils, industrially produced trans-fats would drop to near undetectable levels, precisely as we've seen in presumably authentic extra-virgin olive oil.[113]

Since 2006, the U.S. FDA has allowed American food manufacturers to label their food products with the statement "Contains 0 grams trans fat per serving" if the trans-fat content is below 0.5g per serving.[101] As of 2015, the average serving size of oil in the U.S. is 14 grams, or about one tablespoon.[101] Therefore, as long as the trans-fat content of an oil remains at or below about 3.6% of total fat calories and the serving size is 14 grams or less, a food manufacturer could label an oil containing product with the statement, "Contains 0 grams trans fat per serving." It's trickery and deceitful, in our view, but this is the work of our own FDA, who aims to please manufacturers.

Thus, even today, with Americans consuming an average of around 80 g oils per day (around 5.7 tablespoons), if an oil contained 0.49g of trans-fats per serving, a consumer could conceivably consume

2.8g trans-fats per day, while repeatedly observing labels which read "Contains 0 grams trans fat per serving." It is worth noting, our own FDA has confirmed that there is no level of trans-fat consumption that has been determined to be safe.

PROCESSED FOODS: ADDED SUGARS, REFINED FLOURS, SEED OILS, AND TRANS FATS

By 2009, the USDA found that 63% of the American diet consisted of these four highly processed, nutrient-deficient foods, in the form of added sugars, refined flours, seed oils and trans fats.[4] Thus, 63% of the American diet was made up of ultra-processed food, while 75% of the world's diets in recent years is now considered processed.[114] This is the recipe for metabolic disaster, overweight, and myriad chronic disease. In Chapter Two, we'll examine processed foods, seed oils, and their incomparable contribution to chronic disease in much greater detail.

SUGAR AND PROCESSED CARBOHYDRATES OFTEN PROPOSED AS THE MAIN DIETARY PROBLEM

In 1972, in his book *Pure, White and Deadly*, British scientist and author John Yudkin, exposed the dangers of excess sugar consumption as the leading cause of most nutritionally related disease.[115] Many natural health authorities in more recent decades have chimed in with agreement on Yudkin's hypothesis, espousing sugar and processed carbohydrates (mostly, refined grains) as the leading agents of chronic disease induction and progression.

Nutrition researcher Stephan Guyenet, PhD identified that between the years of 1822 and 1999, sugar consumption in the U.S. increased by 17-fold, from 6.3 pounds per person per year in 1822 to 107.7 pounds/person/year by 1999.[116] And whereas all wheat was typically stone-ground and 100% whole-grain flour up until 1880, by year 2000, Loren Cordain's group had determined that 85.3% of grains were "highly processed refined grains."[117]

Indeed, added sugars and refined grains are nutrient-deficient foods, and these two foods alone now account for approximately 38% to 41% of the American diet in recent years.[3][4] Nutrient deficiency, however, is the primary concern with added sugars and refined grains in the diet, and this is markedly less problematic than the seed oils, which are a far more potent metabolic poisons than sugar. As will be shown subsequently and repeatedly, seed oils exact their destructive effects through pro-oxidative, pro-inflammatory, toxic, and nutrient-deficient effects. As such, we will argue that seed oils are complex biological poisons with a marked proclivity to produce obesity and chronic disease all on their own.

SEED OILS IMPOSED UPON PROCESSED CARBOHYDRATES: A DEADLY COMBINATION

As previously noted, seed oils were introduced to the U.S. in 1866, with cottonseed oil.[37] Prior to that year, cottonseed oil had its use primarily as lamp oil, fertilizer, and cake for cattle feed, with machine oil being a minor use.[37] Going back a few centuries prior to the American Civil War, however, J.L. Flandrin, in a study of diets between the 14th and 17th centuries, wrote, "The dividing line between areas where olive oil and butter are used for cooking obviously has a natural basis: people cooked with olive oil where olive trees grew, and where there were no olive trees they resorted to butter..."[118]

Even by the late 19th and early 20th centuries, however, the only olive trees available for significant distribution on any scale were grown primarily in Europe, with much smaller crops in California.[119] [120] As such, the enormous majority of the world resorted to butter, lard, or beef tallow for cooking oil if needed, although culinary historians have asserted that most cooking in history was completed without oils.[121] Also, given that olive trees were available primarily in California and Italy for most of history, olive oil consumption on a global scale was relatively small.

Total vegetable oil consumption in the U.S. remained very low in the 19th century at no more than approximately 2 g per person per day, until 1909, when soybean oil was introduced.[44] A few years before that, in the year 1900, Valerius Anderson introduced the continuously operated expeller press, which further automated the process of crushing seeds for the mass production of edible oils.[122]

This, along with Proctor & Gamble's use of seed oils (initially, cottonseed oil) as the fodder to produce Crisco, set the stage for 'vegetable oils' to be mass produced, eventually outselling butter, lard, and beef tallow (rendered beef fat), which were almost exclusively the only added fats in the diet in the year 1900. In review of these facts, *The Atlantic* published an article in 2012 written by authors Drew Ramsey and Tyler Graham entitled, "How Vegetable Oils Replaced Animal Fats in the American Diet;" the subtitle appropriately included, "… discover how Proctor & Gamble convinced people to forgo butter and lard for cheap, factory made oils loaded with trans fat."[123]

So while lard, butter, and beef tallow occupied 99% of the added fats in the diet in 1900, by the year 2005, 86% of added fats in the diet were from 'vegetable' oils.[3] [4] In fact, by the year 2010, the average American was consuming about 80 grams of seed oils per day, or roughly 24 to 32% of their diet from seed oils alone![4]

Thus, the introduction of seed oils and the replacement of animal fats by the Edible Oil Industry unquestionably became the single greatest dietary transformation in all of history. The intake of seed oils increased from nearly zero consumption from antiquity up through 1865, to around one-fourth to one-third or more of the American diet, by 2010.[3] [4] Furthermore, the data clearly show that numerous westernized populations are now consuming 15% to 25% or more of their calories from seed oils and this is unprecedented throughout history.

For example, the U.S., Spain, Canada, Greece, Italy, Israel, Australia, Taiwan, Turkey, Czechia, Belgium, and Austria all consume, on average, more than 500 kcal/person/day of vegetable oils while a total of 64 countries are now consuming more than 300 kcal/day.[124] Before 1865, consumption of seed oils per se (e.g., corn, canola, rapeseed, grapeseed, sunflower, safflower, soybean [a legume], etc. and excluding olive oil and the tropical oils), for all of these countries, would have been very close to zero.

Since the late 19th century and in parallel with this drastic increase in seed oil consumption globally, chronic disease conditions of every sort have elevated from the status of medical rarity (or virtually unknown) to become common household terms as well as the leading causes of death.

Coronary heart disease (CHD), cancers, metabolic diseases, overweight and obesity, Alzheimer's disease, age-related macular degeneration, and innumerable and myriad chronic disease conditions of every sort have sprung up out of nowhere to become the leading causes of disease, suffering, and demise.

In native, traditional healthful diets, whether they be near-strict carnivore, like the Eskimos and Inuit, or 66% natural animal fats, like the Maasai tribe of Kenya and Tanzania, or based on seafood, root vegetables and coconut oil, like the South Pacific islanders of Tokelau, all of whom are exceedingly healthy, the primary omega-6 fatty acid, known as linoleic acid, or LA, is generally less than about 2% of total dietary calories.[3]

This is true because in most traditionally raised foods, whether they are animal meats, seafood, or fruits or vegetables, the omega-6 LA content (of total energy) is generally about 2.0% or less. It is important to remember this figure of 2% as it relates to LA content, because it will be one of the most important points in this book. Keeping your LA intake under about 2% of your total calories is one of the most important steps you can take to eliminate or prevent disease.

Seed oils, on the other hand, which are almost entirely unnaturally derived, as well as the processed foods that contain them, generally contain anywhere from approximately 16% omega-6 LA, up to about 79% LA by weight![125] Thus, the traditional American diet, as well as most native, traditional diets with which we are aware, produces omega-6 LA content of less than 2% of total calories, while the American diet, as of 2008, is now nearly 12% omega-6 LA alone!

That's right, this single primary omega-6 fatty acid alone, now accounts for about 8 to 12% of caloric consumption in Western societies. This is, at the very least, 4- to 6-fold too much LA on a percentage basis, and approximately 6- to 12-fold too much LA by weight.

Omega-6 LA accumulates in your adipose (fat) tissue, in your cell membranes, and in your mitochondrial (energy producing) membranes,[126] and as we'll see, this sets the stage for multiple biological noxious threats induced by a highly pro-oxidative, pro-inflammatory, and toxic biological milieu, which ends in metabolic disaster.

This is often associated with rapid and uncontrollable weight gain even in the face of reduced caloric consumption, and finally, an onslaught of chronic disease conditions, such as coronary heart disease, cancers, strokes, hypertension, Alzheimer's disease, and almost every other disease that you can think of.

Combine seed oils, which are nothing short of potent metabolic biological poisons, with marked nutrient-deficiency through consumption of processed (refined) carbohydrates, and the health risks are magnified even more greatly. That is, the harms of seed oils are amplified even further by increasing sugars and refined carbohydrates in westernized diets, which results in even greater nutrient-deficiency.[127][128][129] This is precisely where modernized, processed foods have led us, that is, to grave degrees of nutrient-deficiency, combined with the extraordinarily dangerous and noxious effects of seed oils and trans fats. There are numerous examples of this, which will be reviewed throughout this book.

For example, it has been shown repeatedly that the requirements for vitamin E increase in proportion to the increase in PUFA (again, mostly LA) in the diet.[127][130] It has also been shown that animals and humans with low vitamin E status have been sensitive to PUFA damage in cellular membranes with consequent muscle, neurologic, and embryogenic (i.e., fetal) developmental problems as a result.[131][132][133][134] Currently, vitamin E intake is below the recommended level in more than 90%

of North Americans as well as in some European countries.[135]

Furthermore, at the same time that vitamin E consumption levels are markedly down from processed food consumption (sugar and refined flours contain no and low vitamin E, respectively), most Western populations are being encouraged to consume more polyunsaturated oils, especially those with the greatest degree of unsaturation![136][137] Just briefly, let's examine the nutrient-deficiency of refined flours and sugars and their associated negative effects, versus whole grain flours and sugars, which would naturally accompany whole foods.

According to the University of Minnesota's Nutrition Coordinating Center (NCC), 100g of unenriched whole wheat flour contains 7 times as much vitamin E (0.7mg) as does 100g of unenriched white wheat flour (0.1mg) and the former contains 5 times as much vitamin B1, almost 4 times more B3, 50% more B5, six times more vitamin K1, and markedly more B2 (0.2mg vs. 0.0mg) and B9 (44 µg vs. 26 µg).[138][139] The whole wheat flour also contains more than twice as much calcium (34mg vs 15 mg), four times as much copper (0.4mg vs 0.1mg), three times more iron (3.6mg vs 1.2mg), six times more magnesium (137 mg vs 22mg), six times more manganese (4.1mg vs 0.7mg), three times more phosphorus (357mg vs 108mg), more than three times more potassium (363mg vs 107mg), almost twice as much selenium (61.8 µg vs 33.9 µg), and almost four times more zinc (2.6mg vs 0.7mg) than the unenriched white wheat flour.

Additionally, refined wheat flour loses 83% of total phenolic acids, 79% of total flavonoids, 78% of total zeaxanthin, 51% of total lutein and 42% of total β-cryptoxanthin as compared with whole wheat flour.[140]

Added sugars to the diet, for example, those in sugar-sweetened beverages, contain zero vitamins and almost zero minerals. However, the sugars of fruits, such as bananas and apples, are associated with small but significant amounts of vitamins B2, B3, B5, B6, B9, and a variety of minerals. But the question is, what are the consequences of consuming nutrient-deficient flours and sugars, physiologically, especially in the face of high seed oil diets? The answer to that may follow from both human and animal research.

Epidemiologic studies have suggested that whole-grain cereal consumption, as opposed to refined grain (e.g., white flour) consumption, helps to protect against atherosclerosis, diabetes, and cancer.[141] In fact, the additional nutrients in whole grains are thought to improve bowel physiology, blood lipid status, antioxidant status, and even to suppress tumor growth.[142][143]

It has also been suggested that the antioxidants in whole grains improve the redox status of an individual (i.e., the delicate balance of reactive oxygen species (ROS) produced and the antioxidant system which scavenges those ROS) which, in turn, reduces the risk of associated disorders.[142][144][145] In studies of rats fed whole grain wheat flour versus those fed refined wheat flour, the livers of rats fed the whole grain flour had more glutathione (GSH), glucose, and betaine, than the livers of rats fed refined flour.[146]

The higher levels of glutathione in the whole grain fed animals indicates enhanced antioxidant capability, as glutathione is the master antioxidant in the body.[147] Betaine participates in the conversion of homocysteine to methionine, which in turn, increases glutathione. As such, betaine further enhances antioxidant status.[146]

In summary, what we repeatedly observe is that whole grains, fruits and vegetables, for example, as well as numerous other nutrient-dense foods, which produce (in part) metabolic changes that help protect against oxidative stress, are particularly beneficial in those consuming higher levels of omega-6 fatty acids (mostly LA), the latter of which further increases demand for antioxidants. The greater the vitamin E, B-vitamins, and minerals in the foods, the more metabolically favorable the physiological environment will be.

Thus, it is clear that consumption of highly processed and refined foods, i.e., refined flours and sugars, along with increasing consumption of highly polyunsaturated vegetable oils, is the ultimate recipe for metabolic disaster and physical degenerative disease. On the other hand, a zero seed oil diet combined with nutrient-dense foods, such as wild-caught and/or 100% grass-fed and pastured meats, fowl, fish, eggs, and dairy, as well as organically grown fruits, vegetables, and whole grains, all become the recipe for health and prevention of overweight and chronic disease.

MORE EARLY 20TH CENTURY RESEARCH – E.V. MCCOLLUM – SEED OILS CANNOT SUSTAIN LIFE

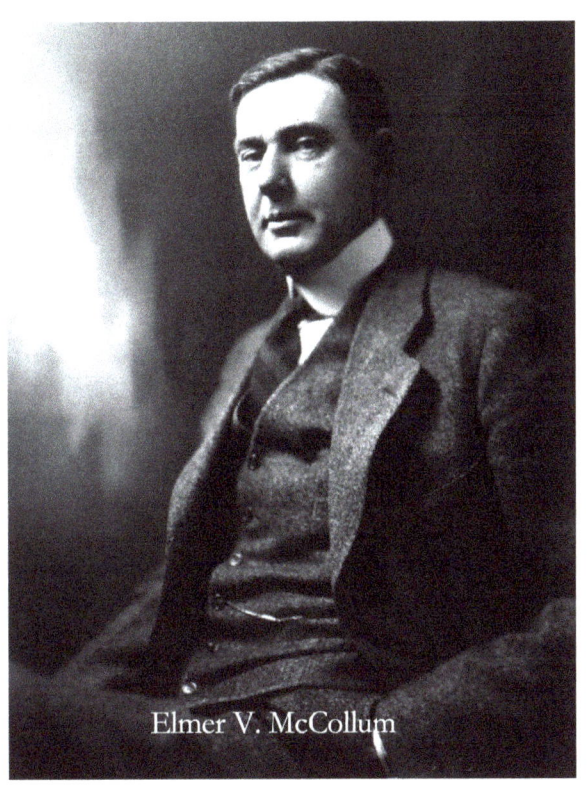

Elmer V. McCollum

Elmer V. McCollum (1879-1967). Image courtesy of the NIH National Library of Medicine, Digital Collections.

By the year 1918, nutrition researcher E.V. McCollum and colleagues had firmly established that if the only fats fed to animals were in the form of 'vegetable oils,' growth of young animals would rapidly come to a halt and they would develop rough coats, crooked and abnormal teeth, red and matted eyes, night-blindness, infections, and then weight loss.[148] If the experiment was continued, the animals would soon wither away and die.

The diet that was first used to establish the nutrient-deficiency of vegetable oils at that time was a diet of 18% purified casein (milk protein), 20% purified lactose (milk sugar), 5% of some type

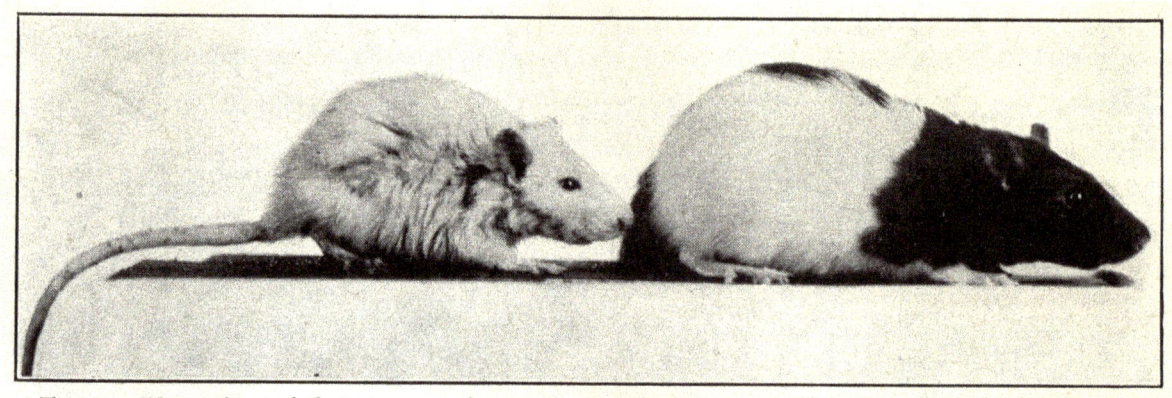

FIG. 5.—The rations of these two rats from weaning time were exactly alike except in the character of the fat which they contained. The one on the left was given 5 per cent of sun-flower seed oil. The one on the right was given 1.5 per cent of butter fat. Butter fat, egg yolk fats and the leaves of plants, contain a dietary essential, the chemical nature of which is still unknown, which is necessary for growth or the maintenance of health. This substance is known as fat-soluble A, and is not found in any fats or oils of vegetable origin. A lack of this substance in the diet causes the development of a peculiar eye disease known as xerophthalmia.

Reprinted from: E.V. McCollum. The Newer Knowledge of Nutrition. New York, The MacMillan Company, 1919. Fig. 5, p. 87. Image in public domain.

of fat, salt mixture, and starch for the remainder. In evaluating the results of this diet based on the type of fat consumed, McCollum wrote,

"With this diet the interesting observation was made that growth could be secured when the fat in the food mixture was butter fat, whereas no growth could be secured when the butter fat was replaced by lard, olive oil, or other vegetable oils."[149]

Similarly, if adult animals were given 'vegetable oils' as the only source of fat, a similarly disastrous outcome was in store for them. They too would develop rough coats, night-blindness, tooth decay, and infections, all of which would be followed by markedly premature death if such diets were continued.[148]

In 1915, Thomas B. Osborne and Lafayette B. Mendel reviewed McCollum's research with regard to such experimental diets wherein young animals were raised consuming vegetable oils or even commercial lard as their only fats, stating,

"…they usually grow normally for about three months, but never attain their full size. Sooner or later nutritive disaster manifests itself by a complete or partial cessation of growth which ultimately (and sometimes precipitately) ends in a decline in body weight, followed by death if a suitable change in diet is not promptly instituted. The disturbance of growth may be attended by symptoms of malnutrition…"[150]

McCollum found, however, that just small amounts of natural butter, egg yolks, whole milk, or cod liver oil would allow healthy growth to continue in the young and would also maintain excellent health in adulthood.[148] Beef fat, they found, was inferior to these other fats in maintaining growth or health in adulthood. Vegetable oils, olive oil, almond oil, and even lard could not sustain growth in the young or health in adulthood. In 1918, McCollum continued,

> *"Both the growth promoting fat [butter, egg yolks, milk, liver, kidney, or cod liver oil]] and the trace of unidentified substance in the alcoholic extract of wheat germ are necessary for the promotion of growth or the preservation of health."*[151]

McCollum also concluded,

> *"The diet must contain two as yet unidentified substances or groups of substances. One of these is associated with certain fats, and is especially abundant in butter fat, egg yolk fats and the fats of the glandular organs such as the liver and kidney, but is not found in any fats or oils of vegetable origin."*[152]

The research was clear. The natural animal fats of butter, egg yolks, whole milk, liver, and cod liver oil, even in amounts as little as about 2 to 4% of the total dietary calories, were able to maintain both growth and health.[148] But, the vegetable oils as the fat source could not. Vegetable oils could not support growth nor support health in adulthood. With vegetable oils as the only source of fat, the fate of animals was certain to be an agonizing physical degeneration followed by an extremely early demise.

At the time, it wasn't clear what was in the butter, egg yolks, whole milk, liver, or cod liver oil, which could sustain excellent growth and health, but which wasn't in the vegetable oils.

During this early era of investigation – the 19-teens – vitamins had just been theorized to exist, as proffered by Casimir Funk in 1911 and later accepted by the scientific community in 1912.[153] [154] However, it was E.V. McCollum who suggested the very first to be named vitamin, which was at the time the presumed single vitamin which would maintain healthy growth in the young as well as

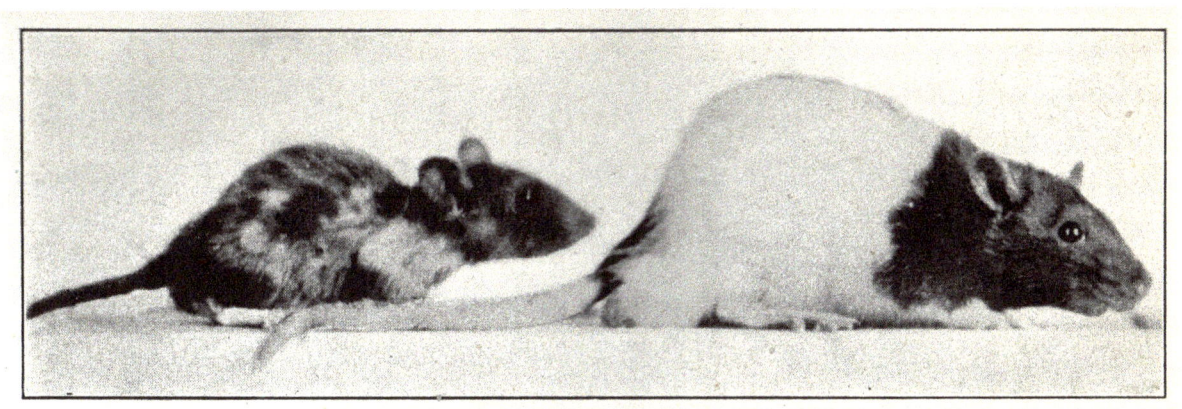

FIG. 6.—From weaning time the rations of these two rats were identical except in the character of the fats which they contained. The rat on the right was given 1.5 per cent of butter fat in its diet, while the one on the left received 5 per cent of bleached cottonseed oil. The former grew at the normal rate, while the latter remained stunted, and suffered loss of hair and emaciation. The small rats in Figures 5 and 6 had not yet developed xerophthalmia when photographed.

Reprinted from: E.V. McCollum. The Newer Knowledge of Nutrition. New York, The MacMillan Company, 1919. Fig. 6, p. 89. Image in public domain.

CHAPTER 1

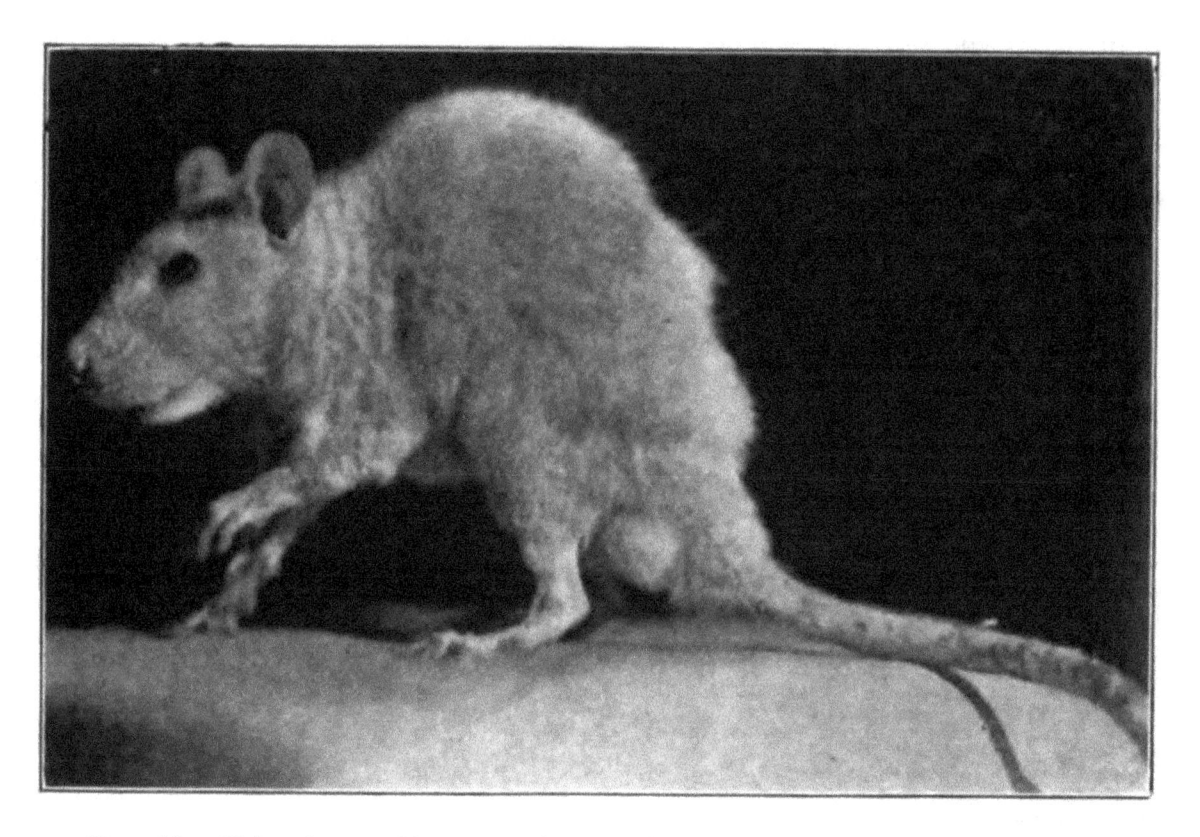

FIG. 13.—This picture illustrates the emaciated appearance of a middle aged rat after being fed about four months on a diet consisting of bolted flour, degerminated corn meal, rice, sugar, starch, pork fat, molasses, sweet potato, and cabbage. Such a diet has been reported by Goldberger to have produced pellagra in man in five and a half months. This diet affords wide variety and consists of wholesome food products, yet fails to maintain normal nutrition because it contains too little of the *protective foods,* milk, eggs and the leafy vegetables.

Reprinted from: E.V. McCollum. The Newer Knowledge of Nutrition. New York, The MacMillan Company, 1922. Fig. 13, p. 293. Image in public domain.

excellent health in adults, and McCollum called this vitamin "fat-soluble A."[155][156] This vitamin, of course, would later become known as "vitamin A."

What no one knew at that time, but which would be discovered over the next several decades, was that grass-fed butter,[157] egg yolks,[158] whole raw grass-fed milk,[157] liver,[159] and cod liver oil[160][161][162] all contain significant amounts of vitamins A, D, and K2 (Exceptions: cod liver oils vary markedly by type in K2 and may not be a reliable source; beef liver is very high in vitamin A but low in vitamin D and K2), whereas vegetable oils,[163][164][165][166] olive oil,[167] and almond oil[168] contain none of these. Even pork lard contains too little of these to sustain growth or health.[169][148]

WHY DOES ALLOPATHIC CONVENTIONAL MEDICINE RECOMMEND SEED OILS?

Shockingly, in recent decades, orthodox, allopathic medicine has ignored all of this fundamental nutrition science, and has promulgated the consumption of vegetable oils for one simple reason: they lower cholesterol levels in the blood.[170 171 172 173 174] But is this of any benefit whatsoever?

Seed oils are rich in LA, which in turn, increases the levels of LA in low-density lipoprotein (LDL); the higher levels of LA in LDL then causes the LDL to become highly susceptible to oxidation, producing higher levels of oxidized LDL (Ox-LDL).[175] Ox-LDL is actively, rapidly, and avidly scavenged by macrophages in the arterial wall, thus beginning and propagating atherosclerotic plaques.[176 177 178 179] That is, seed oils lower LDL cholesterol in the blood, but at the expense of that same LDL (now, Ox-LDL) driving atherosclerosis and coronary heart disease (CHD)![180] And, of course, atherosclerosis, also known as 'hardening of the arteries,' is the very process that we want to prevent!

As if this weren't harmful enough, it appears that the lowering of cholesterol in the blood via seed oil consumption may even be extremely harmful, elevating the risks of memory loss,[181] cancers,[182] overall mortality and cancers in the very elderly,[183] Parkinson's disease,[184] mortality in advanced heart failure,[185] depression,[186] suicide and especially violent suicide,[187] and even a much greater propensity for committing violent crimes.[188] But, once again, allopathic medicine fails to recognize all of this, because the belief system for around six decades has been that cholesterol is evil. Cholesterol per se is harmful.

Confusing isn't it, that a single molecule – cholesterol – found naturally in all animal cell membranes, required for normal physiology, a precursor to numerous natural steroid hormones, a molecule active in a plethora of biological pathways, and which is required for normal growth and life itself, has been vilified as the cause of coronary heart disease?[189 190] Yet, as it turns out, seed oils just so happen to lower the unfairly criticized and vilified cholesterol, and thus was born the core reason for health authorities to recommend seed oils.

Seed oils themselves, on the other hand, were born – not out of a desire to benefit health – but mostly to undersell and outsell lard, butter, and beef tallow, thereby turning big financial profits. And that they have done, to the tune of U.S. $259 billion in 2020, with that number expected to grow to $393 billion by 2027, on a global scale.[191] Growth of seed oil sales and consumption has outpaced any other single 'food' source since the year 1865. In fact, seed oil consumption has grown from almost none in 1865 (on a global scale) to occupy 15% to nearly 30% of calories in many westernized populations.[192] This has been paralleled by a near-infinite increase in numerous chronic disease conditions.

CHAPTER 1: SUMMARY

In the 1930s, Weston A. Price evaluated many thousands of people on five continents as they transitioned from native, traditional diets, to westernized diets which contained the "modernized" processed foods. He found that as the "modernized foods" displaced the natural foods of traditional diets, the children grew up with marked development of dental cavities, crooked teeth, and narrowed faces with numerous physical maladies.

Adults consuming such processed foods developed dental cavities, abscesses, arthritis, cancers, loss of immunity to infectious diseases like tuberculosis, and even mental deterioration and suicidal ideation. Price called the processed foods the "displacing foods of modern commerce," and he defined them as such because they displaced the nutrient-dense natural foods. The "displacing foods" were defined by Price as those containing refined (added) sugars, refined white wheat flour, white rice, canned goods, sweets, and vegetable fats (oils).

Earlier in the 20th century, nutrition researcher E.V. McCollum established that vegetable oils, nut oils, and even pork lard could not sustain growth in young animals or maintain health in adult animals, but that small amounts of butter, egg yolks, milk, liver, or cod liver oil could maintain both.

Vegetable oils and, in fact, all plant-based oils (with the exception of Japanese natto), contain not even a microgram or single international unit (IU) of the fat-soluble vitamins A, D, and K2, unlike the natural fats of butter, eggs, milk, cod liver oil, and the organs of animals such as liver, all of which contain substantial amounts of these vitamins. These vitamins are absolutely critical to both growth and health and are required in substantial amounts from the date of conception through old age.

Processed foods, which are best defined as those foods containing added sugars, refined grains (like white flour), seed oils, and trans fats, have almost exclusively entered the food supply since the end of the American Civil War in 1865. Of the four major processed food components, only sugar was generally available in most diets before 1865, practically on a worldwide basis; seed oils, refined white wheat flour, and artificially created trans fats, all primarily entered the food supply between the years 1866 and 1911.

These four 'foods' have gradually supplanted and replaced the natural foods of fruits, vegetables, animal meats (including beef, pork, chicken, fish, and seafood), whole grains, eggs and dairy, with 63% of the American diet being ultra-processed as of 2009, and 75% of the world's diets in recent years now considered processed.

Seed oils, which entered the food supply in 1866 in the U.S., have gradually displaced the natural animal fats of lard, butter, eggs, beef tallow, and even cod liver oil (once commonly recommended), rising from zero consumption in 1865 to occupy 86% of added fats in the diet in the U.S., by 2005.

During this same interval of time, i.e. 140 years, chronic diseases such as coronary heart disease, heart failure, hypertension, strokes, cancers, Alzheimer's disease, dementia, age-related macular degeneration (AMD), metabolic syndrome, type 2 diabetes mellitus, and overweight, have all gradually risen from medical rarity (or virtually unknown) to the most commonly known chronic disease conditions and causes of death.[3] [4] This has not only induced mass suffering, but also, marked disability and premature death.

In westernized diets, omega-6 LA consumption alone is approximately 8 to 12% of dietary consumption, but we need no more than 0.5% of our diet as LA. Linoleic acid (LA), while an essential fat and needed in exquisitely small quantities, when consumed to excess, induces a marked pro-oxidative, pro-inflammatory, toxic, and nutrient-deficient biological milieu (to be reviewed), which we will argue drives overweight and virtually every chronic disease known to man.

The primary omega-6 fatty acid in diets, known as linoleic acid, or LA, during the period of 1865 to 2008, elevated from about 1% to 12% of the diet in the U.S. So while omega-6 LA occupied a mere 1/100th of dietary calories in the U.S. in 1865, by 2008 it occupied 1/8th of caloric consumption. This increase in omega-6 LA consumption is almost entirely driven by seed oils. In parallel with this increasing omega-6 LA consumption is a marked to infinite increase in overweight, obesity, and nearly every chronic disease known to man, including coronary heart disease (CHD), hypertension, stroke, cancers, type 2 diabetes, metabolic syndrome, Alzheimer's disease, dementia, autoimmune diseases, and age-related macular degeneration (AMD).

CHAPTER 2

Dr. Price discovered the nutritional wisdom of native, traditional cultures. Images from Weston A. Price archives, courtesy of Price-Pottenger Nutrition Foundation. © Price-Pottenger Nutrition Foundation, Inc. All rights reserved

CHAPTER 2

PROCESSED FOODS AND SEED OIL DANGERS

"Life in all its fullness is Mother Nature Obeyed."

— WESTON A. PRICE

ANCESTRAL HEALTH
FOUNDATION

CHAPTER 2

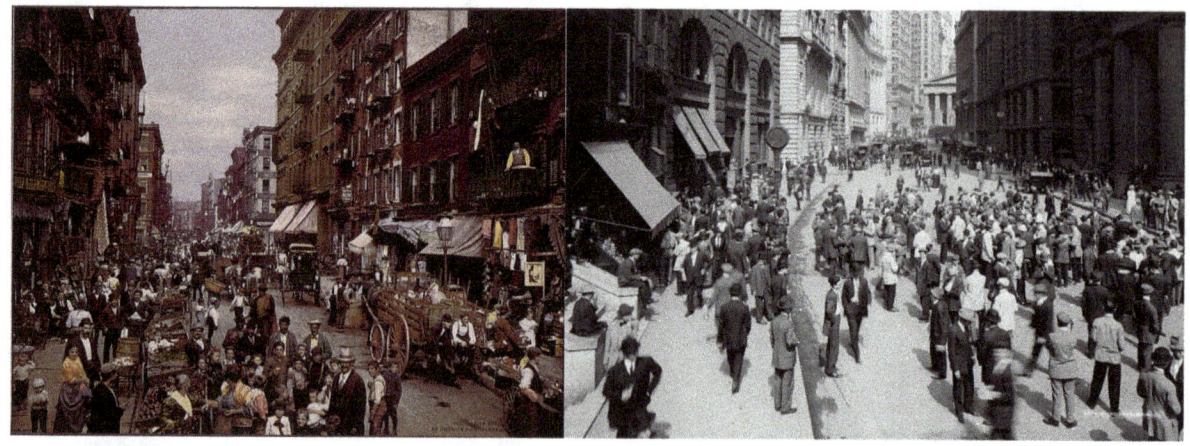

Photo, Left: Mulberry Street, New York City, circa 1900, photo courtesy of the U.S. Library of Congress, in the Public Domain.
Photo, Right: Broad Street, New York City, photo taken between 1910 and 1920, courtesy of U.S. Library of Congress, in the Public Domain.

THE EMERGENCE OF CORONARY HEART DISEASE AND MARKEDLY INCREASING CANCER

During the last few minutes of my recent live presentations, I have run a short vintage film of one of the earliest pieces of cinematography taken in the U.S., which shows people walking in the streets of New York City in 1911. While I let this film run for about 90 seconds, I discuss the fact that no matter how much footage one views of people on the streets, you will rarely find an overweight person, and I have yet to witness an obese person.

Of course, in 1900, only about 1.2% of Americans fell into the obese category,[449] [450] as compared to 42.5% obesity in 2018,[453] which is projected to climb to 48.9% by 2030.[454] I also discuss the fact that, in 1911, virtually none of these people had witnessed a heart attack, as the first documented heart attack in the U.S. occurred in 1912.[276] Only five cases of Alzheimer's disease were on record for the entire world (1 in 1908 and 4 cases in 1910),[193] whereas today, dementia, of which 60-70% of cases are Alzheimer's, affects 55 million people worldwide.[194]

Cancers were relatively unusual, with only one in 17 people dying of cancer in 1900,[271] versus nearly one in three today,[271] type 2 diabetes was virtually unknown,[195] metabolic syndrome (a combination of hypertension, increased blood sugars, insulin resistance, abnormal blood lipids, and visceral obesity) had never been diagnosed, as that would come in 1921-1922,[196] [197] and age-related macular degeneration (AMD), the leading cause of irreversible vision loss and blindness in people over the age of 60 worldwide, was an extreme medical rarity, with no more than about 50 cases diagnosed between 1851 and 1930.[4]

Yet, despite the fact that obesity was a rarity and most of the chronic diseases were virtually unknown, these people knew practically nothing about nutrition. And they probably didn't have much concern to know. Vitamins hadn't even been theorized, as that would come the following year after this film was taken, in 1912, when Casimir Funk published his theory of "vitamines," later to become known as "vitamins."[153] [198]

The people of 1911 had likely never heard of saturated fats, polyunsaturated fats, or monounsaturated fats, and there certainly is no evidence that

56

they feared any specific type of fat.[199] The enormous majority generally had little or no interest in low fat or low carbohydrate diets. They almost certainly weren't interested in extended fasting or intermittent fasting. Exercise for the sake of exercise was indeed a rarity; in fact, the first gym in the U.S. wouldn't be opened until 1936, in Oakland, California, by fitness guru Jack LaLanne.[200]

Of course, we're all curious, what were Americans eating in 1900 or thereabouts? And perhaps more importantly, *what were they not eating*? The late culinary researcher, Lynne Olver (1958-2015), who created an encyclopedic review of culinary history, affirmed that in the early 1900s, the U.S. population was vastly agricultural, many raising their own livestock and poultry, the latter of which were kept mostly for eggs, rather than "broilers" to be consumed.[201] Many cultivated their own vegetables and herbs. Hunting and fishing provided wild game as well. The great majority of food was prepared at home, from scratch.

Livestrong (Livestrong.com), in a recent review of Olver's voluminous works, affirmed:

"Meat was the mainstay of the 1908 American diet. Culinary researcher Lynne Olver lists veal, steak, roast beef, hamburger, ham, oysters, clams, flounder, mackerel, codfish and shad as typical spring menu items... fresh markets were not as easily accessible as they are now... [Refrigeration wasn't invented and available until 1913,[202] however,] It wasn't until the 1930s that the average American family owned an electric refrigerator.

"The typical family ate home-grown, seasonal fruits and vegetables... Milk and dairy foods weren't the focus of the American diet circa 1908, as it was difficult to prevent spoilage... you would have eaten potatoes, of some variety at least once a day... bread making was part of the daily routine... Whole grain cereals were year-round breakfast staples. [They were] much taken with sweets. In 1908, you would have treated your family to homemade muffins, cakes and pies, or bought them at the local bakery."[203]

Around 1908, as reviewed above, wheat was consumed almost daily along with other cereal grains, including oats, rice, corn, etc., which accounted for 37% of the diet (in 1909),[5] although we are not aware of any evidence as to how much was whole grain versus refined grain at that time. Potatoes and, less often, sweet potatoes, were almost daily staples, particularly in meals such as roast beef and potatoes, hash (chopped meat, potatoes, and onions), and side dishes of boiled potatoes, mashed potatoes, creamed potatoes, and fried potatoes, the latter fried in butter or lard.[201] [204] Sugar consumption was actually moderate, with total availability of 65 g/day in 1900 and 81 g/day in 1908 (S. Guyenet data), which is consistent with the review of Olver's work that Americans were "much taken with sweets."[203]

But what were Americans *not eating* around the years 1900 to 1908, when they enjoyed rather profoundly good health – when chronic diseases were almost unknown – and when infectious diseases were the leading causes of death?

We know for a fact, that between 1866 and 1908, Americans had no more than an average of about 1 gram of seed oils per day, that is, for the previous ~ 40 years![4] During those years, only approximately 2 grams of oils per day were available to a typical American, about half of which was olive oil.[4] There were also no artificially created trans fats in the diet, as the first of these – Crisco – didn't hit the market until 1911.[82]

Refined grains, such as white flour, had become available in 1880 via the introduction of roller mill technology,[73] but we have been unable to find any reliable evidence as to the relative consumption of refined grains versus whole grains at that time. We suspect that the bulk of grains were still consumed as whole grains.

Clearly, late 19th and early 20th century Americans were not consuming a low-carbohydrate diet, with 37% of their calories coming from grains (breads, cereals, pastries), along with moderate amounts of tubers (mostly potatoes), and some fruit and vegetables.

In the earliest years of the 1900s, the diet would have had almost no processed foods, but the single most significant difference in the diet between 1900 and anytime in the last 60 years would have been the relative lack of seed oils. In 1900, Americans consumed 2g (18 calories) of edible oils per day, but by 2010, consumption had increased to 80g (720 calories) per day. This is a 40-fold (3,900%) increase in seed oil consumption over a period of approximately one hundred years.

AN EARLY WORD ON DIETARY MANAGEMENT OF DISEASE CONDITIONS

There's an old adage which states, "If you cannot prevent or reverse a condition, you probably don't understand it." There's a great deal of truth in this statement. However, the good news about most chronic disease, whether we're referring to coronary heart disease, type 2 diabetes mellitus (T2DM), cancer, age-related macular degeneration (AMD), overweight or obesity, or a rare chronic disease with unknown origins, the dietary management will generally follow the same fundamental principles. And what kind of diet is that, you ask?

Our dietary recommendation will be any version of an ancestral diet. And such a diet may be of any ethnic origin. Whether the diet is American, French, Chinese, Japanese, Indian, Brazilian, African, Caribbean, or of any other ethnic origin, in all cases we recommend elimination (or extreme reduction) of the processed foods, which will be reviewed next.

PROCESSED FOODS VS. NATURAL ANIMAL AND PLANT FOODS – AND CHRONIC DISEASE OUTCOMES

As presented in Chapter One, we will define processed foods essentially as those foods containing added sugars, refined grains (mostly white wheat flour), seed oils, and artificially produced trans fats. Foods containing these are generally considered processed foods. Whole, natural foods, on the other hand, contain none of these. Natural foods would consist of the meats of any animals, such as beef, chicken, pork, fish and seafood, etc. as well as fruits, vegetables, whole grains, eggs, and raw dairy (e.g., raw milk and cheeses, but not pasteurized, homogenized milk and cheeses from same).

As first documented by Price in the 1930s and 1940s,[28] and more recently by the World Health Organization (WHO),[205] the Pan American Health Organization,[207] and literally thousands of scientific papers, processed foods have often been indicted as potent promoters of chronic disease.

For example, the WHO official website affirms,

"A healthy diet helps protect against malnutrition in all its forms and is a foundation for health and development. It also helps to prevent noncommunicable diseases including diabetes, cardiovascular diseases, some cancers and other conditions linked to obesity."[205] The WHO continues, "Noncommunicable diseases (NCDs) kill 41 million people each year, equivalent to 71% of all deaths globally…

"Unhealthy diets and lack of physical activity may show up in people as raised blood pressure, increased blood glucose, elevated blood lipids and obesity. These are called metabolic risk factors that can lead to cardiovascular disease, the leading NCD in terms of premature deaths."[206] The Pan American Health Organization (PAHO) states, "Consistent with previous findings, sales of ultra-processed products are associated with weight gain and obesity in Latin America."[207]

The PAHO continues, "The most striking change in food systems of high income countries, and now of low- and middle-income countries, is displacement of dietary patterns based on meals and dishes prepared from unprocessed or minimally processed food and drink products… that increase the risk of obesity and other diet-related NCDs."[207] The authors further state, "There is an urgent need to reduce the health risk posed by ultra-processed products by reducing their overall consumption."[207]

But while the WHO and PAHO are careful that their language doesn't vilify processed foods 'too harshly' and thereby offend Big Food manufacturers, numerous scientific researchers are more direct. For example, researcher Artemis Simopoulos, MD, Founder and President of the Center for Genetics, Nutrition and Health in Washington, D.C., states, "the rapid changes in our diet, particularly the last 100 years, are potent promoters of chronic diseases such as atherosclerosis, essential hypertension, obesity, diabetes, and many cancers."[208]

S. Boyd Eaton, MD, who might well be considered the founder of "Paleolithic nutrition" following a paper published under that same in 1985, wrote in a subsequent paper in 1988 "…it [westernized diet] acts as a potent promoter of chronic illnesses: atherosclerosis, essential hypertension, many cancers, diabetes mellitus, and obesity among others."[209]

Loren Cordain, PhD, whom many consider the modern founder of the "Paleo diet," in a paper published in 2005, wrote, "In the United States, chronic illnesses and health problems either wholly or partially attributable to diet represent by far the most serious threat to public health…Although dairy products, cereals, refined sugars, refined vegetable oils, and alcohol make up 72.1% of the total daily energy consumed by all people in the United States, these types of foods would have contributed little or none of the energy in the typical preagricultural hominin diet."[78]

Jasminka Ilich-Ernst, PhD, professor at Florida State University, and colleagues, wrote, "while the modern diet includes more than 70% of energy from refined sugars, refined vegetable oils, and highly processed cereals and dairy products…[this is] promoting the development of many chronic diseases, including obesity and osteoporosis."[210]

Researchers David Stuckler, PhD, MPH of Bocconi University in Milan, Italy and Marion Nestle, PhD, professor emeritus of New York University, stated, "Increasing consumption of Big Food's products tracks closely with rising levels of obesity and diabetes."[211] Jennifer M. Poti, PhD, professor of nutrition at the University of North

Carolina at Chapel Hill, along with colleague researchers, wrote "Recent research provides fairly consistent support for the association of ultra-processed food intake with obesity and related cardiometabolic outcomes."[212]

Westernized dietary consumption has been associated with the development of numerous diseases of civilization, including but not limited to coronary heart disease, atherosclerosis, epithelial cancers, hypertension, type 2 diabetes mellitus, autoimmune diseases, osteoporosis, obesity, metabolic syndrome,[213][214][215][216][217][218] Alzheimer's disease,[219][220][221] dementia,[222] inflammatory bowel disease,[223] depression, dysthymia (persistent depression), anxiety,[224] myopia (nearsightedness),[225] and non-communicable diseases (chronic diseases) in general.[213][226]

The *Lancet NCD Action Group*, whose goal is to promote health and reduce non-communicable disease risk through global reduction of unhealthy commodities, defines ultra-processed and processed foods as "substances extracted or refined from whole foods – e.g., [vegetable] oils, hydrogenated oils and fats [trans fats], flours and starches, variants of sugar, and cheap parts or remnants of animal foods—with little or no whole foods."[227] On a global scale, transnational corporations have reached virtually the entire world with ultra-processed foods, which have now largely replaced traditional dietary patterns.[227]

FIG 2.1

Processed Vs. Animal/Plant Foods U.S. Diet: 1865 Vs. 2009

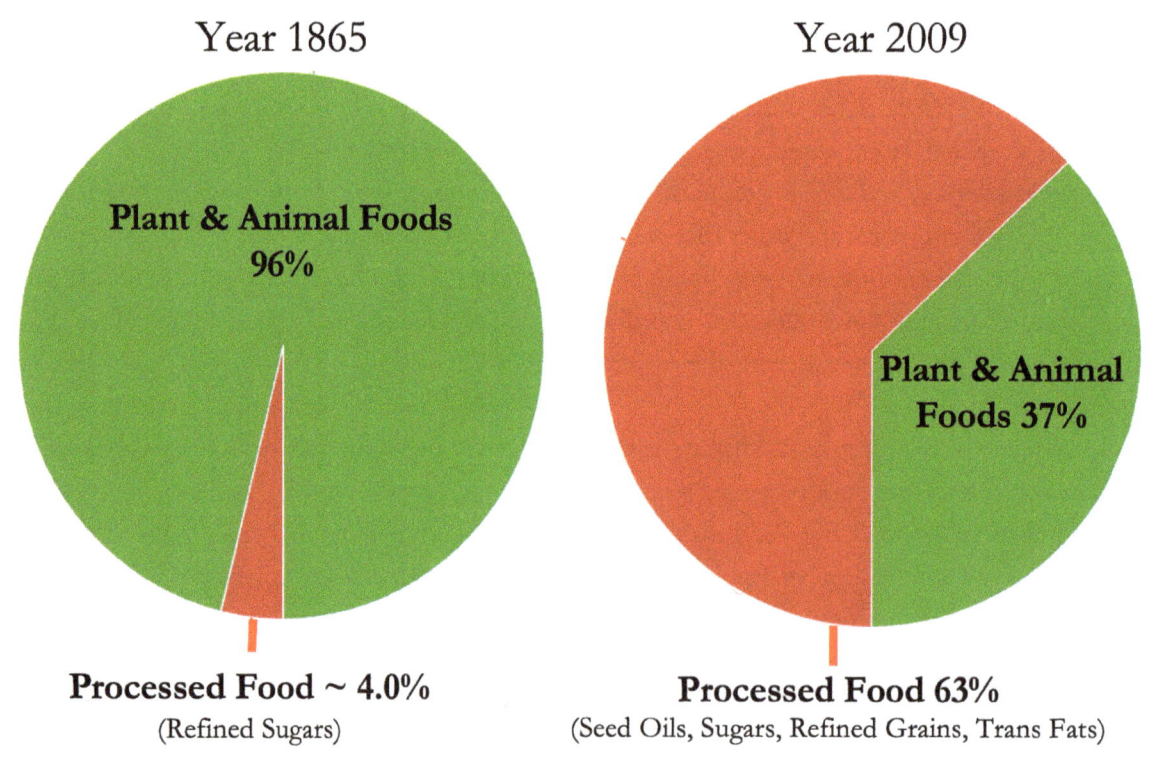

Year 1865

Plant & Animal Foods 96%

Processed Food ~ 4.0%
(Refined Sugars)

Year 2009

Plant & Animal Foods 37%

Processed Food 63%
(Seed Oils, Sugars, Refined Grains, Trans Fats)

Sources: USDA Economic Research Service (ERS), 2009. FAO. US. Dept Commerce. U.S. Census. Knobbe. Medical Hypotheses. 2017;109:184-198.

In the U.S., sugar consumption in the year 1865 was approximately 20g/day, or about 80 calories per person per day (data not shown).[4] [116] If we assume that Americans in 1865 consumed the same number of calories as Americans did in 1971 (NHANES 1971), which was 1955 cal/day, the 80 calories worth of sugar consumed in 1865 was about 4% of the diet and this was virtually the only processed food available at that time. In 1865, there were no seed oils, no refined grains (unless substantially "bolted" [sifted] at home – an extreme rarity), and no artificially produced trans fats.

The USDA and allied data confirm that, in 1889, about 93 percent of food expenditure was on food consumed at home, most of which was made from scratch.[228] [229] By 2010, Americans spent 50% of their food expenditure on food away from home, which was largely full-service restaurants and fast-food restaurants), which was up from 41% in 1984. Energy consumed as food away from home elevated from 17% in 1977-78 to 34% in 2011-12, and fast food expenditure, which was insignificant historically through the 1950s, accounted for 18% of total food expenditure by 2009.[228] The USDA makes a particular notation that food prepared away from home adversely affects the quality of nutrition and health outcomes, reduces levels of many micronutrients (vitamins and minerals), and that fast food, in particular, "is associated with high energy intake, low intake of essential micronutrients, and inferior metabolic outcomes."[228]

Globally, more than 75% of all food sales are now processed foods,[227] virtually none of which existed before 1865. As examples, ultra-processed foods now account for nearly 60% of calories consumed in the USA,[230] 48% in Canada,[231] and 56.8% in the UK.[232] *In 2009, the USDA ERS published data confirming that 63% of the U.S. diet was made up of processed foods, as added fats and oils, sugars, and refined grains* (see Fig 2.1).[233] Once again, just 155 years ago at the time of this writing, diets worldwide did not contain any amount of vegetable oils, trans fats, or refined flours, with only very small amounts of added

CHRONIC DISEASES IN AMERICA

6 IN 10
Adults in the US have a **chronic disease**

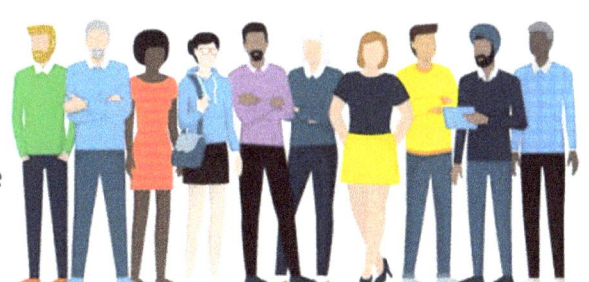

4 IN 10
Adults in the US have **two or more**

THE LEADING CAUSES OF DEATH AND DISABILITY
and Leading Drivers of the Nation's **$3.8 Trillion** in Annual Health Care Costs

Source: CDC. Use of content does not constitute an endorsement or recommendation by the U.S. Government, Department of Health and Human Services, or Centers for Disease Control and Prevention.

Six in ten adults in the US have a chronic disease and **four in ten adults** have two or more.

HEART DISEASE · CANCER · CHRONIC LUNG DISEASE · STROKE · ALZHEIMER'S DISEASE · DIABETES · CHRONIC KIDNEY DISEASE

Source: CDC. Use of content does not constitute an endorsement or recommendation by the U.S. Government, Department of Health and Human Services, or Centers for Disease Control and Prevention.

sugars (about 4% as previously indicated), and were based almost entirely on freshly prepared, unprocessed ingredients.

Today, 6 out of 10 American adults are living with a chronic disease condition, while 4 of 10 adults have two or more chronic diseases.[234] This is driving the enormous bulk of the nation's $3.8 trillion dollar (USD) annual health care costs.[234] In fact, the U.S. Department of Health and Human Services determined that chronic diseases accounted for 86% of all health care spending.[235]

However, the research linking processed food consumption with chronic disease conditions is abundantly clear. Processed, nutrient-deficient, and toxic foods, which are now greater than three-fourths of the global food supply[236] including most pre-prepared foods, packaged foods, canned goods, fast foods, and many restaurant foods, are potently promoting overweight and chronic diseases of almost every type. And on a caloric basis alone, seed oils account for a greater percentage of processed foods than any other ingredient.[4,3]

With regard to the fundamental concept and evidence that processed foods drive chronic disease development, conventional medicine has largely disregarded most all such evidence since 1950.[237,238] In fact, allopathic medicine has divorced itself from the study and discipline of Nutrition, and instead, promotes medicines and procedures for most all chronic disease management.[237,238] Rarely does medication cure or reverse any chronic disease.[239]

Medication certainly does not cure or reverse hypertension, coronary artery disease, atherosclerosis, strokes, diabetes, metabolic syndrome, Alzheimer's disease, dementia, autoimmune diseases, or age-related macular degeneration (AMD), and has had little if any impact on cancer outcomes.[239,240,241] Instead, medical management is simply a "band-aid" for chronic disease as it fails to address the root cause, thereby allowing the precipitating nutritional and lifestyle factors to persist, leading instead to worsening disease.[242]

WESTERNIZED CHRONIC DISEASES ARE RARE OR VIRTUALLY ABSENT IN HUNTER-GATHERERS AND POPULATIONS CONSUMING NATIVE, TRADITIONAL DIETS

The most important question to ask, having observed the ever-increasing prevalence of obesity and chronic disease in the world today, is this: What is the chronic disease burden (development) in populations who do not consume man-made, processed foods? If such populations, either currently or historically, do not develop overweight, obesity, heart disease, strokes, cancers, diabetes, and other chronic diseases, that is the most compelling evidence of all that processed foods drive chronic disease.

Indeed, we find that chronic diseases are either rare or virtually absent in hunter-gatherers, horticulturists, pastoralists (e.g., cattle herders), and other populations that have maintained native, traditional diets and who have virtually no access to, or negligible consumption of, processed foods, refined sugars, refined wheat flour, seed oils, and artificially produced trans fats.[243][244]

In 1981, physician researchers Denis P. Burkitt, MD, FRCS, and H.C. Trowell, MD, in their book *Western Diseases: Their Emergence and Prevention*, were so convinced that westernized diets produced a myriad of chronic disease that they wrote in the Preface of the book, "The Western [chronic] diseases are essentially the 'man-made diseases' and man is almost the only creature who profoundly alters his own environment."[245]

They continued, "...preliminary studies suggest that some of the Western diseases – essential

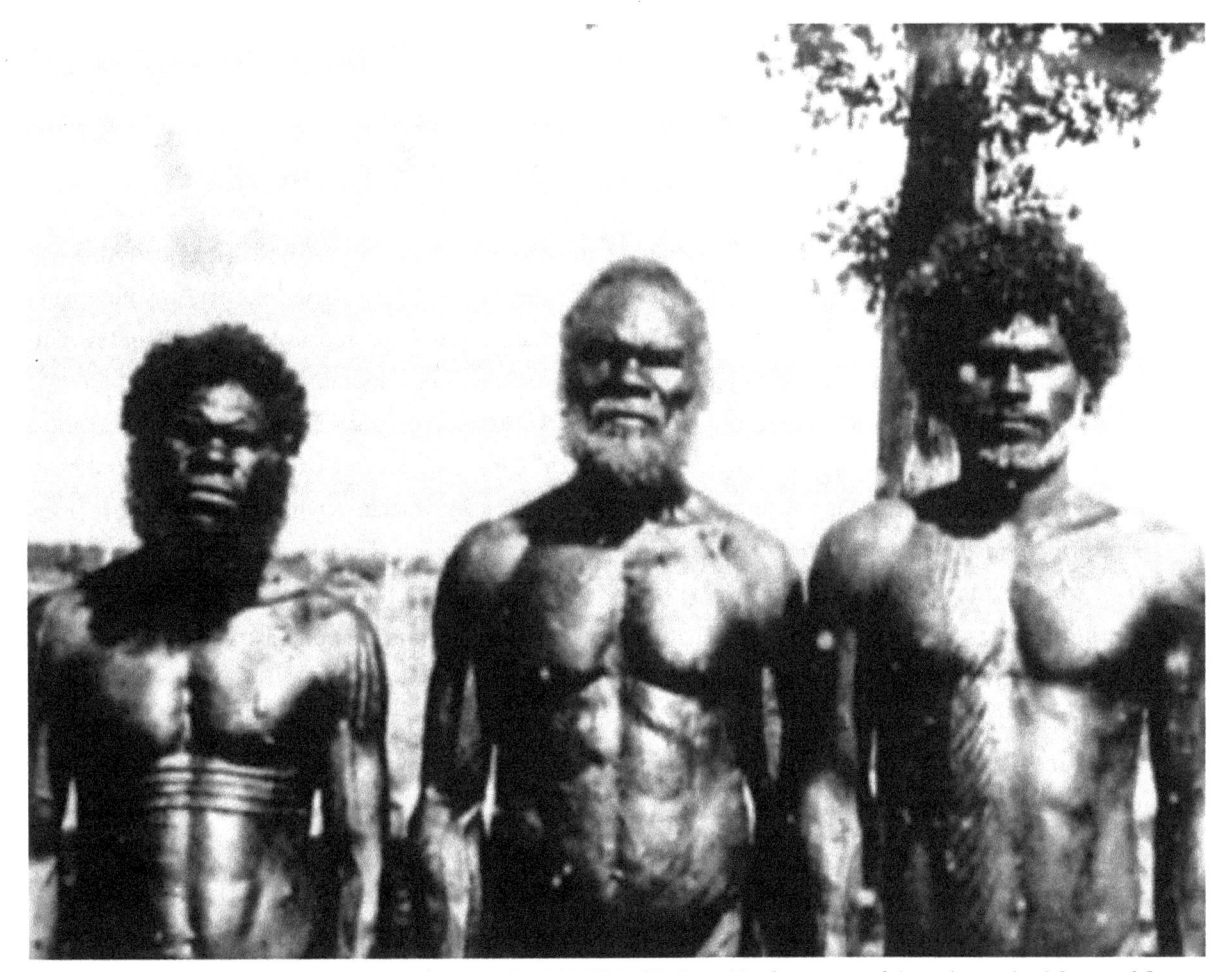

Three Aboriginal Australians on Bathurst Island in 1939. In 1929, 75% of Bathurst islanders supported themselves on local fauna and flora.

hypertension [high blood pressure], angina and diabetes mellitus type II, formerly called maturity-onset diabetes—may regress if patients revert to the diet, and even the physical activity, of early peasant agricultural groups, who have a low incidence of these diseases."[245]

Thus, according to Burkitt and Trowell, not only would native, traditional, ancestral diets generally prevent these diseases, but reverting to such ancestral diets would also cause regression of these same diseases. It's also quite interesting that they refer to such chronic diseases as 'man-made,' i.e., that such diseases are indeed produced by man through modernized diets. Trowell referred to our westernized diets and the associated chronic disease conditions as "affluent malnutrition,"[246] which is precisely evident.

In what should be considered the seminal paper on "Paleolithic Nutrition," S. Boyd Eaton, MD, and Melvin Konnor, PhD, wrote, "Physicians and nutritionists are increasingly convinced that the dietary habits adopted by Western society over the past 100 years make an important etiologic [causative] contribution to coronary heart disease, hypertension, diabetes, and some types of cancer. These conditions have emerged as dominant health problems *only in the past century and are virtually unknown among the few surviving hunter-gatherer populations* whose way of life and eating habits most closely resemble those of preagricultural human beings [italics added]."[624]

Eaton and Konnor continued, "The longer life expectancy of people in industrialized countries is not the only reason that chronic illnesses have assumed new importance. Young people in the Western world commonly have developing asymptomatic forms of these conditions, but hunter-gatherer youths do not. Furthermore, the members of technologically primitive cultures who survive to the age of 60 years or more remain relatively free from these disorders, unlike their "civilized" counterparts."[624]

For example, in 1988, S. Boyd Eaton and colleagues reviewed what they referred to as the "evolutionary mismatch" between modernized diets and our genetic constitution, which fosters numerous westernized chronic diseases, the latter of which were already known to produce 75 percent of all deaths in Western nations.[209]

However, they noted that such diseases are "rare among persons whose lifeways reflect those of our preagricultural ancestors."[209] In 2005, Loren Cordain, PhD, Professor Emeritus of Colorado State University, published a paper in which he reviewed the concept that recent and profound changes in our diet and lifestyle have created "evolutionary discordance" resulting in the current extraordinary prevalence of overweight, obesity, cardiovascular disease, cancer, hypertension, type 2 diabetes, osteoporosis, and osteopenia.[78]

In 2010, researchers Melvin Konnor, PhD and S. Boyd Eaton, MD reviewed the nutritional transition in westernized societies which has resulted in a vast number of chronic diseases, among the list including atherosclerotic cardiovascular disease, most coronary artery disease and cerebrovascular accidents, type 2 diabetes mellitus, chronic obstructive pulmonary disease, lung and colon cancers, essential hypertension, obesity, diverticulosis, and dental caries, all of which are rare among hunter-gatherers.[247]

From their studies of hunter-gatherers, they noted that even older hunter-gatherers "rarely got or died of coronary artery disease, diabetes mellitus, or chronic obstructive pulmonary disease, among other ailments common in societies like ours" while confirming that deaths were overwhelmingly related to infectious diseases for which such populations had neither antibiotics nor medicinal treatments.[209]

Historically, more than 50 hunter-gatherer societies have been substantially studied to a degree that certain dietary and nutritional generalizations can be made about them.[624] Unfortunately, there are only a few remaining hunter-gatherer populations in existence today which have not westernized their diets.[624] One analysis of hunter-gatherer diets, at least for those living in semitropical habitats, found that such groups derive somewhere between 50 and 80 percent of their foods (by weight) from plant sources, with animal foods providing between 20 and 50 percent.[254]

Loren Cordain, PhD, Janette Brand Miller, S. Boyd Eaton, MD, and other colleagues, extracted data on all 229 hunter-gatherer populations from the *Ethnographic Atlas* produced in 1999 by J.P. Gray. The data from this extensive analysis suggests that in the tundra (circumpolar) regions of the Earth, where there is very limited foliage, meat from hunted or fished animal sources contributes approximately 85% of the diet, whereas animal products contribute 42-62% of the diet in grassland ecosystems and 52-80% of the diet in temperate and rain forests.[248] Cordain and colleagues concluded, "Whenever and wherever it was ecologically possible, hunter-gatherers consumed high amounts (45-65% of total energy) of animal food. Most (73%) hunter-gatherer societies worldwide derived >50% (≥56-75%) of their subsistence from animal foods, whereas only 14% of these societies derived more than half (≥56-65%) of their subsistence from gathered plant foods."[248]

With regard to typical hunter-gatherer macronutrient (carbohydrate to protein to fat) intakes, Cordain and colleagues stated, "The most plausible…percentages of total energy would be 19—35% for dietary protein, 22—40% for carbohydrate, and 28—58% for fat. In the United States, the third National Health and Nutrition Survey showed that among adults aged ≥ 20 years, protein contributed 15.5%, carbohydrate 49.0%, fat 34.0%, and alcohol 3.1% of total energy intake."[248]

So while Americans' protein intake is lower and carbohydrates perhaps a bit higher than the typical hunter-gatherer, we will subsequently review populations (e.g., Japanese, Okinawans [a subset of Japanese], and Papua New Guineans) that fall far outside of the typical macronutrient ratios of hunter-gatherers, yet remain very healthy and relatively free of chronic disease.

Furthermore, while the diets of hunter-gatherer populations differ dramatically from one to another, from the almost entirely carnivorous, like the Inuit[249] and Eskimos,[250] to the nearly vegetarian, like the Papua New Guineans of Tukisenta,[251] it is our observation that all ancestral diets have one unifying commonality: They exclude processed foods – and they particularly exclude refined (added) sugars, refined flours (e.g., white wheat flour), and seed oils. The latter, of course, is only true for such populations who have remained traditional and have avoided the modernized, processed foods.

We are not aware of a single hunter-gatherer population that includes any seed oils in their diets whatsoever.[249,250,251,252,253,254,255,256] Some specific examples include the Maasai of Kenya and Tanzania,[257] the Inuit of Greenland,[249] the Eskimos of Northern Canada,[250] Papua New Guineans of Tukisenta,[251] the !Kung San of Southern Africa (Botswana, Namibia, and Angola),[253,256] the Hadza of Tanzania,[255] the Cave-Dwelling Tasaday hunter-gatherers of the Philippines,[258][259] the Aché of Paraguay,[260] and the inhabitants of the Island of Kitava.[261]

It should be quite obvious that no such populations would utilize mechanized high-temperature and pressure seed oil presses, hexane solvent baths, steaming and degumming procedures, followed by chemical alkalinization, bleaching, and deodorization procedures – the complex, mechanized, and chemical-laden technological procedures of modern seed oil production – to produce common 'vegetable oils.' Hence, such edible high PUFA oils are not a part of their dietary regime.

With regard to macronutrient ratios of hunter-gatherers, it is again clear that there are no unifying commonalities, but rather, it is empirically obvious that macronutrient ratios in these populations are all over the board, from as little as 10% or less plant foods – and perhaps 10% or less carbohydrate – like the Inuit[262] and Eskimos (~50 g carbohydrate/day),[263][264][250] to the 66% animal fat diets of the Maasai tribe warriors,[265] to the 3% fat (94.6% carbohydrate) diet of the Papua New Guineans of the Tukisenta highlands.[251] Yet all of these populations remain mostly lean, fit, and virtually free of chronic disease.

Furthermore, all of these aforementioned hunter-gatherer populations were found to have either complete absence of chronic diseases or such conditions were extraordinarily rare. This is extraordinary evidence that neither low-carb nor low-fat diets are necessary to either prevent or treat chronic disease; but rather, it is the quality of the diet – and the fats in particular – which are key. This will be reviewed in greater detail subsequently.

One need not be a hunter-gatherer to benefit from their experience, knowledge, and wisdom, just as Weston A. Price found after evaluating many such populations in the 1930s.[28] Avoidance of processed foods not only results in much higher consumption of all nutrients, but it also results in consumption of a very low level of omega-6 LA, which is obvious by any analysis of traditional foods and/or progressive Westernization of diet.[266][267]

CORONARY HEART DISEASE IS A 20TH CENTURY PHENOMENON

Many people do not realize that in the 19th century, coronary heart disease (CHD) was virtually unknown.[268] Researchers David S. Jones, MD, PhD, and colleagues, wrote a paper that reviewed much of the changing medical landscape over the past 200 years of history, beginning with a "Bill of Mortality" from the city of Boston, Massachusetts, for the year 1811.[271] This actual bill (see figure on page 67) for the city of Boston, Massachusetts, population of ~34,737 at the time, lists no deaths from heart disease. However, it is still possible there were cases of which they were unaware.

As can be viewed from the actual "Bill" shown (see page 67, left hand side of table), there were 942 deaths that year. Of these, a total of 25 (2.6%) suffered sudden death. Ergo, even if we were to presume that all of these sudden-death cases were myocardial infarction (MI or "heart attack") related deaths, that number is still extremely low as compared to today's prevalence of heart-related deaths, which is 32.3% of deaths.[271] Apoplexy, which was possible stroke, accounted for only 13 of the total deaths (1.4% of deaths), while aneurism accounted for one death (0.1% of deaths).

At that time, one can see exactly what Jones and colleagues mentioned with regard to the usual causes of death, that is, "Consumption [tuberculosis], diarrhea, and pneumonia dominated the mortality data…"[271] All three of these conditions are infectious and, interestingly, these are the same top three causes of death in the year 1900 (Jones table below). Thus, it is clear that infectious diseases dominated all of the major causes of death at that time, while cardiovascular diseases played only a diminutive role, accounting for just a few percent of deaths in totality.

It will likely come as quite a surprise to most, but during the entire century between the years of 1800 to 1900, we are only aware of nine scientific papers published documenting myocardial infarction (MI, or "heart attack") or coronary heart disease, with just three of those nine being related to thrombotic coronary disease, that is, specifically MI (see detail below).

Harold Feil, in a review paper entitled *History of the Treatment of Heart Disease in the Nineteenth Century* (published in 1960 by Johns Hopkins University Press), wrote, "Little was said about either hypertensive or coronary heart disease [in the 19th century]… A number of observers, Parry, Scarpa, Hodgson, Lobstein, Leyden, Marie, described coronary artery disease and myocardial infarcts ["heart attacks"], and rare cases of clinical coronary thrombosis were described by Hammer in 1876 and by Dock in 1896."[268] Thus, the first six authors reviewed the presence of coronary artery disease and, as far as we are aware, there were only a few

Causes of Death, Boston, MA, U.S. 1811 – With Notations

The Deaths preceding were caused by Diseases and Casualties as follows, viz.

Abscesses	1	Hernia, or Rupture	3	
Aneurism	1	Jaundice	10	
Apoplexy	13	Inflammation of the bowels	1	
Burns or Scalds	6	—— of the stomach	1	
Cancer	5	Killed by lightning	1	
Casualties	15	Insanity	1	
Childbed	14	Intemperance	2	
Cholera Morbus	6	Locked jaw	2	
Colic	2	Mortification	11	
Consumption	221	Old Age	26	
Convulsions	36	Palsy	12	
Cramp in the stomach	2	Pleurisy	8	
Croup	1	Quinsy	15	
Debility	28	Rheumatism	1	
Decay	20	Rupture of blood vessels	1	
Diarrhœa	15	Small-Pox, (at Rainsford's Island)	2	
Drinking cold water	2	Sore throat	1	
Dropsy	21	Spasms	2	
—— in the head	23	Stillborn	49	
Drowned	13	Suicide	1	
Dysentery	14	Sudden death	25	
Dispepsia or Indigestion	15	Syphilis	12	
Fever, bilious	7	Teething	15	
—— pulmonic	46	Worms	11	
—— inflammatory	24	Whooping Cough	14	
—— putrid	6	White swelling	2	
—— typhus	33	Diseases not mentioned	48	
Flux infantile	57			
Gout	3	Total,	942	
Hoemorrhage	4			

Notations…

Boston, MA Population in 1811: ~ 34,737

Cancer: 5/942 Deaths, i.e. 0.53%

Heart Disease: No deaths listed.

Sudden Death: 25/942 deaths, i.e. 2.6%

Apoplexy (Possible Stroke): 13/942 Deaths, i.e., 1.4%

Aneurism: 1/942 deaths, or 0.1%

Consumption (Tuberculosis): 221/942 deaths, i.e. 23.5%

Adapted from: Jones DS, et al. The Burden of Disease and the Changing Task of Medicine. NEJM. 2012;366:2333-2338. "Notations" per C. Knobbe.
© C. Knobbe, 2022. Ancestral Health Foundation.

papers (e.g., Johanss, 1859 [see below], Hammer, 1876, Dock 1896) documenting heart attacks in that century.

Dr. David S. Grimes, consultant physician in the U.K. at the Royal Blackburn Hospital, published a review paper on coronary heart disease, in which he stated, "The earliest clinic-pathological report of CHD was in 1859, an anecdotal case report of myocardial infarction (MI) presented to the Swedish Medical Society. It defined the clinical features of MI and also the pathological features found at autopsy, linking the two aspects. The report was not known outside Sweden and at the time it did not appear to be important."[269] Swedish physicians contrasted this single case report of known MI during the entire 19th century in Sweden to the fact that the city of Malmo, Sweden, had 770 new cases of MI in 1978 alone (Malmo population 1978, 236,000).[270]

Grimes further wrote, "At the beginning of the 20th century, CHD was effectively unknown in the UK. It received no mention in the earlier writings of Sir James Mackenzie, who was initially a general medical practitioner in Burnley, Lancashire [U.K.] and later the father of cardiology in the UK."[269] He continued, "… it is now clear that in these countries [in particular, the UK, temperate parts of the world, northern Europe, and North America] CHD was an epidemic of the latter half of the 20th century. The onset of the epidemic appears to have been shortly after the First World War [post 1918].... In the early years of the 20th century, the major forms of heart disease were the late results of rheumatic fever and syphilis, and also endocarditis, all of which are caused by micro-organisms and for which penicillin later became an effective treatment."[269]

What Grimes referenced here is the fact that cardiac valvular disease – and not coronary heart disease (CHD) – accounted for the major forms of potentially lethal heart disease up through the late 19th and early 20th centuries.[271]

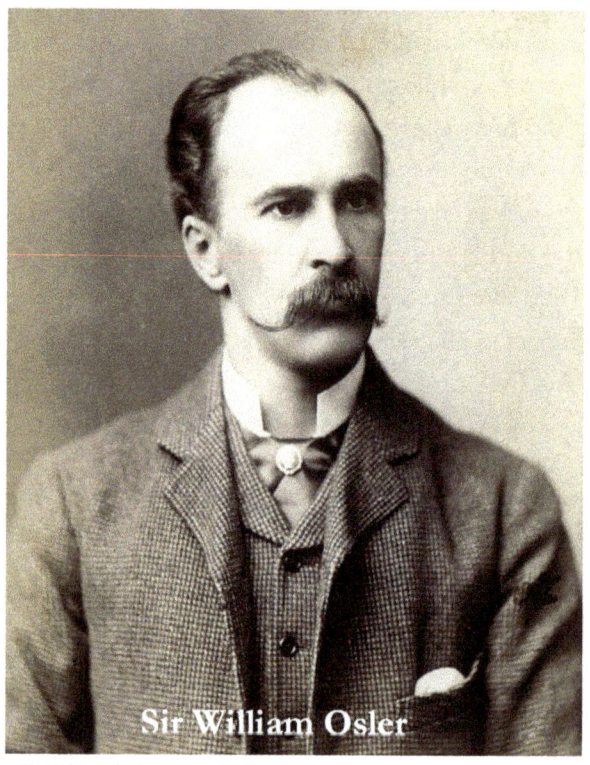

Sir William Osler. Circa 1884 – 1888.

In 1892, famed physician, Sir William Osler, co-founder of Johns Hopkins Medical Center in Baltimore, Maryland, published the first edition of *The Principles and Practice of Medicine*, which is considered the first textbook of medicine.[272]

In this textbook, Osler described numerous cardiac conditions and available treatments at the time, which included chronic cardiac valvular disease with heart failure, mitral valve disease with irregular pulse (another type of valvular disease), pericarditis, endocarditis, arteriosclerosis, aneurysm, angina pectoris (the squeezing chest pain associated with coronary artery disease) and congenital heart disease, but as reviewed in 1960 by Harold Feil, coronary heart disease with heart attack was not a subject of review because "Myocardial infarction ["heart attack"] had not yet been diagnosed clinically."[268] It also is certain that Osler was aware of angina in 1892, at least in rare cases having ended in death, however, as he mentioned "fatal cases of angina."[273]

In 1897, Osler gave a detailed review of the clinical rarity of angina pectoris, when he confirmed:

> *"[A]ngina pectoris is a rare affection in hospital practice… During the ten years in which I lived in Montreal, I did not see a case of the disease either in private practice or at the Montreal General Hospital. At Blockley [Blockley Almshouse, later known as Philadelphia General Hospital] too, it was an exceedingly rare affection. I do not remember to have had a case under my personal care… During the seven years in which the Johns Hopkins Hospital has been opened… there have only been four instances of angina pectoris."*[274]

This record, provided by Osler in 1897, would recount his private practice and hospital experience for the previous 21 years. That is, between 1876 and 1897, Osler documented around half a dozen cases of angina and perhaps not a single myocardial infarction. Most interestingly, the cases of angina virtually all took place in the 1890s and generally not prior.

Some thirteen years later, in 1910, Osler reported having seen an additional 208 cases of angina in the period between 1897 and 1910.[274] In a lecture given to the Royal College of Physicians in London, in review of this increasing trend of angina, he asked the audience,

> *"Has angina pectoris increased in the community? Has the high-pressure life of modern days made the disease more common? There is an impression among consultants in the United States that there has been an increase [during the] late years."*[274]

This collective review by Sir William Osler, which recounted his clinical experience between 1876 and 1910 – a period of 34 years during the late 19th and early 20th centuries – indicates that he had never witnessed a heart attack (MI). Of course, almost no one on the planet had ever seen, heard of, or witnessed a heart attack in that era because the disease condition was practically unknown.

David S. Jones, MD, PhD, and colleagues, who published Boston's "Bill of Mortality" for the year 1811 (see page 67), also published the table on page 70, "United States Top 10 Causes of Death: 1900 vs. 2010."[271] As one can see, "heart disease" was the 4th major cause of death in 1900, however, at that time Jones and colleagues reviewed that heart disease was "chiefly infectious or valvular rather than atherosclerotic."[271]

Indeed, infectious diseases, such as rheumatic fever, endocarditis, and syphilis, for which they had no antibiotics at that time, not infrequently left the heart valves scarred and dysfunctional, resulting in the bulk of fatal heart disease at that time.[269][271][275] In fact, it wouldn't be until after 1940, when penicillin and other antibiotics became available, that rheumatic, syphilitic, and infectious endocarditis-induced heart disease would rapidly decline, thereby resolving the enormous bulk of cardiac valvular disease.[269]

In 1912, James B. Herrick, MD, published a paper followed by a presentation at the Association of American Physicians conference, in which he

United States Top 10 Causes of Death: 1900 vs. 2010

1900 (No. of Deaths/100,000):
- Pneumonia or influenza, 202.2
- Tuberculosis, 194.4
- Gastrointestinal infections, 142.7
- Heart disease, 137.4
- Cerebrovascular disease, 106.9
- Nephropathies, 88.6
- Accidents, 72.3
- Cancer, 64.0
- Senility, 50.2
- Diphtheria, 40.3

Notation: In the year 1900, "Heart disease" was chiefly cardiac valvular disease, not coronary heart disease (CHD)

2010 (No. of Deaths/100,000):
- Heart disease, 192.9
- Cancer, 185.9
- Noninfectious airways diseases, 44.6
- Cerebrovascular disease, 41.8
- Accidents, 38.2
- Alzheimer's disease, 27.0
- Diabetes, 22.3
- Nephropathies, 16.3
- Pneumonia or influenza, 16.2
- Suicide, 12.2

Source: Jones DS, et al. The Burden of Disease and the Changing Task of Medicine. NEJM. 2012;366:2333-2338.

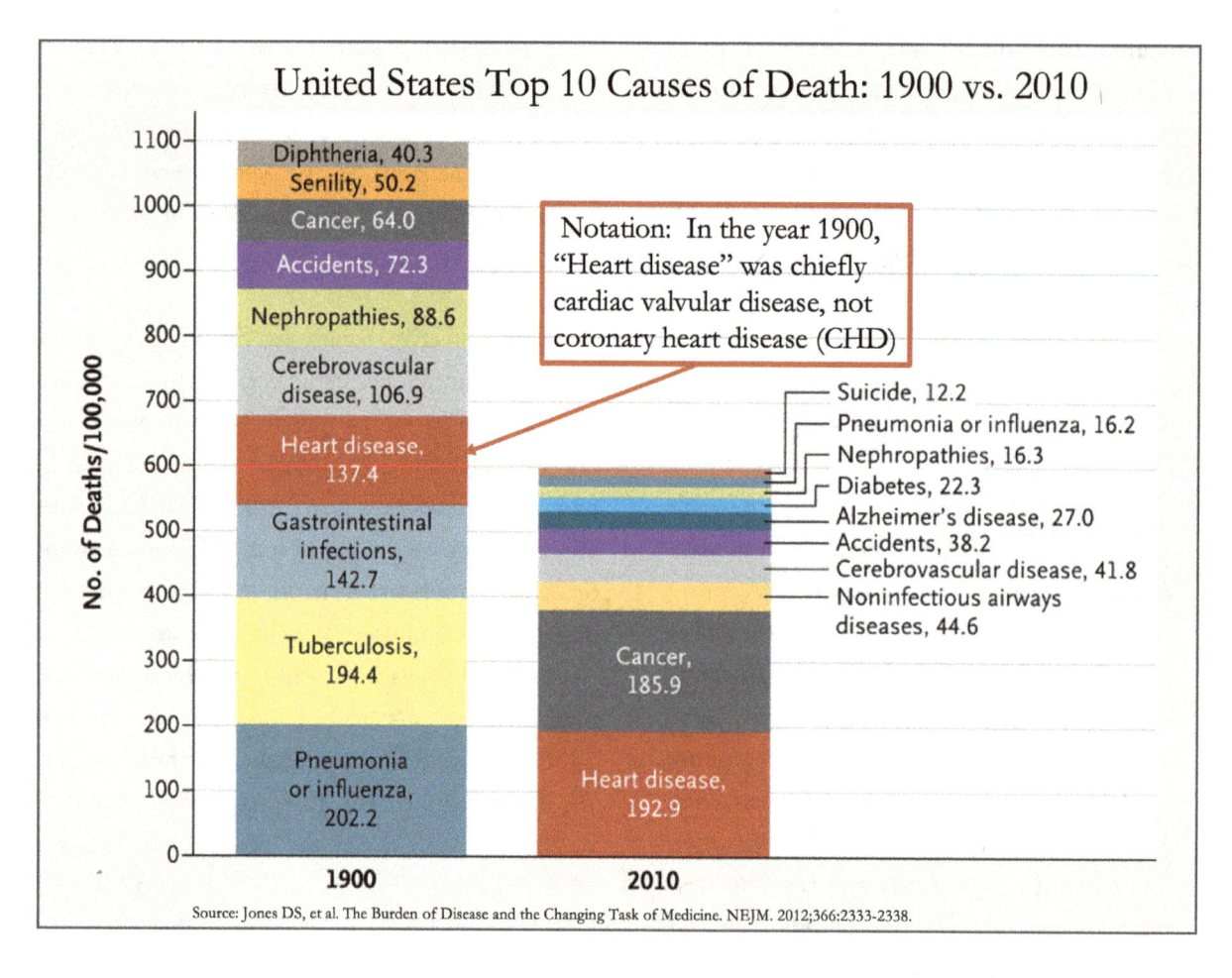

documented the first confirmed case of myocardial infarction in the U.S., associated with autopsy evidence.[276] But no one even took it seriously. In fact, he much later stated:

"In 1912 when I arose to read my paper at the Association [Association of American Physicians], I was elated, for I knew I had a substantial contribution to present. I read it, and it fell flat as a pancake. No one discussed it except Emanuel Libman, and he discussed every paper read there that day. I was sunk in disappointment and despair."[277]

In 1919, Herrick addressed the Association of American Physicians again, and it was then that medical doctors began to seriously consider the diagnosis of myocardial infarction as well as Herrick's original paper.[277] Some medical biographers have concluded that "a full decade passed before the medical profession recognized his [Herrick's] clinical description of coronary thrombosis [coronary artery clot] and myocardial infarction..."[278] Herrick published two more papers regarding coronary heart disease; one on angina in 1918[279] and a second entitled "Thrombosis of the coronary arteries"[280] (heart attack), which began to be accepted by colleague physicians in the UK in the 1920s.[269]

As coronary heart disease (CHD) became more

James B. Herrick, MD, Circa 1910

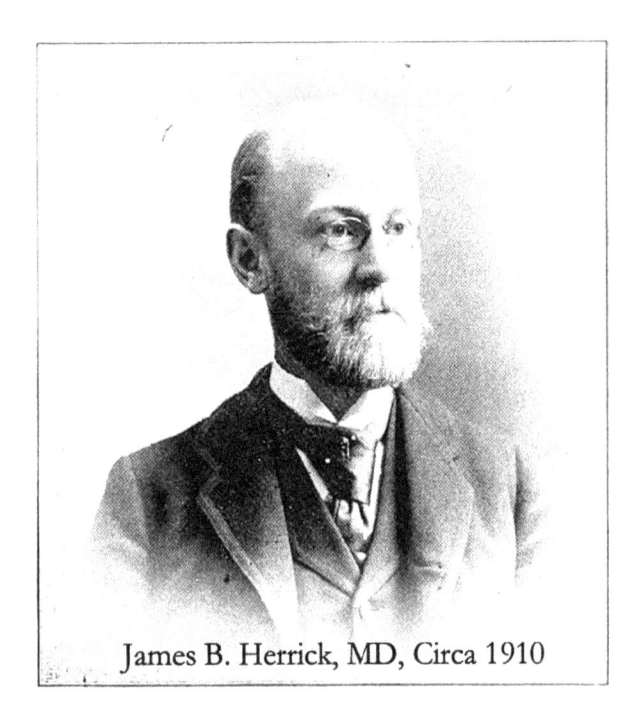

prominent and understood in the early decades of the 20th century, Herrick's pioneering discoveries laid more groundwork for the cardiology profession. In 1930, Herrick received the Kober Medal for his distinguished research in medicine, an honor conferred by the Association of American Physicians, and in 1939, the American Medical Association recognized Herrick with the Distinguished Service Medal.[277]

Whereas Sir William Osler had referred to angina as "a rare disease" in his 1892 text, twenty-three years later, in the 8th Edition of his *Principles and Practice of Medicine* textbook, published in 1915, he wrote, "The disease is not uncommon, about 700 dying yearly of it in England and Wales. In the United States it is more common, the average number of deaths per million of the population being more than double that of England… It [angina] is a rare disease in hospitals; a case a month is the average even in the larger metropolitan hospitals."[281]

In Osler's 1921 edition of *Principles and Practice of Medicine*, he reviewed coronary artery thrombosis (heart attack), stating, "Involvement of the coronary arteries may lead to various symptoms—thrombosis with sudden death, fibroid degeneration of the heart, aneurism of the heart, rupture, and angina pectoris [chest pain]." These documentations appear to clearly indicate that CHD was far more common by 1915 while it was exceedingly rare in 1892.

Osler's statistic of 700 deaths yearly in England and Wales for the year 1911 is worth examining further. The population of England and Wales in the year 1915 was 36,070,000 and there were 562,253 deaths (1.5% of the population).[282] If we apply Osler's statistic of 700 deaths secondary to "angina" in England and Wales, this is approximately 0.12% of deaths, which is only 1 in every 803 deaths! Contrast that to the fact that 32.3%, or nearly 1 in every 3 deaths in the U.S. in 2010 were of CHD,[271] and in 2009 it was confirmed that 64% of cardiac deaths were driven by coronary artery disease.[283]

The U.K. Office for National Statistics recorded almost no male heart disease deaths in either 1915 or 1925, but recorded 7,845 deaths due to "myocardial degeneration" in 1935, and then remarkably, in 1945, a total of 7,198 deaths due to "diseases of the coronary arteries."[282] This trend continued with striking increases in coronary artery disease deaths in 1955, 1965, and 1975, followed by some decline through 2015.

Maurice Campbell, the first editor of the *British Heart Journal*, now known as *Heart*, completed a careful statistical work to better understand heart disease in the U.K.[284] He determined that, between 1876 and 1921, there was little or no change in diseases of the heart, and no specific mention of

CHD.[285] Then, beginning in the years 1922 to about 1924, an epidemic of CHD began to initiate. He noted that the death rate from CHD in England and Wales increased from just 2.9/100,000 in 1921 to 16.6/100,000 in 1931.

Deaths from cerebrovascular diseases increased substantially during this time as well. Campbell noted that the CHD death rate doubled between 1921 and 1927, doubled again by 1929, doubled again by 1933, doubled again by 1939, and again for the sixth time by 1956.[285] He confirmed a geometric increase in CHD that could not have been due to a change in diagnosis, name change in the disease, etc., but affirmed a new factor had presented itself to cause the onslaught of CHD.

Campbell's analysis ended in 1956, but subsequent evidence confirmed that the UK death rate from CHD was 200/100,000 in 1950, which more than doubled by 1960, peaking at 550 deaths per 100,000 in 1970. Thus, we see an increase in CHD deaths in the U.K. from 2.9/100,000 in 1921 to 550/100,000 in 1970.[269 286 287 288]

This analysis confirms an approximate 190-fold (18,900%) increase in CHD deaths during this period. For men aged 55 to 64 years in 1972, the peaks were even higher, with mortality rates from CHD of 730/100,000 in England and Wales, which is a 252-fold (25,100%) increase, and a staggering 960/100,000 in Scotland, the latter of which is a 331-fold (33,000%) increase.[269] Certainly, an 'environmental factor' is at work here, but what is it?

Smoking, of course, has been linked to CHD in many studies.[315] Cigarette smoking only gained prominence in the 20th century, unfortunately, which muddies the picture when it comes to understanding the cause of CHD.[319] In the U.K., smoking peaked in prevalence at a staggering 82% in 1948, and then fell progressively to 45% by 1974, 26% by 2002, and 14.1% by 2019.[289]

We see a very strong correlation between smoking and CHD on a nationwide basis over time, such that when we just look at smoking versus CHD on comparative graphs, the two look well correlated. But, are they? Is smoking the pri-

Total vegetable oil consumption in UK

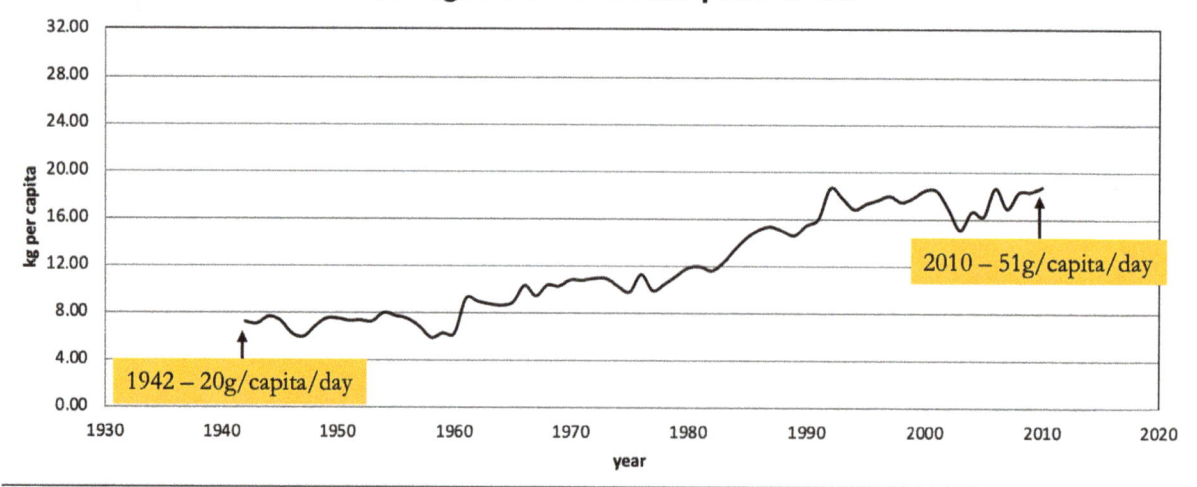

1942 – 20g/capita/day

2010 – 51g/capita/day

Knobbe C, Stojanoska M. The 'Displacing Foods of Modern Commerce' Are the Primary and Proximate Cause of Age-Related Macular Degeneration: A Unifying Singular Hypothesis. Medical Hypotheses: 2017;109:184-198. © C. Knobbe, 2022. Ancestral Health Foundation.

mary cause of CHD? We'll come back to this question after examining the evidence between smoking, seed oil consumption, and CHD in the U.S (below).

While there is much evidence for increasing seed oil consumption on a global scale since the late 19th century, we can be certain that seed oil consumption in the U.K. was virtually zero in 1865, just like the U.S. and most all of the world (reviewed previously). In fact, researchers Martin Pitts, MA, PhD, at the University of Exeter in the U.K., along with colleague researchers, affirmed that there was no significant vegetable oil production worldwide in the year 1900, further stating, "…until the late nineteenth century, the only edible oil-bearing crop grown in Europe was the olive, with the rest of the continent relying on animal fats as the principal source of cooking oil."[290]

The earliest accurately known seed oil consumption data that we have been able to obtain for the U.K. began in 1942, when consumption was already 7.21 kg/capita/year, which is approximately 20g/person/day, and this rather steadily increased all the way through 2010, when consumption was at 18.69 kg/year, which was 51 g/day[4] (see graph, page 72).

Thus, if we estimate that seed oil consumption elevated from perhaps around 1-2 g/day in 1900, which is the same as the U.S., then elevated to 20 g/day by 1940 and climbed all the way to 51 g/day by 2019, we see that CHD has fallen in recent decades while seed oils are still rising. Uh-oh… does this mean seed oils are not causing CHD? Of course not. However, there may be a threshold effect. That is, it may be that, above a certain level of consumption, a greater dose doesn't cause an increasingly negative outcome with respect to CHD, i.e., greater risk of CHD. As we will see subsequently, this is exactly the case with seed oil consumption and cancer.

Clearly, cigarette smoking in the U.K. had an enormous peak prevalence at 82% in 1948, but then rather steadily fell to 14.1% by 2019, while seed oils consumption has had a non-stop ascent at least since 1942, but almost certainly since the late 19th century. Almost without question, we've already observed that CHD was virtually unknown when seed oil consumption was near zero in the 19th century, but cigarette smoking was near zero in the 19th century as well.

Most certainly, CHD, like most diseases, is multi-factorial. With just the evidence we've examined so far, it appears quite clear that CHD did not occur in the U.S., U.K., nor anywhere in the world to any significant degree before seed oil consumption became substantial.

Though only a few heart attacks had ever been witnessed by 1900 all around the world, by the 1930s in the U.S., coronary heart disease (CHD) had risen to become the leading cause of death.[291] Why? What had happened? It was virtually unknown in 1910, just 20 to 30 years previously! By about 1950, atherosclerosis of the coronary arteries, the fundamental cause of CHD, was considered responsible for 25% of all deaths.[292] This was a staggering increase for a condition that was hardly known in 1920.

This trend of markedly increasing CHD and heart attacks continued, seemingly unabated, from the 1920s onward, peaking in about 1968, but with declining age-adjusted CHD death rates in the U.S. thereafter.[293][294][298] Nevertheless, by 2010, CHD still accounted for 32.3% of all deaths in the U.S. and remained the leading cause of death with cancer deaths just slightly behind.[271] Currently, every year around 1,100,000 people in the U.S. experience an acute myocardial infarction (heart attack).[295] Around 35% of those affected will die of sudden death around the time of the heart attack.[296]

Earl Ford, MD, MPH, and colleagues, completed an in-depth analysis of coronary disease deaths in the U.S. between 1980 and 2000, and attributed 47% of the reduction in CHD deaths to medical and surgical treatments and preventive therapies, with another 12% of the decrease based on a reduction in smoking.[297] Assuredly, a massive increase in cardiac medications, anticoagulants ("blood thinners"), clot-busting drugs (thrombolytics), coronary angioplasty and stents, bypasses (coronary artery bypass grafting), and other procedures and drugs have all been developed and implemented primarily since 1980.

Thus, it appears to be quite well accepted that, between the mid-19th century and about 1920, CHD ending in death was virtually unknown. In contrast, about a century later in the U.S., in 2010, nearly one of every three people died of the condition. This cannot be explained by increased longevity alone.[298] Today CHD commonly strikes people in what might be considered the prime of their lives, that is, between the ages of 45 to 64, where researchers found a total of 129,000 deaths occurred in that age group in the U.S., which is precisely half of those dying between the ages of 75 to 84 (258,000 deaths).[299]

Even more disturbing, in 2005 alone, CHD accounted for 26,000 deaths in people 45 years and younger in the U.S.[299] This amounts to an average of 71 deaths per day in people aged 45 and under. The CDC has recently shown that cancer and heart disease are the leading causes of death for middle-aged adults in the U.S., accounting for 50% of all deaths in that age group.[300] By 1999, it was shown that the lifetime risk of CHD for men was 48.6% and 31.7% for women.[301] That means vir-

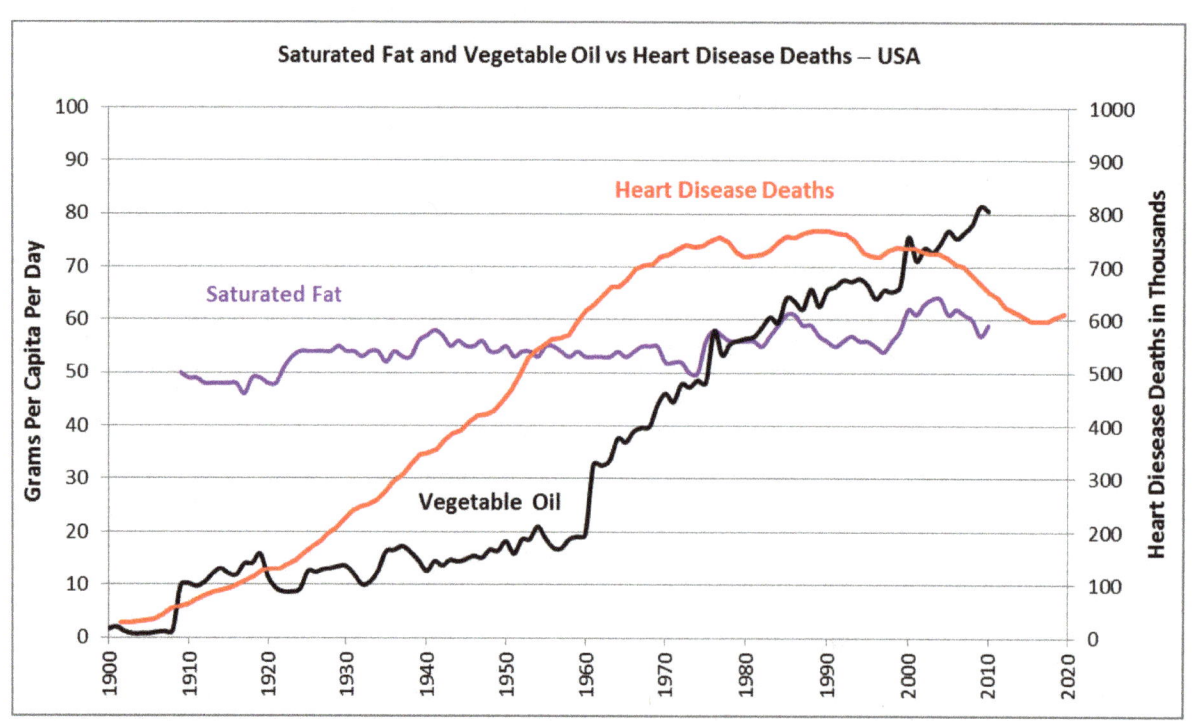

Saturated Fat and Vegetable Oil vs Heart Disease Deaths – USA

Knobbe C, Stojanoska M. The 'Displacing Foods of Modern Commerce' Are the Primary and Proximate Cause of Age-Related Macular Degeneration: A Unifying Singular Hypothesis. Medical Hypotheses: 2017;109:184-198. © C. Knobbe, 2022. Ancestral Health Foundation.

tually half of men and one-third of women in the U.S., if they live to age 40 or beyond, are destined for CHD. This is a staggering statistic, considering that cancer was unusual (1 in 17 deaths) and CHD virtually unknown just 100 years previously, in 1900.

Also, the CDC found that "43.3% of adults diagnosed with CHD, or a stroke, or both reported participating in 150 minutes or more of physical activity (or vigorous equivalent minutes) per week in past 30 days."[302] Thus, nearly half of those affected with CHD or stroke were apparently obtaining moderate degrees of exercise, which suggests exercise is not strongly preventative.

BIRTH OF THE DIET-HEART HYPOTHESIS

While CHD has generally been blamed primarily on saturated fat consumption, it should be noted that between 1910 and 1990, saturated fat consumption increased from about 50 grams/person/day (g/day) to 55 g/day, that is, an increase of about 5 g/day, or about one teaspoon difference.[4] This is an increase of 10%. However, between 1900 and 1990, seed oil consumption elevated from 2g/day to about 66 g/day, which is an increase of 33-fold, or a 3,200% increase![4] (See the graph on page 74.)

This, of course – the recommendation to consume more polyunsaturated seed oils – has been the norm in Western medicine, at least since 1961, when the American Heart Association (AHA), enjoined by physiologist Ancel Keys, PhD, of the University of Minnesota, first recommended a low-fat diet – and even a low saturated fat diet.

In that paper, entitled "Dietary Fat and Its Relation to Heart Attacks and Strokes," published in the *Journal of the American Medical Association (JAMA)*, the authors wrote, "In the usual diet eaten in the United States, a large part of the fat is of the saturated type. Too much of this type of fat tends to increase cholesterol in the blood. Considerable amounts of saturated fat are present in whole milk, cream, butter, cheese, and meat. Coconut oil and the fat in chocolate also have a high content of fats of this saturated type. Most shortenings and margarines have less than half as much saturated fat, and the common vegetable oils have still less. When the intake of saturated fats is reduced, blood cholesterol levels usually decrease."[303]

The authors wrapped up the paper with, "In Conclusion – The reduction or control of fat consumption under medical supervision, with reasonable substitution of polyunsaturated for saturated fats, is recommended as a possible means of preventing atherosclerosis and decreasing the risk of heart attacks and strokes."[303]

Without so much as a single graph to support the contention that saturated fat correlated with coronary heart disease (CHD) *over time*, nor any evidence that CHD had risen in any country *along with increasing saturated fat consumption*, and without any controlled scientific study to suggest CHD was driven by saturated fat, shockingly, with nothing more than an assertion by a group of like-minded colleagues who held positions at the American Heart Association (AHA), the AHA recommended a low-fat, low saturated fat diet, and thus, the "diet-heart hypothesis" was born.

Appallingly, the investigators failed to even examine the history of CHD, which would have proven that, just 50 years earlier, in 1910, there was barely a shred of evidence that CHD even existed. Given all of the history, we would suggest

CHAPTER 2

that, prior to the early 20th century and since time immemorial, CHD was virtually unknown.

Again, a careful historical examination by researchers in the 1950s or 1960s would have proven that the bulk of heart disease in the early 1900s, which ended fatally, was cardiac valvular disease born of infectious etiology, not coronary artery disease. Furthermore, the evidence would have also concluded that meat consumption was much higher in 1910 than it was in the 1930s, when CHD elevated to become the leading cause of death (see graph below).

In fact, in her book *The Big Fat Surprise*, investigative journalist Nina Teicholz chronicled an extraordinary review of the history of heart disease and its relation to both meat consumption and vegetable oils. She wrote:

"The loss of a historical perspective about our food traditions is perhaps the overriding reason that our nutrition policy has gone so far astray. Authorities tell us that there's 'no record' of any long-term 'data' on humans eating a diet high in saturated fats, and by this they mean that there are no clinical trials lasting two or more years on a diet high in animal products.

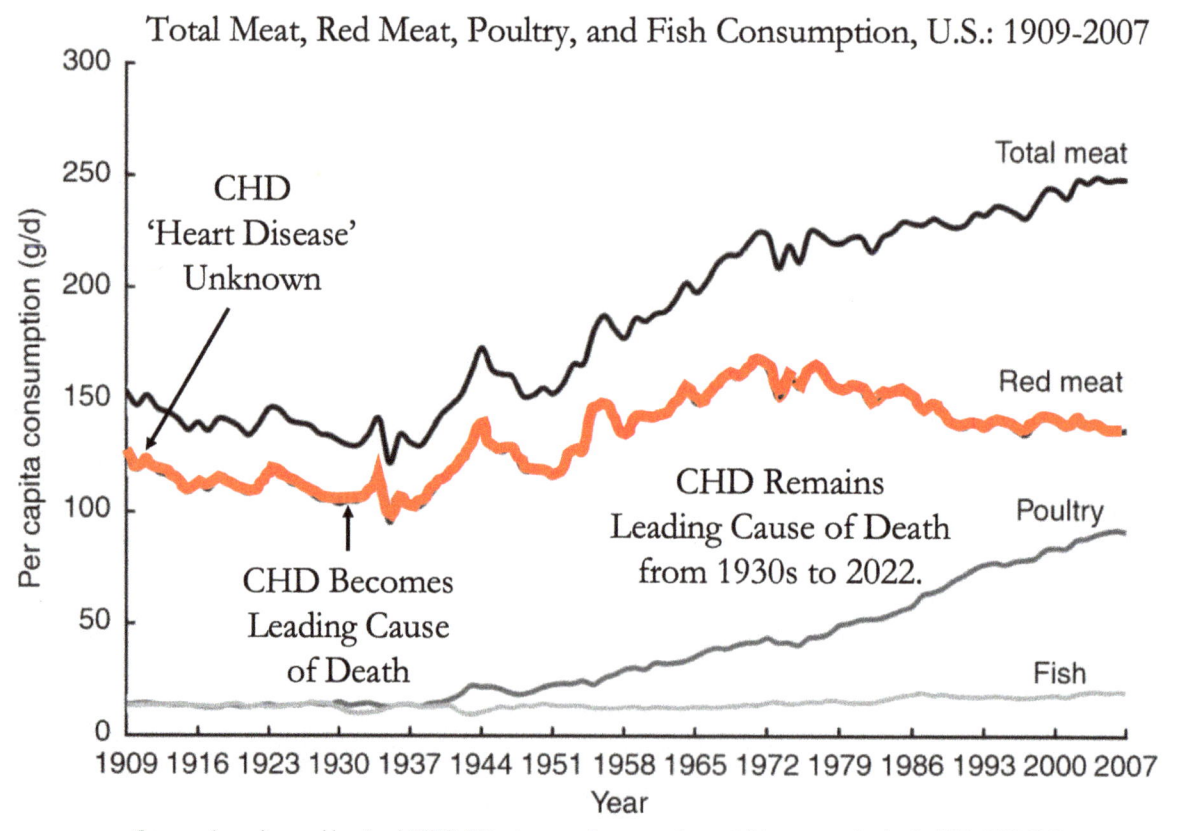

Total Meat, Red Meat, Poultry, and Fish Consumption, U.S.: 1909-2007

Coronary heart disease abbreviated "CHD." Total meat, red meat, poultry and fish consumption in the USA, 1909-2007. Adapted from: Daniel CR et al. Trends in meat consumption in the USA. Public Health Nutrition. 2011;14(4):575-583. Image licensure Cambridge University Press. © Copyright C. Knobbe, Ancestral Health Foundation, 2022.

But there are four millennia of human history that these experts could have consulted. Cookbooks, histories, diaries, memoirs, novels, food logs, or accounts by missionaries, doctors, explorers, and anthropologists—altogether a virtually limitless number of books, from the Bible to the plays of Shakespeare—which make clear how animal foods made up the core of human meals for thousands of years. During these times, people had shorter life expectancy, true, but they died young of infectious diseases. As adults, their lives and deaths were all but free of the chronic diseases of obesity, diabetes, and heart disease that we die from now…"[304]

Despite all of this evidence, along with droves of evidence to the contrary and multiple meta-analyses (summaries of many scientific studies) which have refuted the diet-heart hypothesis for more than 60 years,[305][306][307] the AHA continues to recommend a low saturated fat diet containing no more than 5% to 6% saturated fat.[308] And, of course, the AHA promulgates diets rich in seed oils, stating, "Replacing bad fats (saturated and trans) with healthier fats (monounsaturated and polyunsaturated) is good for your heart. One way you can do this is by choosing healthier nontropical vegetable oils for cooking and preparing food," which is followed by their recommendation to consume "Canola, corn, olive, peanut, safflower, soybean, and sunflower oils."[309]

As we can observe from the USDA Economic Research Service (ERS) data and graph (U.S. per capita availability of beef, pork, chicken, and fish/shellfish—1910-2018, page 78),[310] we see that beef consumption was much higher in 1910, at about 48 pounds/person, when coronary heart disease (CHD) was virtually unknown in the U.S. and worldwide.

Then, at the same time that CHD became the leading cause of death in the U.S. in the 1930s, we see that beef consumption had reached its nadir – truly its lowest point in available history – at a consumption of approximately 33 pounds/person in 1933. From a scientific standpoint, it is disturbing that if this were the only evidence researchers had and literally nothing else was known about the diet, it would have made much more logical sense during the 1930s to indict a *lack of beef* (and therefore, lack of saturated fat) as a major causal factor in CHD! Even in the early 1950s, beef consumption was almost the same – and actually a little lower – than it was in 1909 when CHD virtually didn't exist.

From the early 1950s, we then observe that beef consumption almost steadily increased from a low of about 43 pounds in 1952 to a peak consumption of 88.8 pounds per person per year (before adjustments for losses) in 1976 and has almost steadily fallen ever since. Since 1940 we see more than a 6-fold increase in chicken consumption, a quite stable consumption of pork since the 1950s, and a slight increase in fish and shellfish consumption (approximately 18%) between 1910 and 2000.

If one reviews the graph produced by Tanya Blasbalg and colleagues (Chapter One), we observe that, between 1909 and 1999, butter consumption dropped from 8 kg to 2kg/yr (17.6 lbs to 4.4 lbs), lard dropped from 5.8 kg to 1.2 kg (12.7 lbs to 2.6 lbs), while beef tallow (rendered beef fat) elevated from 0.5kg to 2 kg (1.1 lbs to 4.4 lbs). Thus, most of the primary sources of saturated fat, including beef, butter, and lard, all had marked reductions in consumption during the 20th century.

By far the greatest source of omega-3 fatty acid consumption in the U.S. – fish and shellfish – showed mildly but steadily increased consumption

CHAPTER 2

U.S. per capita availability of beef, pork, chicken, and fish/shellfish–1910-2018

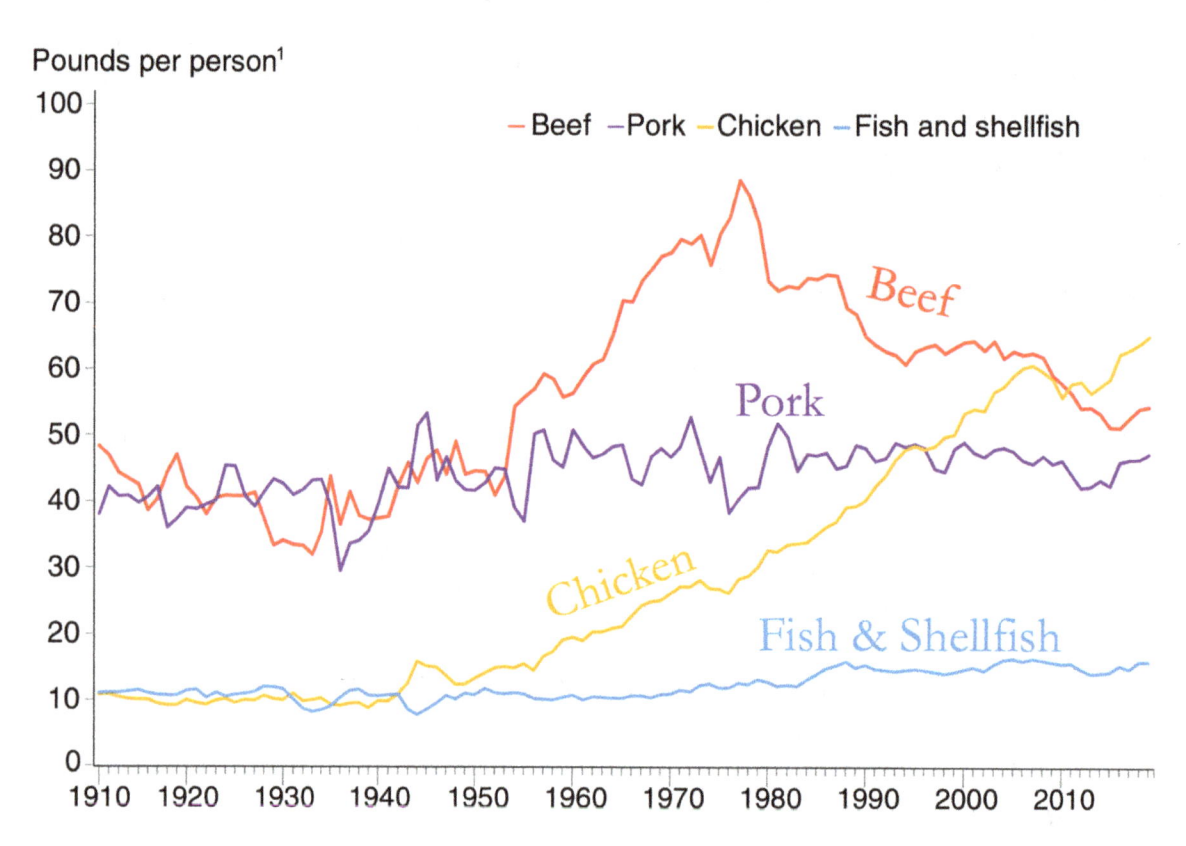

Pounds per person[1]

— Beef — Pork — Chicken — Fish and shellfish

[1]Calculated on the basis of raw and edible meat in boneless, timmed (edible) weight. Excludes edible offals, bones, viscera, and game from red meat. Include skin, neck, and giblets from chicken. Excludes use of chicken for commercially prepared pet food.
Source: USDA, Economic Research Service, Food Availability Data.

over the past century, paralleled by an astounding increase in CHD. This is perhaps the greatest evidence against omega-3 deficiency as a significant cause of CHD and, furthermore, this evidence strongly suggests we're not solving this problem, or perhaps any others, by just consuming more omega-3 fat, whether in food or supplement.

Though we've reviewed animal fat versus vegetable fat (predominantly seed oils) consumption in great detail in Chapter One, the graph on page 79 is presented courtesy of nutrition researcher and author, Stephan Guyenet, PhD, formerly of the University of Washington. The raw data was obtained from the USDA Economic Research Service and is corrected for a waste of 28.8%.

U.S. Added Fat Intake: 1909 – 2009

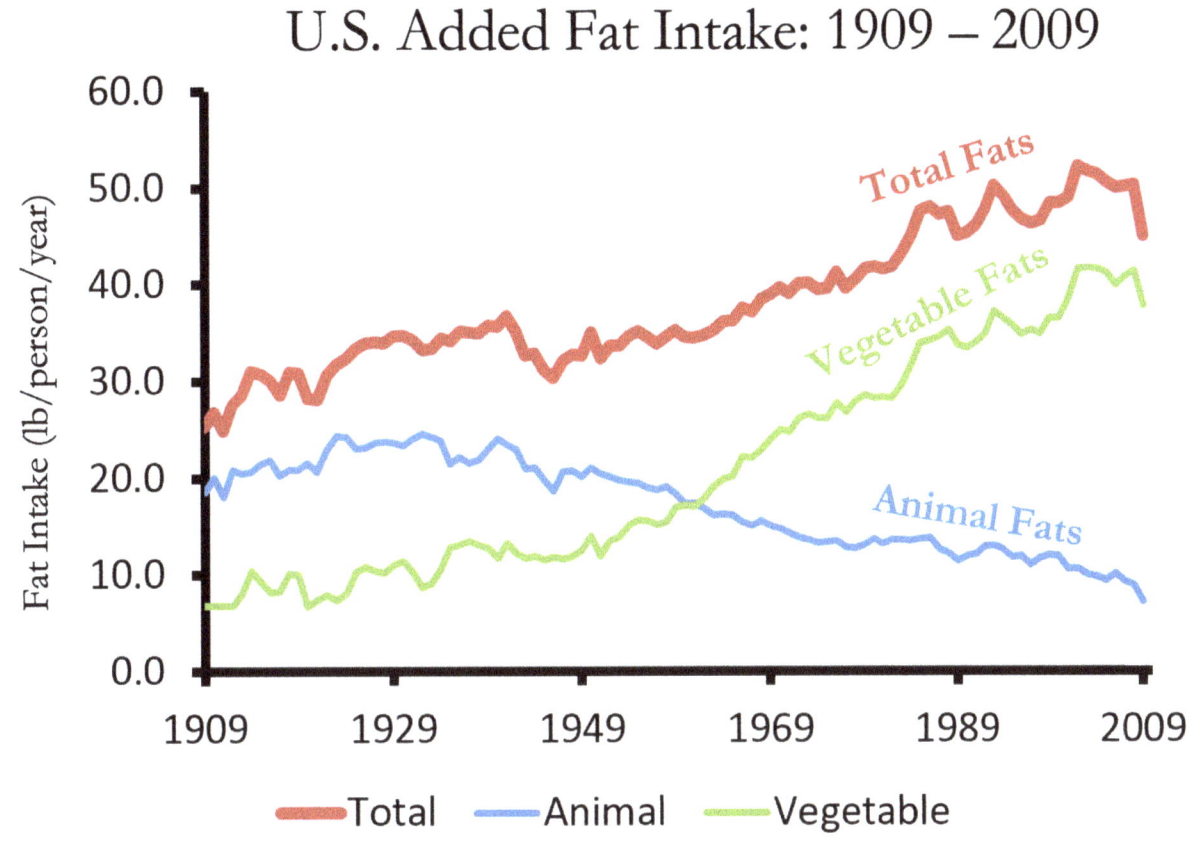

USDA ERS data, roughly corrected for a waste rate of 28.8%. Graph and data courtesy of **Stephan Guyenet, PhD**. *The Hungry Brain*. New York, Flatiron Books, 2017.

Now, if one were to blame animal fats for CHD, please note the relatively stable animal fat consumption between 1909, when CHD was unknown, up through about 1930, which is when the epidemic of CHD began to exact its toll on Americans. This was followed by a *marked decrease in animal fat consumption beginning in the 1930s*, which then continued a downward trend all the way through 2009. From the 1930s through at least 1968, we observe a geometric increase in CHD deaths during the exact same time period that animal fat consumption was falling! However, during this entire period between 1909 and 2009, we see a steady increase in "vegetable fats" (vegetable oils) all the way up to around 2005 (more recent data to be reviewed subsequently).

Regarding total meat consumption in the U.S., Roger Horowitz, in his historical and academic book, *Putting Meat On the American Table*, confirmed, "National estimates deduced from livestock production statistics place per capita meat consumption in the 1830s at 178 pounds [per person per year]. These sources do give us some confidence in suggesting an average annual consumption of 150-200 pounds per person in the nineteenth century."[311]

Using the average consumption of 175 pounds per capita in 1800, we've plotted the graph of total meat consumption in the 19th century and stitched that together with the data and graph from Carrie R. Daniel and colleagues at the Nutritional Epidemiology Branch, National Institutes of Health.[312]

CHAPTER 2

U.S. Total Meat Consumption, 1800 – 2007

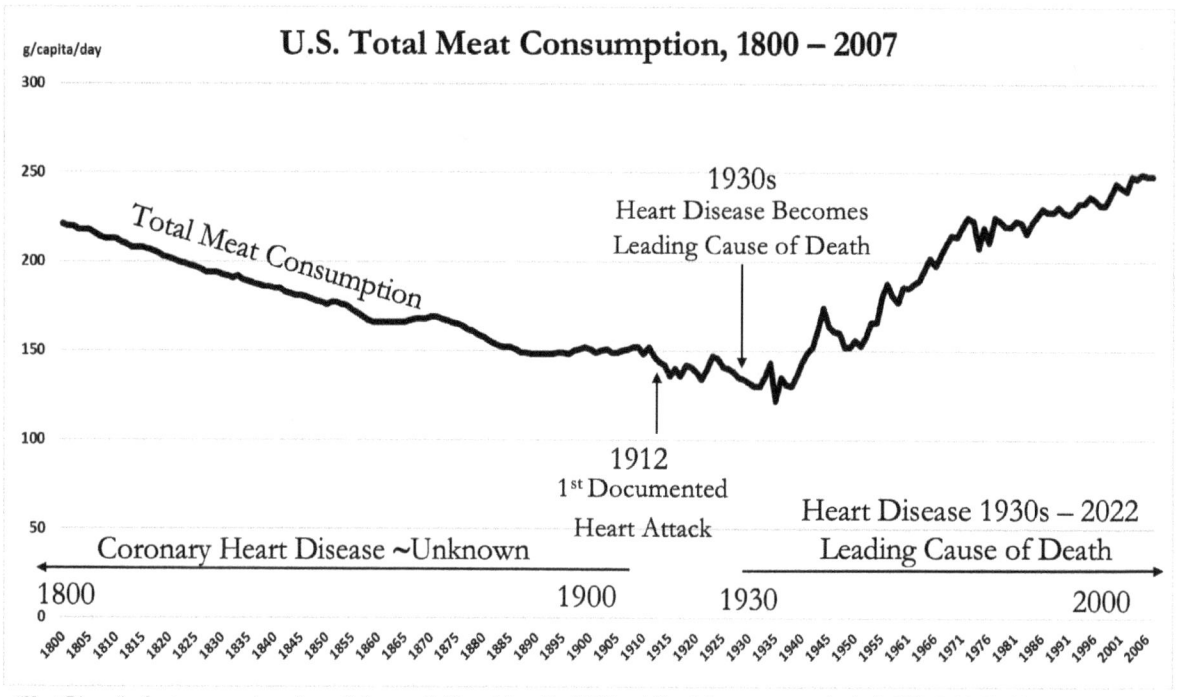

"Heart Disease" refers to coronary heart disease. References: 1) Adapted from: Daniel CR et al. Trends in meat consumption in the USA. Public Health Nutrition. 2011;14(4):575-583. Image licensure Cambridge University Press. 2) Horowitz, R. Putting Meat On the American Table. Baltimore, The Johns Hopkins University Press, 2006, pp.11-12. 3) For CHD, see references cited herein. © Copyright C. Knobbe, Ancestral Health Foundation, 2022.

Please note that we've converted pounds per capita per year to grams/capita/day in order to mesh with the data from Daniel and colleagues at the NIH.

The meat consumption numbers from Horowitz, if anything, are conservative. Historical researcher, Sam Bowers Hilliard, found evidence from a query sent by the U.S. Patent Office in 1848, in which 11 states corresponded with their estimated annual consumption of meat for an adult. Eleven states provided estimates, including Georgia, Illinois, Indiana, Kentucky, Mississippi, New Jersey, New York, Pennsylvania, South Carolina, Tennessee, and Virginia. The average annual consumption was 213 pounds per person per year.[313] Of course, these numbers were for adults, but the numbers are quite consistent with that found by Horowitz.

Historian Maureen Ogle translates U.S. colonialists as "carnivore Americans" stating, "Statistics are hard to come by for an era that predated census bureaus and questionnaires, but the evidence compiled by historians allows a broad generalization: the average white colonial American ate more and more varied food, and especially more meat, than anyone on the planet (aside from queens, czars, and other exceptionally privileged persons). Across Europe, a non-royal was lucky to see meat once or twice a week. A typical American adult male, in contrast, put away about two hundred pounds a year."[314] Thus, meat consumption in the 19th century, by nearly any metric, appears to have been in the 175 to 225 pound per person per year range. With this estimate, that comes to about 0.55 pounds per day, or about 248 g/person/day.

From this evidence, we observe that total meat consumption was very comparable in the 19th century as it was during the 20th century, yet coronary heart disease in the 19th century was virtually unknown. In fact, we observe that, after a period of well over a hundred years (1800 to about 1920) of near silence regarding coronary heart disease, the disease suddenly became the leading cause of death in the 1930s. As mentioned earlier, this hit almost precisely when meat consumption hit its nadir (lowest point) during the entire 200-year period.

SMOKING AND CHD: MUST UNDERSTAND TO GET THE WHOLE PICTURE

In the U.S., how does smoking fit into the picture of CHD causation? Smoking is a known cause of CHD[315] and, therefore, it's crucial to consider smoking in this picture as well, at least briefly. The graph below (courtesy of the CDC), shows that smoking was a rarity in the early 20th century (as was heart disease), and smoking elevated quite consistently with CHD, and then fell with the prevalence of CHD.[316] The graph looks eerily similar to deaths from CHD during the entire 20th century!

The graph on page 82, "Trends in Cigarette Consumption: U.S., U.K., Canada, 1920-2010," shows plummeting numbers of cigarettes consumed in the U.S. and U.K. (as well as Canada), particularly since about 1974.[317] This has been commensurate with falling degrees of CHD death and we can assuredly conclude that reduced cigarette smoking has reduced both the individual and overall prevalence of heart disease.

At first glance, if we examine the prevalence of CHD deaths and the prevalence of cigarette smoking, we might conclude that cigarette smoking caused the bulk of CHD. However, studies have shown that only

Annual adult per capita cigarette consumption and major smoking and health events – United States, 1900 - 1998

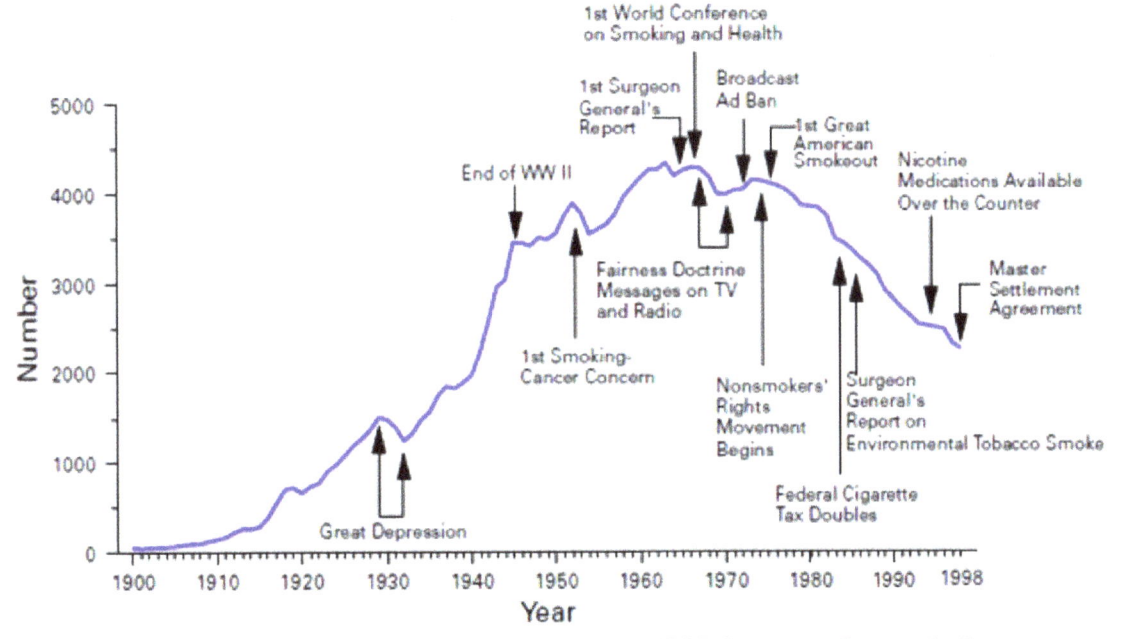

Sources: United States Department of Agriculture; 1986 Surgeon General's Report.

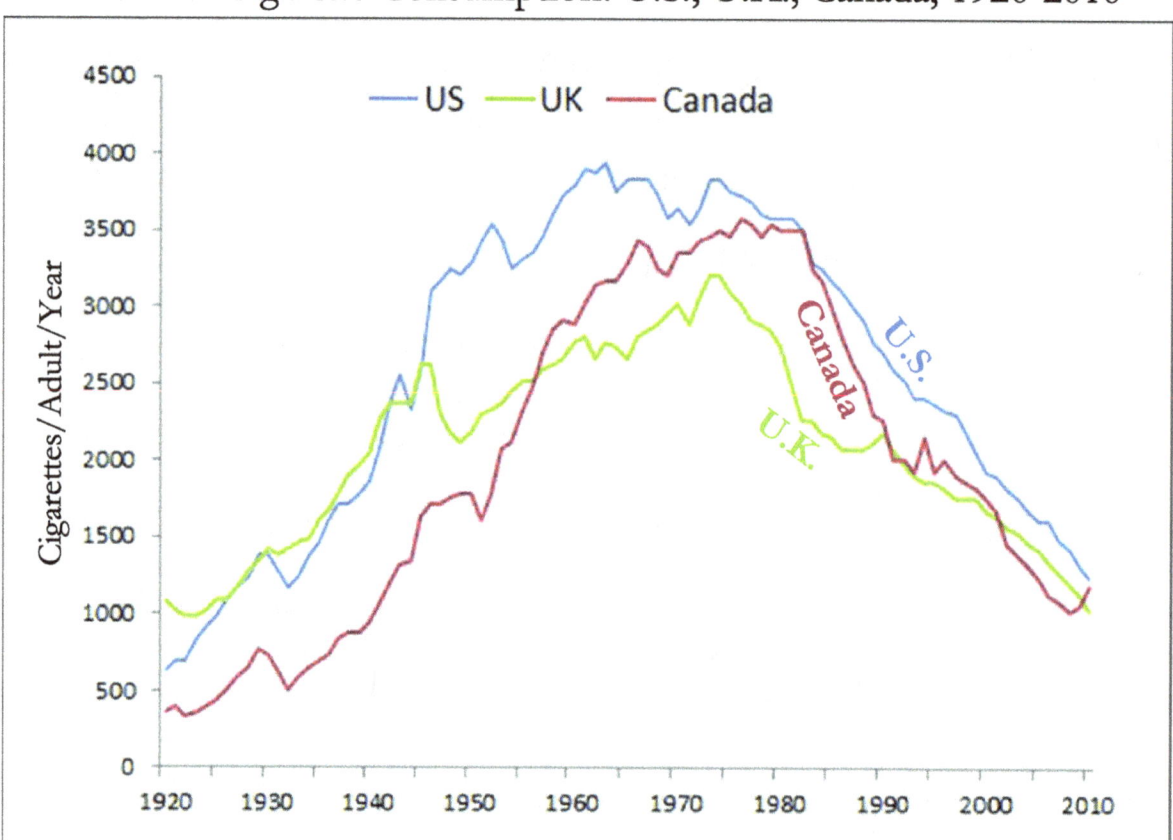

Trends in Cigarette Consumption: U.S., U.K., Canada, 1920-2010

Jha P. The hazards of smoking and the benefits of cessation: A critical summation of epidemiological evidence in high-income countries. eLife Sciences 9. DOI:10.7554/eLife.49979. Creative Commons Attribution 4.0 International, image subject to copyright, title and graph labels modified from original, but not data/trends. Image License availability: https://creativecommons.org/licenses/by/4.0.

about 20% of cardiovascular disease deaths involve people who smoke.[316][318]

Smoking increases the risk of cardiovascular disease, with estimates ranging anywhere from about 20% to 70%, but it is obvious that the bulk of those with CHD – about 70% to 80% – are non-smokers.[319] Unquestionably, smoking contributes to CHD and it's an important and significant part of the picture, but it is absolutely not the primary cause. For that, once again, we'll indict seed oils.

"HIGHLY UNSATURATED FATTY ACIDS" OR HUFA, INCREASE CHD, AND COME FROM LA

As reviewed previously, in the U.S., James Herrick diagnosed the first heart attack-related death in 1912, and his presentation and paper weren't even taken seriously by allopathic medicine for nearly a decade.[276][277] Less than 100 years later, in 2005, some 864,000 cardiovascular-related deaths occurred in the United States.[299]

In 2004, 48% of all deaths in Americans 85

years or older were due to cardiovascular disease, but an astounding 20% of all deaths in people aged 35 to 44 years were also due to cardiovascular disease.[299] From 1909 through 2009, however, we've seen total animal fat consumption drop from roughly 20 lbs/person/year to 8 lbs/year, which is a reduction of 60% in animal fat consumption during this same period (Graph on page 79: "U.S. Added Fat Intake: 1909 – 2009, S. Guyenet).

In the U.S. and most of the world, seed oils have risen infinitely in consumption since 1865 and they've risen at least 40-fold and up to as much as 80-fold between 1900 and 2010 (actual consumption of cottonseed oil versus olive oil in 1900 is unknown, but are estimated to be approximately equal, at 1.0 g/day each).[3][4] Commensurate with that, we've seen what appears to be an infinite increase in CHD and CHD-related deaths since the late 19th and early 20th centuries.

William "Bill" Lands, PhD, American biochemist and Emeritus Professor of Biochemistry in medical schools at both the University of Michigan and the University of Illinois, should be credited with contributing some of the earliest research (1992) on the accumulation of long-chain omega-6 fatty acid derivatives in tissues and their potential displacement by the consumption of omega-3 fatty acids, essentially achieving a better balance of the two.[320]

Lands developed an empirical mathematical formula showing the relationship of accumulated long-chain fatty acids in the tissues, which was strongly reflective of dietary consumption. He called these long-chain omega-6 LA-derived fatty acids (such as arachidonic acid (AA) and dihomo-gamma-linolenic acid (DGLA) "HUFA," which is an abbreviation for "highly unsaturated fatty acids."

In 2003, Lands published a paper in which he showed an extremely strong and linear correlation between these long-chain fatty acids derived from linoleic acid (LA) – the HUFA – stored in body fat and coronary heart disease (CHD) deaths. With studies of multiple populations, Lands showed a correlation so strong that, in his 2003 paper entitled, "Diets Could Prevent Many Diseases," he wrote, "The strong correlation... suggests that making dietary choices that decrease the proportion of tissue HUFA that is n-6 HUFA [omega-6 highly unsaturated fatty acids] can be an effective primary prevention strategy to decrease the risk of fatal CHD events in a population (see graph on page 84)."[321]

Once again, the take-home point is elegant and straightforward – decrease the consumption of seed oils drastically – and many health benefits will be achieved. Lands wrote intelligently but simply once again, "*In maintaining health and preventing chronic disease, the tissue is the issue.*"[321]

THE MUCH BALLYHOOED OMEGA-6 TO OMEGA-3 RATIO: CAN WE FIX IT WITH MORE OMEGA-3S?

George Oswald Burr, Professor in the Department of Botany, University of Minnesota, and his wife, Mildred Burr, established in 1929 that there were *fatty acids in the diet essential to life, which included omega-6 linoleic acid (LA) and omega-3 alpha-linolenic acid (ALA)* [essential fatty acids reviewed in Chapter Four].[636][637]

The discovery that fats were critical to health and life was a paradigm-shifting discovery, and these seminal studies are still considered landmarks in nutrition science.[635] These two polyunsaturated

CHD Mortality and Tissue HUFA

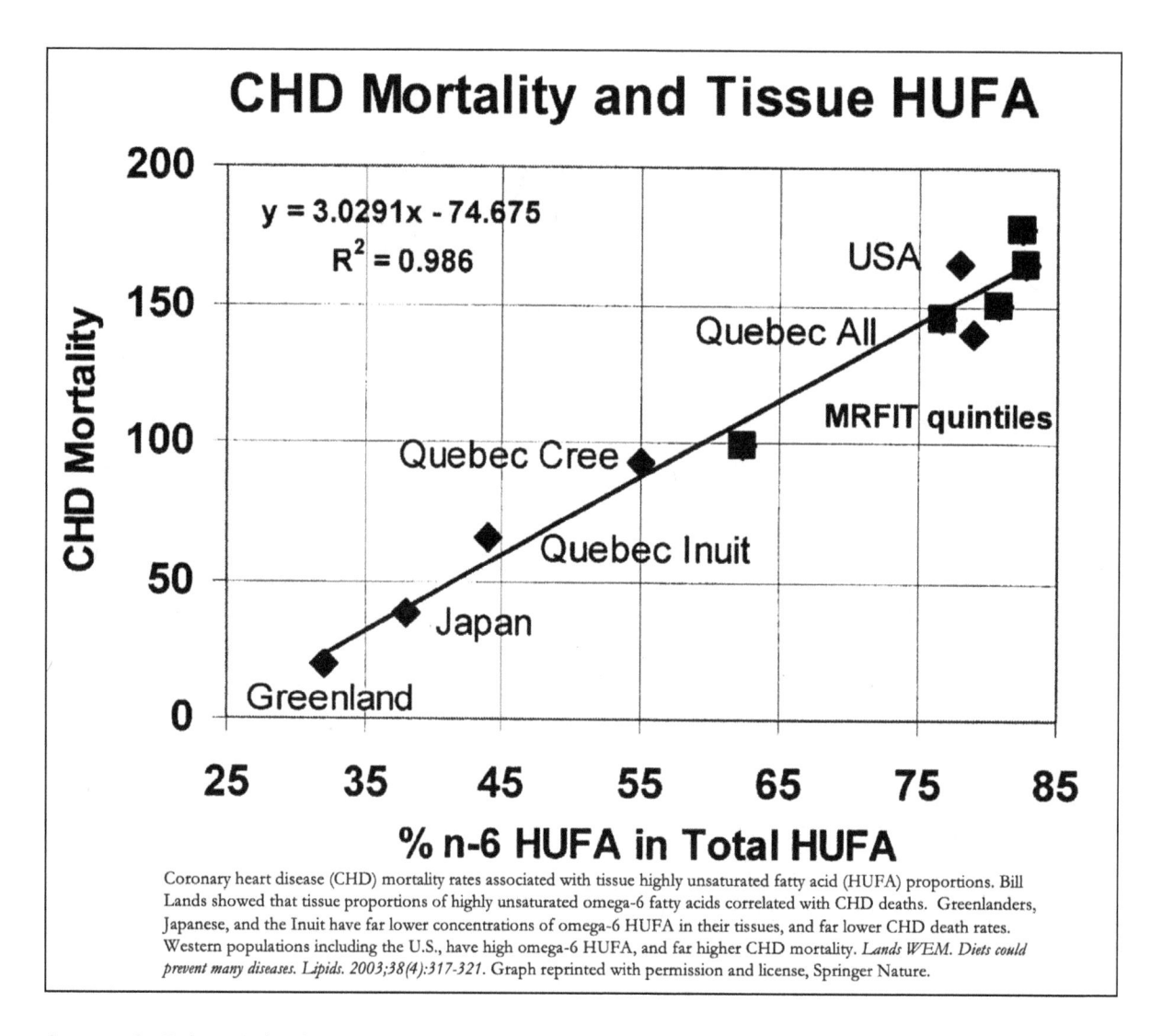

$y = 3.0291x - 74.675$
$R^2 = 0.986$

Data points labeled: USA, Quebec All, MRFIT quintiles, Quebec Cree, Quebec Inuit, Japan, Greenland

X-axis: % n-6 HUFA in Total HUFA
Y-axis: CHD Mortality

Coronary heart disease (CHD) mortality rates associated with tissue highly unsaturated fatty acid (HUFA) proportions. Bill Lands showed that tissue proportions of highly unsaturated omega-6 fatty acids correlated with CHD deaths. Greenlanders, Japanese, and the Inuit have far lower concentrations of omega-6 HUFA in their tissues, and far lower CHD death rates. Western populations including the U.S., have high omega-6 HUFA, and far higher CHD mortality. *Lands WEM. Diets could prevent many diseases. Lipids. 2003;38(4):317-321.* Graph reprinted with permission and license, Springer Nature.

fatty acids, LA and ALA, are precursors of molecules that have almost "hormonal" like actions that affect a myriad of pathways. The general rule-of-thumb is that the omega-6-derived molecules support and amplify inflammatory reactions, platelet aggregation (clotting), and vasoconstriction (vessel narrowing), whereas the omega-3-derived molecules inhibit inflammation and platelet aggregation while enhancing vasodilation (vessel dilation).[322][323]

At first glance, it looks like one would want all omega-3 and no omega-6, but such is not the case. As in all of life and nutrition, it is the balance that is key and this will be reviewed in further detail in Chapter Four. Complete absence of either LA or ALA is either not consistent with life, or may induce a host of biological dysfunctions (see Chapter Four).

Since time immemorial, almost all humans survived without seed oils.[324][78] The industrial revolution, with the advent of mechanized seed oil production, changed all of that.[323] Seed oils, of course, have provided opportunities for enormous consumption of omega-6-rich oils. The overconsumption of omega-6 fats has been strongly implicated, associated with, and causally related to the development of many modern diet-related chronic diseases (as reviewed here and throughout this book).[323]

The ratio of omega-6 to omega-3 fatty acids is also thought to be critical to health and a number of investigators, including Loren Cordain, PhD,[325] S. Boyd Eaton, MD,[209] and Remko S. Kuipers,[326] have shown that during the Paleolithic period, the ratios included about equal amounts of the two (i.e., a 1:1 ratio). Throughout history, but before industrialized seed oil production, the ratio is believed to have been about 1 to 2: 1.[323] That is, traditional foods provided about one to two times more omega-6 than omega-3 in the diet. This is purported to be a "perfect and balanced ratio."[323]

The advent of seed oil production, rich in omega-6 LA, combined with a public admonishment to consume 'vegetable oils,' has resulted in an extraordinary increase in the ratio of omega-6 to omega-3.[323] The ratio between these two has progressively increased right along with increasing seed oil consumption. About 1935-1939, the omega-6 to omega-3 ratio was 8.4 to 1, which increased to 10.3 to 1 in 1985, to 16 to 1 between 2001 and 2011, and by 2021, in westernized populations, the ratio was about 20 to 1, but as high as 50 to 1 in South Asia.[323]

Artemis Simopoulos, MD, Founder of the Center for Genetics, Nutrition and Health, has been instrumental in completing a large body of research supporting the omega-6:omega-3 ratio as critical to human development and health.[327] For more than 30 years, she has helped develop a core of science relating to this entire foundational concept.

In 1999, following the Workshop on the Essentiality of and Recommended Dietary Intakes (RDIs) for Omega-6 and Omega-3 Fatty Acids (at the NIH), Dr. Simopoulos published a paper reviewing the findings and recommendations of the workshop, of which she was a key voice.[328] The workshop participants collectively agreed that the adequate intake (AI) for LA was 2.0% of consumed energy (calories), with an upper limit recommendation of 3.0% of energy. This translates to 4.44 g/day for adequate intake with an upper limit of 6.67 grams LA.

As previously reviewed, in 1865, Americans were only consuming about 1.0% of calories as LA, however, by 2008, Americans were consuming about 29 g LA per day, or 11.8% of energy. Given this and much other evidence to be reviewed in Chapter Four, as well as the many population studies cited herein, the adequate intake for LA is actually much less than 2.0% —actually only about 0.5% — and our recommendation is that the goal for LA consumption should be about 2% of calories or less. Nevertheless, the workshop members' goals of achieving even 3.0% of calories consumed as LA, if adhered to globally, would have achieved immeasurable success.

The U.S. Institute of Medicine (IOM), a division of The National Academies, sets Dietary Reference Intakes (DRIs) which are "nutrient reference values" that are intended to serve as a guide for good nutrition based on all current science. They're based on age, gender, and other factors of life, e.g., pregnancy, nursing, etc.

The IOM has shirked its responsibility to set either an Estimated Average Requirement (EAR) or a Recommended Dietary Allowance (RDA) for healthy individuals, asserting that there is inadequate information to make a determination.[329] In these scenarios, the Adequate Intake (AI) is used.

For both LA and ALA, the IOM bases its decision on "the highest median intake of LA and ALA in United States adults, where a deficiency is basically nonexistent in non-institutionalized populations."[329]

Using nothing more than current average intakes, the IOM set the omega-6 Adequate intake (AI) "requirement" range as 11 to 12 g/day for men and 14 to 17 g/day for adult women who are neither pregnant or lactating, and made the AI for omega-3 fatty acids as 1.6 g/day for men and 1.1 g/day for women.

We would not recommend more than approximately 2.0% of calories as LA, which, on a 2,250 calorie per day diet, would be just 5.0 g/day of LA. As will be reviewed in detail in Chapter Four, only 0.5% of calories as LA is essential [54,56,644] and, therefore, we would advocate that the adequate intake (AI) should be set at no more than 0.5% to a maximum of 1.0% of total calories which would be 1.25g to 2.5 g/day (on a 2,250 calorie/day diet).

With regard to the omega-6 to omega-3 ratio, Dr. Simopoulos has published many papers on the subject since 1999 (not all of which are referenced here).[330,331,332] She is a strong advocate for reducing the omega-6 content of the diet and balancing the ratio in favor of an ancestrally relevant profile, which she suggests would favorably reduce overweight, obesity, coronary heart disease, cancer, diabetes, metabolic syndrome, and chronic disease in general. "It is essential," Dr. Simopoulos writes, "that every effort is made to decrease the omega-6 fatty acids in the diet, while increasing the omega-3 fatty acid intake."[331]

The belief system that increasing omega-3 fatty acids, such as fish oils, flax, perilla, and chia, for example, is born primarily out of the fact that there is competition between the enzymes that convert LA or ALA into their longer chain fatty acid counterparts, which would include the omega-3 fatty acids, eicosapentaenoic acid (EPA) and docosahexaenoic acid (DHA), and the omega-6 arachidonic acid (AA). There is competition for the enzymes that convert LA and ALA to their longer chain counterparts and, therefore, "saturating" the enzymes with omega-3 is thought to favor benefits.[331]

Although there is a very lengthy and extraordinary literature on this subject, in general, there are conflicting findings as it relates to supplementing with omega-3. For example, in trials using omega-3 fatty acids in an attempt to aid weight loss, there have been positive effects[333,334,335] as well as negative effects.[336,337,338]

A meta-analysis that evaluated supplementation with omega-3 fatty acids in the form of "marine omega-3" (typically fish oil), which evaluated more than 127,477 participants, found that the oils reduce cardiac-related deaths significantly. However, the reductions are relatively small, for example, over a mean treatment duration of 5 years, the omega-3 oils reduced myocardial infarctions (heart attacks) by 8%, CHD deaths by 8%, and cardiovascular disease (mostly heart attack and stroke) deaths by 7%.[339]

These are meaningful numbers, but certainly, the goal is a 100% reduction in such conditions, which is essentially what we observe in ancestrally living populations. It is indeed evident in much research that increasing omega-3 fatty acids, with or without antioxidant-rich plant foods, cannot fully moderate the dangerous and even disastrous effects of excess LA consumption.[340]

In general, it appears that omega-3 supplementation or eating more fish may be beneficial, particularly when omega-6 consumption has been high. However, the ultimate goal is to drastically reduce omega-6 consumption by eliminating seed oils, which will ultimately solve the omega-6 to omega-3 ratio issue.

As will be reviewed in Chapter Four, this may take approximately two to three years' time. At that point, concerns about omega-3 supplementation should likely be abolished. However, even small amounts of wild-caught fish or shellfish consumption, for example, even just once a week, may be of benefit. Because of concerns about oxidation of fish oils in supplements, eating wild-caught fish will always be the safest approach.

MID TO LATE 20TH CENTURY: CORONARY HEART DISEASE EMERGES IN AFRICA

For those who might still believe that CHD is a function of age or genetics, evidence from the entire continent of Africa ought to dispel any such myth. In the medical text *"Western Diseases"* written by Denis P. Burkitt, MD and Hugh Trowell, MD, Dr. Trowell wrote the following:

> *"All available evidence suggests that coronary heart disease (CHD) is the last major cardiovascular Western disease to emerge [in Africa}... The emergence of CHD in East Africans is the most clearly documented. First, there was the stage of reported absence: Vint (1936—37) reported no CHD in the first thousand Kenyan autopsies. Second, there was the first report of CHD, made by a pathologist (Davies, 1948a, b); one Ganda woman among 2994 autopsies, dating from 1931 to 1946 at Makerere University Medical School, Uganda, had clear signs of myocardial infarction. Third, there was the first clinical report of CHD, a typical case in a middle-aged Ugandan High Court Judge who ate a partially westernized diet (Trowell and Singh, 1956). There has been usually a competition to report first cases of any Western disease in an East African: Ojiambo (1968) in Kenya and Nhonoli (1968) in Tanzania, reported first cases of CHD in these countries."*[341]

It should be emphasized that only a single "Ganda" (the primary ethnic group in Uganda) woman had CHD (and a heart attack in this case) among 2,994 autopsies, during the entire 15-year period between 1931 and 1946. Even in 1959, physician A.G. Shaper, of Cape Town, in a paper published in The Lancet, wrote, "In the African population of Uganda coronary heart disease is almost non-existent."[342] Standing in stark contrast, recall that currently, CHD affects half of all men and one-third of all women aged 40 and above, in the U.S.,[301] and African Americans have the highest overall mortality from CHD as compared to any other ethnic group.[343]

However, by the year 2016, cardiovascular disease (CVD) had become the single most common chronic disease and cause of death in Uganda, accounting for 10% of all deaths in the country.[344] So while CHD deaths were virtually non-existent in 1959, by 2016, cardiovascular disease-related deaths took the lives of approximately 29,700 Ugandans in that year alone.

With regard to smoking, unfortunately, there is no data until the year 2000. Smoking prevalence in Uganda, however, decreased from 29.2% in 2000 to 17.2% prevalence by 2016.[345]

If we examine the dietary habits of the Ugandans of the 1950s when CHD was almost non-existent, Dr. Shaper's paper of 1959 reviewed that the staple foods were green plantains and sweet potatoes, which were steamed in banana leaves; also, cassava, yams, maize, and millet were considered staples for many groups, while pumpkins, tomatoes, and green leafy vegetable were consumed by all. Pulses, groundnuts, and cereals provided much of the protein, and most meals were served with sauces made of groundnuts (peanuts), beans, and a mixture of vegetables.

Only occasionally did they consume meat or fish, which were typically "fried in very small amounts of fat (fat type not specified)."[342] Dr. Shaper further reviewed the incredibly low-fat diet that they had when he confirmed, "In the typical adult attending Mulago Hospital the daily fat intake is 16—20 g, while well-to-do families on housing estates take up to 40g daily with a total daily intake of about 2000 calories."[342]

A 2,000 calorie diet, with anywhere from just 16g to 40g of fat consumption, indicates a diet ranging from 7% to 18% fat, which is extraordinarily low by nearly any standards. However, notice from the graph on 'vegetable' oil consumption, on page 89, that in 1961, edible oils consumption was only 5.3g/day, which elevated all the way to 22.5g/day by 2016. Put another way, consumption increased from one teaspoon of vegetable oils per day in 1961 to 4.5 teaspoons per day in 2016, which is an increase of 324%, while cardiovascular disease (CVD) deaths elevated almost infinitely (from ~none to ~29,700 deaths per year).

If we entertain the hypothesis that sugars are a substantial driver of CHD and CVD, Uganda is

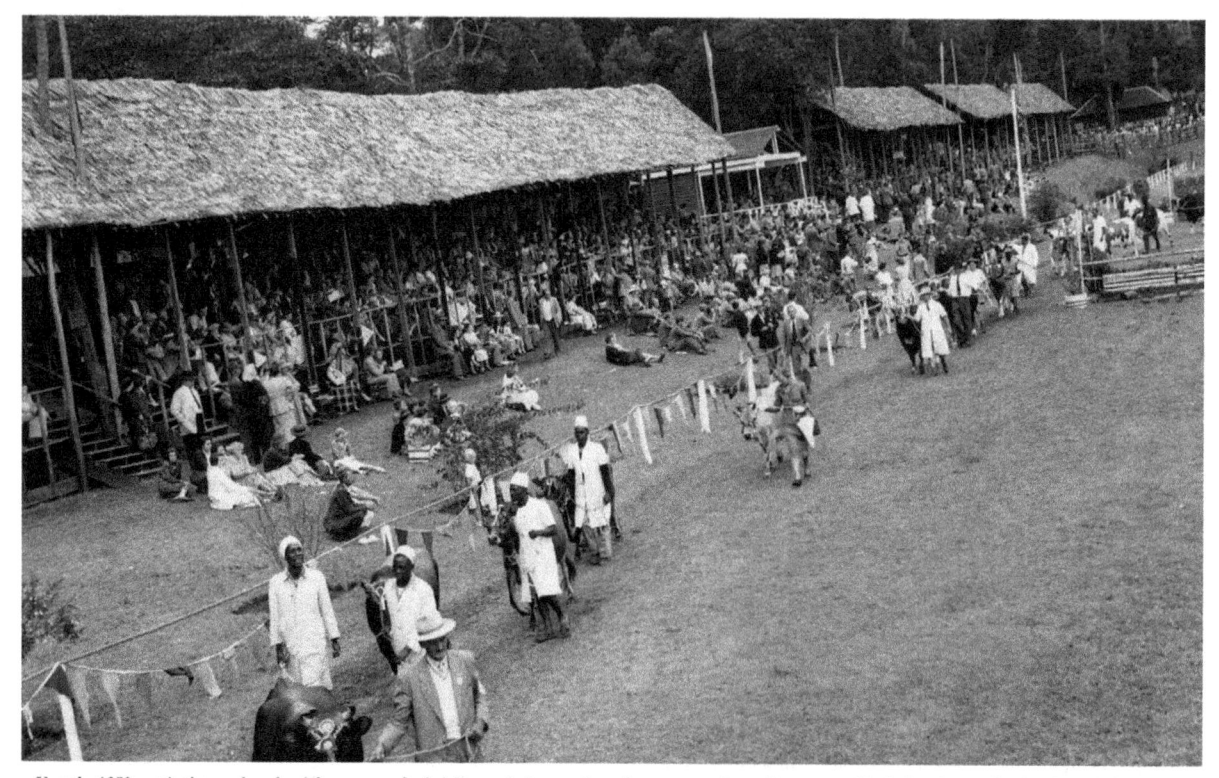

Uganda, 1950s cattle show, where local farmers parade their livestock. Image taken when coronary heart disease was effectively unknown in Uganda, and staple foods were carbohydrate rich, including plantains, sweet potatoes, cassava, yams, maize and millet cereal grains, and pulses, which made up the bulk of the diet, while meat and fish were were only occasional food items. License: Alamy. © Copyright C. Knobbe, Ancestral Health Foundation, 2022.

Uganda: Vegetable Oil & Sugar Vs Cardiovascular Disease (CVD) Deaths, 1959 - 2016

Chart showing vegetable oil consumption, sugar consumption, and % CVD deaths in Uganda from 1959 to 2019. Key data points: 1959 - Cardiovascular Disease "~ Non-Existent", Veg Oils 5.3 g/day; 2016 - CVD 10% of Deaths, Veg Oils 22.5 g/day.

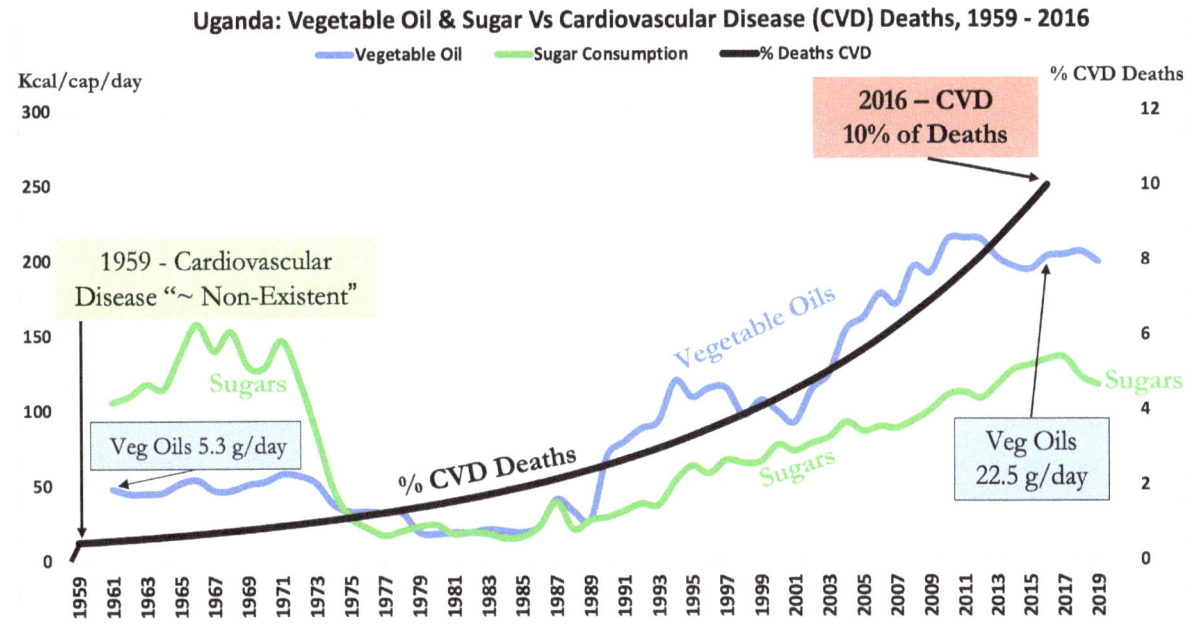

References: 1) 1959 CVD Deaths: Shaper AG. The Lancet. 1959;274(7102):534-537. 2) CVD Deaths 2016: Hearn J. Annals of Global Health. 2020;86(1):85 3). Vegetable oils and sugar data: FAO Food Balance Sheets, Knoema. http://www.fao.org/faostat/en/#data/FBS. © C. Knobbe, Ancestral Health Foundation, 2022. All rights reserved.

a very important country to examine, because over the period between 1961 and 2019, we see that the trend of sugar consumption barely changed. Sugar consumption was 106 cal/day in 1961 and ended at 117 calories in 2019, which is an increase of 10%. We know, however, that there were virtually no CVD deaths in 1959, while CVD deaths in 2016 took the lives of about 29,700 people. We certainly cannot blame sugar.

Yet another reason it is critically important to examine the history of Uganda in regards to CVD and coronary heart disease (CHD) is that, historically, up through about 1960, CHD was virtually unknown when the diet was an estimated 85% carbohydrate, 7% fat, and 8% protein, but seed oils were only about 5.3g/day, (assuming seed oils in 1959 were the same as in 1961). But by the time seed oils had climbed to about 22.5 g/day, in 2016, cardiovascular disease, which includes CHD, was indeed the most common of all chronic diseases and also the most common cause of death in Uganda.

THE MAASAI TRIBE: HIGHEST SATURATED ANIMAL FAT CONSUMPTION IN THE WORLD, BUT VIRTUALLY NO HEART DISEASE

Interestingly, the two populations in the world known to consume the highest percentages of their diets as saturated fats, specifically the Maasai tribe of Kenya and Tanzania and the South Pacific Tokelauans, have been proven in scientific studies to have little or no CHD. Let's look at these populations briefly.

The Maasai tribe of Kenya and Tanzania, Africa, is a population of pastoralists, that is, nomadic cattle herders, who live almost exclusively on the raw milk, meat, and blood, from the cattle (beef) they herd. Consumption of plant foods among the Maasai is uncommon as their collective belief is that green vegetables are meant for livestock feed.[346]

In 1972, George Mann and colleagues rigorously examined the Maasai tribe of Kenya and Tanzania, Africa.[350] This tribe is unique in that no other population on the planet has ever been scientifically documented to consume more animal fat, at least with any rigorous scientific study. The Maasai tribe are pastoralists and their tribal diet is primarily based on the milk, meat, and blood of the cattle they herd.

Consumption of fruits or vegetables among these pastoralists is greatly minimized. In fact, according to George Mann and colleagues, in the Moran cohort of Maasai, which are the warriors from 14 to 30 years of age, they were "bound by tribal tradition to a diet of milk and meat" and they affirmed that "no vegetable products are taken" further stating that it is "among this warrior class that animal fat intake is high."[350]

Consumption of maize (corn), rice, potatoes, and cabbage is becoming more common, but this is a more recent phenomenon and not typical of the traditional diet.[347] Traditionally, the Maasai live mainly on the milk from their cattle, with each individual typically consuming an average of 3 to 5 quarts of raw, unpasteurized milk, per day.[348] In the early 1970s, studies showed that each individual consumed approximately 3,000 calories per day, 66% of which was from animal fat.[348] The saturated fat content of ruminant milk is exceedingly high at 60% to 70% of the total fat.[349] The fat of the milk from the cattle that the Maasai raise is also much higher in fat than typical U.S. cattle, in fact, it is about 84% higher! Thus, a typical Maasai living on this very high milk diet would consume anywhere from about *40% to 46% saturated animal fat!*

If saturated animal fat causes CHD, these nomadic warriors ought to be 'dropping dead like flies,' right? Let's see if that's true.

In the study completed by George V. Mann, MD and colleagues, in 1972, a total of 50 males between the ages of 10 and 65, including 25 men who were at least 40 to 60 years of age or more, underwent autopsy.[350] Not a single case of previous myocardial infarction (MI, or "heart attack") was confirmed. Mann's group then completed 350 EKG's on men over the age of 40, finding evidence of only one previous MI in the entire group. The affected was a 50 year-old man. This was presumably a case of "silent MI" that is, a "heart attack," with little or no clinical symptoms, though we can't be sure. All evidence, in this analysis of 400 Maasai tribal members, concludes that clinically significant coronary heart disease in this population is rare if not absent.

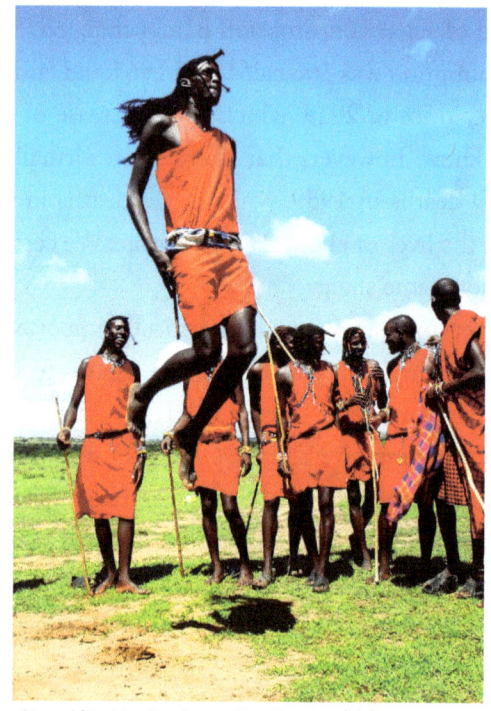

Kenya, Africa, Maasai warriors, traditional jumping cultural ceremony. Photo near Masai Mara National Park Reserve, July 2, 2011.

For those who might question George Mann and colleagues' studies, Kurt Biss, MD, and colleagues also studied the nomadic Maasai in 1971, separately from and actually prior to Mann's published study. Biss's group completed ten consecutive autopsies on Maasai tribe members at the Narok District Hospital, Narok, Kenya.[351] The vasculature of those who underwent autopsy was carefully examined and the authors wrote that, "… the aortas and coronary arteries gave direct proof of the paucity of atherosclerosis… The results demonstrated that the Masai's coronary arteries had much thinner walls than those of whites in the United States matched for age and sex."[351]

The Maasai are also exquisitely lean, fit, and generally slender. In three separate studies from the years 1930, 1989, and 2000, the Maasai have been shown to have average body mass index (BMI) of 21, 19.7, and 19.02, in males, and 22.4, 19.1, and 18.58, in women, for those study years, respectively.[352] The standard deviation for BMI for the years 1989 and 2000 averaged 2.3 and 2.9, indicating that only a small percentage – approximately less than 2.5% -- would have a BMI above 25 (overweight) while a BMI above 30 (obesity) was either exceedingly rare or absent.

With regard to hypertension (high blood pressure), medical consultant, Jex-Blake, in 11 years of practice in Nairobi, Kenya (1923 to 1934), confirmed he had never witnessed a case of hypertension in any Kenyan (genealogically and geographically close relatives of the Maasai).[353] Furthermore, Hugh Trowell, MD wrote about his experience in Kenya in the 1930s regarding diabetes. He confirmed that, in 1933, the medical staff of the Nairobi African Hospital in Kenya had a conference to examine and evaluate a patient with a disease – diabetes – which had not been seen "in an African by most doctors attending the meeting."[354]

The woman, who had apparently developed type 2 (adult-onset) diabetes, according to Trowell, "was a fat African nurse-maid (ayah) living with her British employer."[354] This, perhaps for the first time, convinced Trowell and his colleagues that type 2 diabetes mellitus was a "disease of civilization" which had been induced by something in the Western way of life.[354] They weren't certain of the cause, but obviously, this African woman wasn't consuming her native, traditional diet, but rather was consuming a diet provided by her British employer. As recently as 1989, diabetes prevalence in rural dwellers in Tanzania (genealogically and geographically close to Maasai) was found to be 0.87%.[355]

However, while type 2 diabetes was virtually unknown in Kenyans in the 1930s, by 2012, type 2 diabetes was a staggering 22.9% in urbanized Maasai (in Arusha Municipality, Tanzania) who had westernized their diets and lifestyle,[356] indicating that the Maasai are even far more genetically prone to diabetes with Westernization of the diet than typical white Americans. However, as seen in the graph on page 92, total vegetable oil consumption in Tanzania was only 49 cal/day (5.4g/day) in 1961 and elevated 4.8-fold to 237 cal/day (26.3g) by 2018, while sugar consumption was 67 cal/day in 1961 and elevated 1.6-fold to 109 cal/day by 2018.[357]

Data for "sugar" or "sugar consumption" in all graphs throughout this book, is defined according to both the U.S. FDA and the Food and Agriculture Organization of the United Nations (FAO), who are both in agreement, as follows: "Added sugars include sugars added during the processing of foods (such as sucrose and dextrose), foods packaged as sweeteners (such as table sugar), sugars from syrups and honey, and sugars from concentrated fruit or vegetable juices. They do not include naturally occurring sugars that are found in milk, fruits, and vegetables... For most Americans, the main sources of added sugars are sugar-sweetened beverages, baked goods, desserts, and sweets."[358] [359] Thus, added sugars in the diet include all forms of added sugars, including all forms of granulated sugars, sugar-sweetened beverages (SSBs), corn syrup, high-fructose corn syrup, maple syrup, honey, and all fruit or vegetable juices.

Kurt Biss, MD, and colleagues wrote that the traditional living Maasai have:

"striking physical characteristics – tall, slender bodies (the average male measuring about 173 cm [5'8"] and weighing 61 kg [134.2 lbs])... Milk (raw, unpasteurized) is their main staple, but they are also fond of fresh cow's blood and the meat of cattle, sheep, and goats.

"The cattle are milked directly into a gourd. The milk is drunk either fresh or fermented, since bacterial fermentation takes place in the gourd quite promptly. When enough milk is available, the average Masai will consume 3 to 5 liters of milk daily, divided usually into two meals... The average daily caloric intake

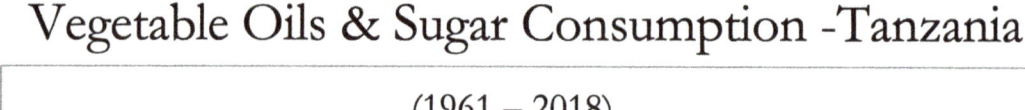

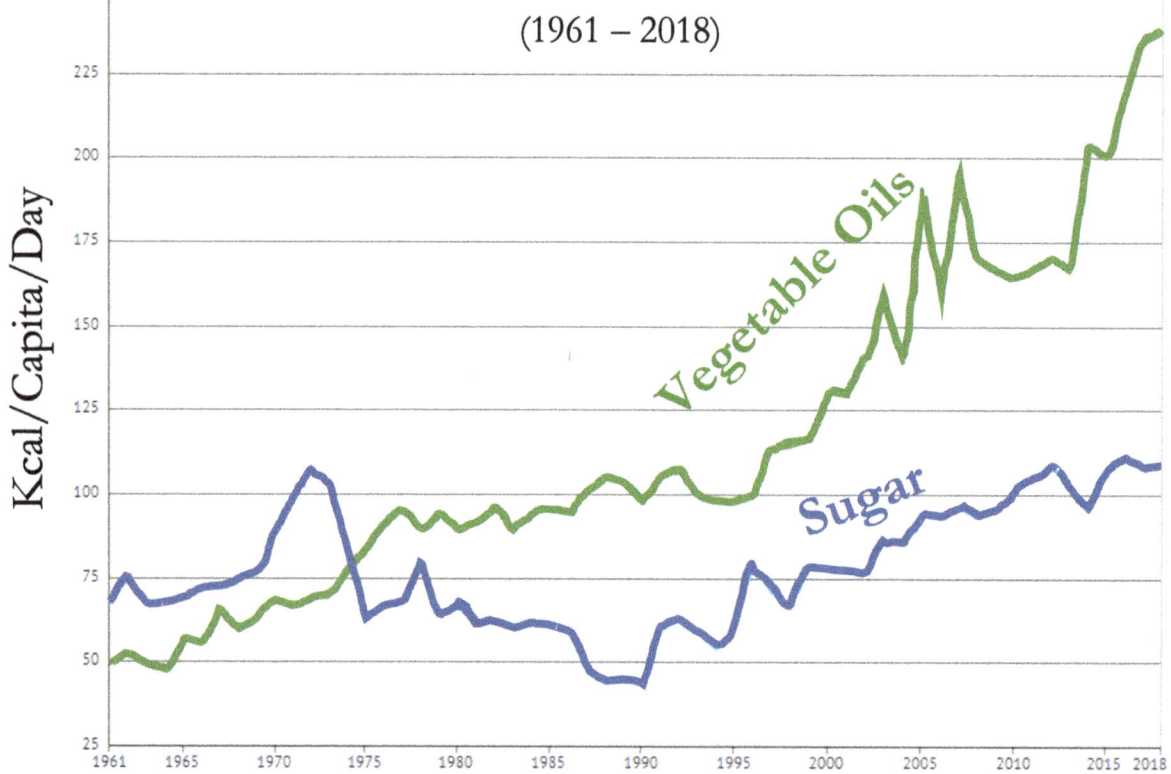

Vegetable Oils & Sugar Consumption - Tanzania
(1961 – 2018)

Data Source: FAO Food Balance Sheets, Knoema. http://www.fao.org/faostat/en/#data/FBS.
© C. Knobbe, 2022. Ancestral Health Foundation. © C. Knobbe, Ancestral Health Foundation, 2022.

was estimated to be about 3000 calories, with 66 per cent derived from fat. The estimated average daily cholesterol intake was 500 to 2000 mg per person, which is comparable to that for the average population in the United States.

"During the dry season, when a thick mixture of milk and blood is drunk and occasionally large amounts of meat are consumed (1814 to 2268 g at one meal), they had a much higher intake of cholesterol and fat than the average intake of the population in the United States."[351]

This amount of meat – 1814 to 2268 grams – translates to 4.0 to 5.0 pounds of meat in one meal! This is a staggering statistic, but the Maasai do not sacrifice their cattle regularly, especially their beloved cows, as cattle are their source of both milk and blood. So perhaps they just occasionally gorge on enormous amounts of meat, but clearly, milk, meat, and blood are the staple foods for the men reviewed in these studies, and they consume almost no plant foods at all.

The most important question to ask, of course, is what was the omega-6 LA consumption in the traditional living Maasai? Cow's milk from cattle grazing on grass, such as the Maasai cattle in Kenya is about 2.57% or less LA.[349] Thus, if we assume that virtually all of the fat in the Maasai diet is from cow's milk, which is a very close approximation, this amounts to 1980 calories worth of animal fat per day (66% fat diet and 3,000 calories per day). 2.57% of the 1980 calories worth of fat indicates that the **omega-6 LA should account for no more than about 1.7% of their total dietary caloric energy.**

Compare the 1.7% omega-6 LA that the Maasai consume to the populations of the Western world who now consume omega-6 LA ranging between 8% to 10% of energy (total calories), as of 2018![180] This Western world level of LA consumption is, therefore, 4.7 to 5.9-fold more LA as a percentage of total dietary calories as compared to the Maasai.

The level of LA consumption in the diet is by far and away the most important consideration,[65] [180] perhaps secondary only to the complete absence of certain vitamins (for example, vitamin B12 deficiency in un-supplemented vegans, which will become fatal within a few years[360] [361]). However, the substitution of edible oils for animal fats in and of itself produces fat-soluble vitamin deficiencies (A, D, and K2), and therein lies a very fundamental aspect of seed oil dangers, as previously reviewed.[148] We will review the pro-oxidative, pro-inflammatory, and toxic effects of seed oils subsequently.

THE TRADITIONAL TOKELAUANS – 50% SATURATED FAT DIET, YET NO CORONARY HEART DISEASE!

In 1992, Albert F. Wessen and colleagues published analyses of the Tokelau Island migrant studies, which documented the negative health transition of the inhabitants of the South Pacific island of Tokelau, which occurred with the westernization of their diet.[362] Wessen and colleagues studied the affected Tokelauans over a period of 20 years. The Tokelauans' traditional diet was based on coconut, fresh fish, starchy tubers, and fruit, the latter of which was mostly breadfruit. Breadfruit is a very starchy staple food of the South Pacific that is seldom eaten raw, but instead is generally consumed after roasting, baking, boiling, or having been fried, or dried and ground into flour.[363]

CHAPTER 2

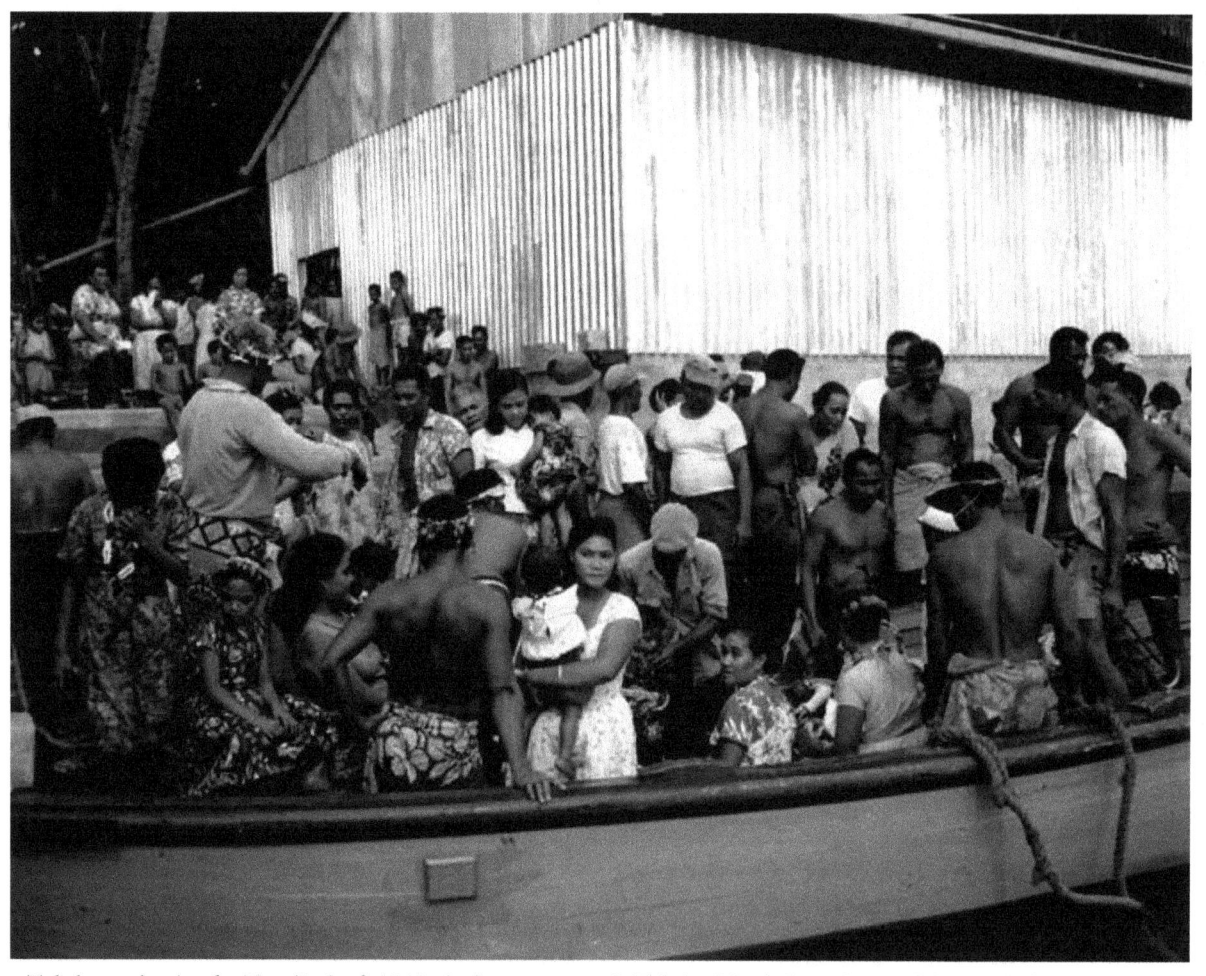

Tokelauans leaving for New Zealand, 1966, via the government's Tokelau Islands Resettlement Scheme. Archives New Zealand, Te Rua Mahar o te Kawanatanga. Reference: AAQT 6539/A81, 257. Carl Wairond. 'Tokelauans – Immigration,' Te Area – the Encyclopedia of New Zealand, http://www.TeAra.govt.nz/en/photograph/728/tokelauans-leaving-for-new-Zealand-1966 (accessed 18 Jan 2022). Creative Commons Attribution 3.0 New Zealand License.

As reported by Ian A.M. Prior, MD, Wessen's colleague, in 1968, the Tokelauans consumed about 56% of their calories from fat (a very high-fat diet), of which coconut oil accounted for some 80% of their total fat.[364] The fatty acid profile of coconut oil is about 91 to 94.5% saturated fat, with another 4.5% being monounsaturated fat, and the remaining 1 to 3 percent being PUFA, that is, omega-3 and omega-6 fats together.[365]

This indicates that the 1968 Tokelauans' saturated fat intake was approximately 40% to 50% of their caloric intake, by our calculations, having been given the types and amounts of foods consumed. However, Ian Prior and colleagues reported on the laboratory analysis of fats and calories for both men and women in Tokelau in 1968, and their saturated fat consumption amounted to a staggering 49% of calories in men and 51% of calories in women![366]

This level of saturated fat consumption is undoubtedly the highest saturated fat intake of any population in the world that has been carefully documented, slightly edging out the Maasai, who consumed 40% to 46% saturated fat. The Maasai, of course, traditionally derive their saturated fat from animal fat, while the Tokelauans traditionally derive saturated fat almost exclusively from the coconut and its oils.

Despite this massive intake of saturated fat intake, studies of Tokelauans in 1982 showed that 0.0% of men aged 40 to 69 years of age had ever had a previous MI (heart attack) based on EKG readings.[362] In fact, Ian Prior and colleagues, who also documented that any form of vascular disease in Tokelauans was very uncommon, asserted, "There is no evidence of the high saturated fat intake having a harmful effect in these populations."[366]

The Tokelauans' diet was proven to contain only 2% total PUFA, which is total omega-3 and omega-6 fats combined.[366] In the well-documented study by Prior in 1968, absolutely none of the PUFA came from seed oils manufactured in a refinery, nor from nuts and seeds; but rather, it came almost exclusively from coconut oil and wild-caught fish from the Pacific ocean,[366] that is, foods from Nature. Coconut oil is about 1.6% omega-6 LA and has negligible omega-3,[367] while wild-caught fish (e.g., Coho salmon) has only 0.06g total omega-6 and 0.90g total omega-3 per 100g raw fillet.[368] Thus, coconut oil is extremely low in LA while many wild-caught fish have negligible LA.

From this knowledge, that is, with 2% of the Tokelauans' diet verified as being total PUFA and, knowing that coconut oil accounted for 80% of the fat, the **estimated omega-6 LA of the diet would have been about 1.6% of total energy**. Once again, contrast that to westernized diets which now contain 8% to 10% omega-6 LA.[180]

PUFA fats, which are primarily omega-6 LA and omega-3 ALA, accumulate in our body fat, and the level in our adipose (body fat) is reflective of the relative amounts in our diets. This will be reviewed in detail in Chapter Four. Three years ago, a little piece of data in the scientific literature was incredibly enlightening to us at the time – the Tokelauans, obviously one of the very few populations still consuming a native, traditional diet without seed oils – also had adipose biopsies completed with fatty acid analysis in 1968, by Ian Prior and colleagues.

Incredibly, their body fat LA was only 3.8%.[17] **Contrast that to Americans, who averaged 9.1% in 1959 and 21.5% by 2008!**[6] Such a low level of LA concentration in the body fat of the Tokelauans is only possible without seed oils and this number – the concentration of LA in the body fat – will become another central theme that we'll keep coming back to as it is reflective of seed oil consumption over a very long period of time.

Despite such evidence of healthy populations consuming 40% to 50% or more of their diets as saturated fats, as of 2013, the American Heart Association continues to advise Americans "to aim for a healthy dietary pattern that achieves 5-6% of calories from SFA [saturated fatty acids]" and to "replace [saturated fat] with MUFA and PUFA [monounsaturated fats and polyunsaturated fats, respectively, i.e., seed oils]."[369]

The 2020 USDA's "Dietary Guidelines for Americans" likewise advises, "For those 2 years old and older, intake of saturated fat should be limited to less than 10% of calories per day by replacing them with unsaturated fats, particularly polyunsaturated fats."[370] Ironically, as unhealthy as Americans are, leading the developed world in obesity[474][475] and with CHD being the leading cause of death,[271] the same "Dietary Guidelines for Americans" affirms that "Current intakes of saturated fat are 11 percent of calories."[370] The Dietary Guidelines continues to advise Americans as follows: "Oils are important to consider as part of a healthy dietary pattern…Strategies to shift intake include cooking with vegetable oil in place of fats high in saturated fat, including butter, shortening, lard, or coconut oil."[370] The World Health Organization (WHO) also continues to assert, "Intake of saturated fat should be less than 10% of total energy intake…"[371]

THE TOKELAUANS DEVASTATING HEALTH TRANSITION – DRIVEN BY PROCESSED FOODS, SUGARS, AND SEED OILS

It's too bad that the story of good health in Tokelau doesn't end there, but food manufacturers' processed food provisions to the Pacific island countries have changed all of that. Historically, the Pacific islanders enjoyed brilliant health, as reviewed by Robert G. Hughes at the University of Queensland, Australia, who wrote, "The geographic isolation and the relative abundance of food provided early Pacific people with the elements of a healthy life. Descriptions by early European explorers provide evidence. The French explorer Louis de Bougainville recorded that the Tahitians were almost God-like and lived in an environment overflowing with natural abundance: 'I never saw men better made' and 'I thought I was transported into the Garden of Eden.'"[372]

Captain James Cook (1728-1779), British explorer famous for his voyages to the South Pacific islands and Australia, logged in his journals, during three voyages to the Pacific islands between 1768 and 1780, very favorable descriptions of the health and diet of the people living in Tahiti, Tonga, Cook Islands, Vanuatu, and New Caledonia, all neighboring islands of Tokelau.[373] Reviews of the writings of Magellan (1521) and Quiros (1606) and many other European explorers of Pacific islands are remarkably consistent, including, "… of a singularly tall, muscular and well-proportioned people."[372]

In 1923, after spending several weeks on Fakaofo, an atoll of Tokelau, author William Burrows, in his descriptions of the inhabitants, wrote, "The natives of the Tokelau Group do not present uniform physical characteristics… They are a big people, but, unlike the Samoans, do not seem to run to fat. It is a rare thing to see either an old man or old woman who has become ungainly, and the women especially keep their figures to an advanced

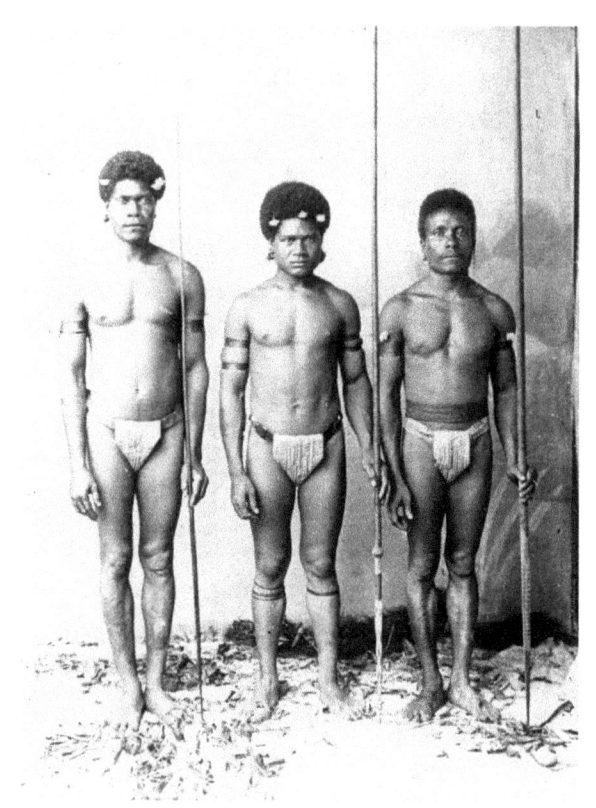

South Pacific Islanders, photo taken in 1900. State Library of Queensland, photo in the public domain, courtesy of Picryl.com.

age. They appear to be a healthy race... One factor in the lives of the people which tends to keep them fit is the fact that they are compelled to put out in their canoes almost daily to obtain fish."[374]

Historically, according to author and researcher, Nancy J. Pollock, Pacific Islanders were vegetarian about 85% of the time.[373] High value was placed on starchy foods, especially starchy root crops such as breadfruit, bananas, plantains, yams, taro, sweet potatoes, and cassava.[375] Coconuts and pandanus (fibrous fruit similar to coconut) were also staples.

Meat and fish – fresh, wild-caught fish – from the ocean were regular fare. Typical fare for the region was large quantities of starchy roots, a side of green leaves, seafood, and coconut. The Tokelauans relied extensively on coconut (and coconut oil) due to poor soils and crop conditions on the islands, which could not support root crops.[376]

However, reminiscent of the words written by Weston A. Price regarding the displacements of traditional foods for processed foods and the consequent devastating outcomes, author Mele Malolo and colleagues, in a review for the Secretariat of the Pacific Community, wrote, "Traumatic changes began to appear in the early 1950s and even prior to the Second World War, when rice, flour, and tinned corned beef began to appear in the daily food of atoll as well as volcanic-island dwellers. Today in the atolls, coconut and pandanus no longer make up a major part of everyday meals. This is due to the increasing availability and use of imported staple foods such as flour, rice, and noodles."[375]

Robert G. Hughes, in a 2002 review for the World Health Organization, entitled, *"Diet, Food Supply and Obesity in the Pacific,"* wrote, "The largest single providers of energy for Pacific countries are cereal products (white flour and rice). However, the largest single increase since 1965 has been in the availability of vegetable oils. Fat availability from all sources except coconuts has increased... Imported fat has been added to and has not replaced existing fat sources such as coconuts."[372]

However, whether coconut oil is still utilized substantially comes into question, as reviewed by researchers Andrew McGregor and Mark Sheehy. In a study prepared for the International Fund for Agricultural Development (IFAD), in which they evaluated grocery stores in nearby Tuvalu, they found that "No coconut oil for cooking was found in any of the shops visited – even though it is the traditional source of cooking oil."[377] However, they suspected local production and sales might account for some coconut oil use. And while 72% of Americans now recognize the health benefits of coconut oil,[378] McGregor and Sheehy noted that "In the Pacific islands coconut oil generally has a reputation as poor man's inferior product compared with the other imported cooking oils."[377] In nearby Fiji, they noted that soybean and canola are the major imported oils.

So while the inhabitants of Tokelau were once reviewed by authorities as "strong, muscular, and mostly in good health,"[372] with an obesity prevalence historically through about 1940 that we estimate at approximately 1% (based on all available evidence) in 2014, obesity (BMI > 30) had skyrocketed to an extraordinary 67% and overweight (BMI ≥ 25.0-30.0) was 23%.[379] This extraordinary degree of obesity and overweight was documented by the WHO STEPS survey and published by the Tokelau National Statistics Office. The combined obesity and overweight was a staggering 90% of the population. We suspect that this is approximately a 90-fold increase in obesity in a period of about 75 years.

In 1969, Tokelauans were also confirmed to

have a relatively low diabetes prevalence of 1.0% in men and 3.3% in women, with an average of about 2.15%.[380] Today, that would be the lowest prevalence of diabetes for any country in the world.[381] Yet, in 2013, Tokelau had the highest diabetes prevalence in the world, at a staggering 37.5%.[382] This is an increase of greater than 17-fold (greater than 1,600%) in a period of 44 years.

Professor Paul Zimmet, MD, Tel Aviv University, and Sunny Whitehouse, colleagues of H.C. Trowell, MD, and Denis P. Burkitt, MD, conducted some of the earliest recorded epidemiological studies in many Pacific Island countries including Nauru, Tuvalu, and Western Samoa, and they confirmed, "Our prevalence studies were the first performed in each country and hospital records indicated that diabetes was virtually unknown prior to 1960. Yet, in each of these countries there has been an increase in the number of cases since then. We were unable to obtain evidence of any cases of diabetes in Funafuti [atoll of Tuvalu], Western Samoa, or Nauru before 1945."[383] Given this data, we might also expect that diabetes in Tokelau was also unknown before 1945.

With respect to CHD, as previously reviewed, Tokelauan men aged 40 to 69 years of age were found not to have any evidence of previous MI (heart attack) based on EKG readings.[362] And while there are no recent studies specifically on the Tokelauans and CHD, currently, it has been well documented that "Pacific people experience a disproportionate burden of cardiovascular disease (CVD), whether they remain in their country of origin or migrate to higher-income countries…"[384] Astoundingly, today, CVD is the leading cause of mortality among Pacific peoples.[384]

Noncommunicable diseases (NCDs), including coronary heart disease (CHD), cancer, diabetes, dementia, and the like, are now the leading causes of death in the Pacific Island countries.[377] For atoll countries, like Tokelau, NCDs range from 67% to 73%.[377] We can be quite certain, however, that chronic disease deaths in Tokelau in the year 1940 were close to zero.

Documentation of seed oil consumption (and other food consumption) in some Pacific Island countries has been difficult if not impossible, as generally the most reliable source of data for food consumption products has been the Food and Agriculture Organization of the United Nations (FAO), utilizing the FAOSTAT database. Data is available from 1961 to about 2010 at FAO (or was until just two weeks ago at the time of this writing).

The FAO data is quite accurate in countries that closely track domestic production, plus imports, and exports, and then carefully calculate and log data, however, this is not the case in many smaller countries. We have found, for example, that seed oil data tracking in Barbados wasn't accurate, and two if not three seed oil manufacturers that provided edible oils to the country failed to report data to the FAO.[4] It is obvious that there are similar issues with FAO data for certain countries, particularly in the South Pacific, both internally at the FAO and by observation of the data.[385] [386]

Fortunately, the Tokelau National Statistics Office carefully tracks the local population, imports, etc., on all three atolls of the country (Atafu, Fakaofo, and Nukunonu), and data for 2014 has been reported. With regard to sugar consumption in Tokelau inhabitants, the office reports, "… they consume high levels of sugar and refined carbohydrate with low fibre content. The calculated sugar intake, including that hidden in other foods and non-alcoholic beverages, averages to a range of 0.83 to 1.35 kg per person per week. This is equivalent to 207 to 336 teaspoons per week."[379]

With respect to vegetable oils, the office reports, "Fat: Cooking oil is the main 'pure' source: 0.29-0.47 litres per week... a much greater source of fat will be hidden in protein sources such as chicken, tinned fish, lamb/mutton, corned beef, and sausages."[379]

They also report on imports for the year 2014 some 25.6 metric tonnes of "Baker's and normal flour," 8.7 tonnes of instant noodles, 15.3 cubic meters of Just Juice (brand name), 49.2 tonnes of milk, 4.7 tonnes of milk powder, and 12.9 cubic meters of Zap chocolate drink, among other processed foods.

They also consumed an average of 1.8 standard drinks (147 calories) of alcohol per day. They imported 8.1 tonnes of mackerel in oil and 5.0 tonnes of tuna in oil. These are tinned fish that are almost certainly packed in seed oils, which are less expensive and produce greater profit for manufacturers. This was for their confirmed population of 1,383 people in the year 2014.

If we use the average consumption for both sugar and seed oils for 2014, as provided by the Tokelau National Statistics Office, we calculate that this equates to 129g sugar/capita/day (517 calories), 50.7 g white flour (203 calories) per day, 17 g (73 calories) instant noodles per day, and 147 calories of alcohol per day; the 0.38 L of vegetable oils (average) per person per week equates to 50g/capita/day (450 calories). The latter number will not include oils in tinned fish, other processed food items, and potentially other sources of oils not tracked.

In 2014, the Tokelauans consumed a minimum total of 1,389 calories per day of processed foods in the form of sugar, white flour, instant noodles, alcohol, and vegetable oils alone. This is perhaps more than half of all calories, and we expect that the seed oils consumption may be under-represented by 10 to 20 grams per day or more. Thus, seed oil consumption in Tokelau may approach that of the U.S. (80g/day in 2010).

We should recall that, in 1968, Ian Prior and colleagues confirmed that the Tokelauans had 21 g (84 calories, 3% of calories) of sugars per day, 20 g "cereals" (80 calories) per day, and absolutely zero consumption of vegetable oils.[366] Thus, total processed food in 1968 was no more than a maximum of 164 calories per day, while the cereal grains may have been whole, unprocessed grains, and there wasn't a speck of seed oils to be found.

Thus, we've observed that the Tokelauans, who once consumed the greatest amount of saturated fat in the world, as far as we know, were documented to have virtually zero coronary heart disease (CHD) in middle-aged men. They were also once quite lean and fit, healthy, and most all appear to have enjoyed freedom from chronic diseases, including diabetes. Then, in a period of a half-century, their health was devastated in perhaps 90% of the people or more.

As is seen in the graph on page 100, this is not only attributable to the transition to a highly processed food diet, but mostly, the initiation and progressive increase in seed oils, primarily over the past 50 years, to which we believe they are particularly vulnerable. In this same graph, we've documented the relationship between the introduction of seed oils, increased sugar consumption, and an estimated 90-fold increase in obesity (1940 obesity estimated at 1%) as well as a 17-fold increase in diabetes between 1969 and 2013.

All of this carefully validated medical evidence

regarding the native, traditional diets of the Maasai and Tokelauans, all proven in scientific studies, confirms extraordinarily high intakes of saturated fat in two populations – about 40% to 46% saturated animal fat in the Maasai and about 40% to 51% saturated fat (mostly from coconut oil) in the South Pacific Tokelauans – yet both populations, while consuming their native, traditional diets, were shown to have little or no coronary heart disease (CHD), obesity, diabetes, or chronic disease, and both were found to be in exceedingly good health. Most importantly, we observe that both the traditional living Maasai and Tokelauans did not consume processed foods, added sugars, refined grains, or seed oils.

CANCER IS ANOTHER 20TH CENTURY PLAGUE – MARKEDLY INCREASING IN PARALLEL TO SEED OILS

In the town of Boston, Massachusetts, in the year 1811, a total of 942 deaths occurred (see the "Boston, Massachusetts, Bill of Mortality, 1811, in Chapter One). Physicians documented all causes of death for the year, noting that just 5 of those 942 deaths were caused by cancer.[271] By 1900, 5.8% of the population in the U.S was found to have succumbed to cancer.[271] Just over a century later, in 2010, 31.1% of deaths in the U.S. were due to cancer.[271]

Thus, in the United States, 1 in 188 deaths was due to cancer in 1811, rising to 1 in 17 deaths in 1900, and finally, rising to 1 in 3 deaths by 2010. Over a nearly 200-year period, this is a staggering 62-fold (6,100%) rise in cancer deaths.

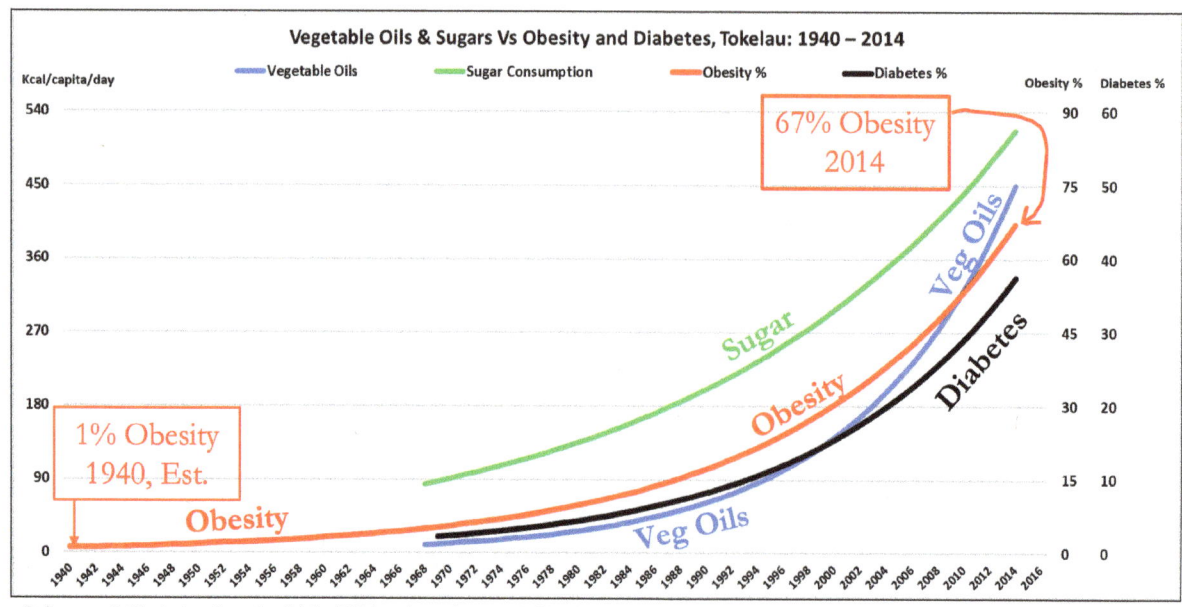

Vegetable Oils & Sugars Vs Obesity and Diabetes, Tokelau: 1940 – 2014

References: 1) Obesity is estimated at 1% for 1940, based on references cited herein. 2) Obesity, 2014: A Study of 2014 Imports by the Tokelau National Statistics Office, 2015/2016, summary version 2. 3) Diabetes: 1969 Data: Trowell & Burkitt. Westernized Diseases, 1981, p.255. 4) Diabetes 2013: IDF Diabetes Atlas, 6th Edition. 2013, p.68. 3) Vegetable oil and sugar consumption: FAO Food Balance Sheets, retrieved from Knoema.com. © C. Knobbe, 2022. Ancestral Health Foundation.

Just as Weston A. Price found that the "displacing foods" induced marked degenerative disease including cancer,[28] we've seen a remarkable correlation between rising processed food consumption since 1865 and steadily increasing rates of cancer and cancer deaths. Are we to believe this is all due to aging and genetics, as conventional medicine would have us believe?

Such a conclusion would not only be inchoate, but entirely unfounded and erroneous. Please view the painstakingly prepared graph below and take note of 1) the drastic increases in sugars and seed oils that parallel this 62-fold increase in cancer deaths in roughly 200 years, 2) the remarkable correlation with both sugars and seed oils, and 3) the fact that both sugars and seed oils are proxy markers for processed foods.[4] It may be shocking to those who believe that the increase in cancer deaths is primarily driven by aging, as that alone will account for only a small percentage of such fatalities. People who survived childhood have commonly grown old throughout all of history, and we'll delve into that detail subsequently.

In 1929, W.M. Strong published research noting that in 20 large American cities, the cancer death rate per 100,000 people (hereafter referred to as the cancer death rate) was 49 for the period of 1881 to 1885, which increased to 89 by 1913.[387] In the U.S. registration for the year 1900, the cancer death rate was 63, which rose to 79 by 1913, indicating an increase of over 25% in a period of just thirteen years. In 2010, the cancer death rate was 185.9.

Thus, the cancer death rate elevated from 49 in 1881 to 185.9 by 2010. As will be reviewed in some detail subsequently, little of this can be accounted for secondary to aging of the population, given that high infant and childhood mortality through the late 19th and early 20th centuries accounts for the large majority of decreased lifespan.

In 2010, the Centers for Disease Control

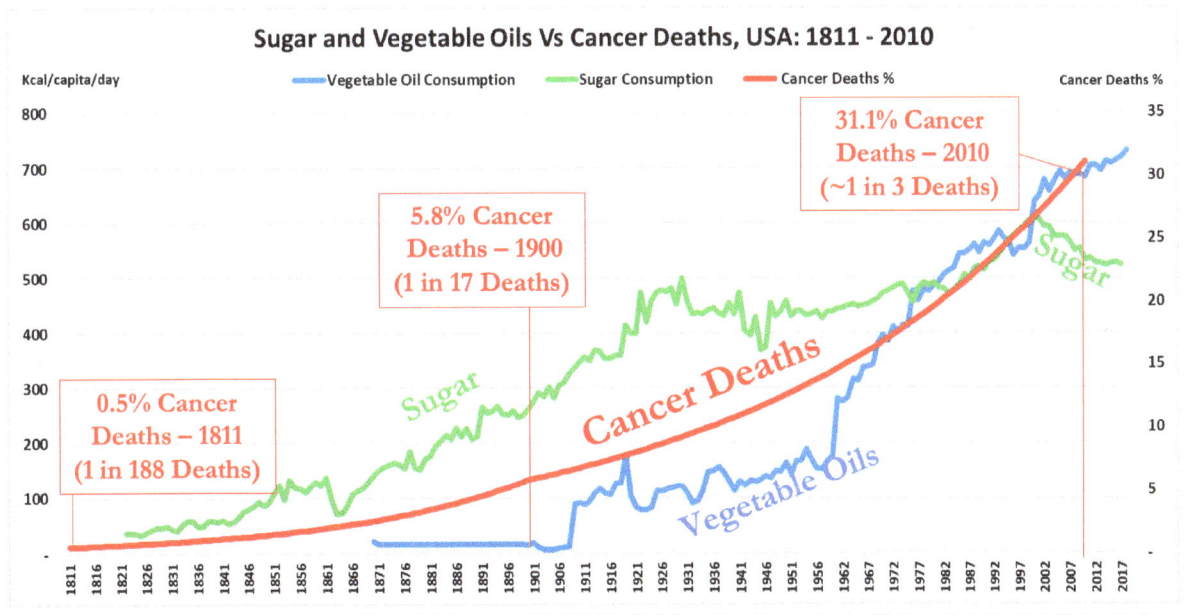

Sugar and Vegetable Oils Vs Cancer Deaths, USA: 1811 - 2010

- 0.5% Cancer Deaths – 1811 (1 in 188 Deaths)
- 5.8% Cancer Deaths – 1900 (1 in 17 Deaths)
- 31.1% Cancer Deaths – 2010 (~1 in 3 Deaths)

References: 1) Vegetable Oil Data: Knobbe, Stojanoska. Medical Hypotheses: 2017;109:184-198 2) Sugar Data: Guyenet, Landen. *The Hungry Brain*. New York, Flatiron Books, 2017. 3) Cancer Death Statistics for years 1811, 1900, and 2010 only for U.S.: See references herein. © C. Knobbe, 2022. Ancestral Health Foundation.

(CDC) found that cancers were the second leading cause of death in the U.S., ranking just slightly behind heart disease, but were by far the leading cause of potential life years lost, accounting for 5.6 million years of life lost in that year alone, as compared to heart disease at 3.8 million years.[388] As with coronary heart disease, diabetes, Alzheimer's disease, dementia, and age-related macular degeneration (AMD), all of which will be reviewed subsequently, cancer was a medical rarity in the early 19th century, causing only about 0.5% of all deaths, but has steadily risen, now causing nearly one of every three deaths in the U.S. as of the early 21st century.

Evidence in recent decades in the U.S. shows marked increases in cancer rates over very short periods of time. For example, the age-adjusted incidence of invasive breast cancer in the U.S. increased nearly 30% in less than 15 years, from approximately 85/100,000 women in the mid-1970s to approximately 110/100,000 women in the late 1980s, based on Surveillance, Epidemiology, and End Results (SEER) data.[389]

In Los Angeles County, California, incidence rates of female breast cancer, in cases per 100,000, rose from 42.5 to 50.8 in Chinese, 69.5 to 114.3 in Japanese, 81.5 to 98.1 in Filipino, and 26.1 to 44.5 in Korean women.[390] For all women in the SEER study, the 1997 incidence rate of 115/100,000 for all ethnic groups combined was found to be the highest annual rate ever historically recorded.[389] Just during the five-year period between 1993 and 1997, the annual increase in invasive breast cancer incidence for Asian women over age 50, in Los Angeles County, was 6.3%, which is an approximate 31.5% increase in that period alone.[390]

On a global scale, the WHO estimated that 18.1 million people developed cancers in 2018, with some 9.6 million deaths attributed to the disease.[391] Worldwide cancer death rates are also increasing markedly, with 11.5% of deaths due to cancers in 1990, which increased to 15.7% of all deaths in 2016 (see graph p. 103).[392] This is a 36.5% increase in the percentage of deaths attributed to cancer in this 26-year period alone. The WHO also determined that one in 8 men and one in 11 women in the world will die from malignant disease. In contrast to global rates of cancer, however, in the U.S. the American Cancer Society confirms that the risk of developing invasive cancer or dying from cancer for males is 39.66% and 22.03%, respectively, and for females, is 37.65% and 18.76%, respectively.[391]

Thus, whereas one in 8 men will die of cancer globally, that risk is one in 5 in the U.S. And whereas one in 11 women will die of cancer globally, that risk is also nearly one in 5 in the U.S. Therefore, both the risk of developing cancer as well as dying from cancer is far higher in the U.S. than the world at large. However, as of 2017, consumption of both seed oils and sugars is higher per capita in the U.S. than in any other country in the world.[124][393]

The incidence of breast cancer in Japanese women in Los Angeles County, California, is the highest reported anywhere in the world.[390] In Japan, the incidence rates of invasive breast cancer more than doubled between 1960 and the late 1980s and rates continue to rise.[394] Multiple studies have shown that subsequent generations of Asian women who migrate to the United States have marked increases in breast cancer risk, which has been strongly correlated to westernized dietary habits.

Our research confirmed that the consumption of highly polyunsaturated seed oils in Japan increased nearly 4.5-fold in a 46-year period, rising

Cancer Deaths by Type, World: 1990 – 2016

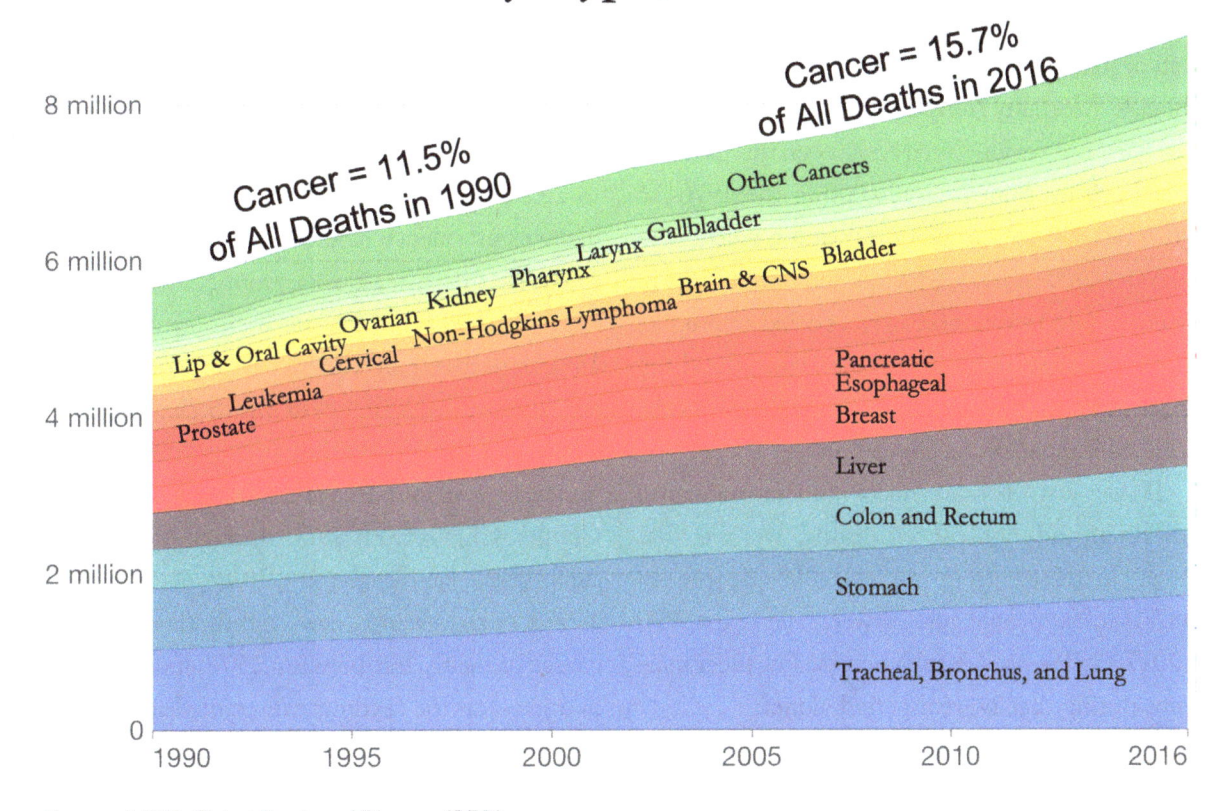

Cancer = 11.5% of All Deaths in 1990

Cancer = 15.7% of All Deaths in 2016

Other Cancers, Gallbladder, Larynx, Pharynx, Kidney, Ovarian, Lip & Oral Cavity, Cervical, Non-Hodgkins Lymphoma, Brain & CNS, Bladder, Leukemia, Prostate, Pancreatic, Esophageal, Breast, Liver, Colon and Rectum, Stomach, Tracheal, Bronchus, and Lung

Source: IHME, Global Burden of Disease (GBD)
Note: All cancer types with less than 100,000 global deaths in 2016 into a collective category 'Other cancers'. OurWorldInData.org. Annual cancer deaths by type, measured as the total number of deaths across all age categories and both sexes.

from 9g/day in 1961 to 39g/day by 2006.[4] Cancer as a cause of death in Japan has been increasing in every single generation since 1890,[395] quite similar to the U.S., with cancer becoming the leading cause of death in 1981.[396] This is all in lockstep with Westernization of the diet, particularly since the late 1940s to 1950s, following American occupation of Japan after World War II.[397] [398]

Next, let's examine cancer in China – the country with the largest population in the world. The escalating rate of cancer there, rather like that of the rest of the world, ought to help support or refute our hypothesis that processed foods and seed oils are the primary drivers of malignancy.

CANCER ESCALATION IN CHINA – ALONG WITH OBESITY, CHD, DIABETES, & OTHER CHRONIC DISEASES – IN PROPORTION TO SEED OILS

In 2010, cancer became the leading cause of death in China, and by 2015, when the population in China reached 1.37 billion, there were an estimated

4,292,000 new cancer cases and a total of 2,814,000 cancer deaths, which corresponds to more than 7,500 cancer deaths per day.[399] Cancer now represents 25% of all deaths in urban areas and 21% in rural areas of China.[400] Mortality from cancer in China has been markedly and steadily increasing over the past few decades, rising from 74.2/100,000 in the 1970s to 108.3/100,000 in the 1990s and most recently, to 135.9/100,000 in 2004, which is an 83% increase in the death rate from cancer over a period of roughly 30 years.[401] From the 1970s to the 1990s, the rising cancer mortality also could not be attributed to the increased lifespan of the population.[401]

If we just look at major cancer incidence in China, and not cancer deaths, we see that cancer increased from 495/100,000 people to 1587/100,000 people, just between the years 1990 to 2017.[402] This is a 3.2-fold increase in cancer incidence during that 27-year period alone!

Lung cancer in China, as of 2009, had increased 465% over the previous 30 years and became the leading cause of death.[401] The WHO estimated that, by 2025, more than one million Chinese will be diagnosed with lung cancer every year.[401] Perhaps surprising to most people, the prevalence of smoking during much of this period of increasing lung cancer has steadily decreased, dropping from 28.65% in 1990 to 20.87% in 2016.[403]

As of 2005, the incidence of breast cancer in China had been rising 3% to 4% per year, with a more than doubling of incidence in the previous 30 years.[404] Also, China now has nearly 50% of the world's liver cancer cases[405] and mortality rates from liver cancer have risen from 17.6 and 7.3 per 100,000 in 1973-1975, to 29.0 and 11.2 per 100,000 in 1990-1992, to 37.55 and 14.45 per 100,000 in 2004-2005, in men and women, respectively.[406] This represents a doubling of liver cancer-related deaths in both men and women in China in a period of just 30 years.

But it isn't just an explosion of cancer that is the problem in China, the incidence of hypertension in adults increased from 13.6% in 1991 to 23.2% by 2015.[407] [408] Between 1990 and 2017, diabetes prevalence rose from 3.7% to 6.6%[409] and cardiovascular disease rose from 5266/100,000 to 6037/100,000,[410] which are increases of 78% and 15%, respectively, over that 27-year period alone. In urban areas, the incidence of metabolic syndrome in China was 8.0% in 1992, 10.6% in 2002, and estimated to be about 15.5% in 2017.[411] In Shanghai County, China, from 1960 through 1962, cancer, cerebrovascular disease, and heart disease ranked as the sixth, seventh, and eighth most common causes of death, but between 1978 and 1980, they had become the leading causes of death for that region.[412] [413]

Overweight and obesity in China rose from 13.9% and 1.4%, respectively, in 1991, to 34.9% and 7.1%, respectively, in 2015.[414] If we tally up the totals, we observe that the percentage of overweight and obese elevated from 15.3% in 1991 to 42% by 2015 – truly, a staggering increase over a very short period of time. As always, we need to examine what they've been eating (see the graph on page 105).

As one can see from the same graph, which represents seed ('vegetable') oils and sugar consumption in China, between 1961 and 2018, we observe **that seed oil consumption has increased remarkably,** from a very low 30 cal/day (3.3g/day) in 1961 to 204 cal/day (23g/day) in 2018, which is a 7-fold increase in seed oils during this time.[415] **Sugar consumption was and remains among the lowest in the world,** at just 22 cal/day (5.5g/day) in

1961, rising slightly but still remaining extremely low at just 78 cal/day (19.5g/day) in 2018. According to combined data from the Food and Agriculture Organization (FAO) (accessed through Knoema), out of 169 countries for which the data exists, only seven countries have less sugar consumption per capita than China.[416]

Sugar consumption in China, therefore, averaged just a bit over one teaspoon per day in 1961 and elevated to just about four teaspoons per day by 2018. Even at the highest level in 2018, sugar consumption in China was still a mere 2.5% of total calories (this assumes caloric consumption in 2018 was the same as 2013, which was 3,108 cal/day of total available calories, with neither sugar nor total calories corrected for losses).[417] The WHO recommends that sugar consumption remain below 10% of calories[418] and, for comparison, the most recent data shows people in the U.S. are consuming approximately 21% of calories as sugar.[4]

Thus, we observe that, while sugar consumption remains among the lowest in the world in China, seed oil consumption has risen 7-fold between 1961 and 2018, which has been paralleled by a 3.2-fold increase in major cancer incidence, a 465% increase in lung cancer during a period marked by progressively less smoking, a doubling of liver cancer deaths, a near tripling of overweight and obesity between 1991 and 2015, a near doubling of diabetes during the same period, and marked increases in cerebrovascular disease and coronary heart disease.

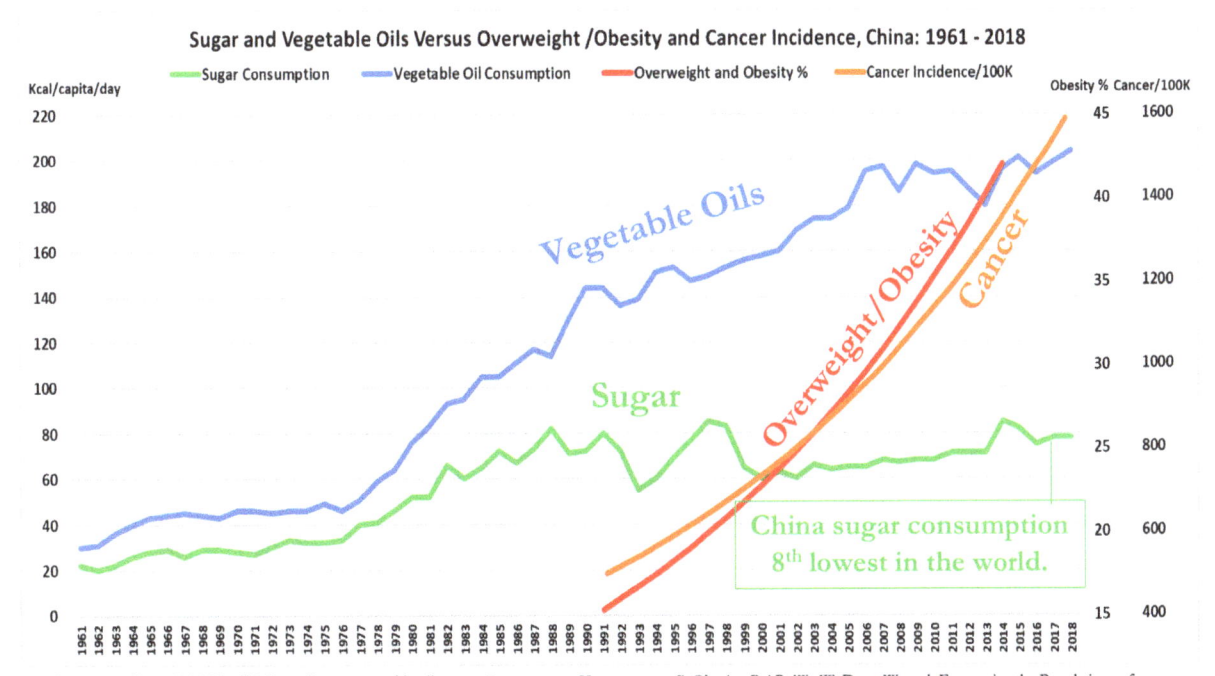

Sugar and Vegetable Oils Versus Overweight /Obesity and Cancer Incidence, China: 1961 - 2018

China sugar consumption 8th lowest in the world.

References: 1) China: FAO Food Balance Sheets, vegetable oils, sugar & sweeteners. Knoema.com. 2) Obesity: Bai R, Wu W, Dong W, et al. Forecasting the Populations of Overweight and Obese Chinese Adults. Diabetes Metab Syndr Obes. 2020;13:4849-4857. 3) Cancer Incidence: Global Burden of Disease Cancer Collaboration. Global, regional, and national cancer incidence, mortality, years of life lost, years lived with disability, and disability-adjusted life-years for 29 cancer groups, 1990 to 2017: a systematic analysis for the global burden of disease study. JAMA Oncol. 2019;5(12):1749-1768. © C. Knobbe, 2022. Ancestral Health Foundation.

RODENT STUDIES SHOW SEED OILS INDUCE FAR HIGHER CANCER RATES – WITH A THRESHOLD EFFECT

Beginning mostly in the 1940s and 1950s, rodents fed high-fat diets were consistently found to be more prone to develop cancers than rodents fed low-fat diets. This was observed both with spontaneously occurring tumors as well as those induced by carcinogens.[419][420] However, there was then and remains relatively little interest in distinguishing between different types of fats (e.g., seed oil versus animal fats) with respect to this susceptibility.[421]

Kenneth K. Carroll, DSc, and colleagues, at the University of Western Ontario, published some of the first evidence linking omega-6-rich diets as promoters of cancer in 1970. These studies showed that high corn oil diets (corn oil is approximately 59% LA) stimulated tumors after rats were treated with a carcinogenic agent (7,12-dimethylbenz [a] anthracene, i.e., DMBA), whereas lower omega-6 fat diets were more resistant to cancer promotion.[422]

Carroll suggested at the time that the corn oil was acting as an active promoter of cancer, but not necessarily an initiator directly since a carcinogen was being given. In 1971, Carroll published another paper in which he and fellow researcher, H.T. Khor, found that 0.5% and 5% corn oil diets produced fewer breast cancers in rats treated with the carcinogen DMBA than rats fed 10% or 20% corn oil diets.[423] Carroll and Khor wrote, "Experiments with 10 different fats and oils fed at the 20% level indicated that unsaturated fats enhance the yield of adenocarcinomas [cancers] more than saturated fats."[423]

In a subsequent study (1979), Carroll found that, following a carcinogen, rats fed diets containing 3% sunflower oil (about 68% LA) and 17% beef tallow or coconut oil (approximately 2.0% and 2.5% LA, respectively) developed at least twice as many tumors as those fed diets containing 20% saturated fat alone, again, strongly implicating higher omega-6 in cancer promotion.[424]

In 1975, Carroll also reviewed the fact that feeding entirely natural diets to animals produced lower tumor yields,[425][426] with their own experience in agreement with such evidence.[427] All-natural diets would never contain seed oils or processed foods, of course.

Since the 1970s, a very large and striking body of scientific evidence has accumulated which indicates that when the intake of omega-6 polyunsaturated fats (PUFA) is above 4.0 to 5.0% of caloric energy intake, which practically only occurs with seed oil consumption, the induction of cancers increases in direct proportion to the total fat in the diet.[428][429] In fact, dozens of experimental studies have consistently shown that omega-6 fat – primarily LA from seed oils – is the main and primary promoter of cancers of the breast, colon, and pancreas, while saturated and monounsaturated fats do not promote carcinogenesis.[429][430][431][432]

Researcher Montserrat Solanas, of Autonomous University Barcelona in Spain, who has been investigating the effects of edible oils on cancer induction for decades, recently wrote, "The dietary lipids [fats] effects not only depend on the quantity but also on the type of fat… In general, n-6 polyunsaturated fatty acids (PUFA), especially linoleic acid (LA; 18:2n-6), have strong tumor-enhancing effects."[433] In carcinogen-induced cancers, extra-virgin olive oil (approximately 10% LA), for example, produced tumors that were far more benign, as compared to tumors from rats fed corn oil (approximately 59% LA), which were much more aggressive.[433]

Eduard Escrich, a colleague researcher of Solanas, also at the Autonomous University Barcelona, reviewed numerous studies which confirm that diets high in omega-6 PUFA are associated with tumors in experimental animals that appear sooner, grow larger, and occupy more volume than in animals on low omega-6 diets.[434] A number of animal studies have shown that diets enriched in seed oils, such as corn oil and safflower oil, which are rich sources of omega-6 LA, promote the development of mammary (breast) cancers[435][436][437] and lung tumors.[438] Further evidence also implicates high PUFA diets, rich in corn oil, as potent promoters of prostate cancer growth with increased mortality.[439]

Clement Ip, PhD, Distinguished Member and Head of Cancer Chemoprevention at Roswell Park Cancer Institute in Buffalo, New York, completed one of the most compelling rodent studies in history, which documented the progressively increasing risk of cancer promotion with higher omega-6 LA-containing diets.[440] Dr. Ip fed female rats diets that contained different levels of LA, beginning at 0.5%, but also at 1.1%, 1.7%, 2.2%, 3.5%, 4.4%, 8.5%, and 11.5%. Each diet contained a total

Breast Tumors Vs Dietary Linoleic Acid (LA) Percentage

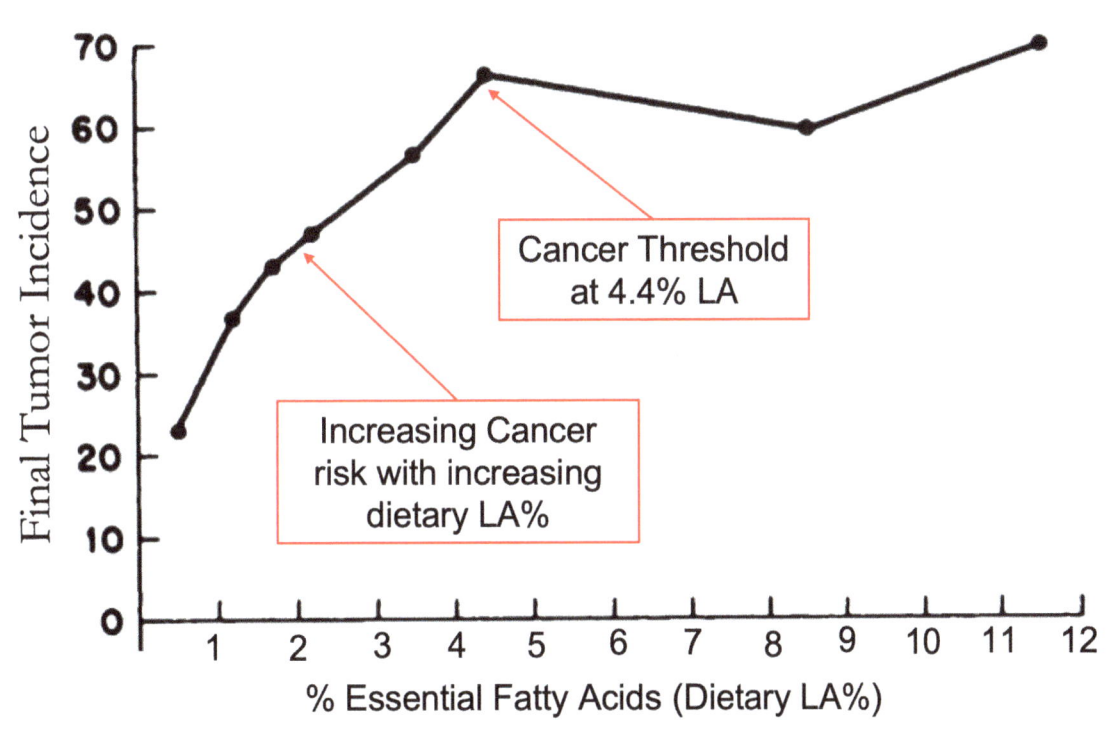

FIG 1. Final incidence of mammary tumors (percent of rats with tumors) and total tumor yield of rats fed diets containing different levels of EFA. Each group included 30 rats. Reproduced with permission (14).

Ip, C. Fat and essential fatty acid in mammary carcinogenesis. Amer Journal of Clinical Nutritional. 1987;45(1):218-24. With permissions.

of 20% fat by weight, and the fat was mixtures of corn oil (about 59% LA) and coconut oil (about 2% LA), in proper proportions to produce the linoleic acid levels. The rats were treated with the carcinogen DMBA and then were begun on the respective diets beginning three days later and remained on such diets until being sacrificed.

With respect to dietary LA percentage and cancer outcomes in these rodents, Dr. Ip wrote, "It can be seen that mammary tumorigenesis [tumor production] was very sensitive to linoleate [LA] intake and increased proportionately in the range of 0.5—4.4% of dietary linoleate [LA]."[440] Above 4.4% of LA, Ip continued, "tumor development appeared to level off,"[440] which strongly suggests that there is a threshold effect, and increasing the LA percentage above about 4.4% makes little difference in terms of increasing cancer risk, as seen in the graph on page 107.

Dr. Clement Ip's research, as well as others, all strongly indicate that cancer induction and/or promotion is sensitive to omega-6 LA consumption, with a threshold at about 4.4% of dietary energy, above which almost no further increases in cancer risk occur. This knowledge would essentially nullify almost all studies that have attempted to find epidemiologic (population-wide) studies that correlate seed oil consumption and cancer risk, since virtually all developed countries are now consuming above 5% of caloric energy as omega-6 LA alone.[441]

In another aspect of Dr. Ip's classic research, rats given a carcinogen were maintained on so-called 'natural ingredient diets' versus "purified diets," however, in these studies, the primary fat provided to modify the fat intake for all diets was none other than soybean oil, which, we would submit is an entirely processed ingredient. Nevertheless, at the 5% level of fat in the diet, the animals provided the 'Natural Ingredient Diets,' which were certainly much less processed, developed half as many tumors as those on the "Purified Diets" (see the graph below, reproduced with permissions).[440]

Mammary (Breast) Tumors on Purified (Processed) Vs. Natural Diets

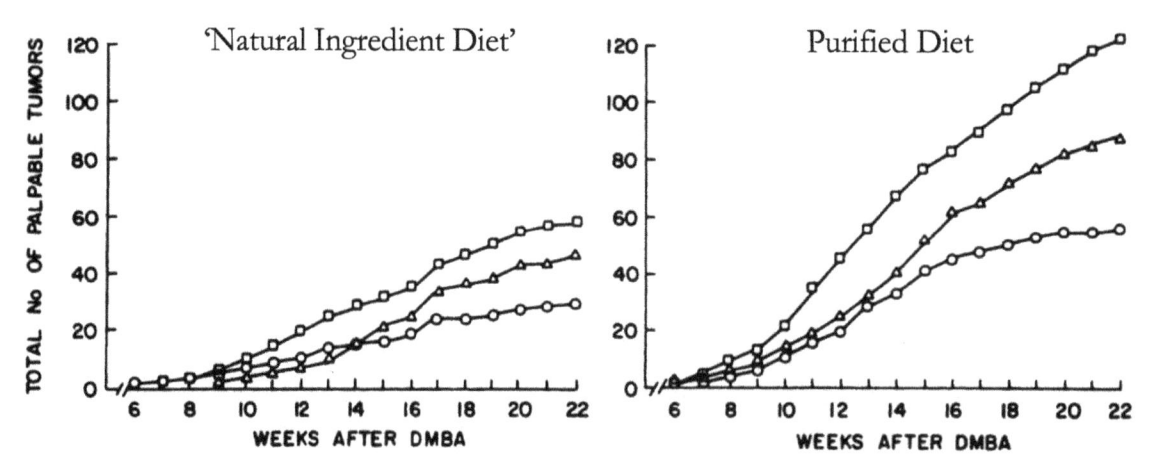

FIG 5. Effect of fat level in natural-ingredient vs purified diets on mammary tumorigenesis. Each group included 30 rats.

Ip, C. Fat and essential fatty acid in mammary carcinogenesis. Amer Journal of Clinical Nutritional. 1987;45(1):218-24. Reproduced with permission.

In Clement Ip's research, it's interesting that, despite the fact that both diets were quite processed in character, the 'Purified Diet" caused animals to develop twice as many tumors as the 'Natural Ingredients Diet.' However, even in the 'Natural Ingredients Diet,' the animals were consuming seed oils, dried skim milk, ground No. 2 yellow-shelled corn, and fish meal,[440] none of which we would consider natural. Yet even this diet protected the animals far more than the purified diet, which, by its very definition, is highly refined (processed).[442] Processed food diets are substantially like purified diets and should be avoided, of course. The natural diets of rodents, which are omnivores, would include insects, worms, meat, poultry, snails, other rodents, carrion (decaying flesh), fruit, vegetables, grains, seeds, and more.[443] We can only wonder how well the rodents would have fared had they consumed an all-natural, wild-type diet, which would have provided the ultimate in nutrition while preventing toxicity.

In the French Nutrinet-Santé Cohort Study, which was a large prospective analysis lasting from 2009-2017, researchers found that for every 10% increase in ultra-processed foods in the diet, an associated 12% increase in overall cancer and an 11% increase in breast cancer occurred.[444] However, as we've reviewed previously, ultra-processed food is defined at the macro-level by the presence of refined sugars, refined flours, and seed oils, but the bulk of processed foods on a caloric basis, is none other than seed oils.

Westernization of the diet invariably comes with seed oil consumption. As we've reviewed repeatedly, seed oils had virtually no place in perhaps 99.8% of the world's diets from antiquity through the end of the American Civil War in 1865. And with progressively increasing seed oil consumption at the individual, country, and global levels, we've seen skyrocketing rates of cancer incidence. We've seen cancers claim the lives of only 1 in 188 people in the year 1811 when seed oils weren't in the food supply, sugar consumption was negligible, and processed foods did not exist.

Cancer deaths escalated to one in 17 people in the year 1900 after sugars and seed oils had entered the food supply, but consumption was still very low. Within another century, when seed oils, sugars, and processed foods accounted for 75% of the diet in the U.S., cancers claimed a staggering 1 in 3 lives by 2010. With a boatload of evidence in support, which could fill an entire medical textbook, we will submit that a return to an all-natural, whole foods-based diet, rich in nutrient-dense foods, with zero edible oils and low in refined sugars, would well be expected to nearly eliminate cancer risk for almost all people.

CHAPTER 2: SUMMARY

Processed food is most simply defined as food that has added sugars, refined white flours, seed oils, and trans fats. These foods have risen in the food supply from the year 1865, when they occupied nothing more than trivial amounts of sugar on a worldwide basis, to the past decade, when processed foods elevated to 75% of the world's food supply.

During the same time frame, the chronic diseases of coronary heart disease (CHD), heart attack, cancers, metabolic syndrome, type 2 diabetes, Alzheimer's disease, dementia, age-related macular degeneration (AMD), overweight, obesity, and autoimmune diseases have risen from rarity to the leading causes of suffering and death (only CHD, heart attack, and cancers reviewed in this chapter).

During this same time frame, that is, from about 1866 to 2010 and even more recently, the single greatest change (even on a caloric basis) in all of the world's diets, was none other than seed oil consumption. Consumption of seed oils elevated from almost zero in 1865 globally (China had exceedingly low levels of sesame oil consumption at that time), to occupy somewhere between one-seventh and one-fourth of caloric consumption by 2010 in 76 countries.[124]

Due to the fact that such oils are massive sources of omega-6 fatty acids, the omega-6 being about 90% linoleic acid (LA), and the fact that excess LA consumption drives a pro-oxidative, pro-inflammatory, toxic, and nutrient-deficient biological milieu, we will submit that this is by far and away the single greatest cause of overweight and chronic disease.

We have observed that the Maasai tribe of Kenya and Tanzania, with an ancestral diet based almost entirely on raw milk, meat, and blood from the cattle they herd, have the greatest saturated animal fat consumption ever analyzed, at approximately 40% to 46% of total calories, and yet have little or no heart disease. They also consume a very high-fat diet, with about 66% of calories coming from animal fat, yet they are exceedingly lean and fit, with an average BMI in males and females of 19.4 in 1989. Historically, the Kenyans, which are close relatives of the Maasai, have been shown to be virtually free of hypertension and diabetes.

The Tokelau Island Migrant Studies completed by Wessen (1992) confirmed that the Tokelauans have the greatest saturated fat consumption in the world. However, in this case, their saturated fat is derived from the tropical oil of the coconut. The Tokelauans were confirmed to consume a diet based almost exclusively on coconut, fish, starchy tubers, and fruit, the latter being mostly breadfruit. About 56% of Tokelauans' calories came from fat, of which coconut oil accounted for some 80%. Coconut oil is about 91 to 94.5% saturated fat; thus, the diet is approximately 50% saturated fat, which appears to be the highest documented saturated fat intake in the world. Yet, studies in 1982 found that none of the men aged 40 to 69 years of age had any previous heart attacks. Furthermore, diabetes and obesity were practically unknown.

Virtually all known chronic diseases have risen

in direct correlation to processed food consumption. The "proxy markers" of processed foods, that is, the most easily tracked "markers" of processed foods, are primarily seed oils and sugars.[4] Sugar, however, is toxic only when processed and consumed in excessively large quantities.[445][446]

In contrast, seed oils begin to induce toxicity at very low levels of consumption, and this metabolic toxicity progressively rises as their consumption increases. In Chapters 4 and 5, we'll examine in more detail how seed oils and increasing omega-6 LA consumption drive massive destruction at the cellular level – and we are comprised of a massive collection of cells – which leads to a plethora of chronic diseases and premature death.

Seed oils are poisons to the vascular system, liver, central nervous system, and retina (retinal pigment epithelium) of the eye. Indeed, seed oils are poisons to every cell of the body through powerfully pro-oxidative, pro-inflammatory, toxic, and nutrient-deficient pathways, which synergistically result in widespread destruction.

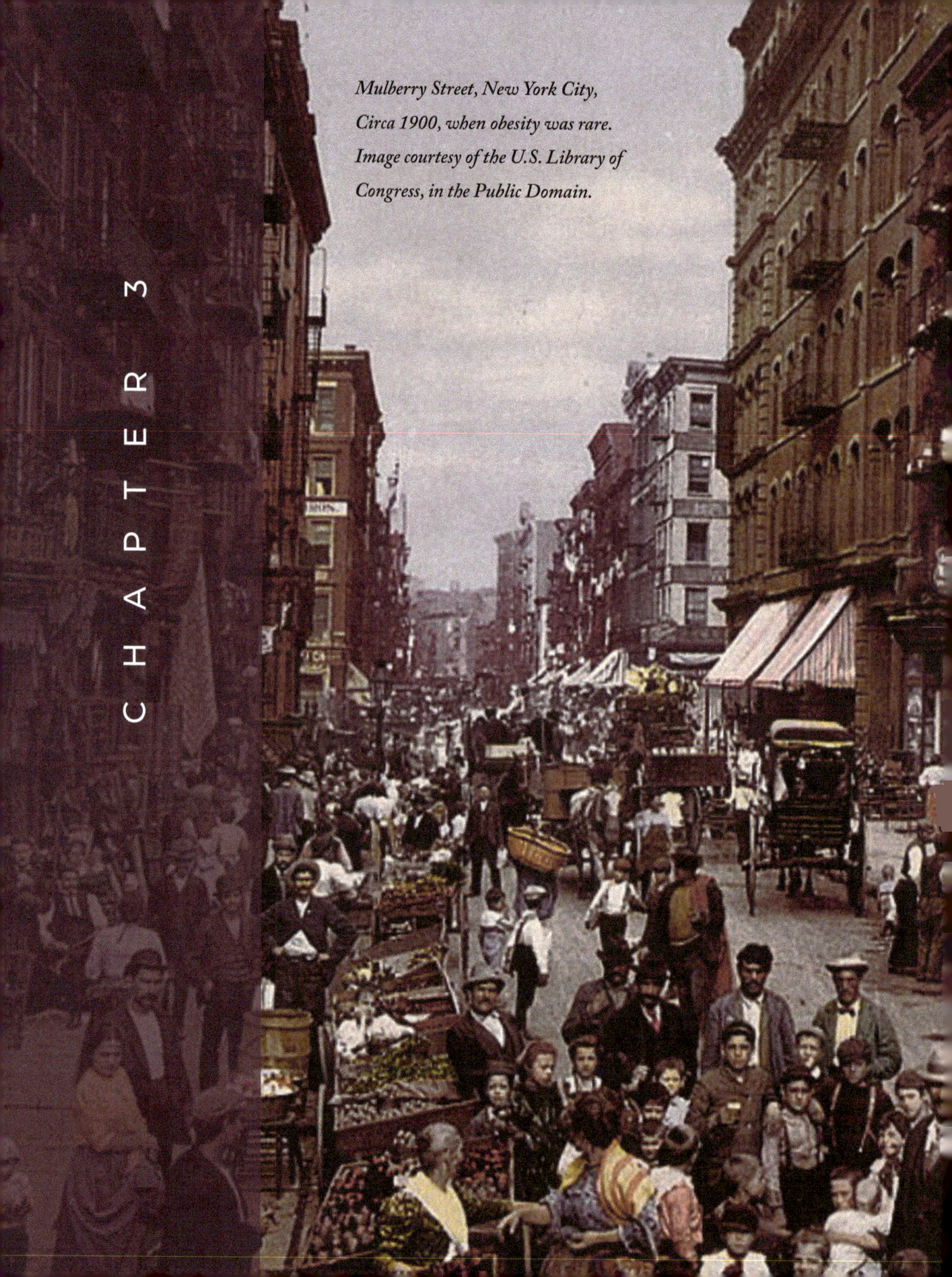

CHAPTER 3

Mulberry Street, New York City, Circa 1900, when obesity was rare. Image courtesy of the U.S. Library of Congress, in the Public Domain.

CHAPTER 3

MORE ON PROCESSED FOODS AND SEED OIL DANGERS

"Whenever I meditate on a disease, I never think of finding a remedy for it, but rather a means of preventing it."[447]

— LOUIS PASTEUR

ANCESTRAL HEALTH
FOUNDATION

CHAPTER 3

EPIDEMICS OF OBESITY, DIABETES, METABOLIC SYNDROME, ALZHEIMER'S DISEASE, AUTOIMMUNE DISEASES, MACULAR DEGENERATION, AND MORE – ALL ALIGNED WITH SEED OIL CONSUMPTION

It wasn't just CHD, heart attacks, and cancers that were once rare and which elevated exponentially with processed foods and seed oil consumption. Unquestionably, almost every chronic disease known to man today appears to have been either markedly unusual, rare, or virtually unknown, until about the turn of the 20th century. Of course, most all chronic diseases also are either rare or virtually unknown among hunter-gatherers who do not consume processed foods and seed oils.

OBESITY IS LARGELY A RESULT OF THE INTRODUCTION OF SEED OILS

British physician and nutrition researcher H.C. Trowell, MD, who completed numerous anthropological medical and nutrition studies in Kenya and Uganda (from 1929 to 1958) wrote in his 1981 book *Western Diseases*, "Obesity emerges as a new disease, rare in peasant agriculturists, but common in modern society...hunter-gatherers ate 'primitive food' and remained slim; modern man eats 'super-market food' and often gets fat."[448] As we will see, Trowell's observation and statement, based on a lifetime's worth of work, is not only profound but empirically obvious. No matter where you look, this simple truth rings true.

Researcher Scott Alan Carson analyzed a mountain of data gathered from late 19th and early 20th century U.S. prisoners in Texas and Nebraska, where both the height and weight of American men, ages 18 to 80, were documented upon incarceration. Carson found that in a several decade period around the year 1900, only 1.2% of men met the current definition of obesity, which is a BMI (body mass index) of greater than or equal to 30.[449,450]

The NHANES studies show that the combined total for both obesity (BMI ≥ 30) and extreme obesity (BMI ≥ 40) was 13.4% in 1960-1962, 15.0% in 1976-1980, 23.2% in 1988-1994, 30.9% in 1999-2000, 36.1% in 2009-2010,[451] 39.8% in

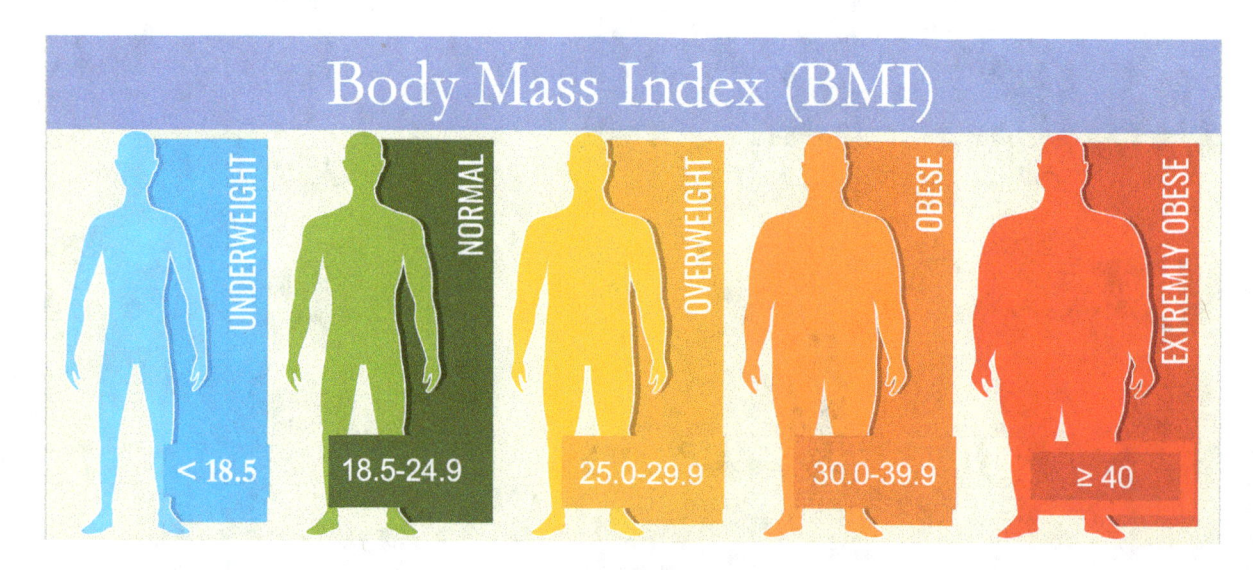

Body Mass Index (BMI)

UNDERWEIGHT	NORMAL	OVERWEIGHT	OBESE	EXTREMELY OBESE
< 18.5	18.5-24.9	25.0-29.9	30.0-39.9	≥ 40

114

— MORE ON PROCESSED FOODS AND SEED OIL DANGERS —

Body Mass Index (BMI)

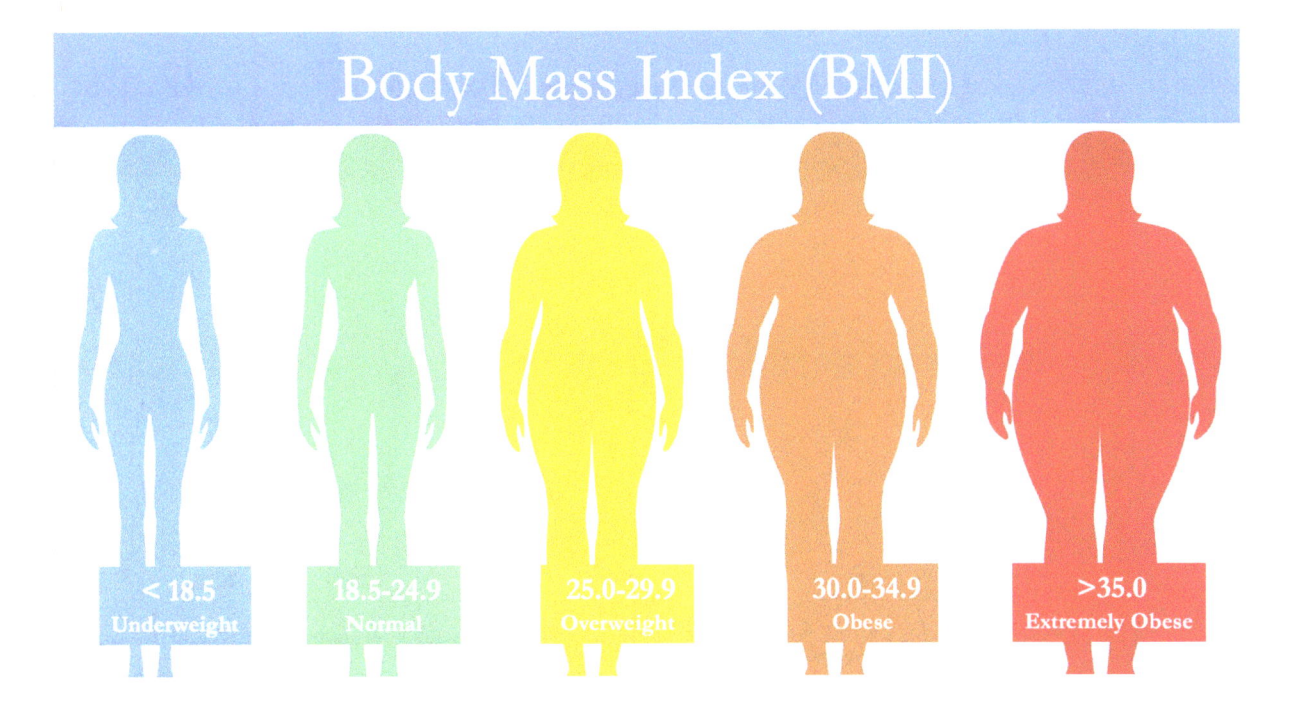

< 18.5	18.5-24.9	25.0-29.9	30.0-34.9	>35.0
Underweight	Normal	Overweight	Obese	Extremely Obese

2015-2016,[452] and 42.5% in 2018.[453] And while we Americans often look back at our recent ancestors of 1960 and marvel at how lean they were, obesity that year was 13% and had already risen 11-fold since approximately 1900.

By 2018, with 42.5% of Americans over the age of 20 being obese and another 31.1% overweight (BMI 25.0-29.9), the most recent total for adult Americans who are either overweight or obese is 73.6% (see graph on page 116).[453] Projected obesity for adults in the U.S. is 48.9% by 2030, with nearly one in four (24.2%) adults having severe obesity.[454]

Based on "WHO (World Health Organization) Expert Consultation" and further consensus, between 2004 and 2014, leaders agreed to adjust the cut points for the categories of overweight and obesity in Asians, to 23-27.4 kg/m² and ≥ 27.5 kg/m², respectively, as compared to the remainder of the world, which defines overweight as 25.9 kg/m² and obese as ≥30 kg/m².[455] [456]

BODY MASS INDEX (BMI) INCREASING SINCE THE 19TH CENTURY IN ALL AGE GROUPS!

The Centers for Disease Control (CDC) of the United States has propagated the official view that the epidemic of obesity began suddenly, beginning in the 1980s or 1990s.[457] This view has been disseminated by numerous diet 'authorities and even the diet "dictocrats" of major institutions, many tying it to the Dietary Guidelines for Americans of 1980, which promulgated low-fat dietary advice.[458] Whether intentional or not, this view is not only inaccurate, it is misleading.

John Komlos, Professor Emeritus of Economics, University of Munich, and Marek Brabek, Statistician for the NIH, in a review article published at VoxEU.org regarding the "Evolution of BMI values of US adults: 1882-1986," wrote the following:

CHAPTER 3

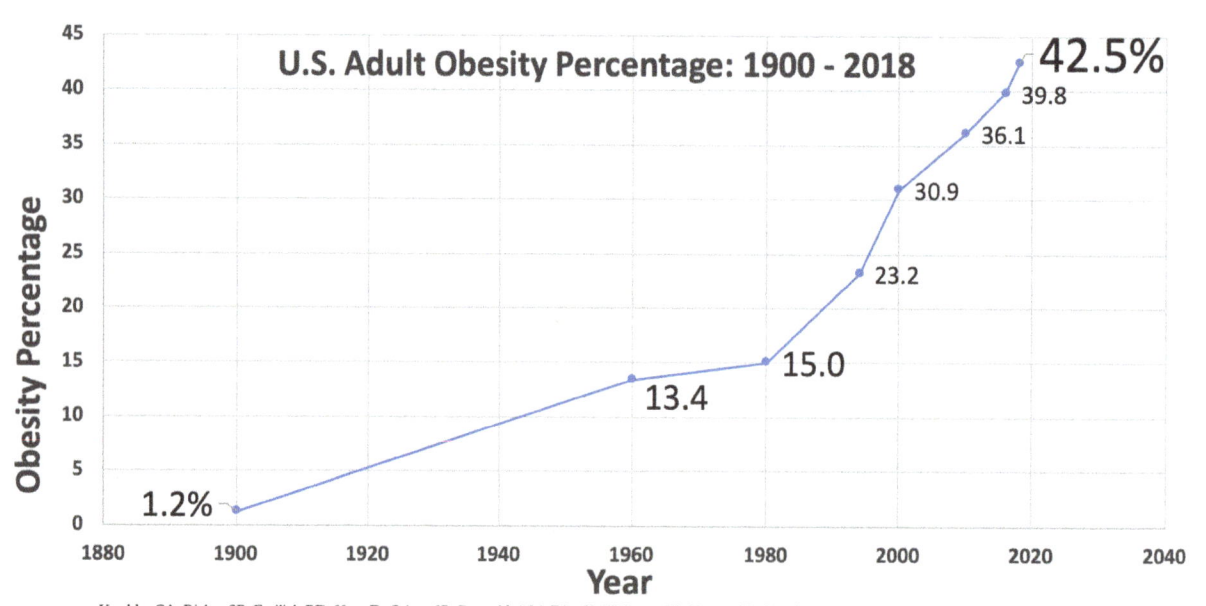

U.S. Adult Obesity Percentage: 1900 - 2018

- 1900: 1.2%
- 1960: 13.4
- 1980: 15.0
- ~1994: 23.2
- 2000: 30.9
- 2010: 36.1
- ~2015: 39.8
- 2018: 42.5%

Knobbe CA, Richer SP, Freilich BD, Kent D, Cripps JR, Reynolds TM, Dito JJ, Walgama JP, Hunter JD, Henderson T, Stojanoska M, Barry JT, Kiwara AL, Sommer R, Ross RD, Kaushal S, Luff AK. Westernized Diet, Omega-6 Rich Vegetable Oils, and Nutrient-Deficient Diets: Epidemiologic Evidence and Pathophysiologic Mechanisms for Age-Related Macular Degeneration and Associated Chronic Diseases. Manuscript submitted for publication. University of Texas Southwestern Medical Center, Dallas, U.S., 2022. © C. Knobbe, 2022. Ancestral Health Foundation.

"There is ample historical evidence that the roots of the obesity pandemic do reach much further back in time than is commonly asserted. For the 19th century, we have samples from the West Point Military Academy revealing that by today's standards BMI values were amazingly low: 19-year-old white cadets had an average BMI value of 20.5, i.e., about the 18th percentile of today's standards. About 90% of the cadets were below today's median reference value. In addition, these data indicate that there was very little change in weights in the 19th century.

However, another sample from The Citadel Military Academy in Charleston, SC indicates that a true surge in BMI values took place among those born after the First World War. Note that 18-year-old men increased by some 13 kilograms (28.5 pounds) during the course of the 20th century, but half of that increase took place among those born before World War II. Hence, this data indicates that a considerable increase in weight had already taken place by the time the first national survey was taken in 1959-1962 (John Komlos, Marek Brabec © VoxEU.org)."[459]

At this point, we must ask ourselves what is so ubiquitous in our food supply that has caused our prevalence of obesity to elevate 35-fold, from 1.2% in the year 1900 to 42.5% by 2018? This is a 3,400% increase in obesity in a period of approximately one century. And the average 18-year-old male today is 13 kg (28.5 pounds) heavier than our ancestors of just over a century ago. How can we explain this?

As one can see from the graph above, our obesity epidemic didn't begin in 1980 and, in fact, it didn't even begin in 1960. It began in the late 19th century or early 20th century, as seed oils and their

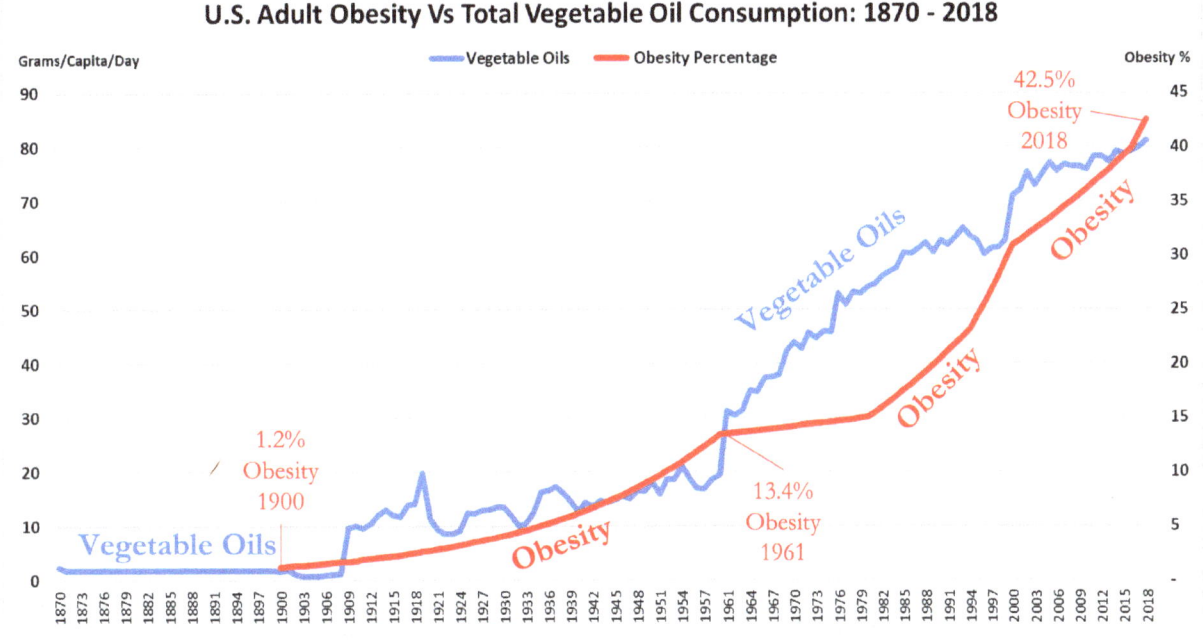

U.S. Adult Obesity Vs Total Vegetable Oil Consumption: 1870 - 2018

References: 1) Knobbe C, Stojanoska M. The 'Displacing Foods of Modern Commerce' Are the Primary and Proximate Cause of Age-Related Macular Degeneration: A Unifying Singular Hypothesis. 2) Obesity Statistics: See references herein. © C. Knobbe, 2022. Ancestral Health Foundation.

derivatives – Crisco and margarines, i.e., industrially produced trans fats – entered the food supply, gained market share, and gradually displaced natural animal fats.

If we observe the increase in seed oil consumption in the U.S. in the graph above, it shows that seed oil consumption was about 2 grams per day in 1900, about half of which was olive oil, and that consumption gradually and steadily elevated to 80 g per day by 2018.[4] Furthermore, as is evident from any reliable data, seed oil consumption in the U.S. has continued an unmitigated ascent since 1909, with the Knoema database revealing that seed oil consumption, for example, was 70g/day (639 cal/day) in 2000 and elevated to 80 g/day (710 cal/day) by 2018.[124]

The FAO Food Balance Sheets confirm that the U.S. has the highest consumption of seed oils on a per capita basis of any country in the world.[124] Data from the FAO shows seed oil consumption at 80g/day even earlier, by 2010, in the U.S.[4] In 2010, total caloric consumption was 2,501 cal/person/day,[460] and with seed oil consumption at 80g/day (720 cal), this indicates that seed oils accounted for 29% of calories. That's correct, nearly one-third of calories in the U.S. in recent years are from seed oils. However, seed oil consumption in the U.S. in the year 1865 would have been exactly zero.

In the next graph on page 118, we observe seed oil and sugar consumption versus obesity in the U.S. between 1822 and 2018, with sugar data provided by nutrition researcher Stephan Guyenet, PhD and his colleague, Jeremy Landen, and vegetable oil consumption provided by myself and colleague nutrition researcher, Marija Stojanoska, MSc (Skopje, Macedonia).[4] Note that there is a fairly strong correlation in this data between obesity and vegetable oil consumption, but a fairly poor correlation with sugar consumption.

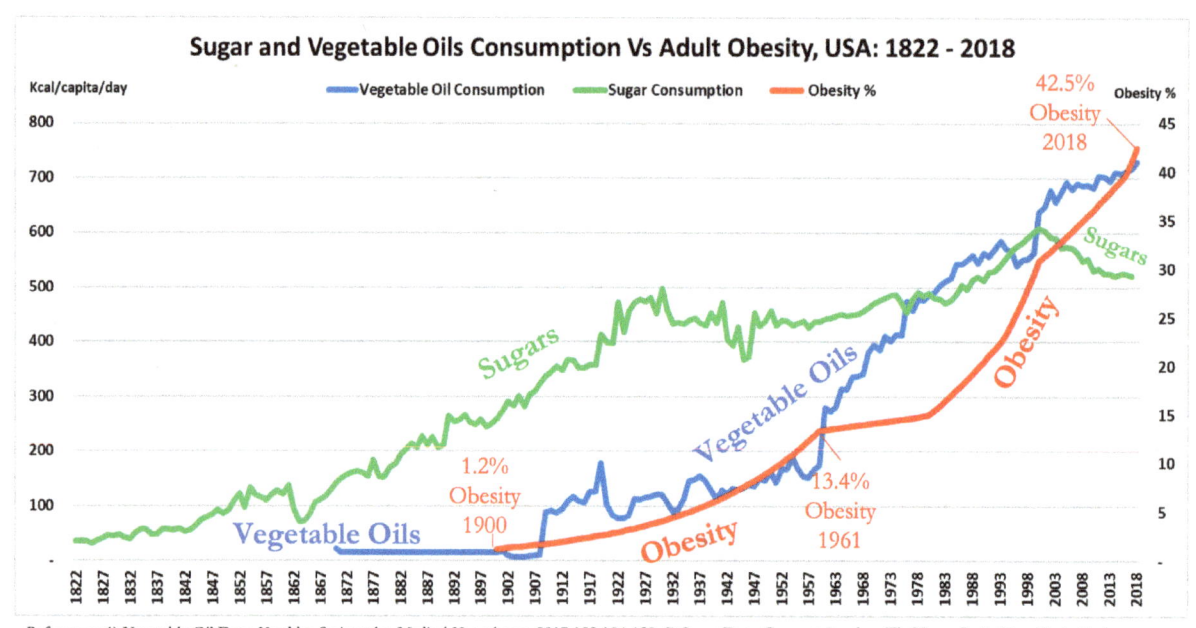

Sugar and Vegetable Oils Consumption Vs Adult Obesity, USA: 1822 - 2018

References: 1) Vegetable Oil Data: Knobbe, Stojanoska. Medical Hypotheses: 2017;109:184-198 2) Sugar Data: Guyenet, Landen. *The Hungry Brain*. New York, Flatiron Books, 2017. 3) Obesity statistics, see references herein. U.S. © C. Knobbe, 2022. Ancestral Health Foundation. All rights reserved.

For example, sugar consumption had already exceeded 200 cal/day by the early 1880s and more than 300 cal/day just after 1907, but obesity was still rare (around 1%). Of course, up until that time, seed oil consumption was still just 1-2 grams/day. It would be hard to tease apart causation if we only had data in the early to late 20th century as both sugars and seed oils increased while obesity increased. However, we then observe an almost vertical ascent in obesity after 1999, precisely while sugar declines! Seed oil consumption during this time, however, continued to climb after 1999, quite precisely in correlation to increasing obesity prevalence (see the graph above, "Sugar and Vegetable Oils Consumption Vs Adult Obesity, USA: 1822 – 2018").

Because this question arises recurrently, we will review once again the definition of "sugar consumption" as used throughout this book. The data (since 1961) are derived directly from the FAO and are corrected for post-production losses using the USDA's current loss estimate of 28.8%. The FAO and U.S. FDA definition of "added sugars" is as follows: "Added sugars include sugars added during the processing of foods (such as sucrose and dextrose), foods packaged as sweeteners (such as table sugar), sugars from syrups and honey, and sugars from concentrated fruit or vegetable juices. They do not include naturally occurring sugars that are found in milk, fruits, and vegetables... For most Americans, the main sources of added sugars are sugar-sweetened beverages, baked goods, desserts, and sweets."[358] [359] Data before 1961 are derived from The Department of Commerce and the USDA (continuous yearly sweetener sales from 1822 to 2005), as published by Stephan Guyenet, and are also corrected for losses.[116]

In a slightly different set of data from Knoema, total sugar and total carbohydrate consumption (reviewed separately) has decreased since 2004, but seed oil consumption has continued to increase unabated, perhaps under the promotion of seed oils as 'heart healthy' by numerous authoritative institutions, including the American Heart Association,[461] Harvard School of Public Health,[462] Tufts University Department of Nutrition,[463] and Mayo Clinic Department of Nutrition.[464] In fact, a recent boldly headlined article from Harvard Health Publishing, Harvard Medical School, asserts, "No Need to Avoid Healthy Omega-6 Fats."[462]

In the graph below, "Vegetable Oil and Sugar Consumption Vs Adult Obesity, USA – 1999-2018," we've focused in on the period of time between 1999 and 2018. Notice that, since 2004, sugar consumption almost steadily fell from 660 calories per day (165g) in 2004 to 589 calories per day (147g) in 2018, while obesity very steadily increased during that same interval from about 33% to 42.5%, thus rising 29% in this 14-year period alone. However, note that during this same interval of time, seed oil consumption increased from 665 calories per day (73.9g) to 719 calories per day (79.9g). For those who wish to blame obesity on sugar consumption, a fourteen-year period of substantial sugar decline in the U.S. while obesity escalates 29% presents an unwieldy paradox.

In the graph on page 120, we've plotted total vegetable oil and total sugar consumption (refined sugars, caloric sweeteners, high-fructose corn syrup, and other added sweeteners) versus severe obesity (BMI ≥ 40). Once again, notice that sugar consumption fell between 2004 and 2018 (same data, of course), while severe obesity elevated from 4.7% to 9.2% (approximately 2-fold) between 1999 and 2018. Yet again, during this interval of time, we see sugars falling by 8%, vegetable oil consumption up 30%, and severe obesity approximately doubling.

With this data, defending the hypothesis that sugar is the primary driver of obesity (and diabetes, Alzheimer's disease, or other chronic diseases still on the rise) becomes more and more difficult.

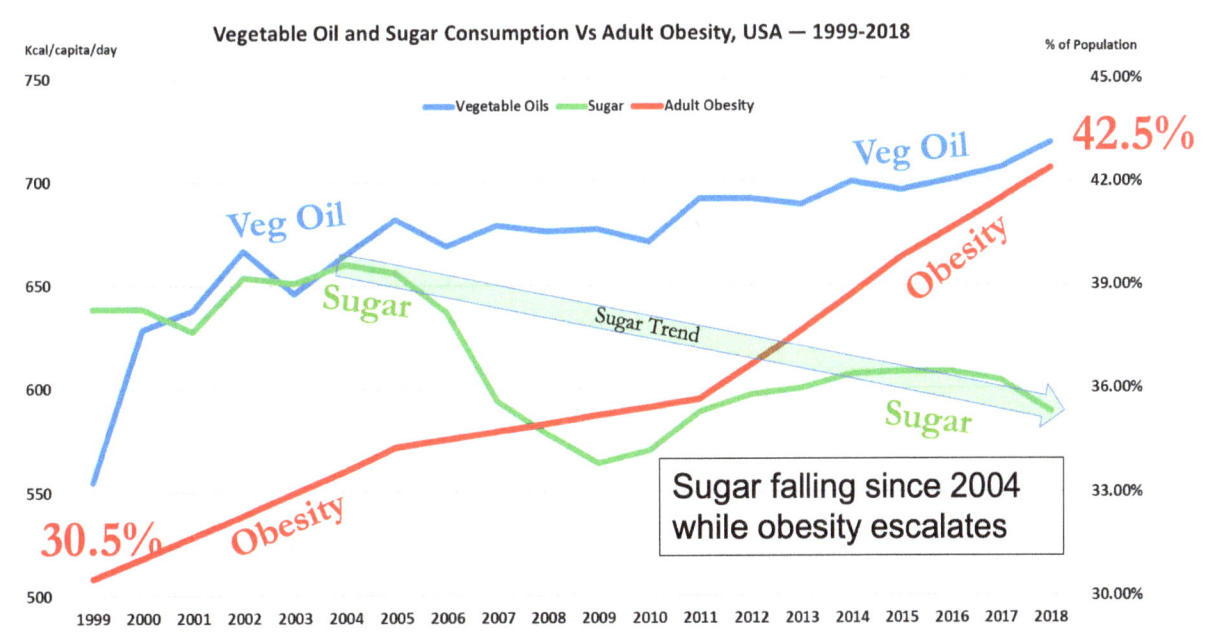

Vegetable Oil and Sugar Consumption Vs Adult Obesity, USA — 1999-2018

References: 1) Food and Agriculture Organization (FAO) FBS, Retrieved 2 Sep 2021. Available: http://knoema.com/FAOFBS2017/food-balance-sheets 2) Obesity statistics: see references herein. U.S. © C. Knobbe, 2022. Ancestral Health Foundation. All rights reserved.

CHAPTER 3

Vegetable Oil and Sugar Consumption Vs Adult Severe Obesity, USA — 1999-2018

Kcal/capita/day — % of Population

- Vegetable Oils
- Sugar
- Adult Severe Obesity

Veg Oil
Veg Oil — 9.2%
Severe Obesity
Sugars: Down 8%
Sugar Trend
Sugar
Sugar
Veg Oils: Up 30%
Severe Obesity
4.7%
Severe Obesity: Up 96% (~2-fold)

References: 1) Food and Agriculture Organization (FAO) FBS, Retrieved 2 Sep 2021. Available: http://knoema.com/FAOFBS2017/food-balance-sheets 2) Obesity statistics: see references herein. U.S. © C. Knobbe, 2022. Ancestral Health Foundation. All rights reserved.

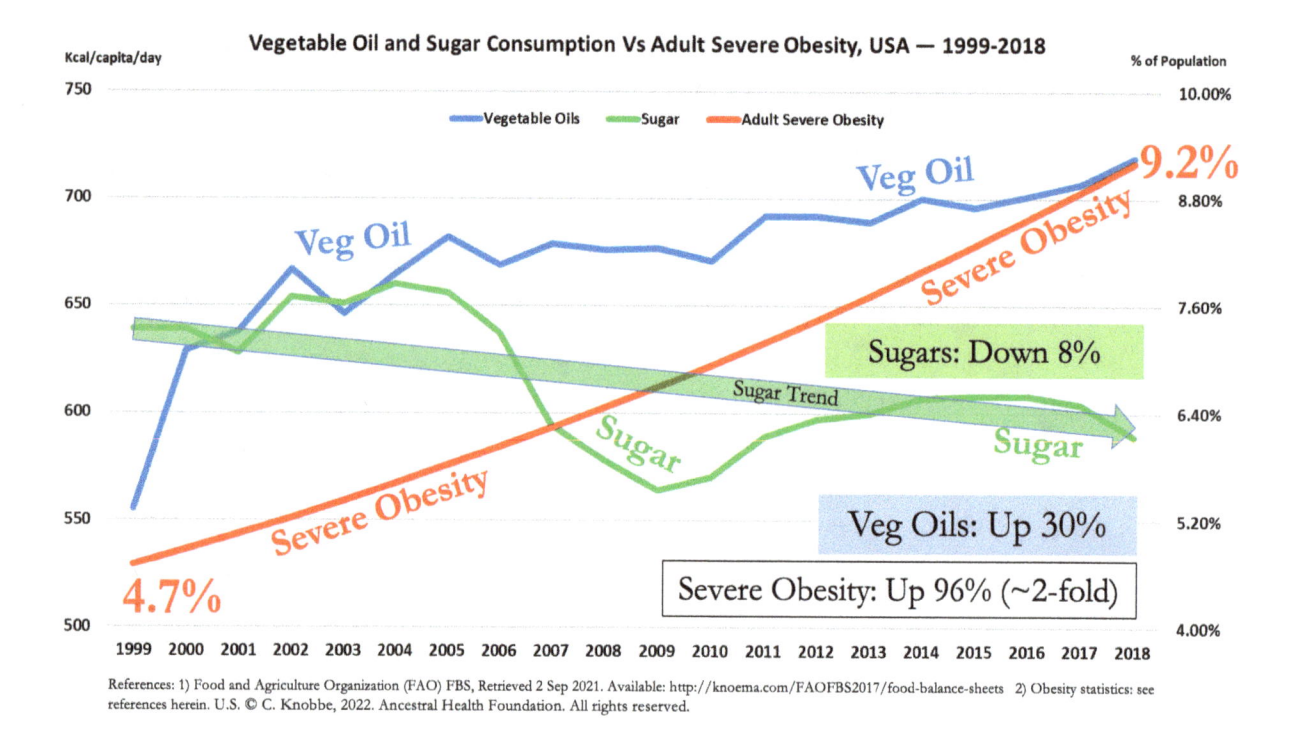

Those that would defend the 'sugar is the villain' hypothesis will need to explain why sugar could be on the decline while overweight, obesity, severe obesity, type 2 diabetes, and metabolic syndrome (we'll cover all of these subsequently) all continue to rise, at least since 2004.

But others will defend the hypothesis that sugar consumption may be declining while the 'dreaded carbs' (carbohydrates) are still the problem. Hence, as I have mentioned in many recent presentations, the pendulum has swung, and instead of a nation obsessed with low-fat, as we were in the 1980s and 1990s, we've now become obsessed with being "low-carb." But are carbs per se really the problem?

In recent decades, there has been an extraordinary resurgence of "low-carb" dietary advice, which was first popularized by Robert Atkins in the early 1970s, with his book *Dr. Atkins' Diet Revolution*.[465] In a recent PubMed (PubMed.org) search for papers including the term "low-carbohydrate," there were 3,489 results, many of which are papers on low carbohydrate or ketogenic diets for weight loss, metabolic disease, seizure disorders, and much more. The enormous bulk of those have been published since 2004.

But, we must ask, are macronutrient ratios (ratios of carbs to protein to fats) even all that important? Let's examine this further, beginning with the U.S. (while other examples will be presented subsequently throughout this book). As you will see, and as has been shown in numerous population studies, macronutrient ratios vary from extreme low-fat to high-fat (or alternatively, low-carbohydrate to high-carbohydrate), and populations are still supremely healthy as long as the foods are ancestral (unprocessed) in nature.

In most of the countrywide data that we've observed, if sugar increases, carbohydrates increase, and if sugar declines, carbohydrates decline. Not always, but usually. The great investigators at Our World In Data (OurWorldInData.org) analyzed the FAO (FAOSTAT) database and completed painstaking calculations to determine the total protein, carbohydrate, and fat consumption in the U.S., for the years 1961 through 2013.[466] We've downloaded their data and plotted total carbohydrate and fat consumption against obesity prevalence as a percentage of adults in the U.S. (graph below, "U.S. Macronutrients Vs. Obesity: 1961-2013").

One can see that calories from fat almost steadily increased from 1961 through 2004, before leveling off, and carbohydrate consumption rather steadily increased from 1961 until a peak in 1997 at 1941 calories per day (data for total food availability), and then began to decline until the end of available data in 2013, at 1790 calories. Because this data is for total carbohydrates, we're counting native, traditional ancestral carbohydrates, such as organic sweet potatoes, white potatoes, whole grain rice, whole grain wheat, etc., the same as refined "junky" carbohydrates, such as the "carbs" in potato chips, french fries, cakes, cookies, candies, and sugar-sweetened beverages.

And because this data is also for total fat, we're counting excellent sources of fat, such as pasture-raised, 100% grass-fed meats, pasture-raised, ancestrally-fed chicken eggs, grass-fed butter, etc., the same as the worst fats, which would be refined seed oils, including soybean, corn, canola, cottonseed, rapeseed, grapeseed, sunflower, safflower, and rice bran oils, as well as the industrially produced trans fats, like the original Crisco and many trans-fat laden types of margarine. In this graph, no distinctions on carbohydrate or fat quality or derivation are made.

Knowing this, the graph ("U.S. Macronutrients Vs. Obesity: 1961-2013") below doesn't separate out the dangerous, nutrient-deficient foods from

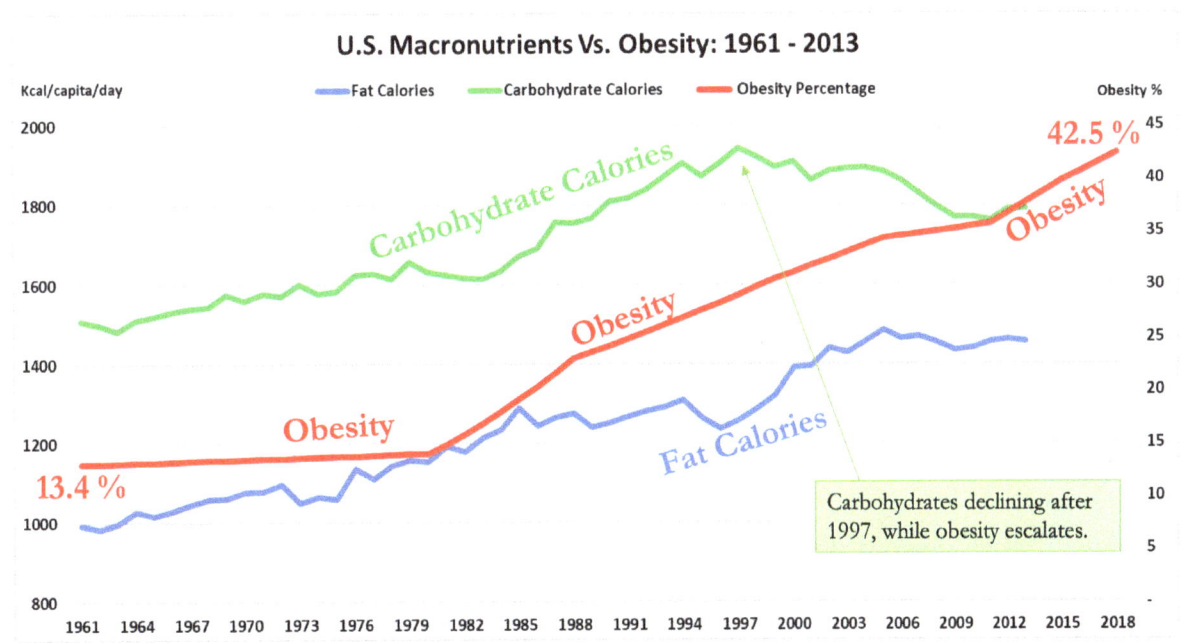

U.S. Macronutrients Vs. Obesity: 1961 - 2013

Carbohydrates declining after 1997, while obesity escalates.

References: 1) UN Food and Agriculture Organization FAOSTAT food balance sheets: http://www.fao.org/faostat/en/#home. 2) Calculation of Energy Content of Foods, http://www.fao.org/docrep/006/Y5022E/y5022e04.htm. 3) Daily Caloric Supply Derived from Carbohydrates, Protein, and Fat, United States, 1961 to 2013. Our World In Data.org. Retrieved: https://ourworldindata.org/grapher/daily-caloric-supply-derived-from-carbohydrates-protein-and-fat?country=~USA. U.S. © C. Knobbe, 2022. Ancestral Health Foundation. All rights reserved.

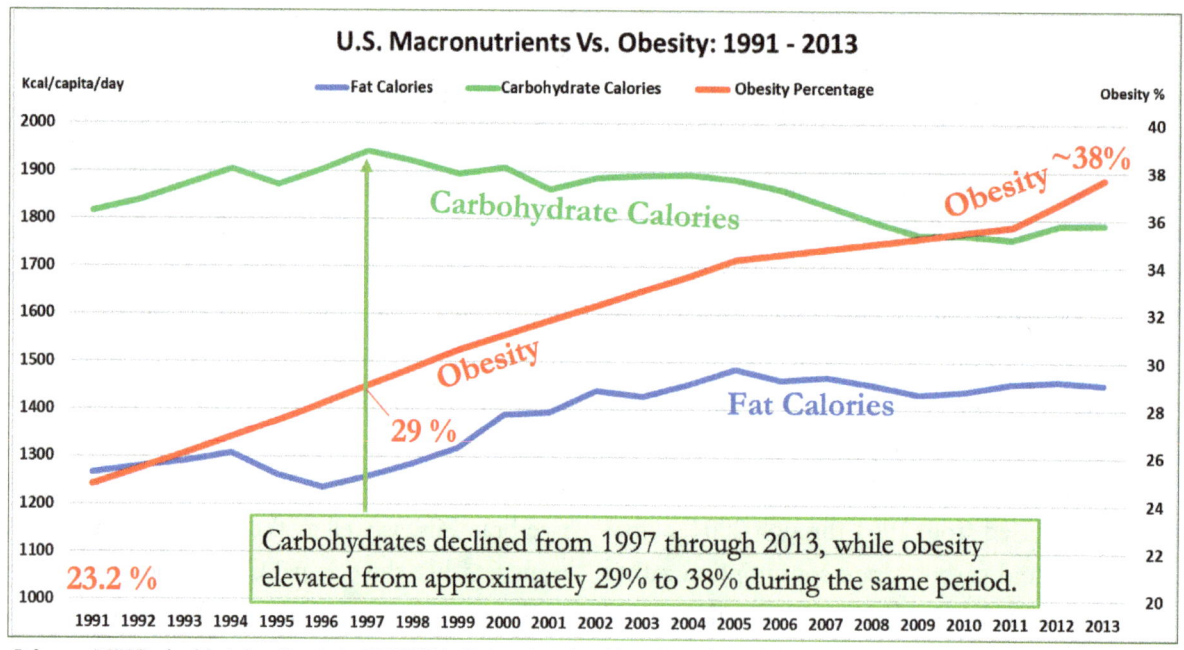

CHAPTER 3

U.S. Macronutrients Vs. Obesity: 1991 - 2013

Carbohydrates declined from 1997 through 2013, while obesity elevated from approximately 29% to 38% during the same period.

References: 1) UN Food and Agriculture Organization FAOSTAT food balance sheets: http://www.fao.org/faostat/en/#home. 2) Calculation of Energy Content of Foods, http://www.fao.org/docrep/006/Y5022E/y5022e04.htm. 3) Daily Caloric Supply Derived from Carbohydrates, Protein, and Fat, United States, 1961 to 2013. Our World In Data.org. Retrieved: https://ourworldindata.org/grapher/daily-caloric-supply-derived-from-carbohydrates-protein-and-fat?country=~USA. U.S. © C. Knobbe, 2022. Ancestral Health Foundation. All rights reserved.

the healthy whole food options. So from this, we mostly just see that, up until 1997, food consumption is rising overall, which could in and of itself account for the obesity epidemic. However, we must ask, why would everyone, especially over just a few decades of time, begin eating up to a couple hundred or more calories per day? But take notice of this: Beginning in 1997, carbohydrate consumption began to decline, right along with sugar, but obesity (and metabolic syndrome, diabetes, etc.) continued to rise, in fact, even faster!

In the graph above ("U.S. Macronutrients Vs. Obesity: 1991-2013"), we've focused in on the last three decades, which clearly shows that carbohydrate consumption peaked at 1,941 calories/day in 1997 and thereafter declined, down to 1,790 calories by 2013, which is a 7.8% decline in carbohydrate consumption during that period. During the same time span, obesity elevated from about 29% in 1997 to about 38% by 2013. Thus, obesity increased just during this 16-year interval of time by an astonishing 31%.

We've observed in the U.S. that sugar consumption has been on the decline since 2004 and carbohydrate consumption has declined since 1997, and yet, we continue to see marked increases in overweight, obesity, type 2 diabetes, and metabolic syndrome (evidence for the latter two presented subsequently). However, what we observe is that seed oil consumption continues to climb while healthy animal meats and fats continue to decline. This is yet another example of the "displacement" of a healthy, nutrient-dense, non-toxic food – animal meats and fats – for a dangerously refined, processed toxic food – seed oils.

Obesity has often been attributed to excess energy consumption, i.e., the energy balance hypothesis. In support of this hypothesis, as seen in the graph below, "U.S. Total Caloric and Macronutrient Availability (1909-2010)," we observe a substantial increase in calories from about 1975 until about 2002, while obesity markedly elevates. However, we then observe that energy consumption declines after 2002, at the same time that obesity continues to rise dramatically.

Thus, we have observed that in recent years, obesity and diabetes (see next section below) continue to steeply increase in prevalence while calories, carbohydrates, and sugar all decline. But what continues to rise? Seed oils, of course.

Obesity, it should be understood, is not a disorder of being 'over-nourished,' as physicians often euphemistically label their overweight patients. It is a disorder, in part, of malnourishment, which may be better termed undernourishment. That is, people who are overweight are nearly always suffering from a lack of nutrients (vitamins and minerals).[467 468 469 470 471 472]

This has been documented in numerous studies. In fact, the lack of nutrients may be severe, which leads to hunger and more food consumption in a physiological attempt to secure the deficient nutrients. This may lead to extraordinary over-eating in terms of calories. However, when the food consumed continues to be lacking in the nutrients the body craves for optimal function, 'over-eating' will continue, often persistently, as the body attempts to correct the missing nutrients.

This is a vicious cycle and, in part, explains why we have a nation consuming approximately 10% more calories per day now than we did in 1980.[473] The substitution of vegetable oils for animal fats is a major aspect of this nutrient deficiency,[467] as this further contributes to vitamins A, D, and K2 deficiency and an inability for the body to properly utilize minerals, even if they're present. There are further mechanisms behind obesity, which we'll review in Chapter Five.

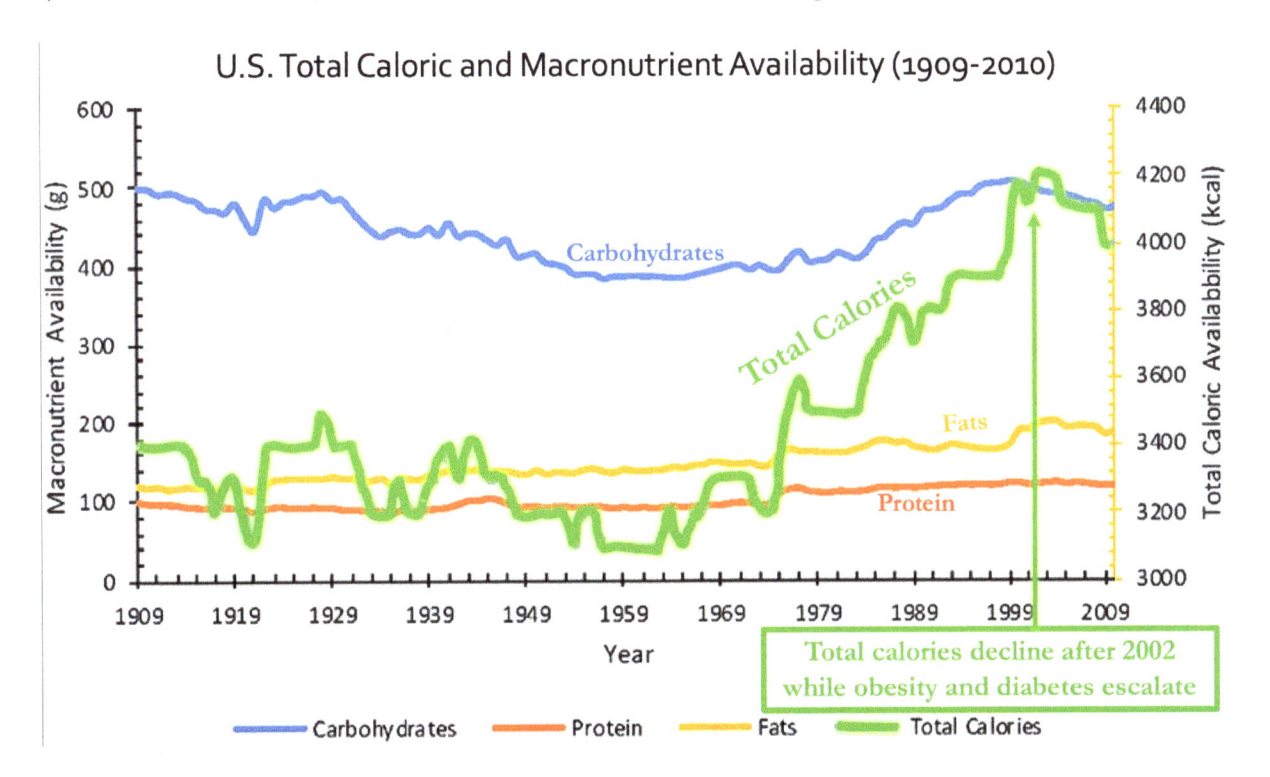

U.S. Total Caloric and Macronutrient Availability (1909-2010)

Total calories decline after 2002 while obesity and diabetes escalate

SEED OIL CONSUMPTION AND OBESITY IN THE WORLD, DEVELOPED AND DEVELOPING COUNTRIES, THE U.S. AND VIETNAM – CIRCA YEAR 2000

In the graph below, entitled "Seed Oil Consumption Per Capita & Obesity %: Year 2000," seed oil consumption for the United States, Vietnam, developed countries, developing countries, and the world was plotted for years 1991 to 2021 with obesity percentage (in parentheses) at the approximate year 2000.

One can see that the U.S., which has the highest seed oil consumption per capita in the world,[124] also has the highest prevalence of obesity in the world, if we consider only the OECD (developed) countries.[474] [475] Vietnam, which has the lowest obesity in the world,[476] at 0.2% prevalence in 2000,[477] has the 2nd lowest seed oil consumption of any country in the world.[124]

Given that the most recent data for obesity in developed and developing countries was only available for the late 1990s approximately, we plotted the closest year's obesity data for the year 2000 as follows: U.S. (36.1% obesity), Vietnam (0.2% obesity), and the world (8.7% obesity).[478] Obesity prevalence for representative developed and developing countries for the closest year to 2000 available (most in the late 1990s) averaged 13.1% and 8.4%, respectively, as graphed below.[479]

Thus, we see in descending order, from highest to lowest seed oil consumption: the U.S.A. at

Seed Oil Consumption Per Capita & Obesity %: Year 2000*
World, Developed Countries, Developing Countries, U.S. & Vietnam

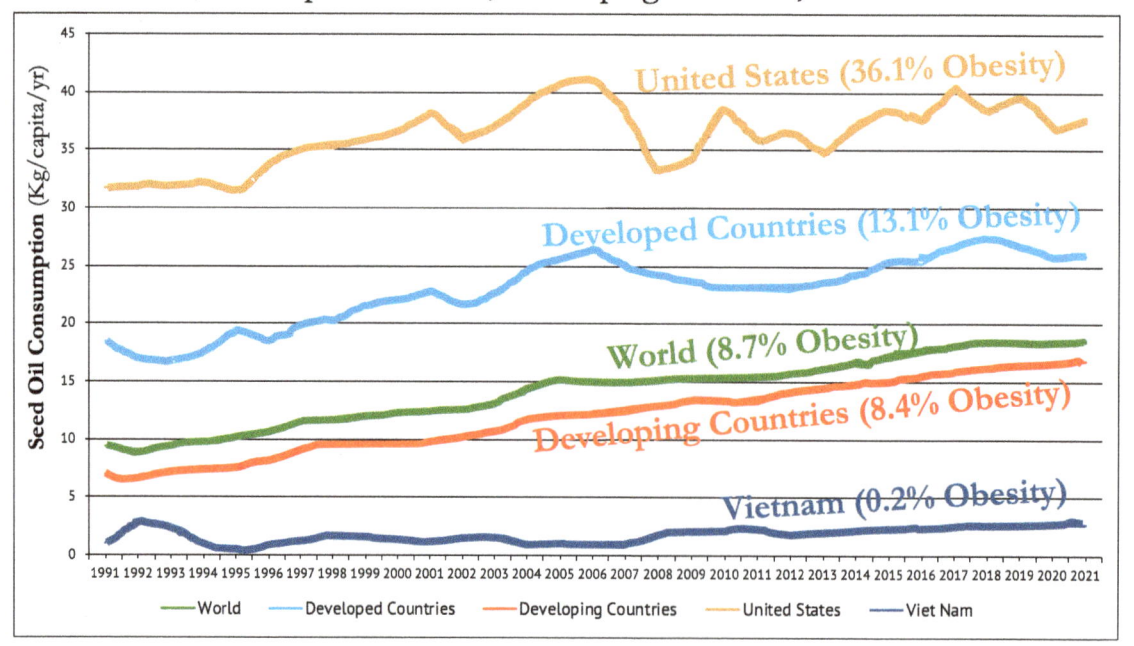

*Obesity Percentage for year 2000 for the World, U.S. and Vietnam, and closest year to 2000 available for Developed and Developing Countries. See references herein. Vegetable oils data: FAO Food Balance Sheets, Knoema. http://www.fao.org/faostat/en/#data/FBS. © C. Knobbe, Ancestral Health Foundation, 2022. All rights reserved.

36% obesity, developed countries at 13.1% obesity, the world at 8.7% obesity, developing countries at 8.4% obesity, and Vietnam at 0.2% obesity, all with obesity prevalence close to year 2000. In alignment with the hypothesis that seed oils are the primary driver of obesity, each of these categories successively runs from highest to lowest in seed oil consumption, broadly representing the entire world.

Obesity, we will assert, is not the cause of other westernized chronic diseases, such as hypertension, coronary heart disease, type 2 diabetes, stroke, etc., but rather, simply runs with these diseases because they're all caused by the same thing, namely, a westernized diet. And what is the single greatest contributor to obesity? Seed oils, as we have observed over and over.

TYPE 2 DIABETES IS A DISEASE ALMOST ENTIRELY OF SEED OIL CONSUMPTION – ESCALATING EVEN WHILE SUGAR DECREASES!

Diabetes has been recognized in antiquity through Egyptian manuscripts that date back to 1500 B.C.[480] However, it has also been confirmed that diabetes of any type was exceedingly rare before the 20th century.[481] One of the earliest clinical descriptions of diabetes was by Aretaeus, who practiced in Cappadocia, Turkey, around 120 AD. He wrote that the disease was "fortunately rare," and "short will be the life of the man in whom the disease is fully developed."[482]

In 1893, Sir William Osler published the First Edition of what would become a classic in the history of medicine, his 1130-page textbook, *The Principles and Practice of Medicine*.[483] Osler devoted ten pages to the subject of diabetes but confirmed that diabetes was an extremely rare disease. He wrote,

"In comparison with European countries diabetes is a rare disease in America. The last census [in 1890] gave only 2.8 per one hundred thousand of population, against a ratio of from five to nine in the former. In this region the incidence of the disease may be gathered from the fact that among thirty-five thousand patients under treatment at the Johns Hopkins Hospital and Dispensary there were only ten cases."[483 484]

By today's standards, this is an unthinkable rarity of the disorder, at just 2.8 per 100,000. This makes the population prevalence of diabetes in 1890 an extraordinarily low 0.0028%! The U.S. population in 1890 was just under 63 million people. At 0.0028% prevalence, there would have only been about 1,764 diabetics in the entire U.S.A, and perhaps nearly all of those would have been type 1 diabetics. Of course, against the backdrop of rarity of all chronic diseases in the 19th century, the rarity of diabetes was, just like coronary heart disease, normal for that time.

The U.S. National Health Interview Survey (NHIS), conducted for the first time in 1935-1936, determined that the prevalence of diabetes that year was 0.37%, which is an increase of 132-fold compared to the 1890 figure given by Osler.[485] In reference to 1890, diabetes continued to rise 325-fold to 0.91% by 1960, 1061-fold to 2.97% by 1991-93,[485] 2,482-fold to 6.95% by 2010,[486] 3,357-fold to 9.4% by 2015,[487] and 3,750-fold to 10.5% by 2020.[488]

However, in a separate analysis, the CDC's latest (2016) evidence confirms that total diabetes prevalence (both diagnosed and undiagnosed) was 34.1 million adults, which was 13.0% of the population.[489] Using the CDC's latest statistics, diabetes prevalence of 13.0% indicates a 4,643-fold increase in diabetes in the 126-year period between 1890 and 2016! (See the graph below.)

For the sake of completeness and for the purposes of an additional table and graph to be revealed subsequently, one analysis showed U.S. adult diabetes prevalence to be 7.7% in 1999-2000 and 13.3% in 2015-2016.[490]

For further historical perspective, it is astounding that there were approximately 1,764 diabetics in the entire U.S. in 1890 when the population was just under 63 million people. If those ratios of diabetics to total population had persisted, with a population of 323.1 million people in 2016 (an increase of 5.1-fold since 1890), there would have been just 9,047 people with diabetes. Instead, there was a total of 34.1 million people with diabetes in 2016, which is more than 34 million people with diabetes greater than expected had the 1890 prevalence persisted.

Of all diabetes, about 95% of cases today are of the type 2 diabetes mellitus (T2DM) type,[487] which was formerly referred to as "Adult-Onset Diabetes," however, the term has now fallen into disfavor since the unthinkable has occurred – yes, even our young children are developing T2DM, a possibility unfathomable just 30 years ago.[491]

Beyond the 34.1 million American adults already diagnosed with diabetes, another 88 million Americans aged 18 or older had prediabetes in 2018, which is 34.5% of all adults.[489] Prediabetes is based on abnormally high fasting glucose or Hemoglobin A1C levels, the latter of which is an accurate marker of average blood sugars over the previous 90 days.

Of those American adults with diabetes, 89.0% were overweight or had obesity (BMI 25.0 kg/m² or

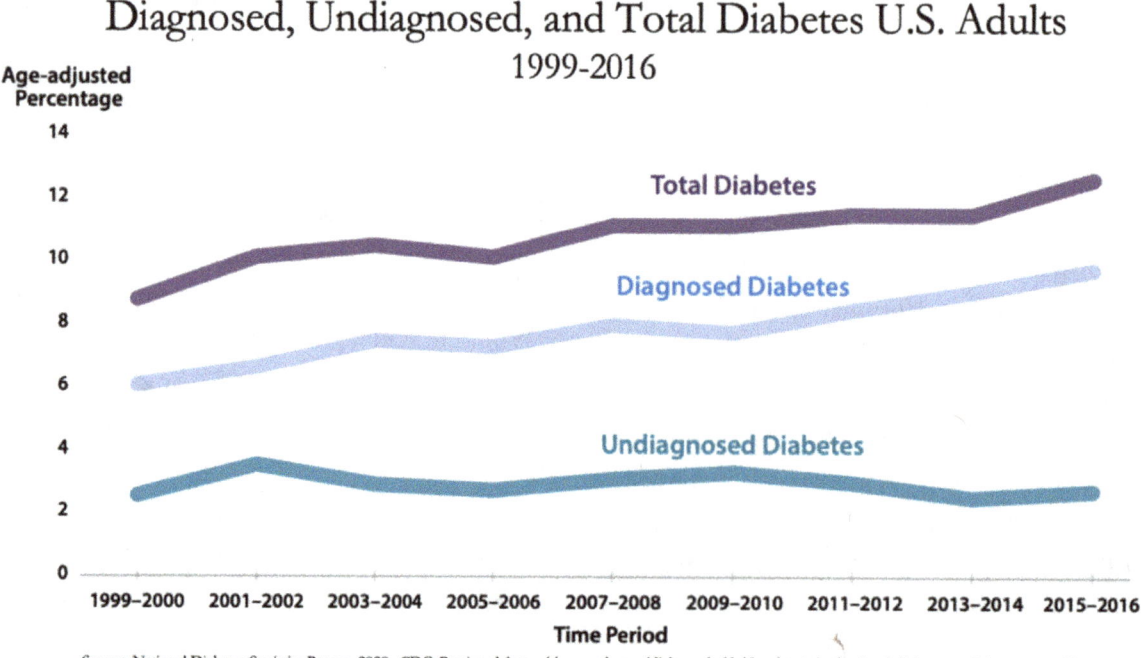

Diagnosed, Undiagnosed, and Total Diabetes U.S. Adults
1999-2016

Source: National Diabetes Statistics Report, 2020. CDC. Retrieved: https://www.cdc.gov/diabetes/pdfs/data/statistics/national-diabetes-statistics-report.pdf

higher), 27.6% were overweight (BMI 25.0 to 29.9), 45.8% were obese (BMI 30.0 or higher), and 15.5% had extreme obesity (BMI of 40.0 or higher).[489] 38.0% of adults with diabetes were physically inactive, 68.4% had high blood pressure, 21.6% were tobacco users, and 37.0% had chronic kidney disease.

With a 35-fold (3,400%) increase in diabetes just during the 80-year period between 1936 and 2016, which is nearly identical to the increase in obesity during this same approximate period, we should certainly expect allopathic medicine to indict something in the 'environment' for both conditions, of which the food supply should generally be the most important factor.

However, in this case, as to the cause of type 2 diabetes, the CDC indicts "insulin resistance" as the primary "cause" with "risk factors" including prediabetes, overweight, age 45 or older, family history, less than ideal physical activity, gestational diabetes, and being of various non-white races, for example, but not a single reference to diet as being causative.[492]

The NIH's National Institute of Diabetes and Digestive and Kidney Diseases attributes the cause of type 2 diabetes to "several factors, including lifestyle factors and genes," including being physically inactive, overweight, or obese, as well as having insulin resistance, described as "a condition in which muscle, liver, and fat cells do not use insulin well."[493] Again, however, there is not a single mention or indictment of processed foods, sugars, seed oils, or trans fats as causes of diabetes.

It is our assertion that type 2 diabetes is virtually entirely driven by processed food consumption, of which seed oils are by far the leading cause, perhaps even the sole cause. In the graph below ("Sugar and Vegetable Oil Consumption Vs Diabetes, USA: 1870-2016"), we've plotted data for total sugar consumption (which would include cane and beet sugar, high fructose corn syrup, corn syrup, other syrups, honey, and other added sugars

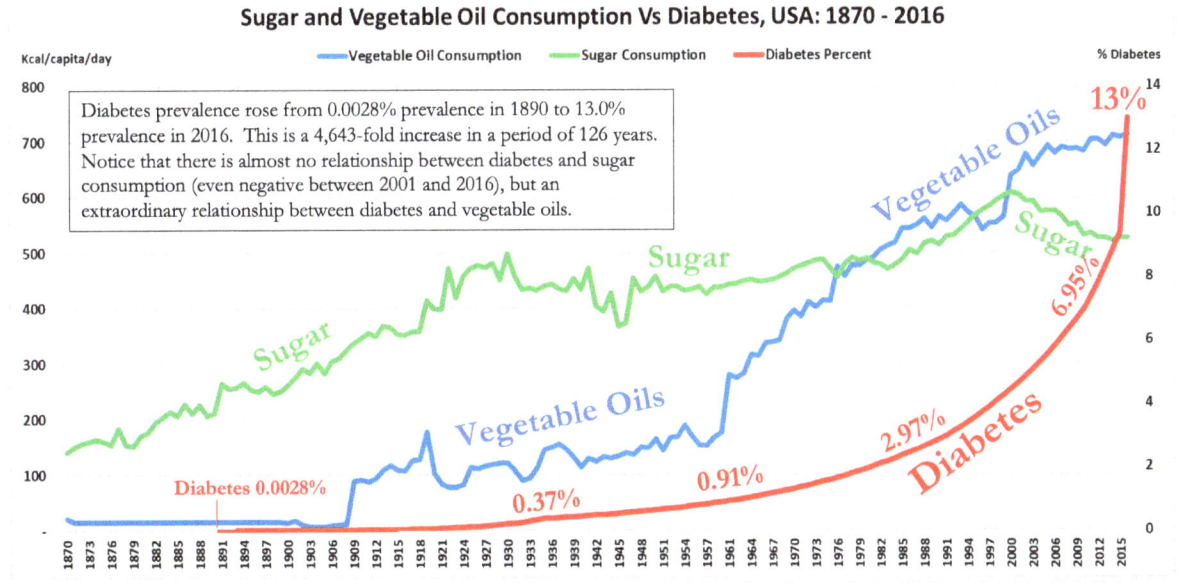

Sugar and Vegetable Oil Consumption Vs Diabetes, USA: 1870 - 2016

Diabetes prevalence rose from 0.0028% prevalence in 1890 to 13.0% prevalence in 2016. This is a 4,643-fold increase in a period of 126 years. Notice that there is almost no relationship between diabetes and sugar consumption (even negative between 2001 and 2016), but an extraordinary relationship between diabetes and vegetable oils.

References: 1) Vegetable Oil Data: Knobbe C, Stojanoska M. Medical Hypotheses: 2017;109:184-198 2) Sugar Data: Guyenet, Landen. *The Hungry Brain*. New York, Flatiron Books, 2017. 3) Diabetes statistics: See references herein. U.S. © C. Knobbe, 2022. Ancestral Health Foundation. All rights reserved.

to the diet, but never the naturally present sugars in fruit) and 'vegetable' (seed) oils, against adult diabetes prevalence in the U.S.[116,4]

Notice the extraordinary increase in diabetes percentage, from 0.0028% in 1890 to 0.37% in 1935, to 13.0% in 2016, which precisely parallels our marked increase in seed oils, but has almost no relation to sugar consumption.

In fact, there is even a negative correlation after about 2001, with sugar consumption falling and diabetes prevalence escalating severely. Note the steep ascent in diabetes prevalence over the past 15 years, particularly as seed oils have escalated incessantly, but sugars have fallen.

In the table and graph on page 129, both entitled "U.S. Sugar Consumption Vs Diabetes Prevalence: 1890 – 2016," we observe the correlational data between sugar consumption – often touted as the cause of diabetes – and diabetes prevalence. In this table and graph, sugar data was obtained from the research of Stephan Guyenet[126] and diabetes prevalence data was reviewed previously. Sugar, as a percentage of total energy, was calculated based on the National Health and Nutrition Examination Survey (NHANES), which found the total average U.S. energy intake to be 1,955 calories/person/day for the years 1971-1975, 2,214 calories for years 1988 to 1994, 2,221 calories for years 1999-2000, and 2,195 calories for years 2009-2010.[494] It is assumed that for all years prior to 1971, total energy intake in the U.S. was the same as in 1971, which is 1,955 cal/day.

Notice that, by 1890, sugar consumption in the U.S. was already 211 calories per day, which is 10.8% of total energy. This level of sugar consumption already exceeded the current WHO recommendation to consume less than 10% of calories as sugar (and less than 5% "for added health benefits").[1095] Yet, diabetes prevalence was only 0.0028%. Sugar consumption then elevated to 15.8% of energy by 1907, but we have no known indication that diabetes prevalence was markedly on the rise.

In 1935, sugar consumption was 440 calories/day, which was 22.5% of energy, but diabetes prevalence was still only 0.37%, which is one in 270 people.

Notice then that sugar consumption, both in total quantity and as a percentage of the diet, didn't change that much over the next 81 years (1935-2016). It was 22.5% of energy in 1935, 22.6% in 1961, 23.9% in 1991, 27.4% in 2000, and finally, 24.0% in 2016. Yet, relative to 1890, diabetes was up 137-fold in 1935, 325-fold in 1960-61, 1,061-fold in 1991, 2,750-fold in 2000, and 4,643-fold in 2016.

That is, just between the years of 1935 and 2016, diabetes prevalence elevated an additional 4,506-fold, as compared to the 1890 prevalence, while sugar consumption (as a percent of total calories) increased just 1.5% (from 22.5% to 24.0%).

In the table on p. 130, "U.S. Sugar Consumption Vs Diabetes Prevalence: 1935 – 2016," we observe that sugar consumption was 440 calories/day in 1935, which is 22.5% of total energy consumed, and consumption increased just 86 calories/day by 2016, up to 24.0% of total energy consumed. Thus, the absolute increase in sugar consumption as a percentage of energy was only 1.5%. However, diabetes prevalence elevated from 0.37% in 1935 to 13.0% in 2016, which is an increase of 3,400%.

Can we possibly indict sugar as a cause of diabetes with an absolute caloric increase (as a percentage of total energy consumed) of just 1.5%, while diabetes increased 3,400%? And if we want to blame the rise in diabetes on the actual sugar

U.S. Sugar Consumption Vs Diabetes Prevalence: 1890 – 2016

Year	Sugar Consumption (cal/capita/day)	Sugar % of Energy	Diabetes Prevalence	X-Fold Increase in Diabetes Relative to 1890
1890	211	10.8%	0.0028%	1
1907	310	15.8%	?	?
1935	440	22.5%	0.37%	137-Fold
1960-61	443	22.6%	0.91%	325-Fold
1991	529	23.9%	2.97%	1,061-Fold
2000	609	27.4%	7.7%	2,750-Fold
2016	526	24.0%	13.0%	4,643-Fold

References: Sugar Data: Guyenet, Landen. *The Hungry Brain*. New York, Flatiron Books, 2017. Diabetes statistics: See references herein. U.S. © C. Knobbe, 2022. Ancestral Health Foundation.

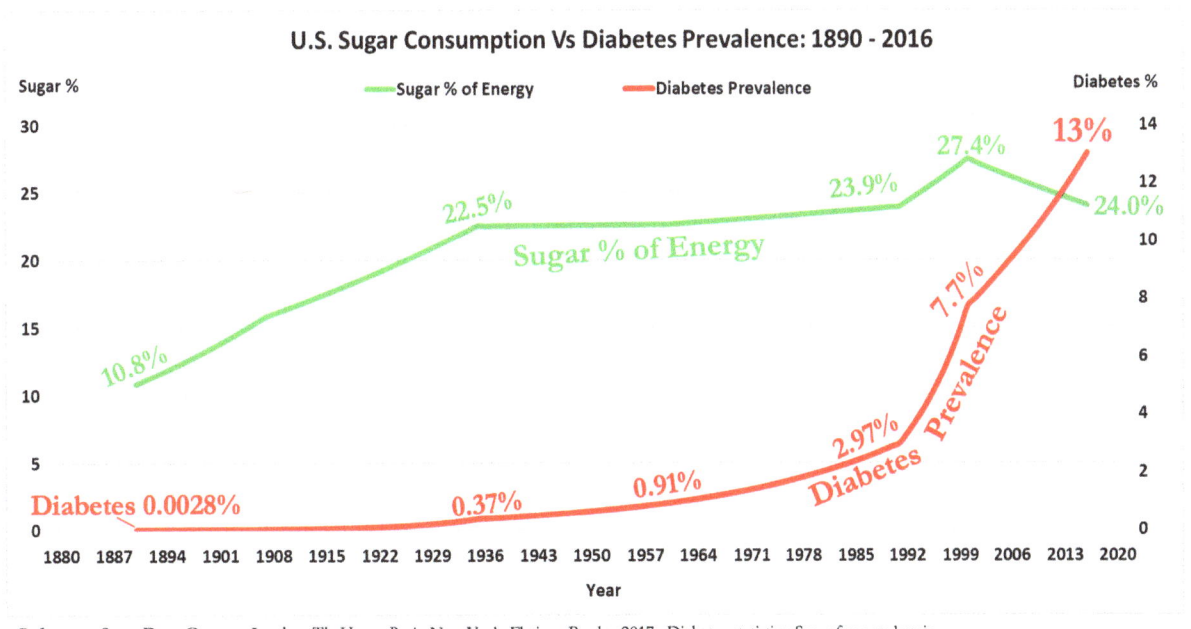

U.S. Sugar Consumption Vs Diabetes Prevalence: 1890 - 2016

References: Sugar Data: Guyenet, Landen. *The Hungry Brain*. New York, Flatiron Books, 2017. Diabetes statistics: See references herein. U.S. © C. Knobbe, 2022. Ancestral Health Foundation.

consumed, the increase was only 86 calories, which is the equivalent of five teaspoons of sugar.

However, let's further examine the relationship between vegetable oil consumption and diabetes in the U.S. Notice that vegetable oil consumption increased from 146 cal/day in 1935 to 713 cal/day

CHAPTER 3

U.S. Sugar Consumption Vs Diabetes Prevalence 1935 - 2016

Year	Sugar Consumption (cal/cap/day)	Absolute Increase in Sugar (Relative to 1935)	Sugar % of Energy	Absolute % Energy increase in sugar	Diabetes Prevalence	% Increase in Diabetes (Relative to 1935)
1935	440	—	22.5%	—	0.37%	—
2016	526	86 cal	24.0%	1.5%	13.0%	3,400%

References: Sugar Data: Guyenet, Landen. The Hungry Brain. New York, Flatiron Books, 2017. Diabetes statistics: see references herein. U.S. © C. Knobbe, 2022. Ancestral Health Foundation.

by 2016, which is an increase of 567 calories. Vegetable oil as a percentage of total caloric energy consumed was 7.5% in 1935 and 29.0% in 2016, which is an absolute increase of 21.5%. Thus, diabetes prevalence was 0.37% when vegetable oils occupied just 7.5% of dietary calories but increased to 13.0% when vegetable oils had increased to 29.0% of calories (see table below).

This, however, is an enormous increase in vegetable oil consumption, equaling more than an additional one-fifth of all *calories* being consumed in 2016, as compared to 1935.

To even further simplify, in the histogram graph on page 131 ("U.S. Sugar and Vegetable Oil Relative Consumption Vs Diabetes Prevalence: 1935 – 2016"), we are able to visualize, side-by-side, the absolute increase of both sugar and vegetable oils, as a percentage of total calories, between the years of 1935 and 2016, versus the increasing prevalence of diabetes. Notice the relatively trivial

U.S. Vegetable Oil Consumption Vs Diabetes Prevalence 1935 - 2016

Year	Vegetable Oil Consumption (cal/cap/day)	Absolute Increase in Veg Oils (Relative to 1935)	Veg Oils % of Energy	Absolute % Energy increase in Veg Oils	Diabetes Prevalence	% Increase in Diabetes (Relative to 1935)
1935	146 cal	—	7.5%	—	0.37%	—
2016	713 cal	567 cal	29.0%	21.5%	13.0%	3,400%

References: Vegetable oil data: Knobbe C, Stojanoska M. The 'Displacing Foods of Modern Commerce' Are the Primary and Proximate Cause of Age-Related Macular Degeneration: A Unifying Singular Hypothesis. Medical Hypotheses: 2017;109:184-198. Diabetes statistics: see references herein. © C. Knobbe, 2022. Ancestral Health Foundation.

MORE ON PROCESSED FOODS AND SEED OIL DANGERS

US Sugar and Vegetable Oil Relative Consumption Vs Diabetes Prevalence 1935-2016

	Sugar absolute % Energy increase relative to 1935	Vegetable Oils absolute % Energy increase relative to 1935	% Increase in Diabetes (Relative to 1935)
(Year 2016)	1.5%	21.5%	3400%

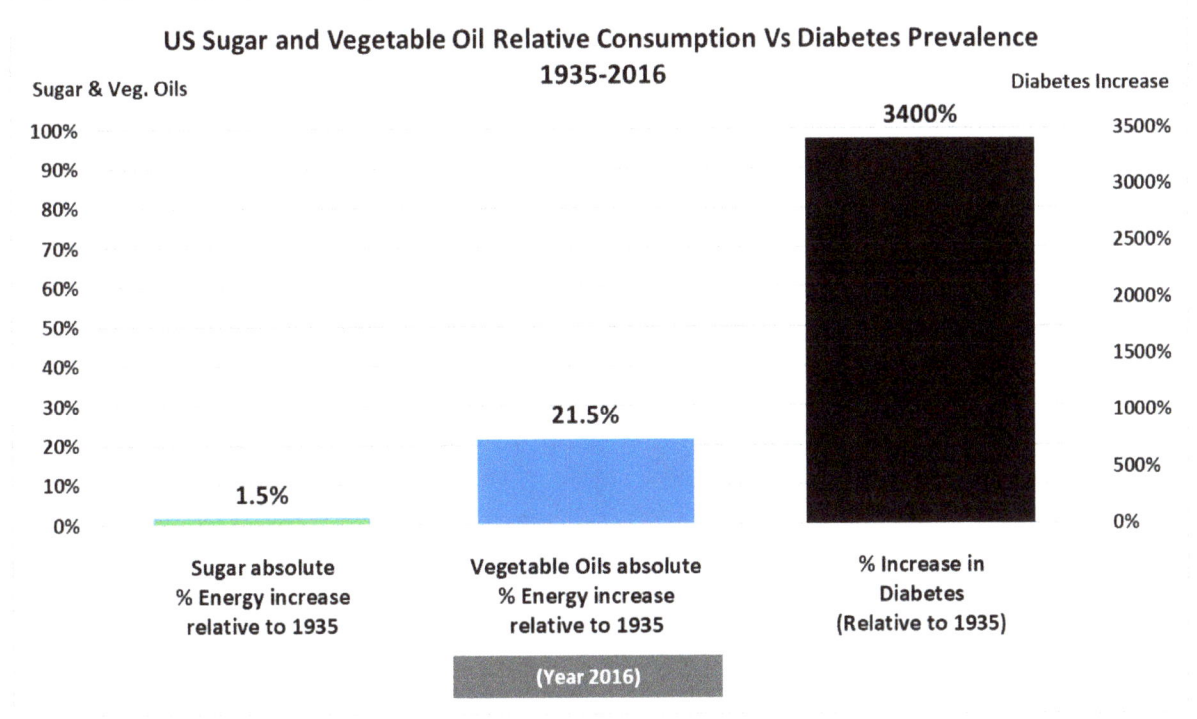

References: Sugar Data: Guyenet, Landen. The Hungry Brain. New York, Flatiron Books, 2017. Vegetable oil data: Knobbe C, Stojanoska M. The 'Displacing Foods of Modern Commerce' Are the Primary and Proximate Cause of Age-Related Macular Degeneration: A Unifying Singular Hypothesis. Medical Hypotheses: 2017;109:184-198. U.S. © C. Knobbe, 2022. Ancestral Health Foundation.

increase in sugar, of just 1.5%, versus the extremely large increase in vegetable oils, at 21.5% (more than one-fifth of all calories), paralleled by a 35-fold (3,400%) increase in diabetes prevalence.

For those who prefer a table rather than a histogram, as above, we present the following (see table "U.S. Sugar and Vegetable Oil Relative Consumption Vs Diabetes Prevalence 1935 – 2016").

U.S. Sugar and Vegetable Oil Relative Consumption Vs Diabetes Prevalence 1935 - 2016

Year	Sugar absolute % Energy increase relative to 1935	Vegetable Oils absolute % Energy increase relative to 1935	% Increase in Diabetes (Relative to 1935)
2016	1.5%	21.5%	3,400%

References: Sugar Data: Guyenet, Landen. The Hungry Brain. New York, Flatiron Books, 2017. Vegetable oil data: Knobbe C, Stojanoska M. The 'Displacing Foods of Modern Commerce' Are the Primary and Proximate Cause of Age-Related Macular Degeneration: A Unifying Singular Hypothesis. Medical Hypotheses: 2017;109:184-198. U.S. © C. Knobbe, 2022. Ancestral Health Foundation.

CHAPTER 3

Sugar and Vegetable Oil Consumption Vs Diabetes, USA: 1991 - 2016

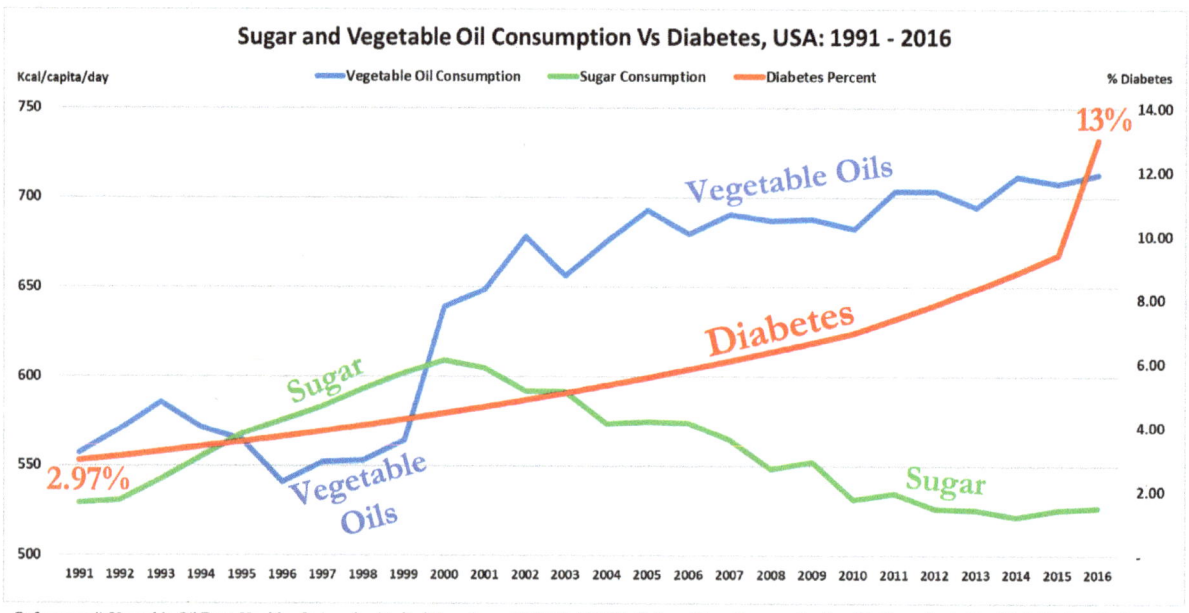

[Chart showing Vegetable Oil Consumption, Sugar Consumption, and Diabetes Percent from 1991 to 2016. Vegetable Oils rise from ~550 to ~710 Kcal/capita/day. Sugar rises then falls from ~570 to ~535. Diabetes rises from 2.97% in 1991 to 13% in 2016.]

References: 1) Vegetable Oil Data: Knobbe, Stojanoska. Medical Hypotheses: 2017;109:184-198 2) Sugar Data: Guyenet, Landen. *The Hungry Brain*. New York, Flatiron Books, 2017. 3) Diabetes Statistics: See references herein. U.S. © C. Knobbe, 2022. Ancestral Health Foundation. All rights reserved.

With this evidence, we can already (there is much more evidence to come) be nearly certain that sugar consumption has little, if any, contribution to diabetes, whereas vegetable oils appear to have an extraordinarily strong, if not the sole, contribution.

In the next graph above, entitled "Sugar and Vegetable Oil Consumption Vs Diabetes, USA: 1991-2016," we've focused on the last three decades. Both sugar and vegetable oil data are plotted against diabetes prevalence, again, of which approximately 95% is type 2 diabetes. Notice the extraordinary increase in diabetes prevalence, which was 2.97% in 1991 but skyrocketed to 13.0% by 2016.

Perhaps the most intriguing characteristic for most observers, however, is the fact that sugar consumption dropped substantially from years 2000 to 2016, during the exact same interval that type 2 diabetes prevalence elevated from about 5% in 2000 up to 13% by 2016 (sugar data provided by S. Guyenet). This is an increase in type 2 diabetes of approximately 2.5-fold in a 16-year period, while sugar consumption progressively and substantially declined. However, during the exact same interval, seed oil consumption continued the ascent, which, of course, is the primary cause of diabetes. We'll review the pathophysiologic (biological) mechanism subsequently.

Throughout the remainder of this book, we will observe five different countries – the U.S. (reviewed), U.K., Australia, Israel, and Japan – with substantial decreases in sugar consumption over decades of time, while diabetes prevalence simultaneously increases. Indeed, in these countries, there is actually a negative correlation between sugar consumption and diabetes. That is, as sugar consumption declines, diabetes prevalence climbs and sometimes, dramatically.

Furthermore, in the U.S., Australia, and Japan, we observe declines in both sugar and carbohydrate consumption while diabetes prevalence increases. And in the U.S. and Japan, we observe declines in sugar, carbohydrates, and total calories consumed, while diabetes prevalence skyrockets. This evidence strongly suggests that caloric consumption, sugar, and carbohydrates have little or no role in the development of diabetes.

In all five previously mentioned countries, that is, the U.S., U.K, Australia, Israel, and Japan, however, we see marked increases in seed oil consumption as diabetes prevalence increases. It is our opinion that seed oils are nearly the exclusive cause of type 2 diabetes, while sugar, carbohydrates, and total calories generally deserve to be exonerated.

This does not indicate that sugar is not problematic in other respects. As reviewed repeatedly, added sugars and refined carbohydrates, such as refined flours, contribute greatly to nutrient deficiencies, which lead to degenerative conditions, just as Weston A. Price showed.[28]

If you do not have diabetes, but instead have pre-diabetes, elevated blood sugars, high triglycerides, low HDL cholesterol, high blood pressure, or belly fat (visceral fat), all of which are conditions of metabolic syndrome (which we'll discuss next), be aware – you may well be headed for type 2 diabetes. And diabetes is a dangerous condition. In the West, evidence shows that 44% of patients with type 2 diabetes mellitus (T2DM) die within ten years of diagnosis.[495] Most of those individuals die of "macrovascular disease," such as heart attacks, strokes, and the like; in fact, those with T2DM are two to three times as likely to die of cardiovascular disease as people in the general population.[496]

Wish to prevent or reverse type 2 diabetes? Stop all seed oils and follow a very low LA diet. Even if you have type 2 diabetes, a low LA diet should soon result in success, perhaps within a few months to a year, but the details of the diet are critical. If taking medication for diabetes, work with your healthcare practitioner to gradually eliminate that medicine as the condition abates. Further details on a low LA diet will be found in the final chapters of this book.

METABOLIC SYNDROME – ANOTHER CHRONIC DISEASE DRIVEN BY SEED OILS

In 1981, physician Markolf Hanefield, MD, PhD, coined the term "metabolic syndrome" and described the condition as a clustering of obesity, abnormal blood lipids, type 2 diabetes, gout, and hypertension, all combined with an increased risk of cardiovascular disease, fatty liver, and gallstones.[497]

In 1988, Gerald "Jerry" Reaven, MD, gained international recognition when he, according to Stanford Medicine, argued "for the existence of insulin resistance, [which is] a diminished response to the hormone insulin," as the critical link in the development of a "cluster of other metabolic abnormalities that together greatly increase the risk for cardiovascular disease, which he called Syndrome X."[498][499]

Syndrome X, which gained attention due to the theory that insulin resistance was a key and unifying condition, was both previously and subsequently referred to as "metabolic syndrome." Metabolic syndrome is indeed a cluster of metabolic disorders that includes hypertension, dyslipidemia (abnormal blood lipids such as high triglycerides and low HDL cholesterol), insulin resistance with elevating blood sugars, and in at least 90% of cases, visceral (organ and 'belly') fat accumulation along with generalized overweight or obesity.[500]

Vascular disease that is characterized by atherosclerosis is central to the condition, as those with metabolic syndrome have a much higher risk of cardiovascular diseases in general.[501] The reason that metabolic syndrome is so concerning is that it is strongly linked to a markedly higher risk of type 2 diabetes mellitus (T2DM), cardiovascular disease including heart attacks and strokes, pro-thrombotic (blood clot-related) disorders, pro-inflammatory conditions, non-alcoholic fatty liver disease (steatohepatitis), reproductive disorders, cancers, and higher all-cause mortality.[502] [503]

However, in contrast to the belief system that Hanefeld and Leonhardt, in 1981, or Reaven, in 1988, were the first to describe metabolic syndrome, recognition of components of the disorder date back to the early 20th century. During the First World War, in Vienna, Austria, two physicians, Karl Hitzenberger and Martin Richter-Quittner, made clinical observations in patients that had metabolic abnormalities, vascular hypertension, and a notable relationship between hypertension and diabetes.[504] [505] The physicians were not able to publish their results until after WWI, in 1921.

Just about the same time that Hitzenberger and Richter-Quittner published their reviews, two other physicians – Eskil Kylin from Sweden and Gregorio Marañón from Spain – independently published two papers with extremely similar titles: "Hypertension and Diabetes Mellitus" (Hypertonie and Zuckerkrankheit).[506] [507]

But the metabolic syndrome cluster of conditions appears to have been a medical rarity, for example, with a rare description in 1936 by acclaimed British physician and scientist, Sir Harold Percival Himsworth, MD. Himsworth made many advances in understanding metabolic disease, including that there were two types of diabetics: one, insulin-sensitive (juvenile-onset) and another insulin-insensitive (adult-onset), which was a major step in understanding the disease.[508]

In 1939, Himsworth wrote:

"The sensitive [type 1] diabetics tend to be younger and thin and to have a normal blood pressure and normal arteries, and as a rule their disease is of sudden and severe onset… The insensitive diabetics [type 2], on the other hand, tend to be older, obese, to have hypertension and frequently to exhibit pronounced arteriosclerosis, and in these patients the onset of the disease is insidious…"[509]

Himsworth's work gave birth to the terms type 1 and type 2 diabetes.[510] [511] In 1947, French physician Jean Vague noted that upper body adiposity (fat accumulation), termed "android obesity" characteristically increased cardiovascular risk in distinction to a "gynaecoid" or "gynoid" type of obesity, which is lower body obesity that is more characteristic of the fat accumulation in women.[512] [513] [514]

The National Health and Nutrition Examination Survey III (NHANES III), completed between 1988 and 1994, determined that approximately 24% of the U.S. adult population had metabolic syndrome.[515] The NHANES II also found that 44% of Americans age 50 and above had the condition.[516] The NHANES study of 1999-2006 found that 34.1% of adults had metabolic syndrome.[517]

And finally, using the International Diabetes Federation (IDF) criteria, between 1999 and 2002 in the U.S., approximately 40% of adults met the definition of metabolic syndrome.[515] Even more concerning, the NHANES III data confirmed that 4% of all adolescents and 29% of overweight adolescents met the criteria for metabolic syndrome.[518] [519]

The most recent analyses for metabolic syndrome in the U.S. found that, between 2009 and

2016, only 12.2% of Americans could be defined as having optimal levels of five factors of metabolic health, including blood glucose, triglycerides, high-density lipoprotein cholesterol, blood pressure, and waist circumference, without the need for related medications (see graph below).[520]

That is, 88% of Americans have at least one or more characteristics of metabolic dysfunction, and this broadly implicates the ubiquitous nature of processed foods and, of course, seed oils, which have been shown to rapidly induce metabolic dysfunction (to be reviewed subsequently).

As of 2017-2018, the NHANES studies found that only 6.8% of Americans had optimal cardiometabolic health, based on adiposity (body fat composition), blood glucose, blood lipids, blood pressure, and clinical cardiovascular disease (CVD).[521]

On a global scale, metabolic syndrome has also escalated dramatically in proportion to global seed oil consumption. In a paper published in the journal Lancet, in 2005, researchers Robert Eckel, MD, and colleagues, wrote, "Over the past two decades, a striking increase in the number of people with the metabolic syndrome has taken place. This increase is associated with the global epidemic of obesity and diabetes" (see adapted graph on page 136, "Prevalence of Metabolic Syndrome Various Countries: ~2005").[522]

So while metabolic syndrome appears to have been a medical rarity up through the mid-20th century, in the last five decades, the disorder has developed to pandemic proportions on a global scale. As can be seen in the figure below, with 88% of Americans not being able to meet 5 criteria of metabolic health, again, we must ask ourselves, 'What is so ubiquitous in our food supply, that only 12% of us

Timeline for Metabolic Syndrome/Metabolic Dysfunction: U.S. Adults
(Combination of Hypertension, Abnormal Lipids, Insulin Resistance, Hyperglycemia, & Visceral Obesity)

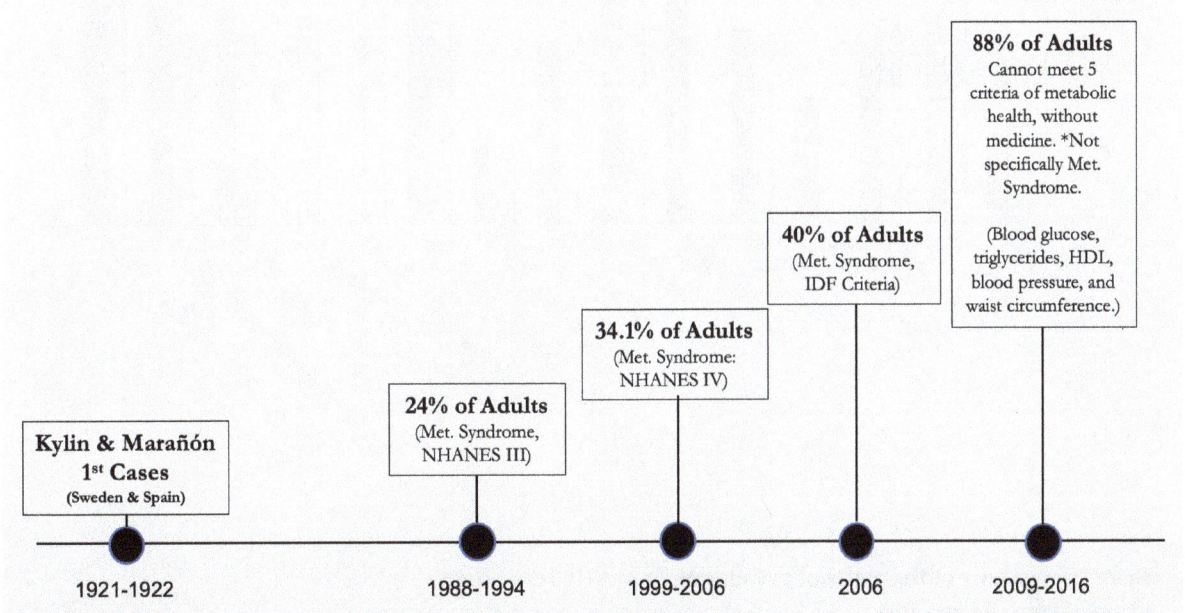

1921-1922	Kylin & Marañón 1st Cases (Sweden & Spain)
1988-1994	24% of Adults (Met. Syndrome, NHANES III)
1999-2006	34.1% of Adults (Met. Syndrome: NHANES IV)
2006	40% of Adults (Met. Syndrome, IDF Criteria)
2009-2016	88% of Adults Cannot meet 5 criteria of metabolic health, without medicine. *Not specifically Met. Syndrome. (Blood glucose, triglycerides, HDL, blood pressure, and waist circumference.)

References: 1) Kylin E. Zentralblatt für Innere Medizin.1921;42:873-877 2) Marañón G. Zentralblatt für Innere Medizin. 1922;43:169-176. 3) Ford ES, Giles WH, Dietz WH. Prevalence of the metabolic syndrome among US adults: findings from the Third National Health and Nutrition Survey. JAMA. 2002;287:356-359. 4) Mozumdar A, Liguori G. Persistent Increase of Prevalence of Metabolic Syndrome Among U.S. Adults: NHANES III to NHANES 1999-2006. Diabetes Care. 2011;34(1):216-219. 5) Araújo J, Cai J, Stevens J. Prevalence of Optimal Metabolic Health in American Adults: National Health and Nutrition Examination Survey 2009-2016. Metab Syndr Relat Disord. 2019;17(1):45-52. Copyright C. Knobbe, 2022. Ancestral Health Foundation.

are avoiding enough of it, to remain metabolically healthy?' The short answer is processed foods, but as will be seen in upcoming chapters, it is the seed oils that induce mitochondrial dysfunction, leading to metabolic syndrome and the components of metabolic disease.

According to the International Diabetes Federation (IDF), the global prevalence of diabetes is 8.8% as of 2015 and is expected to reach 10.4% by 2040.[523] Metabolic syndrome, which is far more difficult to quantify, is known to be about three times more common than diabetes.[411] As such, the global prevalence of metabolic syndrome is currently estimated at about one-fourth of the world's population,[411] which would be in the range of two billion people affected.

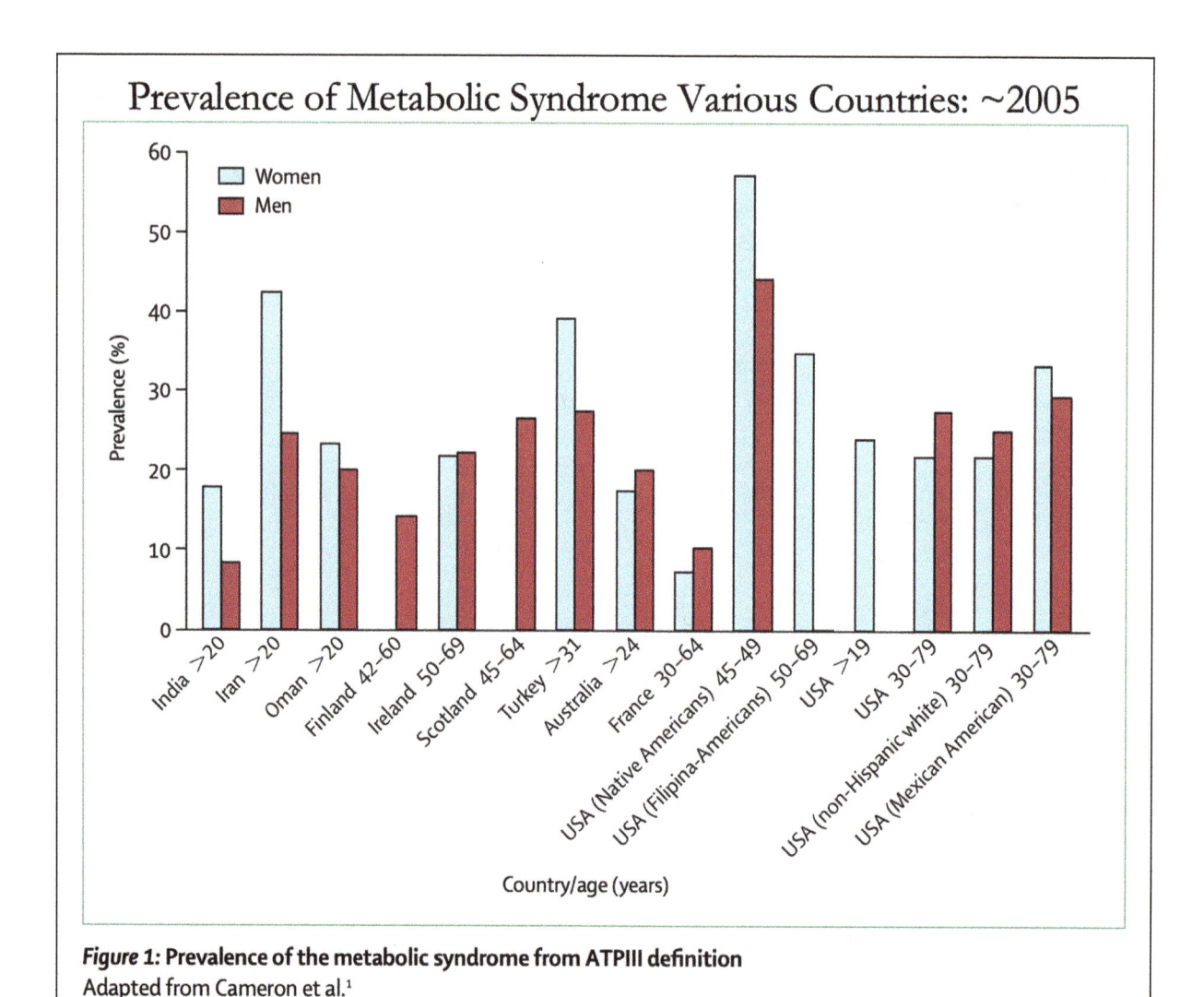

Figure 1: Prevalence of the metabolic syndrome from ATPIII definition
Adapted from Cameron et al.[1]
Eckel RH. The metabolic syndrome. Lancet. 2005;365:1415-28. Reprinted with permission.

ALZHEIMER'S DISEASE AND DEMENTIA – PARALLEL RISE WITH SEED OILS

In 1906, German physician, psychiatrist, and neuropathologist, Alois Alzheimer, gave a case presentation at the 37th Meeting of South-West German Psychiatrists in Tubingen, entitled "A peculiar severe disease process of the cerebral cortex."[524] He described the then remarkable case of Auguste D., a 50-year-old woman who had been admitted to the Frankfurt Psychiatric Hospital "for paranoia, progressive sleep and memory disturbance, aggression, and confusion, until her death 5 years later."[525]

Alois Alzheimer. Circa 1909.

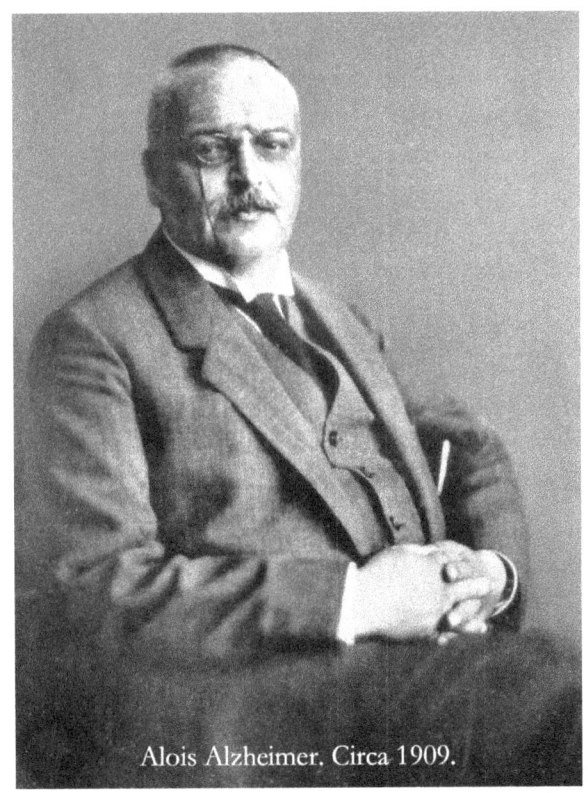

Photo courtesy of Archive for History of Psychiatry, Department of Psychiatry University of Munich. With permission. Hippius H. The discovery of Alzheimer's disease. Dialogues Clin Neuroscience. 2003;5(1):101-108. Creative Commons Attributions License (http://creativecommons.org/licenses/by-nc-nd/3.0/).

Following her death, Dr. Alzheimer examined her brain and found "distinctive plaques and neurofibrillary tangles in the brain histology."[525] There was little interest in this remarkably unusual case, but Alzheimer's mentor and colleague, Dr. Emil Kraepelin, named the "new disease" after its discoverer, calling it "Alzheimer's disease."[525]

In the 8-year period between the admission of Auguste D. in 1901 and 1909, Alzheimer discovered an additional three cases of such dementia, which he published in 1909, and he noted a "plaque only" variant of the disease, in 1911.[525] Alzheimer himself died in 1915 and did not publish any further cases other than those five patients.

According to researchers Waldman and Lamb, in established medical literature worldwide, there was one case of Alzheimer's disease published in the year 1908, 4 cases published in 1910, 13 in 1927, 5 in 1936, 150 in 1948, 250 in 1953, 382 in 1962, 368 in 1970, and 648 in 1978.[526] They wrote, "Alzheimer's disease has become more and more common – to the point that today the dementias of aging are considered the norm rather than the exception."[526] But these researchers also confirmed that, in the not too distant past, the famed physicians Sir William Osler and Sigmund Freud, "the greatest medical observers of all time did not even mention it."[527]

As of September 2, 2021, the World Health Organization reports that, "Currently more than 55 million people live with dementia worldwide, and there are nearly 10 million new cases every year."[528] "Dementia is currently the seventh leading cause of death among all diseases…"[528] on a global scale. WHO statisticians also affirm that "Alzheimer's disease is the most common form [of dementia] and may contribute to 60-70% of cases."[528]

Thus, while the first reported case of Alzheimer's disease was in 1908, with only a few hundred reported cases in the medical literature by the

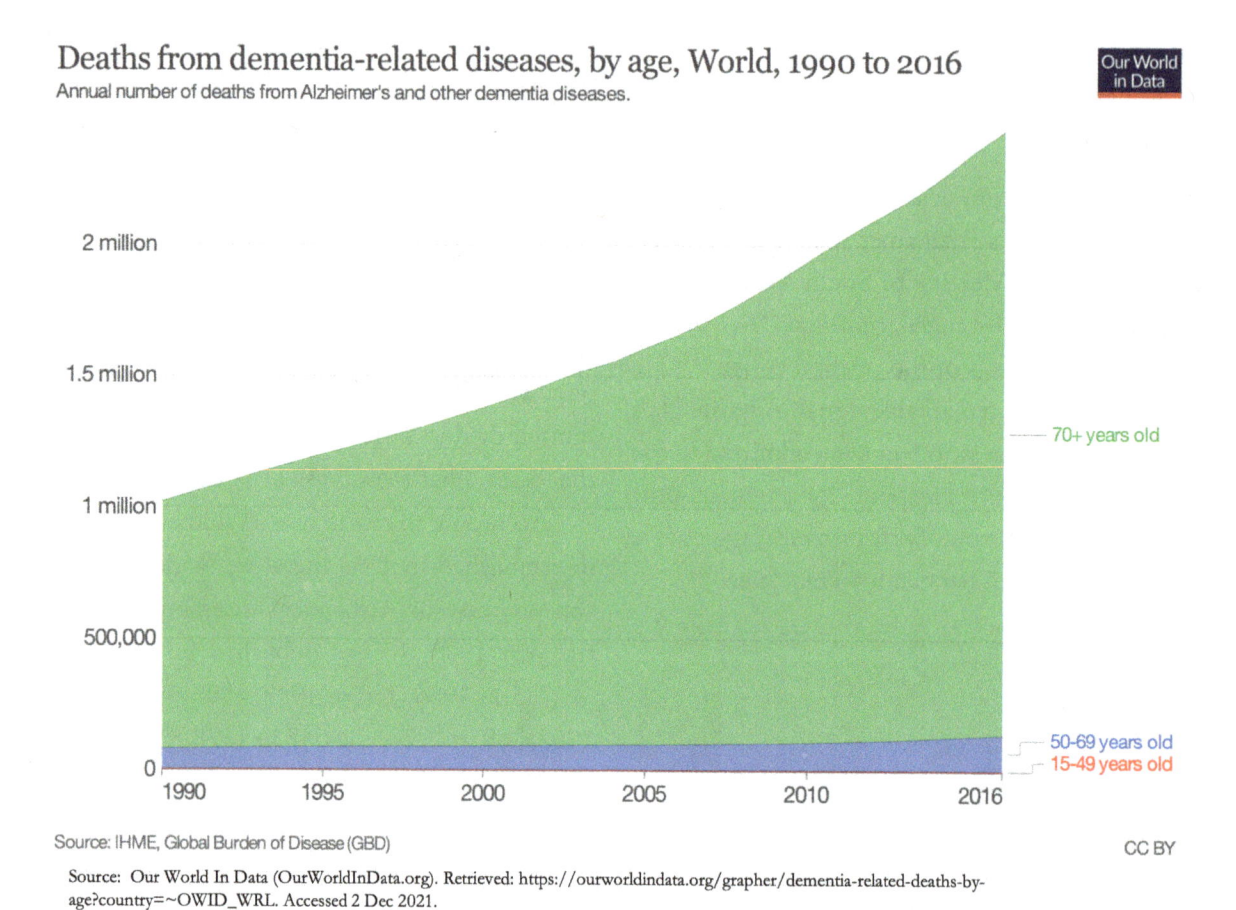

Deaths from dementia-related diseases, by age, World, 1990 to 2016
Annual number of deaths from Alzheimer's and other dementia diseases.

Source: IHME, Global Burden of Disease (GBD)

Source: Our World In Data (OurWorldInData.org). Retrieved: https://ourworldindata.org/grapher/dementia-related-deaths-by-age?country=~OWID_WRL. Accessed 2 Dec 2021.

1950s, today we have 55 million cases of dementia with 50% of those older than 85 having Alzheimer's disease,[529] and on a global scale, one new case of dementia every three seconds.[528] As with most all of the other chronic diseases, we've observed an infinite increase in Alzheimer's disease since the late 19th century, in parallel with an infinite increase in vegetable oil and processed food consumption.

AUTOIMMUNE DISEASES – ONCE MEDICAL RARITIES – HAVE EXPLODED IN THE 20TH AND 21ST CENTURIES

In a scientific paper published in 2015, the title reads, "The World Incidence and Prevalence of Autoimmune Diseases is Increasing."[530] Indeed it is – and severely so. But it wasn't always this way, and like the rest of the chronic diseases reviewed here, the prevalence of autoimmune diseases has taken a near-vertical trajectory in recent decades.[530]

Sir William Osler, famed physician of the late 19th and early 20th centuries, published two papers in The American Journal of Medical Sciences that were some of the earliest writings on systemic lupus erythematosus (SLE). The first paper was published in 1895 and another in 1904, which described 29 cases of patients who presented with skin disorders ("erythema," referencing red, inflamed skin lesions) that connected the skin disease to systemic disease (organ involvement).[531, 532] Osler published another paper in 1900 in the British Journal of Dermatology on SLE, connecting the skin disease to organ involvement.[533]

More than a century later, two physicians proposed that only 2 of the 29 subjects reviewed by Osler actually had systemic lupus erythematosus (SLE), while the majority had other skin disorders.[534] Nevertheless, Osler made a tremendous contribution to medical science in 1904 by tying the erythematous skin disease (skin rashes and "discoid lupus," the latter of which represents coin-shaped skin lesions) to SLE. Systemic lupus erythematosus (SLE), often referred to as "lupus," is the prototypical autoimmune disease because patients develop antibodies to their own cells, which can affect virtually any organ system, including life-threatening involvement of the kidneys, brain, heart, and lungs.

In 1902, dermatologist physicians J.H. Sequira and H. Balean published perhaps the largest series of SLE patients' studies prior to 1950, which included 71 cases.[535] In 1923 and 1924, physicians E. Libman and B. Sacks reported on two patients with a malar (facial) rash and endocarditis (inflammation of the heart), which appeared to be SLE.[536] Thirty years after Osler's 1904 paper, additional patients with apparent SLE were described.[537, 538] In 1935, physician G. Baehr published a paper reviewing 23 patients with SLE type skin features, thirteen of whom had heart lesions.[539]

PubMed shows no papers published on SLE between 1942 to 1944, and then in 1945, a total of 14 papers were published, which increased to 178 papers by 1960, 1,239 by 2000, and 3,765 by 2021. This is indicative of an explosion of cases producing an avalanche of research over the past 60 years (see figure below, "PubMed Timeline for Papers with 'Systemic Lupus Erythematosus' in Title).

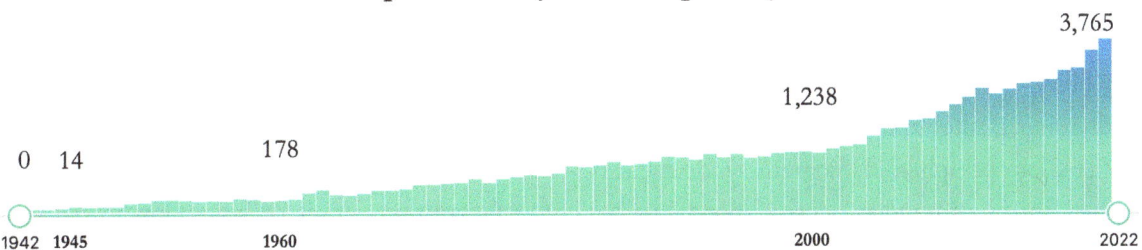

PubMed Timeline for Papers with 'Systemic Lupus Erythematosus' in Title

0 — 1942
14 — 1945
178 — 1960
1,238 — 2000
3,765 — 2022

In New York City, between 1956 and 1965, the prevalence (total existing cases) of SLE was 14.6 per 100,000,[540] however, a study of U.S. Medicare patients between 2003 and 2008 reported a prevalence of 300 per 100,000 population.[541]

The Lupus Foundation of America estimates that 1.5 million Americans are currently affected with lupus, with at least 5 million people worldwide affected.[542] Ninety percent of those affected are women, most of whom develop the disease between the ages of 15 and 44.[542] Unfortunately, one in every three patients with lupus suffers from multiple autoimmune diseases.[542] Clearly, while SLE dates back to antiquity, the incidence and prevalence have skyrocketed over the past 70 years.

MORE THAN 100 AUTOIMMUNE DISEASES SKYROCKETING IN INCIDENCE AND PREVALENCE

The NIH Autoimmune Association lists more than 100 recognized autoimmune disorders today, with 24 million Americans affected, while another 8 million have auto-antibodies (e.g., anti-nuclear antibody, or ANA).[543] They further confirm that 5 to 10% of Americans have more than one autoimmune condition and that 80% of all patients diagnosed with an autoimmune disease are women.

Some of the most common autoimmune diseases include type 1 diabetes (insulin-dependent diabetes mellitus, IDDM), multiple sclerosis, SLE, rheumatoid arthritis (RA), inflammatory bowel diseases (e.g., Crohn's disease and ulcerative colitis), primary biliary cirrhosis, myasthenia gravis, Hashimoto's thyroiditis, autoimmune hepatitis, celiac disease (CD), bullous pemphigoid, Sjogren's syndrome (dry eyes and dry mouth), and ankylosing spondylitis, but there are scores of others. For a complete list, consult the Autoimmune Association (AutoImmune.org) and search "Disease Information."

MULTIPLE SCLEROSIS (MS) RISES IN PARALLEL TO SEED OILS.

Multiple sclerosis (MS), another prototypical autoimmune disease, is the single greatest cause of neurological disability in young adults worldwide; the disease typically presents in the third or fourth decade of life.[544] Individuals affected with MS typically develop central nervous system (CNS) disturbances secondary to demyelination, wherein the "insulating" myelin sheath that surrounds nerve fibers in the brain, optic nerves, and spinal cord, undergoes loss or destruction thus affecting nerve transmission.

This ultimately may affect mobility, gait (walking), hand function, vision, cognition, bowel and bladder function, and sensation, while potentially resulting in pain, depression, spasticity, fatigue, tremors, and coordination abnormalities.[545]

The earliest documented case of MS was that of Lidwina the Virgin (1380-1433), a 16-year-old girl who lived in Schiedam, Holland, documented to have developed acute illness, blindness in one eye, weakness, and pain, with progression of symptoms that led to a very premature death at approximately 54 years of age.[546] The famous Jean-Martin Charcot (1825 – 1893), French neurologist and professor of anatomical pathology, said that multiple sclerosis seemed rare.[547]

According to physician and author, T. Jock Murray, MD, "Thought to be a neurological curiosity in the mid-19th century worthy of single case reports in the journals of the day, by the turn of the 20th century, it was recognized as one of the most common causes of admission to neurology wards…"[547] Murray continued, "At the turn of the

Autoimmune disease

- Heredity
- White blood cells
- Lifestyle
- Hormone influence
- Environmental factors

- Multiple sclerosis (Damaged myelin)
- Systemic lupus erythematosus
- Rheumatoid arthritis

Symptoms:
- Myocarditis
- Skin rash
- Impaired vision
- Pulmonary fibrosis
- Joint pain

Image courtesy of the NIH, NIEHS, "Autoimmune Diseases," with Adaptations.
https://www.niehs.nih.gov/health/topics/conditions/autoimmune/index.cfm

21st century, MS is recognized as the most common serious neurological disease in young adults living in temperate climates."[547] Today, MS affects more than 2 million people worldwide, with meta-analyses showing that the incidence of MS is clearly increasing over time.[544]

MS seems to be a disease that strikes those living within temperate zones outside of the tropical territories and, therefore, is thought to be related significantly to lack of sun exposure which, in turn, relates to poor vitamin D status (i.e., less sunlight, reduced vitamin D production) and other ramifications.[548] The disease is, therefore, very unevenly distributed across the globe, being very prevalent where white people of Nordic origin live, in Northern latitudes, and in high-income countries.

Conversely, MS is very uncommon in tropical regions that receive much sunlight, in non-whites, and in low-income countries.[548] More than half of the global population of people diagnosed with MS reside within Europe.[549]

However, in a global analysis of MS, Danish neurology researchers established "an almost universal increase in prevalence and incidence of MS over time…"[548] which should "challenge the well-accepted theory of a latitudinal gradient of incidence of MS in Europe and North America, while this gradient is still apparent for Australia and New Zealand…" This suggests, according to the authors, "a general, although not ubiquitous, increase in incidence of MS in females."

In other words, it's not just latitude, sunlight exposure, and geography at work here regarding the increasing prevalence of MS. There's something else at play here. The authors continue:

"These observations should prompt epidemiologic studies to focus on factors in western female lifestyle that have changed over recent decades…"[548]

Could it be the ever-increasing consumption of seed oils?

In the graph on page 143, if we can assume that the diagnosis of MS has been quite accurate since approximately 1950, which seems very reasonable, there has been an extraordinary increase in both the incidence and prevalence of MS as documented by this example in Sweden.

Clearly, by every possible account, MS has been increasing over the last century, and apparently, particularly since about 1950. However, the one thing that is increasing worldwide since about 1950 is processed foods and, particularly, seed oils.

INFLAMMATORY BOWEL DISEASE: ULCERATIVE COLITIS AND CROHN'S DISEASE

In 2016, Chinese researchers reported alarming increases in inflammatory bowel diseases (IBDs), which include ulcerative colitis (UC) and Crohn's disease (CD), which are known chronic inflammatory and probable autoimmune diseases.[550] [551] The researchers report that "IBD has become more common in Asia over the past few decades" and that "the incidence of UC and CD are rising in parallel with rapid urbanization."[550]

The phrase "rapid urbanization" is used repeatedly in scientific jargon and might well be replaced with either "Westernization of the diet" or "processed food consumption," as that is exactly what the researchers are referring to. However, as will be seen throughout this book, Asian countries have been among the last to adopt seed oils in place of traditional fats. In Europe, Increased omega-6 LA consumption has also been linked to an increased risk of developing UC.[552]

In a study published in 2020, researchers examined 14,211 participants' blood for the most prominent telltale laboratory indicator of autoimmunity, which is the presence of antinuclear antibodies (ANA).[553] However, in order to determine if autoimmunity was increasing, they analyzed the blood from individuals in three time periods from the National Health and Nutrition Examination Sur-

Multiple Sclerosis (MS), Sweden: 1946 – 2005

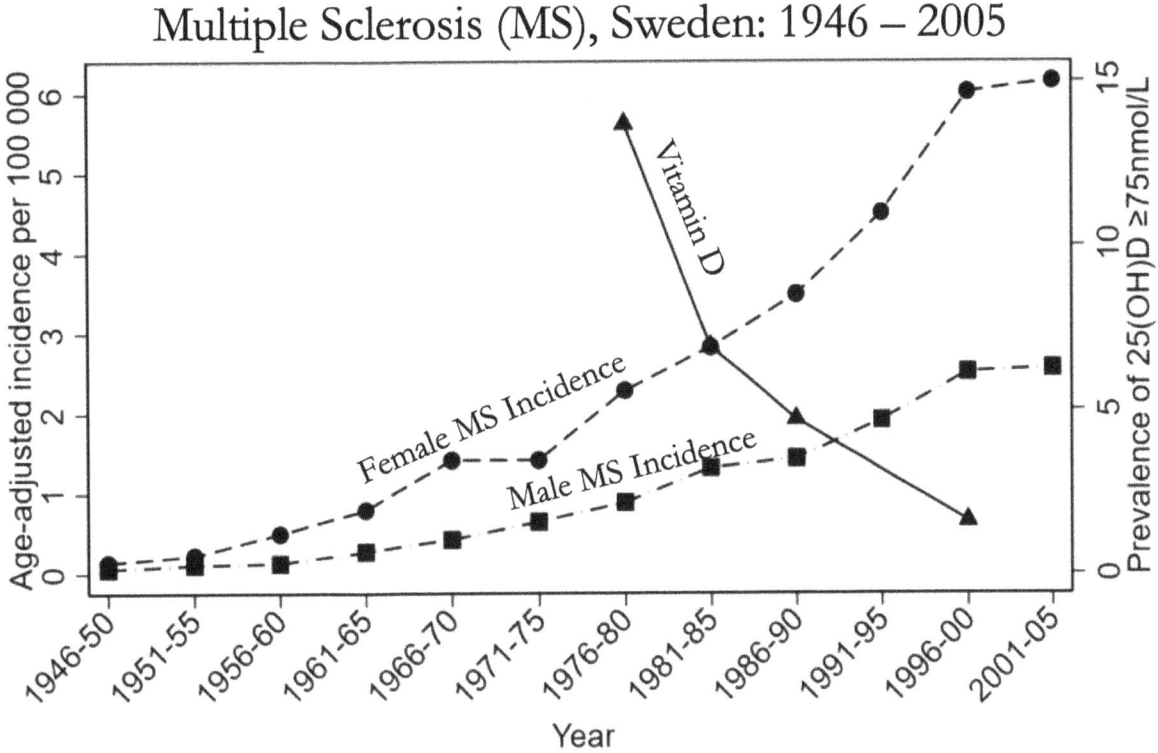

Lucas RM, Harris R. On the Nature of Evidence and 'Proving' Causality: Smoking and Lung Cancer vs. Sun Exposure, Vitamin D and Multiple Sclerosis. Reprinted with permission under Creative Commons Attribution, license: http://creativecommons.org/licenses/by/4.0/.

veys (NHANES). They found that the prevalence of ANA from 1988 to 1991 was 11.0%, rising slightly to 11.5% between 1999 and 2004, and finally rising to 15.9% by 2011 to 2012. These percentages corresponded to estimates that 22 million, 27 million, and 41 million Americans had autoimmune conditions for each of those time periods.[553] In the 2011 to 2012 analysis, this corresponds to about one out of six adults already having evidence of an autoimmune disease, diagnosed or undiagnosed.

AUTOIMMUNE DISEASES SKYROCKET GLOBALLY IN CORRELATION TO SEED OILS

Professor Aaron Lerner, MD, and colleagues, at the B. Rappaport School of Medicine, in Haifa, Israel, conducted what appears to be the most comprehensive analysis of the incidence and prevalence of autoimmune disorders on a worldwide basis, between the years of approximately 1985 and 2015. The results show worldwide net percentage increase per year of 12.5% prevalence (total existing cases) and 19.1% incidence (new onset cases), which are very high rates of escalation (see figure on the top of page 144), with increasing incidence approaching nearly 100% over each 5 to 6 year period.[530]

Lerner and colleagues also examined and categorized groupings of autoimmune diseases, finding that during the same 30-year period, the net percentage increase per year for rheumatologic conditions was 7.1%, endocrine conditions 6.3%, gastrointestinal conditions 6.2%, and neurological conditions 3.7%.[530]

Net Percentage Increase Per Year in Autoimmune Diseases: Worldwide

- Prevalence: 12.5%
- Incidence: 19.1%

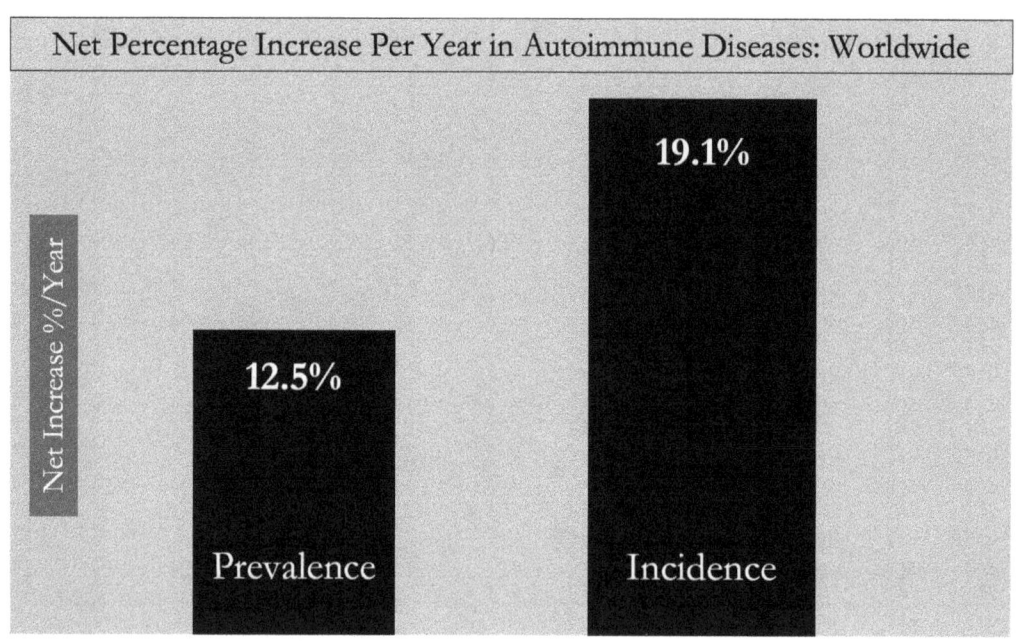

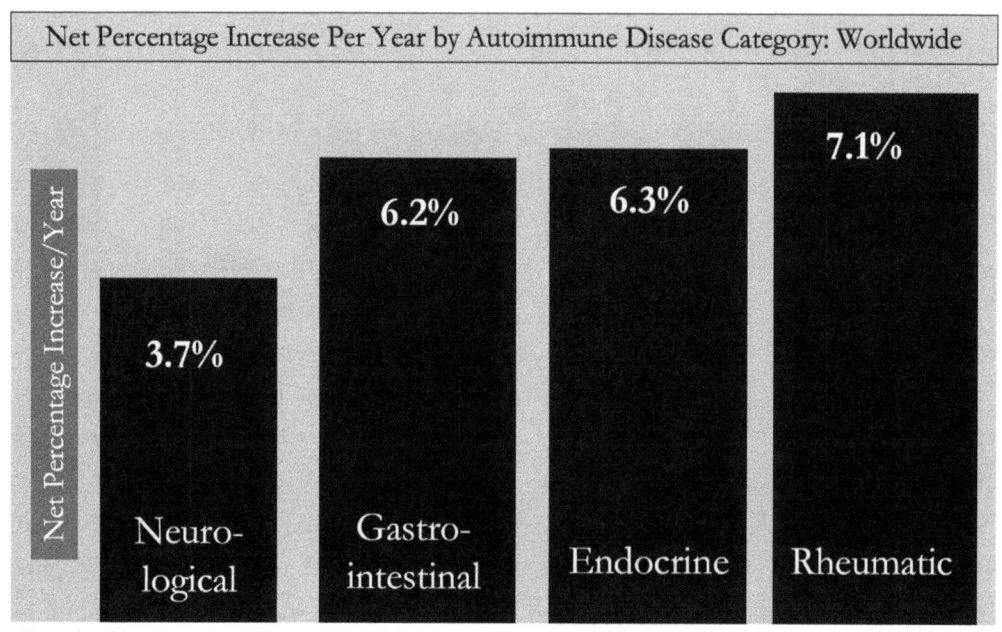

Figure adapted from: Lerner A, et al. The World Incidence and Prevalence of Autoimmune Diseases is Increasing. Int J Celiac Dis. 2015;3(4):151-155.

The National Institute of Health (NIH) affiliate, the National Institute of Environmental Health Sciences' authorities state, "Autoimmune diseases are affecting more people for reasons unknown. Likewise, the causes of these diseases remains a mystery."[554]

Though we'll cover mechanisms of disease in upcoming chapters in much greater detail, suffice it to say here that, once again, we observe these conditions to be spiraling out of control in the face of extraordinary degrees of processed food consumption

Net Percentage Increase Per Year by Autoimmune Disease Category: Worldwide

- Neurological: 3.7%
- Gastrointestinal: 6.2%
- Endocrine: 6.3%
- Rheumatic: 7.1%

Figure adapted from: Lerner A, et al. The World Incidence and Prevalence of Autoimmune Diseases is Increasing. Int J Celiac Dis. 2015;3(4):151-155.

− 75% on a global scale − and dramatic increases in seed oil consumption. Just as with overweight, obesity, diabetes, metabolic syndrome, Alzheimer's disease, dementia, and age-related macular degeneration (see below), we see geometric increases in autoimmune diseases in parallel with westernized diets.

At this point, we might mention that we believe it is fair to say that most autoimmune diseases have at least one unifying factor at the pathophysiologic (biological mechanism) level, and that is intestinal hyperpermeability, also known as "leaky gut."[555][556] Leaky gut, in the simplest terms, is an abnormal condition which allows bacteria, bacterial products, viruses, toxins, partially digested food, etc., all of which may act as antigens, to pass through the gut barrier and, thereafter, through molecular mimicry (antigens that have molecular structures similar to "self") may induce an autoimmune response.[557]

Researchers have clearly linked westernized diets and autoimmunity, in one paper stating,

"The rationale is that the nutritional composition of ultra-processed foodstuffs can induce gut dysbiosis [abnormal gut flora], promoting a pro-inflammatory response and consequently a 'leaky gut.' These factors have been associated with increased risk of autoimmunity in genetically predisposed children... In contrast, unprocessed and minimally processed food-based diets have shown the capacity to promote gut microbiota eubiosis [healthy gut microbiome], anti-inflammatory response, and epithelial integrity..."[558]

It has been shown that high levels of omega-6 fat consumption induce gut dysbiosis leading to chronic inflammation, which sets the stage for leaky gut and autoimmunity.[559] However, even in diets presumably 'high in saturated fat' consistent with so-called "westernized diets," studies typically utilize saturated fat levels that are relatively low by ancestral diet standards (e.g., 11% saturated fat) and omega-6 PUFA (mostly LA) that are very high (e.g., 11% LA), which are strongly associated with leaky gut, and therefore may lead to autoimmunity.[560]

We are not aware of any studies that have compared truly ancestral diets (with naturally raised meats, organic fruits and vegetables, low omega-6, etc.) and compared those to processed food diets in terms of inducing leaky gut.

It has also been shown that the origins of autoimmunity may lie substantially in defective mitochondria[561][562] (the energy powerhouses of the cell), and we'll show how seed oils are the primary cause of mitochondrial dysfunction.[3] However, no matter what the biological mechanisms behind autoimmunity, available science has produced quite strong links between westernized diets and the induction of autoimmunity,[563] with food choices quite strongly linked to autoimmune symptoms.[564] Seed oils, through many mechanisms, are believed to play a substantial role here as well.

MAJOR CAUSE OF BLINDNESS – AGE-RELATED MACULAR DEGENERATION – IS YET ANOTHER SEED OIL CATASTROPHE

Age-related macular degeneration (AMD) is a degenerative condition of the central retina known as the macula, which leads to central vision loss as the disease progresses. This disease is the leading cause of irreversible vision loss and blindness in people over the age of 60 worldwide.[565] In developed countries, AMD is the leading cause of irreversible vision loss in people over the age of 50.[566]

But could vision loss be caused by westernized diets and, particularly, seed oils, as well? This is the question that changed my life. After studying AMD and related chronic diseases in relation to diets for more than a decade, the short answer is, yes. In fact, a resounding yes. And I'm an ophthalmologist who has treated many thousands of patients with macular degeneration. But, before we dig further, let's pause for a moment and – if you're not familiar with the profoundly devastating disease of AMD – take a look at what this tragic disease may do to the vision of those afflicted (see the simulation below).

AMD is currently rampant in the U.S., with approximately 27.9% (nearly 1 in 3) of those over the age of 75 to 80 having the condition, while about 8.8% (1 in 11) of those over age 52 have the disease.[567] However, much like coronary heart disease, in the United States, AMD became increasingly more common after about 1930, elevating to epidemic proportions by the 1970s to 1990s.[4]

The clinical hallmarks of the disease are now recognized in at least one-third of persons over the age of 75 in developed countries.[569] In the year 2020, it was estimated that 196 million people in the world were affected with AMD, with that number expected to rise to 288 million by 2040.[568] Prior to 2006, the WHO had already conservatively estimated that, globally, at least 14 million individual people were already either bilaterally blind or severely visually impaired due to AMD.[569]

Orthodox, allopathic medicine holds that AMD is primarily a disease of aging and genetics,[570] with one estimate suggesting that 46% to 71% of the disease may be attributed to genetics alone.[571] And as written in a recent paper, "Currently, there is neither a cure nor a means to prevent AMD."[569]

We beg to differ. We believe that AMD, just like all of the other chronic diseases, is virtually entirely preventable, and it is also treatable with ancestral diets.

If AMD were a disease of aging and genetics, which is the theory that allopathic medicine and ophthalmology have espoused since at least the mid-20th century, then we should observe that the prevalence of disease, on a per capita basis and for individuals of the same age, should be roughly the same today as it were 100 years ago, correct?

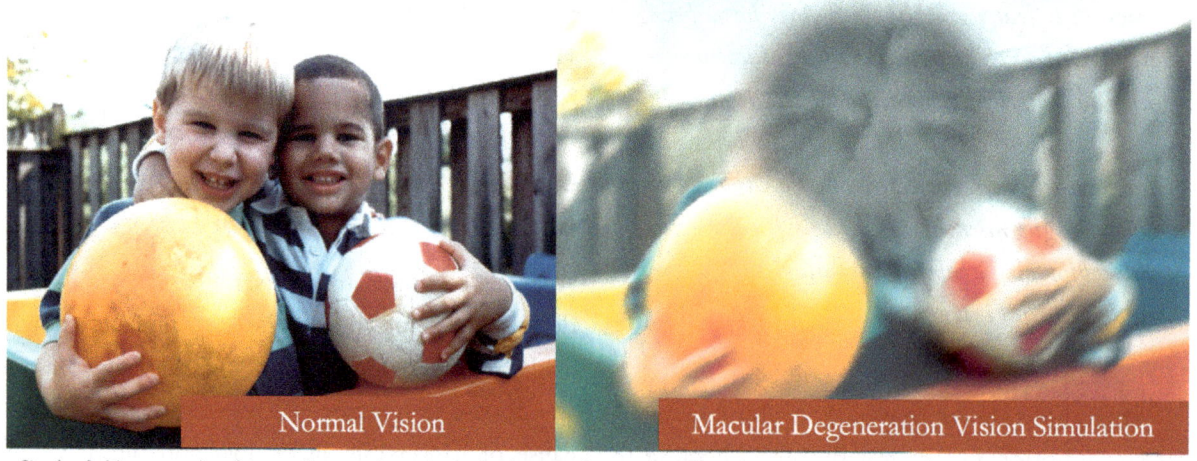

Simulated vision comparison for normal versus advanced age-related macular degeneration (AMD). Image courtesy of the NIH, National Eye Institute Media Library, https://medialibrary.nei.nih.gov/. © C. Knobbe, 2022. Ancestral Health Foundation. Cure AMD Foundation.

Even the most aggressive analysis suggests that only around 7 percent of our genes have undergone any degree of evolvement over the past 5,000 years.[572] This is only an "evolution" of about 0.14% of our genes per century of time, or as little as 0.07% per 50 years. And perhaps a substantial degree of this is within the realm of epigenetics, which is the "turning on" or "turning off" – regulation – of genes, which can generationally affect our offspring.[573] With that said, let's look very briefly at the history of AMD, as we have many other chronic diseases.

Standing in stark contrast to the epidemic proportions of AMD today, an intensive historical review of medical literature from the 19th and early 20th centuries shows that AMD was a medical rarity, with cases of the condition rarely to have been reported despite common reviews of numerous other retinal disorders.[4, 574, 575, 576, 577, 578, 579, 580] In fact, between the years of 1851, when the ophthalmoscope was first introduced (and AMD and other retinal diseases became discoverable), and 1930, there were no more than about 50 cases of AMD in all the world's literature.[4, 575] That's right. No more than about 50 cases in an 80-year period of time. Yet there are 196 million cases today.[568]

While AMD was rare before 1930, prevalence began to noticeably rise in the U.S. and U.K. beginning in the 1930s,[581, 582] and subsequently elevated to epidemic proportions by the 1970s and beyond.[583, 584, 585, 586] Most developed countries have followed suit in recent decades with sharply rising prevalence of AMD.[4, 568, 587]

In our research, we've tracked the consumption of sugar and highly polyunsaturated seed oils (mostly soybean, corn, canola, cottonseed, rapeseed, grapeseed, sunflower, safflower, rice bran, and a few others) over time and tracked the prevalence of macular degeneration. In general, what we've noted in every nation that consumes seed oils to any significant extent, particularly beyond 25 years of consumption, AMD prevalence rises in parallel to increasing seed oil consumption.[4, 591]

In the South Pacific island countries of Samoa, Solomon Islands, and Kiribati, high PUFA seed oil consumption has remained very close to zero since 1961, and AMD remains an extreme medical rarity – approximately 0.2%, or 1 in 500 people over the age of 60.[4, 591] Kiribati, an island country in the central Pacific with a population of about 115,000, had virtually zero high-PUFA seed oil consumption but moderately high sugar consumption, ranging from about 80 to 120 grams/day (320 to 480 cal/day) since 1961, yet still had about 0.2% AMD prevalence (about 1 in 500 people over age 60).[4, 591] Again, contrast this to AMD prevalence rates of at least 1 in 11 people in the U.S. over the age of 52[567] and comparable numbers in most developed countries.

In the graph on p. 149 ("AMD Prevalence vs. PUFA Oil Average Consumption"), prepared by my colleague researcher, Ronnie Sommer, MSc, engineering physicist from Stockholm, Sweden, we observe that there is a strong correlation between seed oil consumption and AMD prevalence. In statistical language, the *Pearson correlation coefficient for our data on seed oil consumption in countries versus AMD prevalence is: r(34) = 0.78, which we would call strong.*[3]

A perfect positive correlation of 1.0 represents a 1:1 relationship, which would exist, for example, when an antibiotic is given in a dose which cures 100% of the treated population. In this case, there is a perfect correlation that moves in lockstep between the two variables. On the other hand, a perfect negative 1.0 correlation would exist when two variables move in lockstep but opposite directions. In medicine, we rarely see positive or negative correlations that approach a perfect +1.0 or -1.0; they're usually somewhere in between. A correlation of zero (0.0) means there is no relationship between the two variables.

To give further credence to the strength of this correlation between high PUFA seed oils and AMD, government statisticians in England made correlations between smoking and lung cancer, and a scatterplot (same as shown in the graph on p. 149, "AMD Prevalence vs. PUFA Oil Average Consumption), found a moderately strong linear correlation, with a correlation coefficient of 0.716.[588] The strongest correlations between cigarette smoking and lung cancer have reached values up to 0.989, which is exceedingly strong.[589] These values, however, require at least 24 to 26 years of lag time between smoking onset and lung cancer, which is exactly what we see with "exposure" to substantial seed oil consumption and AMD development.[4]

With this data in mind, we suggest that the correlation between increasing consumption of vegetable oils and the development of AMD is at least a "moderately strong positive correlation," if we base this on the statisticians' characterization for this degree of correlation.[590] Unquestionably, there are other factors, even though seed oil consumption likely accounts for 80% or more of the risk, in our opinion. Where does the other risk come from? This is where many other factors of the diet come into play, including protection via vitamin and mineral nutrient-density, protective factors against seed oil consumption (e.g., carnosine, vitamin E, etc.), not smoking, exposure to the sun (for vitamin D), genetic susceptibility factors, and many other potential factors, both known and unknown.[3,4,591]

With five years of anecdotal evidence, we've observed that the great majority of patients who adopt strict ancestral diets will enjoy the benefit of halting progression of the dry form of AMD disease (Note: for those with wet AMD, anti-VEGF injections are critical to prevent devastating vision loss and we strongly advise each individual to follow their ophthalmologist's advice on medical/surgical management). For those with further interest in preventing or treating AMD, I have published a book under the title, *Ancestral Dietary Strategy to Prevent and Treat Macular Degeneration*,[591] as well as scientific papers on the subject (and additional manuscripts in the works pending publication).

A final word on AMD before we move on... if you think that your diet could not affect your eyes, your vision, and thus, your life, think again. If you follow a typical 'Standard American Diet' (SAD), and you live to be 52 years of age, your chance of developing AMD is 1 in 11. And if you follow a SAD diet and are still fortunate enough to be alive at age 75 to 80, your likelihood of developing AMD and losing at least some vision to this disease is nearly 1 in 3. Don't take the chance. Severe and irreversible vision loss and blindness are generally the most devastating loss of all, worse than losing a limb or two.

Every shred of evidence that I have uncovered over nearly 11 years of research and investigation leads me to believe that AMD is entirely preventable with any ancestral diet.[3,4,591] Furthermore, the anecdotal evidence continues to mount that instituting an ancestral diet once dry AMD has begun may hold progression in check. There is no other truly worthwhile treatment for dry AMD, including any known supplement on the planet.[3,4,591]

AMD Prevalence vs. PUFA Oil Average Consumption

AMD values based on consumption data 25 or more years back.
Demonstrably faulty points removed.

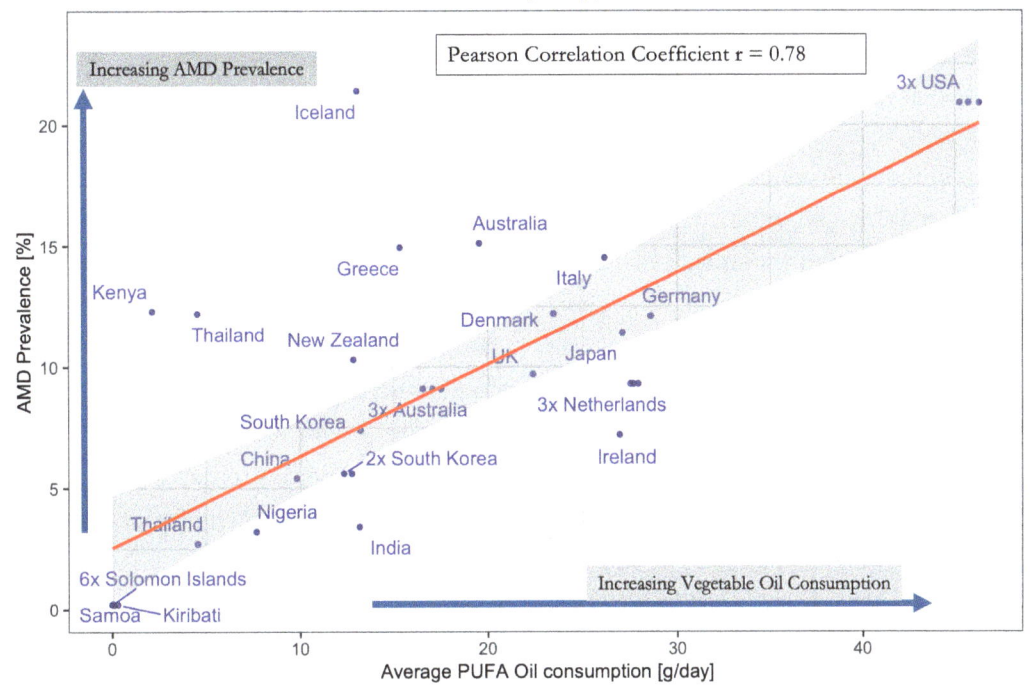

Pearson Correlation Coefficient r = 0.78

Knobbe CA, Sommer R, Richer SP, Freilich BD, Kent D, Cripps JR, Reynolds TM, Dito JJ, Walgama JP, Hunter JD, Henderson T, Stojanoska M, Barry JT, Kiwara AL, Ross RD, Kaushal S, Ham K, Jaffery SMA, Luff AK. Westernized Diet, Vegetable Oil, Nutrient Deficiency and Omega-6 Apocalypse: Can We Explain Age-Related Macular Degeneration and Associated Chronic Diseases – Coronary Heart Disease, Cancers, Metabolic Disease, Diabetes, Obesity, and More – With a Unifying Dietary Hypothesis? Manuscript submitted for publication. University of Texas Southwestern Medical Center, Dallas. Data wrangling, statistical analyses, and graph courtesy of Ronnie Sommer, MSc., Stockholm, Sweden. U.S. Copyright C. Knobbe, 2022. Ancestral Health Foundation.

ARE RARE DISEASES BECOMING MORE COMMON DUE TO PROCESSED FOODS AND SEED OIL CONSUMPTION?

Rare diseases are classified by the National Institutes of Health (NIH) as conditions affecting fewer than 200,000 people in the U.S.[592] This definition was created by the U.S. Congress at the time of the Orphan Drug Act of 1983. In the European Union, a disease is defined as rare if it affects less than 1 in 2,000 people.

There may now be as many as 7,000 rare diseases or even more.[592] In fact, there are now 25-30 million people in the U.S. living with so-called rare diseases. Today, 1 in 17 people is affected by a rare disease, which amounts to 3.5 million people in the U.K. and 30 million people across Europe. The Orphanet database, which maintains comprehensive records on the incidence of rare diseases, affirms that somewhere between 263 to 446 million people (3.5-5.9%) globally are living with any one of these rare diseases.[593] For the enormous majority of these diseases, there is no treatment.[592]

Many of these rare diseases, including numerous birth defects, rare cancers, childhood cancers, and a number of autoimmune diseases, are known to have no genetic inheritance.[592] However, 71.9% of rare diseases are known to be secondary to changes in genes or chromosomes.[593] The suggestion that these diseases are relatively new to humanity lies in the fact that 69.9% of such rare diseases are of pediatric-onset.[593]

And in the cases with a known genetic influence, the underlying cause of the genetic alterations remains obscure. In fact, Orphanet researchers in France have concluded that "Rare diseases are numerous, heterogeneous in nature, and geographically disparate. Few are preventable or curable, most are chronic and many result in early death."[593] They refer further to the glut of rare diseases as "an emerging global public health priority."[593]

Thus, the question becomes, are many or most of these rare disorders relatively new to the human race? Could these disorders have emerged almost entirely in the face of the combined nutrient deficiencies and toxicities of modernized, processed foods? It is our belief that this is not only likely, but exceedingly so. Furthermore, just as E.V. McCollum and Weston A. Price both found in the early 20th century, substitution of 'vegetable fats' for healthy animal fats led to birth defects, abnormal growth, and early demise. The same situation likely holds true for the thousands of rare diseases that seem to be emerging 'out of nowhere.'

BUT DOESN'T LOW LIFE EXPECTANCY IN THE 19TH AND EARLY 20TH CENTURIES ACCOUNT FOR LOW CHRONIC DISEASE PREVALENCE DURING THAT ERA?

Consider a hypothetical population in which 40% of the children die at two years of age, but the other 60% of the population survives to age 80; for this population, the life expectancy at birth (LEB) is only 48.8 years. This example is strongly indicative of the situation in most of the world in the 19th century, including the U.S. Consider another example in which a man lives to be 70, his wife lives to age 80, but their only child dies in infancy; the average lifespan of this population of three people is just 50 years. This represents a common family tragedy in the 19th century all around the world.

We have heard many intelligent physicians, health practitioners, and even a few experts in epidemiology mistakenly conclude that populations with an average LEB of 50, to have very few old people. Yet nothing could be further from the truth. In fact, we are not aware of even a single population at any point in history in which people just mysteriously became old and died around age 50 or even before age 60.

To understand this concept, we must first understand the difference between lifespan, perhaps better termed "maximum lifespan," and "life expectancy at birth" (LEB).[594 595] LEB is the average for all people in a population including those who die just after childbirth, those who die in childhood, those who die in early adulthood, as well as death in old age.

Maximum lifespan is an individual-specific concept, and represents an upper bound rather than an average. The oldest confirmed age for any human is currently 122 years and 164 days, which was the age at death for the French-born Jeanne Calment, who lived from 1875 to 1997.[596] This is likely the absolute maximum lifespan for humans.

In the year 1900, the average age of death in the U.S. was 49.3 years. To this, many people mistakenly assert that 'people didn't live long enough to develop heart disease, cancers, Alzheimer's disease, and other chronic diseases back in the 19th century.' Having understood the examples set forth in the beginning of this section, perhaps now the following will quickly dispel the myths that people somehow mysteriously 'became old and died around age 50.'

In the year 1800, 43.3% of children worldwide

did not survive the first five years of life.[597] A century later, surviving childhood wasn't much better. In 1900, 36.2% of children didn't survive to see their fifth birthday.[597] In the U.S. in 1800, 46.3% of children died before their 5th birthday, but the rate of early childhood death dropped in half by 1900, to 23.9%.[598] Even in France, 22.5% of children born in 1900 did not survive to their 5th birthday.

In 1800, the average woman gave birth to 5 to 7 children, but could expect to lose 2 or 3 of those children in the first few years of life, as this was the norm across the world.[597] In the U.S. in 1900, the risk of death in childbirth was about 0.85% per birth;[599] therefore, if a woman gave birth to five children, the risk of death in childbirth for that mother would have been about 4.25%.

Thus, in the U.S., in the year 1900, if only including early childhood mortality (death before age five years) and young mothers' death in childbirth, about 28.15% of the population died very young. But as can be seen in Figure 3.1, as of 2019, global childhood morality (death before five years of age) has dropped to 3.9%.[597] In the U.S. childhood mortality dropped to 0.65% as of 2019.[597]

Researchers Anthony Volk and Jeremy Atkinson examined 20 hunter-gatherer populations and broad historical data for infant and child mortality, finding that "approximately 27% of infants failed to survive their first year of life, while approximately 47.5% of children failed to survive to puberty.."[600]

Researchers Michael Gurven and Hillard Kaplan published a scientific review that examined the "mortality profiles obtained from small-scale hunter-gatherer and horticultural populations from around the world," and determined that the typical "adaptive" lifespan of our human ancestors was 68 to 78 years.[601] They also determined that the modal (most common) age of death for hunter-gatherers who survived past the age of 15, was 72 years.

In the graph on p. 152 from Our World In Data, we see the survival curve for England and Wales, with graph lines for years 1851 to 2011.[602] As one can see, between the years of 1851 and 1931, there is an extremely high mortality in the first three years of life, but for those who survive past age 5, mortality begins to level off dramatically. We also observe that in the years 1851, 1871, and 1891, almost exactly 20% (one out of five) people survived past the age of 73 years. In 1911, 30% of the population (nearly one in three) survived past the age of 73 and 20% survived past the age of 77.[602]

While life expectancy in Great Britain in 1900 was about 47 for a man and 50 for a woman,[603] it is a great fallacy that many people dropped dead around age 50. In fact, as can be seen in the graph on p. 152 ("The survival curve for England & Wales"), even in 1891, 50% of the population was still alive past age 52, 30% past age 66, 20% past 73, and about 5% past age 85. In 1911, about 64% of the population was alive past age 50, 53% past age 60, 36% past age 70, and about 15% past age 80.[602]

Much further evidence from Our World In Data confirms that, during the 70-year period between 1850 and 1920, many, many millions of people survived past age 65 and, in fact, well into old age both in the U.S. and the U.K.[602] This was a time, of course, when infectious diseases took the lives of most people, but also when obesity, overweight, coronary heart disease, and many other chronic diseases were medical rarities.

All of this evidence should shatter any belief system that lack of chronic diseases in the late 19th and early 20th centuries was due to low life expectancy.

CHAPTER 3

FIG. 3.1

Global child mortality
Share of the world population dying and surviving the first 5 years of life.

Share of people surviving past age 5 years

Share surviving first 5 years of life

Share of children dying before age 5 years

Share dying in first 5 years

Source: Gapminder and the World Bank

OurWorldInData.org/a-history-of-global-living-conditions-in-5-charts/ • CC BY-SA

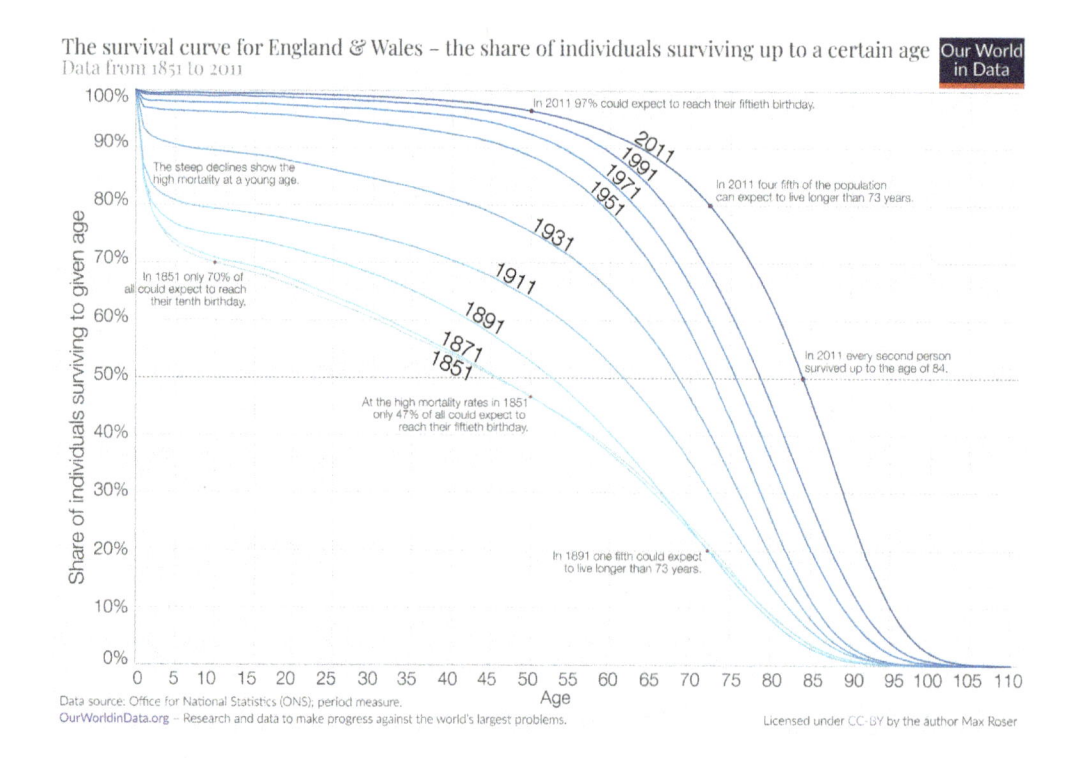

The survival curve for England & Wales – the share of individuals surviving up to a certain age
Data from 1851 to 2011

The steep declines show the high mortality at a young age.

In 2011 97% could expect to reach their fiftieth birthday.

In 2011 four fifth of the population can expect to live longer than 73 years.

In 1851 only 70% of all could expect to reach their tenth birthday.

At the high mortality rates in 1851 only 47% of all could expect to reach their fiftieth birthday.

In 2011 every second person survived up to the age of 84.

In 1891 one fifth could expect to live longer than 73 years.

Data source: Office for National Statistics (ONS); period measure.
OurWorldInData.org – Research and data to make progress against the world's largest problems.
Licensed under CC-BY by the author Max Roser

CAN WE BLAME "BAD GENES" FOR INCREASING CHRONIC DISEASE?

There has obviously been a near obsession within the scientific community relating to the genetics of chronic disease.[604] As of 2016, more than 566,000 papers had been published related to the genetics of chronic disease, and about 72,000 papers related to the relationship between "exposure" and chronic disease.[604] That's a ratio of about 8 to 1 in favor of genetics as the primary concern of chronic disease.

The Human Genome Project (HGP), which was launched in 1990, took 13 years to complete at an estimated cost of $2.7 billion U.S. dollars.[605] The lofty major goal of the National Human Genome Research Institute (a division of the NIH), which completed the genome project, was "to discover the genetic basis for health and the pathology of human disease."[605]

Yet today, while some researchers laud "the incredible impact on the elucidation of the genetic architecture of disease,"[606] a New York Times article appropriately confirms that the "genetic map yields few new cures."[607] Interestingly, in 1991, one published researcher accurately predicted the outcome of the Human Genome Project when he wrote, "Genome mapping and sequencing projects are inappropriate and wasteful expenditures of precious research funds."[608]

Theodore Friedmann, MD, physician, researcher, and director of the University of California-San Diego Program in Gene Therapy, has been deeply involved in the study of "gene therapy" since its inception a few decades ago. Gene therapy is a field of study which seeks to alter or replace abnormal or dysfunctional genes or induce production of proteins that defective genes cannot produce. However, "cures" with gene therapy are practically nonexistent.

In a review article published in the journal Biotechnology Healthcare in 2005, senior contributor author, Jack McCain, wrote, "Friedmann sees gene therapy today at a point comparable to the early days of organ transplantation, when successes were scarce and failures frequent.

Even the first clear successes of gene therapy, he notes, have "been muted by the emergence of three cases of leukemia (including one death) among the 18 children who were treated."[609] In the same paper, McCain also stated, "… you can count the number of clearly effective gene therapies in nonexperimental clinical use with your nose. That's right – there's one [a gene therapy for head and neck squamous cell cancer, available in China]. And you have to go halfway around the world to get it."[609]

As of 2015, in the most extensive review of trials for gene therapy that we are aware of, a total of approximately 164 patients had been treated with gene therapy and remained under review.[610] It remains obvious still today, in 2022, that little benefit has been produced by the vast amount of genetic research.[611] It is our view that the obsessive interest, expenditure, and research in gene therapy has primarily served to further distract allopathic medicine from the true underlying cause of the vast majority of chronic disease, which is processed food consumption.

In college and medical school, we physicians are taught that, for the most part, our genes are our destiny.[612] In other words, our genotype or DNA "blueprint," controls our phenotype, which is our body habitus, development, and destiny for disease. But this is far from the truth. As Weston A. Price showed in the 1930s and 1940s, our genes are not our destiny.[28]

Our genetic blueprint is indeed critical, but as Price found, even when the parents were genetically normal, the consumption of processed foods by the parents produced birth anomalies (defects), while consumption of processed foods in infancy and childhood produced abnormal growth and physical development and, of course, the same modernized, processed, nutrient-deficient foods produced physical degeneration in adults. Thus, the belief that genes per se directly control destiny is fatally flawed. A more accurate description is that genes control destiny, to a degree, but are subject to control, i.e., being turned on or off (expressed), by the presence of various nutrients – primarily vitamins.

This fundamental concept is the study of epigenetics, and it is critical to understand that the regulation of genes – often termed expression – has not only been implicated "in all major chronic diseases affecting humans," but that "the epigenetic signal is heritable," which means that our nutrition can positively or negatively impact our children.[613] Epigenetics is a factor from before conception, during embryogenesis, fetal development, infancy, childhood, and every step of the way through old age and death.[614]

Epigenetics characterizes the process of genes becoming active or inactive in response to needs, stresses, environment, growth, and particularly, the presence of nutrients, for example, vitamins and mineral co-factors. In other words, our bodies are not pre-destined from birth; in fact, in many ways, it's nearly the opposite. Our genetic expression is greatly under our control – and how do we control that in the most beneficial way? With proper nutrition, that is, the proper and abundant supply of vitamins, minerals, and a full complement of amino acids.[615] [616]

For example, folate (vitamin B9), has been extensively studied for its effects on DNA methylation, which acts to affect gene expression.[617] Deficiency of folate in mothers during gestation is known to create much higher risk of neural tube defects, such as spina bifida.[615] Infants born with spina bifida have defects of the spinal cord, which may result in permanent weakness or paralysis of the legs, among other complications.

Other examples of nutrients that are important in epigenetic expression of DNA include vitamin B12, methionine, choline, and betaine.[615] Poor nutrition and socioeconomically disadvantaged parents have been shown to be more likely to give birth to infants with abnormal phenotypes (physical characteristics), birth defects, and greater risk of diabetes and heart disease.[618] [619] [620] [621] [622]

However, if chronic diseases are a product of our DNA and we're genetically programmed to develop chronic disease, then the chronic diseases should have been just as prevalent a century ago, on an age-adjusted basis, right? However, as we've seen, most every chronic disease and perhaps even many of the rare diseases have all had a major onslaught since the 19th century.

Supporting this argument, Stephen Rappaport, PhD, Professor Emeritus of the University of California Berkeley, analyzed genetic factors in chronic disease, finding: "Since heart disease and cancer are the two leading causes of mortality in Western Europe (and worldwide)... then 0.25 million of the 1.53 million cancer and heart-disease deaths (16.4%) can be attributed to G-related [genetic-related] factors."[623] The genetics of cancers, in fact, tended to have the lowest genetic risk (about 8.26% genetic risk with "exposure" accounting for more than 90% of the risk), leading Rappaport to state that the totality of evidence casts "further doubt on the notion that our inherited genomes are the primary causes of chronic diseases."[623]

Ignoring such evidence as above, others might

ask, could our DNA blueprint have changed in the past century? Could new genetic mutations have developed that were passed down through the generations, programming us to develop chronic disease? Let's examine this possibility even further, disregarding the evidence of such low genetic risk in chronic disease as discovered by Rappaport.

S. Boyd Eaton, MD and Melvin Konnor, PhD, in their scientific paper entitled "Paleolithic Nutrition" published in 1985, wrote the following:

"The human genetic constitution has changed relatively little since the appearance of truly modern human beings, Homo sapiens sapiens, about 40,000 years ago. Even the development of agriculture 10,000 years ago has apparently had minimal influence on our genes."[624]

The distinguished paleontologist, Stephen Jay Gould, boldly stated, "There's been no biological change in humans in 40,000 to 50,000 years. Everything we call culture and civilization we've built with the same body and brain."[625]

However, some evolutionary biologists strongly oppose this position, arguing that "human evolution has accelerated in the past 10,000 years, rather than slowing or stopping, and is now happening about 100 times faster than its long-term average over the 6 million years of our existence."[626] But to our knowledge, no reputable scientists have argued that our DNA "blueprint," without the effects of epigenetics, has changed in the last century, which is precisely the time frame that obesity and chronic diseases have increased exponentially.

David Grimes, MD, of the Blackburn Royal Infirmary, may have summed it up best in regards to the onslaught of chronic diseases when he wrote, "… it is obvious that an epidemic [of coronary heart disease] cannot be due to faulty genes, which have a stable prevalence over a long period of time. However, genes can have an influence on susceptibility…"[269]

This is precisely the case with what we observe with CHD, cancers, type 2 diabetes, obesity, Alzheimer's disease, age-related macular degeneration, and so on. It's been our "environment" that has caused epidemics of chronic disease and by far and away, the most important component of our environment is our food.

So, where does seed oil overconsumption fit into all of this? Though every single vitamin and mineral in appropriate amounts is critical to our growth, development, and maintenance of health in adulthood, it is perhaps the fat-soluble vitamins A, D, and K which are the most important to us during all stages of life.[28][627]

The substitution of seed oils for animal fats, as we've reviewed, has substantially displaced the consumption of these fat-soluble vitamins, thereby leaving large percentages of populations undernourished and on the brink of depletion of these critical nutrients. Furthermore, high omega-6 LA consumption drives a pro-oxidative, pro-inflammatory, and toxic biological milieu, markedly promoting a dangerous biological environment. This is the recipe for birth defects, anomalous growth and development, and, of course, physical degeneration in adulthood.

CHAPTER 3: SUMMARY

Between 1900 and 2018, obesity has risen from 1.2% to 42.5% in the U.S., which is an increase of 35-fold. During this same period of time, seed oil consumption elevated from 2 g/day in 1900 to 80g/day by 2010. And while it's been fashionable to blame sugar for obesity and chronic disease in the last few decades, sugar consumption in the U.S. has been on the decline since at least 2004, while obesity rose from 33% at that time to 42.5% in 2018.

"Low-carb" diets have also been greatly espoused in recent decades, however, carbohydrate consumption has been on the decline since 1997 in the U.S., while obesity has escalated markedly. There is similar evidence in the U.K., Australia, and Japan (to be reviewed).

In the year 2000, the U.S. had (and still has) the highest obesity (36.1%) of all developed (OECD) countries and we have the highest seed oil consumption on a per capita basis of any country in the world. Vietnam has the lowest obesity in the world (0.2% in 2000) and has the 2nd lowest seed oil consumption in the world.

Developed countries have higher obesity than developing countries, on average, at 13.1%, and have much higher seed oil consumption than developing countries, who have an average obesity of 8.4%. The world, at large, falls neatly in between these two.

Diabetes in the U.S. rose from 0.0028% in 1890 to 0.37% in 1935 and then progressively elevated to a staggering 13.0% by 2016, an increase of 4,643-fold in the 126-year period between 1890 and 2016. During this same period, seed oil consumption continued an unmitigated ascent. Sugar consumption, however, as a percentage of total calories, increased from 10.8% in 1890 to 22.5% in 1935, to a high of 27.4% in 2000, and then dropped to 24.0% in 2016.

With this evidence, we see, for example, in 1935, that sugar consumption was 22.5% of total calories, but diabetes was only 0.37%. And in 2016, when sugar consumption was just 1.5% higher (as a percent of total calories), the prevalence of diabetes had increased to 13.0%, which is a 3,400% (35-fold) increase compared to 1935.

Furthermore, carbohydrate consumption in the U.S. has been falling since 1997 and sugar consumption falling since 2004, as previously reviewed, while diabetes elevated from 2.97% in 1993 to 13.0% by 2016. Thus, diabetes correlates very strongly with seed oil consumption as seen here, however, there is little to no evidence that carbohydrate consumption is associated with type 2 diabetes.[628][629][630][631]

There are mixed results between sugar consumption and diabetes in the scientific literature, with correlations in studies ranging from positive (more sugar, more diabetes) to negative (higher sugar intake and lower diabetes risk).[632] Still we see little if any correlation in our studies and, in fact, even negative correlations (sugar falling while diabetes escalates), which has been observed elsewhere. Once again, seed oils deserve the enormous bulk of the blame for the diabetes epidemic and perhaps all of it.

Metabolic syndrome, which is generally described as a cluster of disorders that includes hypertension, abnormal blood lipids, insulin resistance, abnormal blood sugars, and visceral (organ-related) obesity, was first described in 1921. The disorder escalated to affect 40% of Americans by 2006 and by the years 2009-2016, 88% of Americans could not meet five criteria of metabolic health: blood sugar, triglycerides, HDL, blood pressure, and waist circumference, without medications.

Autoimmune diseases, while we cannot be certain were rare a century ago, appear to have been dramatically less common. Since the 1980s, evidence that autoimmune diseases have risen dramatically is undeniable, currently with about one out of six adult Americans affected by an autoimmune disorder.

Age-related macular degeneration (AMD), which is the leading cause of irreversible vision loss and blindness in people over the age of 60 worldwide today, was documented in no more than about 50 cases worldwide between the years 1851, when it was first discoverable, and 1920. Currently, AMD affects around 196 million people and is expected to affect 288 million by 2040. Around 14 million people worldwide today either have severe vision loss or are bilaterally blind due to AMD.

It is clear that many, many millions of people lived well into their elder years in the 19th and early 20th centuries and, therefore, we cannot blame low life expectancy on the lack of chronic disease at any point in our past. Nor can we blame our DNA, which is relatively immutable over long periods of time. However, to a degree, we can indict abnormal gene function, i.e., epigenetics, but we must understand that our own individual epigenetic condition is greatly influenced by nutrition.

Certainly, all of us have genetic predispositions that make us more susceptible to the development of one disease condition or another, but for perhaps 99.9% of all chronic disease conditions, we only inherit susceptibilities to those conditions, not the condition itself.

The genetic susceptibility to chronic disease requires an "environmental factor" to produce the disease, and that environmental factor almost always rests within the nuances of a westernized diet and lifestyle. More than anything genetically inherited, what we "inherit" from our parents is a way of eating, and we should recognize this and modify our diets accordingly.

In each and every chronic disease condition that we've reviewed, there is a strong correlation with seed oil consumption. There is also generally no correlation with carbohydrate consumption and mixed results with sugar consumption. So while it is clear that processed foods are to blame for chronic disease, we must indict and convict seed oils for the great majority of such disease.

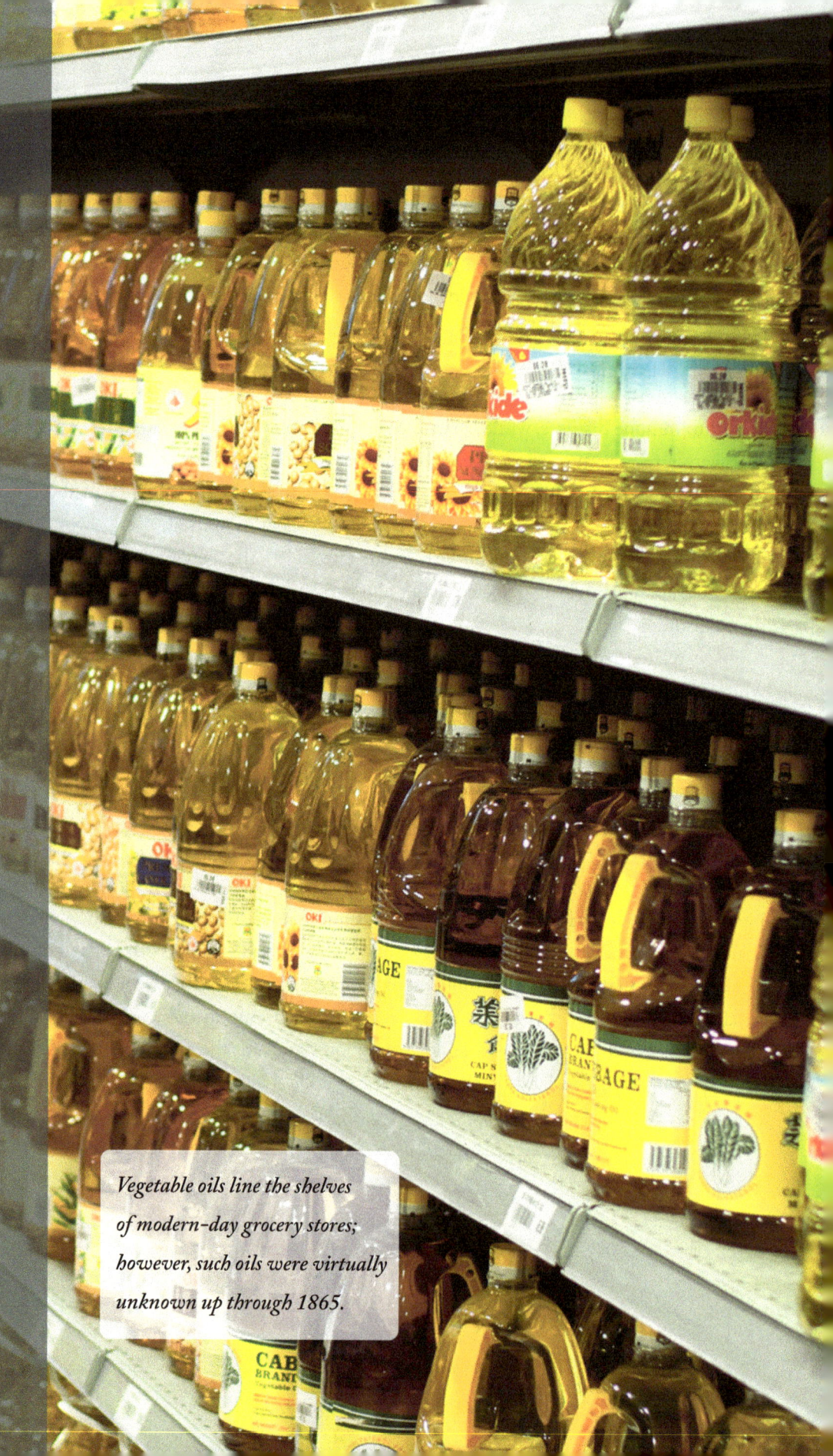

CHAPTER 4

Vegetable oils line the shelves of modern-day grocery stores; however, such oils were virtually unknown up through 1865.

CHAPTER 4

THE DISCOVERY – HOW AND WHY LINOLEIC ACID MAY BE HARMING YOU

"The history of modern knowledge is concerned in no small degree with man's attempt to escape from his previous concepts."

— SIR HAROLD HIMSWORTH

CHAPTER 4

Eleven years ago this year, I had a remarkable, but incomplete recovery of my own arthritis following relatively minor dietary tweaks that removed some food groups. For the moment, I won't mention the foods I removed as it might unintentionally vilify foods that are blameless. Today, following more than ten years of investigation, research, and experience, I have now been enlightened as to a fundamentally critical concept in nutrition: Removal of foods is virtually always associated with the addition of other foods – and the latter can be just as, or more important, than the former.

Concerning my own diet and arthritis and my own personal experience beginning eleven years ago at the time of this writing, in a period of ten days on a partial Paleo type diet, the relentlessly progressive arthritis I'd suffered with for 16 long years, improved by about 80 percent – and off of my usual arthritis medications. This was so shocking – so transformative – it literally changed the entire course of my life. At that point, my journey to understand nutrition began.

Within a couple of years from that point in time, I began to understand with much deeper comprehension how processed foods are the root cause of so many forms of chronic disease. I had also discovered the works of Weston A. Price. As an ophthalmologist, that finally led me to a plaguing question in my own mind: Could westernized diets be the primary cause of age-related macular degeneration (AMD)?

AMD is the leading cause of irreversible vision loss and blindness in people over the age of 60, worldwide. I investigated the plaguing question in my mind for the next 18 months while still practicing ophthalmology, and in February of 2015, when I felt that my hypothesis "held water," I left my clinical practice as an eye surgeon (ophthalmologist, or "Eye MD") to pursue AMD research full-time.

Over the next 18 months, my team and I researched data that correlated processed food consumption to AMD prevalence in 25 nations. Our data turned out to entirely support the hypothesis and, with that, I finally went public with the theory and research in August of 2016. My debut presentation of the hypothesis and data was at the Ancestral Health Symposium (AHS) 2016, which was held at the University of Colorado Boulder.

My thesis held that, in general, processed foods were the major driver of AMD, but the most relevant, reliable, and consistent finding of our research wasn't that sugars, refined white wheat flour, or even trans fats had the most impact on the development of AMD, but instead, it was that seed oil consumption was by far the greatest culprit (of course, trans fats are derived from and are part and parcel of seed oils). This wasn't unexpected, however, as I had already developed a strong impression (in my previous five years of investigation) that this was indeed also the case for coronary heart disease (CHD), obesity, type 2 diabetes, and many other chronic diseases.

ESSENTIAL FATTY ACIDS: OMEGA-6 LA AND OMEGA-3 ALA: MUST HAVE, BUT IN SMALL AMOUNTS!

There are two fats in your diet, which are referred to as "essential." They are considered essential because these fats (fatty acids) are required for optimum health, and your body cannot synthesize them *de novo*.[1, 633, 634]

The first of the essential fats is omega-6 linoleic acid (LA) and the second is omega-3 alpha-linolenic acid (ALA).[1] In the early 20th century and up through at least the end of the 1920s, fat was known as a valuable source of energy, but it was not known that fats were required for life.[635] **E.V. McCollum had shown that animals provided with 100% vegetable oils as their only source of fat would soon fail to grow, begin to degenerate physically, and death would subsequently follow.**[148] However, the fact that fats per se were specifically required by the body was still unknown.[635]

In the early 20th century researchers 'knew' that proteins and carbohydrates were essential to the diet (based on the science of the era), but fat was not believed to be essential because it was known that fats could be synthesized in mammals from carbohydrates.

Even by the end of the 1920s, it was the opinion of the leading experts that fats were not considered essential nutrients.[635]

Then, in 1929, a relatively young and unknown assistant professor of plant physiology, George Oswald Burr, of the University of Minnesota, reported that young rats fed a fat-free diet developed a deficiency disease, which he held was caused by the absence of certain fats in the diet, and specifically not because of something else associated with fats that was missing (e.g., vitamins).[636]

Burr then clearly demonstrated that additions of just tiny amounts of the polyunsaturated fat, linoleic acid (LA), given in very small quantities of fat, cured the deficiency disease.[637] He thus termed LA an "essential fatty acid," and the term stuck. The two seminal papers, to this day, remain classics in biochemistry.

Burr's findings and evidence that supported a belief that animals could not synthesize their own omega-6 LA wasn't readily accepted. However, by the end of the 1930s, proof came that this was, in fact, true through complex (deuterium isotope radiolabeling) studies.[638][639]

Then, in 1931, Burr published another paper which reported that the omega-3 fatty acid, alpha-linolenic acid (ALA), was not synthesized in the rat, making it a second essential fat. Numerous investigations followed over the next 50 years, and today, more than 90 years later, the evidence still supports Burr's findings.[635] National Institutes of Health (NIH) researchers, Arthur Spector and Hee-Yong Kim reviewed 96 scientific papers that were related to LA and ALA as being essential fats, and concurred with Burr's original thesis.[635]

It is presently clear that in nearly any individual consuming virtually any foods prepared outside of a lab (which could potentially, but not unintentionally, create a 100% fat-free preparation), deficiency of LA will not occur.[640] In fact, it appears that essential fatty acid deficiency is essentially unknown in anyone who consumes food. This is true because, with rare exceptions, nearly all plant fats[1] and all animal fats will contain LA[641] in sufficient amounts to prevent LA deficiency on any diet in which natural foods are consumed by mouth.

In the animal experiments in which deficiency of essential fats was in question, lipid chemists James F. Mead, PhD and Armand J. Fulco, PhD, commented, "The usual procedure is to start weanling animals on an otherwise nutritionally adequate diet from which all traces of fat have been carefully removed. This is no easy task since many carbohydrates and proteins contain traces of fatty acids sufficient to supply the EFA [essential fatty acid] requirements. The problem was originally solved by Burr and Burr via the use of [alcohol] extracted casein [milk protein] as the protein and pure sucrose [sugar] as the dietary carbohydrate. Other carbohydrates such as starch can be used, however, if their fat content is completely removed."[642]

The process of removing all fat content from starches and other foods – even foods that one might think have little or 'no fat' – is a complex and intensive procedure. Even the removal of all fat and, therefore, all essential fats, from fruits, vegetables, grains, tubers (potatoes), etc., requires extraction with organic solvents such as alcohols, hexane, ethyl ether, or petroleum ether.[643] The point here is that it is extraordinarily difficult to prepare foods and remove all fats in order to create essential fatty acid deficiency. This literally can only be accomplished in a research lab. It should be clearly evident that deficiency of essential fats requires extreme circumstances.

Essential fatty acid deficiency has occurred exceedingly rarely, for example, in some infants consuming only skimmed milk, in a few individuals with chronically severe fat-malabsorption, and in those receiving parenteral (intravenous) nutrition (which has been prepared with little or no fat).[640] In such cases, when LA intake is less than about 1% of total calories in infants, the result is poor growth, a scaly dermatitis (skin rash), and an impaired immune response.[640]

Infants appear to require a bit more LA in their diet due to rapid growth, however, even in deficiency, the addition of 1% LA to the diet cures the deficiency signs and symptoms; likewise, just 1% of the diet as LA will prevent deficiency symptoms.[640]

The requirements for LA are even lower in children and adults, where only 0.5% LA is considered essential,[644] [54] and it may be as low as 0.35%.[56] LA consumption prior to the introduction of edible oils into the diet would have been based primarily on the fat of natural plants and animals, with the bulk of LA derived from the consumption of pasture-raised animals (which fed upon plants in the case of ungulates), and pork and fowl (which fed upon both plants and animals). In the U.S., the bulk of LA before the introduction of seed oils would have been provided by the consumption of beef, pork, lamb, chicken, butter, eggs, and milk.[3]

In an assessment of the lower limits of LA consumption that would still prevent LA deficiency, anthropologists John D. Speth and Katherine A. Spielmann analyzed grass-fed ungulates, including cattle, bison, deer, antelope, elk, caribou, moose, Dall sheep, and Bighorn sheep, finding that they contained an average LA content in their fat tissue of 2.3%, which would have provided the typical hunter-gatherer with an estimated 0.35% of total calories as LA.[56] Yet, there's no current evidence that even this low level of LA consumption has resulted in LA deficiency in hunter-gatherers.

For comparison, the LA content of grass-fed beef, for example, is as low as 2.01%. Thus, consumption of 100% grass-fed beef as the only source of fat in the diet should provide one with enough LA to prevent deficiency, but would also emulate the fat consumption of a typical hunter-gatherer.

Without the two essential fats, LA and ALA, in the diet of a growing mammal, which is nearly impossible to achieve except in a lab-prepared 100% fat-free diet, health begins to suffer within a few weeks, depending on age.[645] However, our current problem is not too little LA, it is entirely too much.

PARACELSUS PARAPHRASED: 'THE DOSE MAKES THE POISON'

The Swiss physician, natural philosopher, alchemist, and reformer of medicine, Theophrast Paracelsus, wrote, "All things are poison and nothing is without poison; the dose alone makes sure that a thing is not poison."[646] This is commonly reduced to, "The dose makes the poison."

Paracelsus was indeed correct: for every known nutrient required for life, there is a "dose" that falls into a "sweet spot," which is neither too high nor too low.[647] For example, we must have water – but too little or too much – and you will soon die.[648]

Oxygen, of course, is an absolute necessity for life. Just a few minutes without oxygen – and life comes to an end. But, hyperbaric oxygen therapy for more than 24 hours will likely produce oxygen toxicity ending in central nervous system damage, lung failure, and death.[649] There is, without question, an appropriate dose for all of life's requirements, whether those be nutrients, gases, or even sunlight.

When it comes to linoleic acid (LA) for an adult, the practical minimum daily requirement of 0.5% of calories equates to around 11 calories worth, or precisely 1.25 grams, which is only about one-fourth of a teaspoon! Certainly, an argument for 1% LA would be more than enough by any standards. One percent of a day's worth of calories is only about 22 calories worth of LA, or about 2.4 grams. And that is about one-half of a teaspoon.

As previously noted, we modeled American diets for the year 1865 (no seed oils available) and calculated that Americans of that era only consumed about 2.2 g of LA per day, which is rather precisely 1% of calories, i.e., 1/100th of the diet.[3] Yet today, we are consuming 29 g of LA per day in the U.S. as of 2008, which is 1/8th of the diet. This is far beyond the dose that will make LA a toxin – a poison, if you will – which will devastate our health in incomprehensible ways (see figure on page 164).

Using the 1% LA as the minimum, we could achieve the required LA consumption for one day's

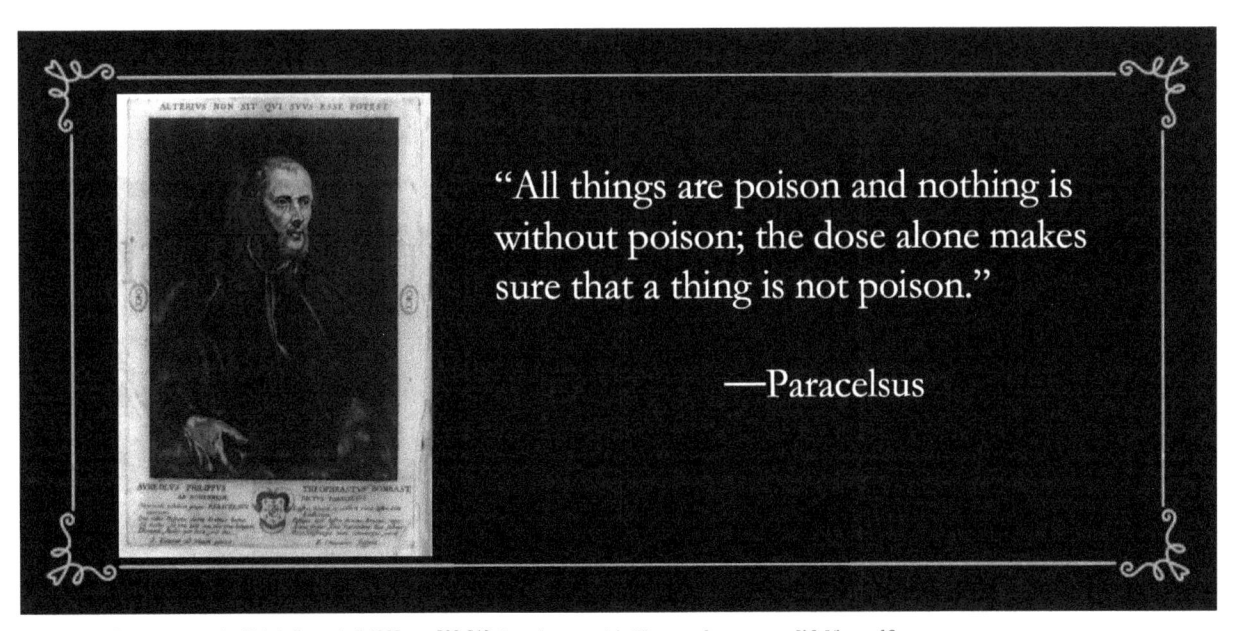

> "All things are poison and nothing is without poison; the dose alone makes sure that a thing is not poison."
>
> —Paracelsus

Theophrast Paracelsus: works. Vol. 2, Darmstadt 1965, pp. 508-513. Paracelsus, portrait by Tintoretto. Image courtesy U.S. Library of Congress.
© C. Knobbe, Ancestral Health Foundation, 2021. All rights reserved.

U.S. Om-6 LA Consumption 1865 to 2008: Optimal ≤ 2% of Energy

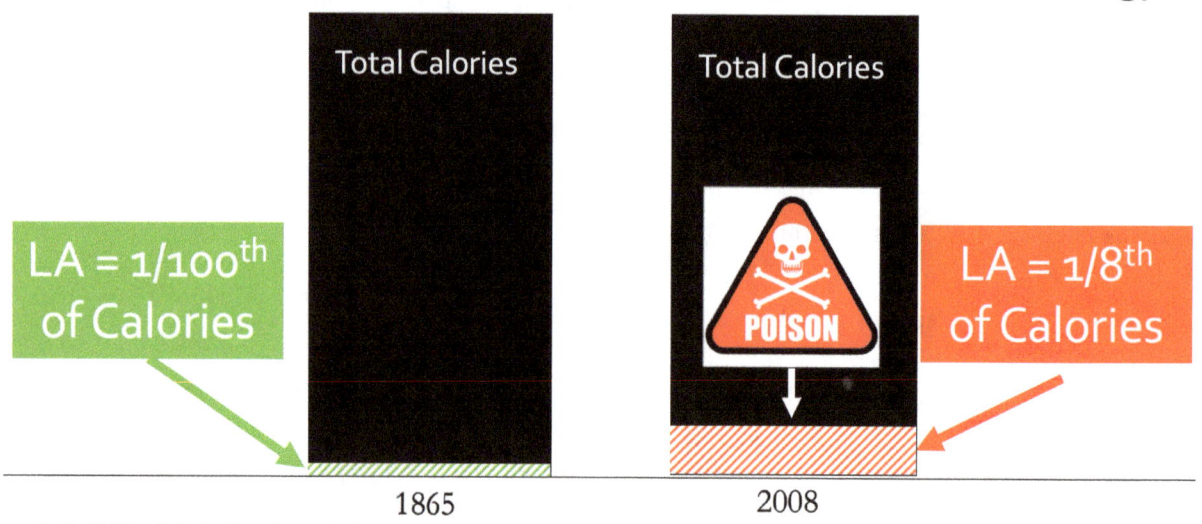

[Figure: Bar chart comparing Total Calories in 1865 (LA = 1/100th of Calories) vs. 2008 (LA = 1/8th of Calories, marked with POISON symbol)]

Knobbe CA, Richer SP, Freilich BD, et al. Westernized Diet, Omega-6 Rich Vegetable Oils, and Nutrient-Deficient Diets: Epidemiologic Evidence and Pathophysiologic Mechanisms for Age-Related Macular Degeneration and Associated Chronic Diseases. Manuscript submitted for publication. University of Texas Southwestern Medical Center, Dallas, U.S., 2022. 2) Guyenet SJ, Carlson SE. Increase in Adipose Tissue Linoleic Acid of US Adults in the Last Half Century. Advances in Nutrition. 2015;6(6):660-664.
© C. Knobbe, Ancestral Health Foundation, 2021. All rights reserved.

worth of calories (assuming 2250 calories/day) with just 5 grams of soybean oil (about 51-56% LA by weight), which is about one teaspoon worth of oil. This is true, even if this was the only fat consumed in the entire diet and the fat of every other food was entirely removed with alcohol extraction. However, it would require more than 100 grams (more than 3 ounces) of grass-fed beef fat (at 2.01% LA), for example, to achieve the daily requirement of LA.

The requirement for omega-3 ALA is even less than LA, but how much less is uncertain. If a diet is deficient in both LA and ALA, which generally requires a 100% fat-free diet, providing ALA in the diet will stimulate growth in a young animal, but it will not cure the dermatitis and infertility (and likely other problems that LA deficiency produces), as that can only be cured by LA.[650]

In a study of numerous rodents on many diets ranging from zero to 3.85% LA and 0.01% to 3.91% ALA, researcher and biochemist, Ralph T. Holman, PhD, and colleagues, at the University of Minnesota, determined that females only need about 0.5% LA and males 1.3% LA, while the requirement for ALA was deemed to be 0.5% of calories.[651] This appears to have been one of the most robust studies to determine essential requirements.

Thus, we would estimate that humans may only need about half as much omega-3 ALA as LA – perhaps just 0.5 to 1.0 grams per day in adults – in order to fulfill the body's needs. Greater amounts of omega-3 ALA in the diet may have benefits when omega-6 LA in the diet has been too high but, in general, historical evidence, ancestral living population studies, and experimental evidence in animals suggests that omega-3 requirements are very minimal.

So let's review the big picture. LA and ALA, the essential fats for mammals, can be found in nearly all plant fats, which includes natural fruits, vegetables, grains, nuts, and seeds[1] and both LA and ALA are found in all animals, as they either consume these fatty acids by eating plants or by eating the flesh of other animals (e.g., mammals) or, in some cases, they synthesize their own (some insects, nematodes, and mollusks).[641]

Whether consuming plants or animals, we're consuming LA and ALA in sufficient amounts, as long as we're eating food. It's almost impossible to get too little. But again, mammals, including humans, cannot make LA and ALA.[1] We require it, from plants. But we also don't actually need to eat plants to get LA and ALA, since we can get these fats by eating animal-based foods, including meats, organ meats, eggs, milk, butter, and every single animal-based food there is, as they all contain LA and ALA.

In summary, the LA and ALA are both moved up the food chain. But, whether one is a strict vegan, a strict carnivore, or the far more typical omnivore who consumes both plants and animals, it is practically impossible to consume too little LA or ALA and produce an essential fatty acid deficiency.

It appears that, in general, the only way to get too little LA or ALA, while still eating food, is to consume a 100% fat-free diet. By all accounts, the latter has only been accomplished in laboratory settings, for example, by creating diets of purified protein (e.g., 100% whey or casein) and pure sugar. Even commercial protein powders, for example, all contain fats that will contain LA and ALA.[652]

Thus, deficiencies of the essential fats, LA and ALA, are practically unknown. But, just because these fats are essential does not mean we should get more. The fact that these fatty acids are essential has led many to consume them in supplemental form in the belief that more is better, not realizing that LA in excess of 2% of total calories may very well cause disease - not prevent it.

WHY SEED OILS ARE FAR MORE DEVASTATING THAN SUGAR OR PROCESSED CARBS

When we eat carbohydrates, the ultimate fate of those carbohydrates is either to be burned for energy by first being converted to pyruvate and then acetyl-CoA (called cellular respiration),[653] stored as glycogen, or converted to fat (triglycerides) for storage as body fat, a process called *de novo* lipogenesis, DNL.[654][655] However, whether in health or disease states, excess carbohydrates in the diet are primarily converted to saturated fats, with monounsaturated fats being secondary.[656][657][658]

The human body will not and cannot convert excess carbohydrates (or proteins or even other fats) to the two essential fats, omega-6 LA or omega-3 ALA (alpha linolenic acid).[633][634] Isn't it interesting that, when the body needs to convert and store excess carbohydrates consumed, even when greatly overfeeding carbohydrates, it chooses primarily to make saturated fat? Indeed, monounsaturated fats (mostly oleic acid) are second in line for conversion when carbohydrates are overconsumed, but omega-6 linoleic acid (LA) cannot be synthesized.[633][634]

On the other hand, when we consume fats, if those fats are not burned for fuel they must be stored in fat cells or incorporated into cell membranes and other cellular structures and, more importantly, may directly alter cellular membrane fat composition, structure, and function.[659] This process has been implicated in numerous pathological conditions including cancer, diabetes, hypertension, Alzheimer's and Parkinson's disease.[659] Fats are components of all cellular membranes, they are integral in the transport of the fat-soluble vitamins (A, D, E, and K), act as signaling molecules, supply energy, and are known to have numerous other roles and effects.[660]

CHAPTER 4

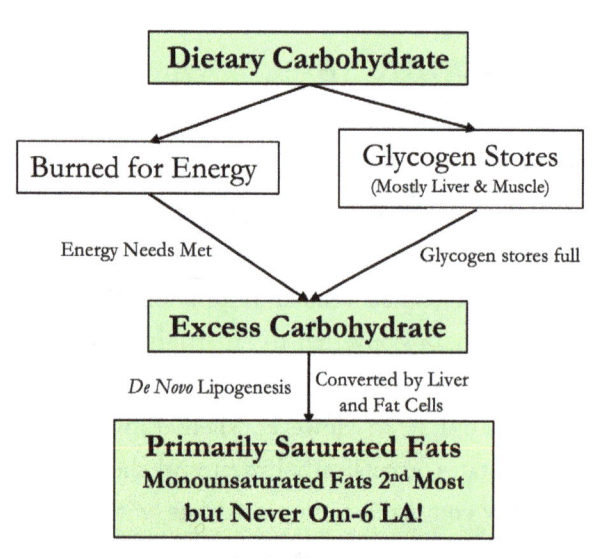

Dietary Carbohydrate
→ Burned for Energy
→ Glycogen Stores (Mostly Liver & Muscle)

Energy Needs Met / Glycogen stores full
→ **Excess Carbohydrate**

De Novo Lipogenesis / Converted by Liver and Fat Cells
→ **Primarily Saturated Fats**
Monounsaturated Fats 2nd Most
but Never Om-6 LA!

References provided herein. © C. Knobbe, 2022. Ancestral Health Foundation.

The important point here is that when we consume carbohydrates, even to excess, our body will convert those carbohydrates into safe fats and the fats that it desires (even when our body fat is in excess). But when we consume fats, the type and amount of fats, at least with respect to the PUFA (omega-6 and omega-3 fats) and trans fats, is directly reflected in the stores of our body fat and in all of our cellular membranes.[661][640]

In fact, there is such precision between the type of dietary fat consumed and the type of fat stored in our bodies that it can be defined in a mathematical relationship.[661] The strongest correlations between the types of fat consumed and the fatty acid profile in the body fat is for omega-6 LA, omega-3 ALA, and trans-fats, all of which are the types of fats that cannot be synthesized by the body.[662] However, the composition of saturated and monounsaturated fats in the diet is not reflected in the body fat, since these fats can be synthesized in both liver and fat cells.[640]

What this means is that, for those who have been fearing the consumption of saturated fat because it's 'dangerous and causes heart disease,' the fact is, the body so desperately needs and desires saturated (and monounsaturated) fats that, if you don't consume these, it will make them from the carbohydrates we consume anyway.

Saturated fats do not cause coronary heart disease, which should be obvious from the studies of the Maasai and the Tokelauans, both of whom consume around half of their diets as saturated fat and yet have little or no coronary heart disease. Furthermore, this should be plainly evident based on many population studies from around the world, including those of 19th century American, British, and European populations. Nevertheless, we'll review further details on the safety of saturated fats subsequently.

Unquestionably, when processed carbohydrates – added sugars and refined flours (instead of wholegrain flours) – are consumed to excess, these displace nutrient-dense foods, which can have a devastating impact on health. Again, the landmark studies of Weston A. Price made this apparent. However, as is (or will be) evident throughout this book, even processed, nutrient deficient carbohydrates will generally not induce the metabolic derangement and physical degenerative disease induced by high seed oil containing diets.

SEED OILS ARE RICH IN OMEGA-6 LA, WHICH ACCUMULATES IN OUR BODY FAT

Please recall for a moment the evidence for vegetable oil consumption in the U.S., reverting back to its introduction in the food supply in 1866. And do you recall that there has been an ever-increasing consumption of seed oils, high in omega-6 LA, which has not ceased to increase to this very day?

Knowing that the type of consumed fat influences what is stored in our bodies and that omega-6 and omega-3 fats are ultimately critical to practically every cellular process known,[640] the question is, 'What do you suppose this is doing to our body fat (and cellular membranes, cell functions, etc.)?'

To answer that question, let's examine the evidence of the increasing omega-6 LA in our diets versus the omega-6 LA in our body fat, from a landmark paper published by our friend and colleague, nutrition researcher, Stephan Guyenet, PhD, formerly of the University of Washington, and his colleague, Susan E. Carlson, PhD, Professor of Nutrition at the University of Kansas. Dr. Guyenet and Dr. Carlson's paper is appropriately entitled, "Increase in Adipose Tissue Linoleic Acid of US Adults in the Last Half Century."[6]

Guyenet and Carlson collated and analyzed the body fat fatty acid analyses from 37 different studies in the U.S., between the years of 1959 and 2008, verifying that there were no further studies of body fat composition published in the U.S. after 2008. Let's first look at the graph entitled, "U.S. Percentage LA in Body Fat Vs. Year," which shows the increase in body fat (adipose) LA between the years 1959 and 2008. We see that the average body fat LA percentage averaged 9.1% in 1959 and elevated to 21.5% LA by 2008.[6]

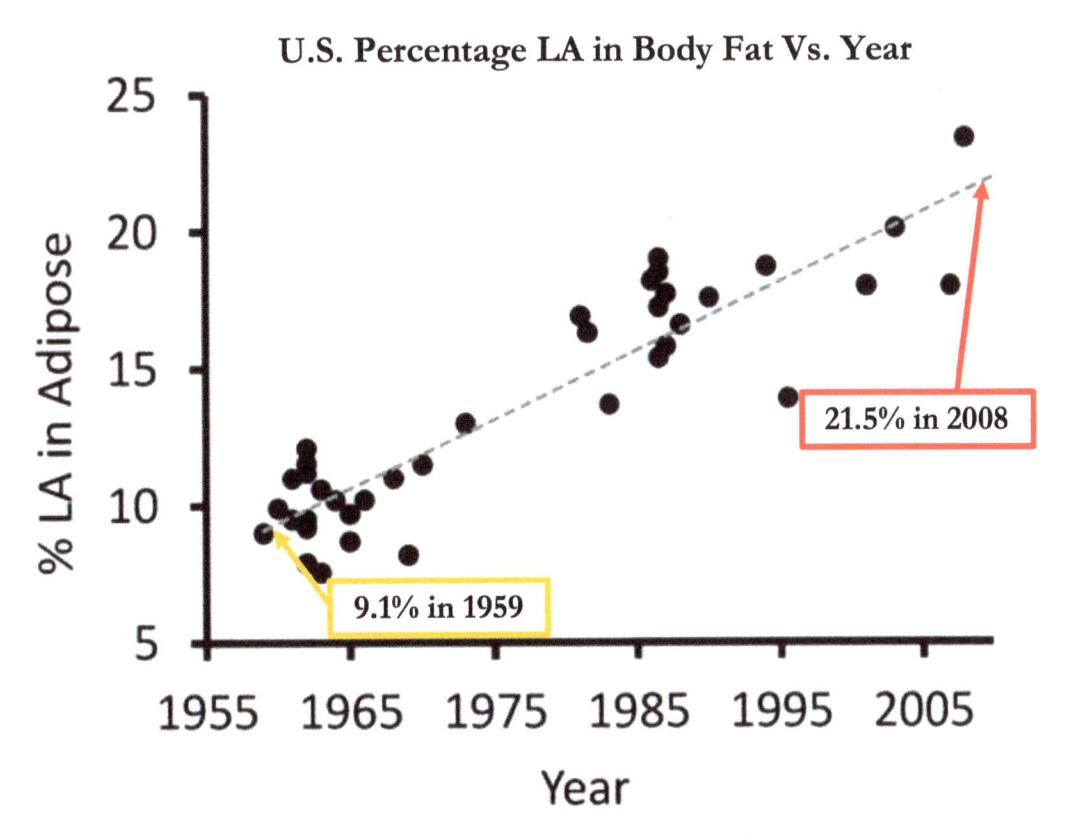

U.S. Percentage LA in Body Fat Vs. Year

Guyenet SJ, Carlson SE. Increase in Adipose Tissue Linoleic Acid of US Adults in the Last Half Century. Advances in Nutrition. 2015;6(6):660-664. U.S. Adipose tissue LA concentration, 1959-2008, including studies of all subcutaneous sites. Reprinted with permission.

U.S. Om-6 Linoleic Acid Intake vs % LA in Body Fat

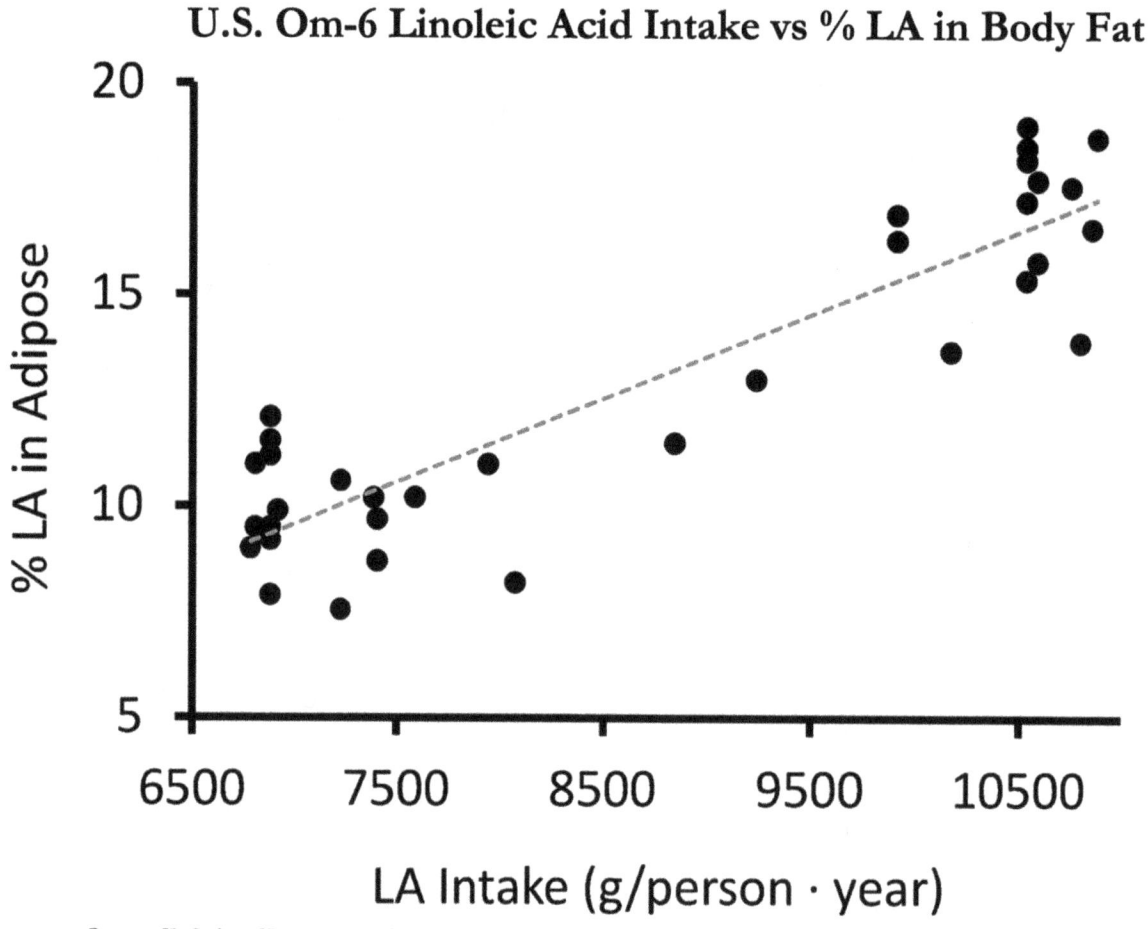

Guyenet SJ, Carlson SE. Increase in Adipose Tissue Linoleic Acid of US Adults in the Last Half Century. Advances in Nutrition. 2015;6(6):660-664. U.S. correlation between adipose tissue LA and dietary LA intake. Reprinted with permission.

In the next graph from Dr. Guyenet and Dr. Carlson, we observe their correlation between LA% in body fat versus LA consumed in the diet per year (see "U.S. Om-6 Linoleic Acid Intake vs % LA in Body Fat" above).

Thus, we see that not only has the omega-6 in the body fat increased by 2.36-fold (136%) just since 1959, but we also see an extremely strong correlation between body fat LA percentage and dietary LA intake (for the statistically minded, R^2= 0.81; P <0.001).[6] Now, can you imagine what the typical omega-6 LA percentage would have been for most Americans back in the 1800s before seed oil consumption was available?

As previously reviewed, we've estimated that LA consumption in the U.S. in 1865 was about 2.2 grams/day or 1% of consumed energy; LA consumption then gradually elevated to 2.23% of energy in 1909, which translates to about 4.84 g/day, 18.0 g/day or 7.21% of energy in 1999, and to 29g/day or 11.8% of energy by 2008.

So, we could create a linear correlation and estimate how low the body fat LA was in 1865 and 1909, but the mathematical model may falter slightly at the lowest levels of consumption, since our bodies must store and utilize LA and perhaps may increase storage when consumption levels are very low. Nevertheless, as an approximation, we would estimate that 1865 Americans' body fat LA was in the 2.5% - 3.0% range.

For a comparison of body fat LA percentage, we should review the Tokelauans, who are one of only about three known ancestrally living, non-westernized, non-processed food, non-seed oil consuming populations with whom we are aware, who have also had adipose biopsies completed.

As reviewed in Chapter One, the **Tokelauans** had a high-fat diet of approximately 56% fat, with 40% to 50% of fat as saturated fat, and only about 1.6% LA as a percentage of calories consumed. We should recall that they had no heart disease whatsoever and obesity and diabetes were virtually unknown.

So what was their body fat LA percentage? An extraordinarily low 3.8 percent! Again, compare this to Americans' LA percentage in body fat at 9.1% in 1961 and 21.5% by 2008 and, once again, recall that typical westernized populations consume 8 to 10% dietary LA.[180] [173]

OMEGA-6 LA IS STORED IN OUR BODY FAT WITH A HALF-LIFE OF NEARLY 2 YEARS!

In the 1960s, Jules Hirsch, MD, who had a long career at Rockefeller University in New York, along with colleagues, completed the seminal studies which determined that fatty acids, like LA, were very slow to change in the body fat.

He wrote, "In adults in caloric balance, dietary effects on adipose tissue are produced only slowly; in short term studies no effects are seen…" He continued, regarding one particular subject, "After ten weeks on a formula containing forty per cent of calories as corn oil (~59% LA) the adipose tissue of this subject was normal in fatty acid composition."[663]

Hirsch continued, "Then, after thirty-eight days on a fat-free high carbohydrate formula, the adipose pattern was still unaffected. During ten weeks on high intakes of corn oil, this patient ingested more than 3.5 kg [7.7 lbs] of linoleic acid, an amount roughly three times that present in his entire adipose [fat] tissue. Yet, the adipose linoleic concentration did not rise… When formulas rich in corn oil are fed over extremely long periods, slow changes in adipose composition are seen eventually, and they continue until an adipose pattern is evolved which is very similar to that of the fed corn oil [fatty] acids."[663]

Hirsch and colleagues established a mathematical relationship between the LA (and other PUFAs) turnover in the fat and determined that **the half-life of LA (and other PUFAs) was about 350 to 750 days.**[663]

Twenty years later, researcher A.C. Beynen and colleagues also established a mathematical relationship between "the average fatty acid composition of the habitual diet and that of the lipid stores of subcutaneous adipose tissue."[664] Beynen determined that the **half-life of LA was on the "order of 600 days,"** asserting that the body fat stores qualitatively reflected the PUFA fats consumed over **"a period of 2 to 3 years."**[664] Beynen also found that the fractional rate of turnover for fatty acids in body fat was just 0.12% of the body fat per day, asserting, "The total body fat of men would thus completely be replaced in 800 to 900 days."[664]

By 2008, some 15 studies further verified the findings of Hirsch in 1960 and Beynen in 1980, establishing that the consumption of PUFA – omega-6 LA and omega-3 ALA – has a strong positive correlation with the PUFA in the body fat.[665] In other words, high omega-6 LA in the diet will produce a high level of LA in the body fat and a low omega-6 LA containing diet will produce a low level of LA in the body fat. In the low range, the relationship is almost linear, that is, a one-to-one ratio. In any case, adipose fatty acid analysis is not a standard or typical procedure completed by physicians, as such procedures have only commonly been completed for the purpose of scientific investigations.

The good news is that we can control the deposition of LA into our body fat by what we consume. The bad news is that it takes a long time to turn over. How do we lower the LA percentage in our body fat and cell membranes? Simple. Do not consume seed oils. Also, greatly minimize or eliminate most nuts and seeds and nut oils, as they're mostly all very high in omega-6 as well. We must also avoid the consumption of certain animal foods high in LA (e.g., CAFO-raised chickens and pigs), as those that have been fed an inappropriate diet of corn and soy will develop high body fat LA just like humans. We'll get into more detail on this with general dietary advice, in Chapter Six and beyond.

NEW ZEALAND MĀORI – ONCE BRILLIANTLY HEALTHY, WITH THE LOWEST ADIPOSE LA% EVER DOCUMENTED – NOW SUFFER DEVASTATING HEALTH EFFECTS OF SEED OILS

The Māori are yet another population in which 'urbanization,' as it is so often euphemistically termed in scientific journals, has had disastrous consequences. According to Marcus Hawkins, in a paper published in the *Journal of Primary Health Care*:

> *"The Pacific region became colonized by Europeans from the early nineteenth century onwards and, as a consequence, 'European' foodstuffs were introduced to New Zealand Māori… obesity is now common among New Zealand Māori, who suffer disproportionately from the chronic diseases…"*[666]

The WHO, in a 2003 publication, stated, "Before European contact, the food behavior of the people of the Pacific region may have remained the same for millennia. The main staples were root crops. Upon European contact, Pacific people were described as strong, muscular and mostly in good health (see image of Māoris on Waikato River, Circa 1960s)."[372]

Early European explorers had quite unified voices in their descriptions of the Māori of New Zealand. In 1769 – 1770, Captain James Cook described the Māori as "A Strong, rawboned, well-made, Active People, rather above than under the common size, especially the Men."[667] Joseph Banks, ship-mate of Cook, noted that "men are of the size of the larger Europaeans, Stout, Clean Limnd [sic] and active, fleshy but never fat," "vigorous, nimble…"[668] Banks also reported that the Māori women were "rather smaller than Europaean women."

P.H. Buck, in a paper published in 1927 in the *Medical Journal of Australia*, described "pre-European Māori among the tallest races of the world and the muscular development of the legs was the finest known. The standard of physique was very high," further commenting, "These factors cannot be considered apart from diet in the aetiology [cause] of the Māori physique."[669]

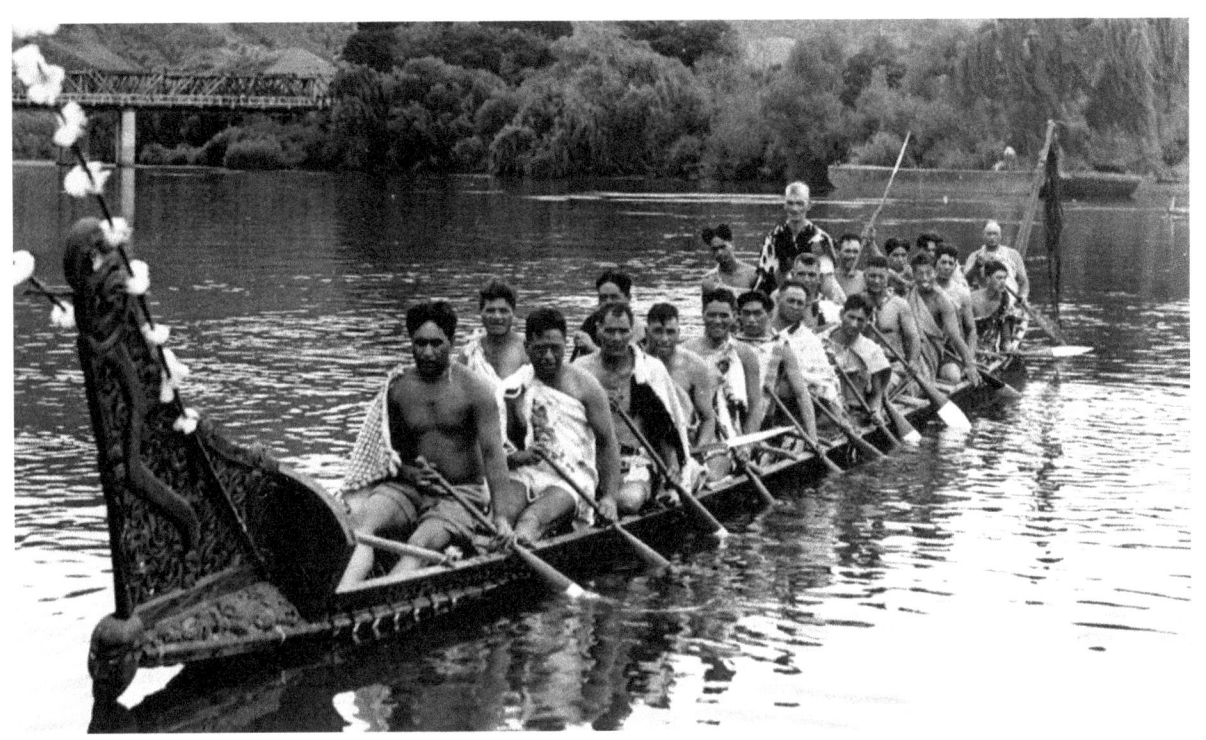

New Zealand Maoris on the Waikato River, Circa 1960s. Photo representative of the typical health of Maoris in the 1960s.

Curiously, despite Joseph Banks' comment regarding the Māori as being "among the tallest races," a study published in 1854 by researcher A.S. Thomson, in the *Journal of the Statistical Society of London*, reviewed the measured heights and weights of 147 Māori men, which showed that they averaged 5 feet 6³/⁴ in (1.63 m), weighed an average of 140 pounds (63.6 kg or ten stone), and had an average BMI of 22.8 kg/m²; this affirms that they were very lean, but not generally tall, at least by current American standards.[670] The tallest man was 6 ft 4 in (1.94 meters) and the heaviest men (2) were 185 pounds (84.1 kg). This strongly suggests that not a single individual approached obesity in this group of 147 men.

Interestingly, in his 1854 paper, Thomson wrote the following excerpt:

"The New Zealanders, like all men in a savage state, are indolent and lazy, working only when an absolute necessity for so doing exists [sic]. A few days' labour will enable them to plant enough potatoes to sustain life for a year, and to rear a few pigs to exchange for blankets and tobacco. The greater part of their time is spent in a dreamsy [sic] state of indolence, smoking, talking, and reading. The latter is a newly-acquired taste, but is very common."[670]

In the 1930s, Weston A. Price evaluated the Māori quite extensively, stating, "The reputation of the Māori for splendid physiques has placed them on a pedestal of perfection. Much of this has been lost in modernization."[671] Price noted that the traditionalists used seafoods liberally, including fish and shellfish, edible kelp, and large quantities of fern root.

And while those who had already westernized their diets were developing tooth decay, which Price attributed to "the foods of modern civilization, foods consisting largely of white flour, sweetened goods, syrup and canned goods,"[672] Price also found that the Māori who lived near the sea maintained their traditional diet and remained healthy and robust.

Price wrote, "these people maintain excellent figures to old age."[671]

Following Price's expedition to study the Māori of New Zealand, the greatest nutrition transition was still yet to come and, in fact, began to take effect somewhere between about 1950 and the 1970s apparently, as the book *Normal Nutrition* described that the New Zealand average diet in 1969 already had too much sugar, cakes, biscuits, and confectionery.[673] By the 1980s, many concerns were beginning to be raised regarding the risk factors for chronic diseases such as CHD and diabetes, with the often blamed "dietary imbalance and energy excess."[673]

In 1966, however, the New Zealand Government Statistician determined that the total fat intake of New Zealanders at that time was 150.7 g/day, 56 g of which came from meat, 41.2 g from butter, and 27.6 g from milk and cheese.[674] The total fat intake was 39.1%, which was approximately the same as Americans at that time. They reported no edible oils, however, the FAO database records just 2.5 g/day (24 calories) of oils for that year, which is virtually the same level of consumption Americans last had in 1908.[4]

Consumption of vegetable oils for New Zealand (which would include most Māoris), based on FAO data, gradually and fairly steadily rose from 2.5g/day (24 calories) in 1966 to 28 g/day (246 calories) by 2008, with a drop-down to 24 g/day (220 cal) by 2019 (see graph on page 175 entitled, "New Zealand Māori: Obesity, Body Fat LA%, Veg Oils & Sugar, 1961-2019"). One should bear in mind the potential for under-reporting of food consumption data to the FAO, particularly in smaller countries.[385] [386]

In 1969, physician Ian Prior, MD and colleagues, completed adipose biopsies for fatty acid analysis on **New Zealand Māoris, proving, as far as we are aware, the lowest recorded percentage of LA in the fat of humans anywhere, at an average of 2.6%**.[674] This extraordinarily low level of LA in the body fat (adipose) is truly indicative of an extremely low omega-6 LA diet and, of course, their near-complete lack of vegetable oil consumption up to that time. Indeed, it appears they still had relatively good health by the late 1960s but, of course, not nearly the health and fitness that they enjoyed in the early 20th century.

The extremely low LA in the Māori of New Zealand also wasn't peculiar to their ethnic group, as the Europeans of New Zealand in the same study (1969) had nearly identical body fat LA, at an average of 3.02%.[674] [673] The Pukapukans also had nearly identical body fat LA, at an average of 3.22% for Pukapukans residing in Pukapuka, and an average of 2.6% for Pukapukans living on the island of Raratonga.[674]

Body fat LA climbed to 10.5% by 1981 in New Zealand men, indicative of substantial seed oil consumption by then, but unfortunately, we are not aware of any more recent studies on body fat LA analyses.[675]

The Māoris of the island of Pukapuka, in a study completed in 1962-1963 by Ian Prior, MD and colleagues, showed that 7% of the males were obese and one subject (out of 188 total) was grossly obese (however, he was afflicted with elephantiasis), while 23% of the females were obese and an additional 2% grossly obese.[676] At that time, Prior wrote that the Pukapukans:

> "were still living largely on their basic diet of fish, taro, coconuts in many and varied forms, with modest supplements of flour, rice, and sugar."[676]

This statement, along with their extremely low LA% in their body fat, both strongly suggest that the Māori are highly susceptible to obesity, even without seed oils, when the traditional diet is substantially displaced by refined, processed foods. This appears to be rather unlike most other populations worldwide, but seems to be common among the Pacific Islanders.

Nancy Pollock, an author with vast knowledge of the history and diets of Pacific Islanders, wrote the following:

> "...we must also bear in mind the irregularity of their food supply – that vast amounts were eaten when available, and that abstinence for two or three days was commonplace. So the argument has been made that a store of fat would have enabled those people to survive longer than their thin counterparts."[677]

It generally seems to be recognized that Pacific Islanders tend to become "fleshy" more easily than most other populations. In 1962, geneticist James V. Neel proposed the "thrifty gene hypothesis" to explain this observation in South American populations, suggesting that a genetic predisposition to diabetes (which is most always associated with overweight or obesity) existed in certain indigenous peoples.[678]

The idea was soon expanded to include obesity, even in common rhetoric. Several others, including Paul Baker in 1981,[679] Ian A.M. Prior in 1977,[680] and Paul Zimmet in 1980,[681] have applied this hypothesis to Pacific Islanders.

In view of this hypothesis and its relation to either processed food and or food abundance, even when the diet is ancestral, we have personally reviewed the thousands of photos in the archives of Weston A. Price's work at Price-Pottenger Nutrition Foundation (as well as Price's books). This historical evidence reveals that, while physical degeneration was obvious and often profound in those consuming the most processed foods (refined flours, sugars, canned goods, etc.), overweight and obesity appeared to be quite rare. However, at that time (the 1930s) seed oils were of very minor consumption, unlike today.

Regarding Māoris on the island of Pukapuka in 1962-1963, despite obesity having already increased significantly at that time, their health was still very good. Only 3% of males and 7% of females had hypertension, a relatively small 1.3% had "diabetic abnormality," and none had any EKG abnormalities, suggesting cardiovascular disease was quite rare if not absent (although the sample size was small).[676]

Regarding obesity in the Māori of New Zealand, the earliest data available came from the New Zealand Health Survey in 1977, and this was for all of New Zealand, not specifically just the Māori. The survey found an obesity prevalence of 10% at that time.[682] Obesity specifically in adult Māori of New Zealand then rose to 19.6% in 1989, 26.7%

CHAPTER 4

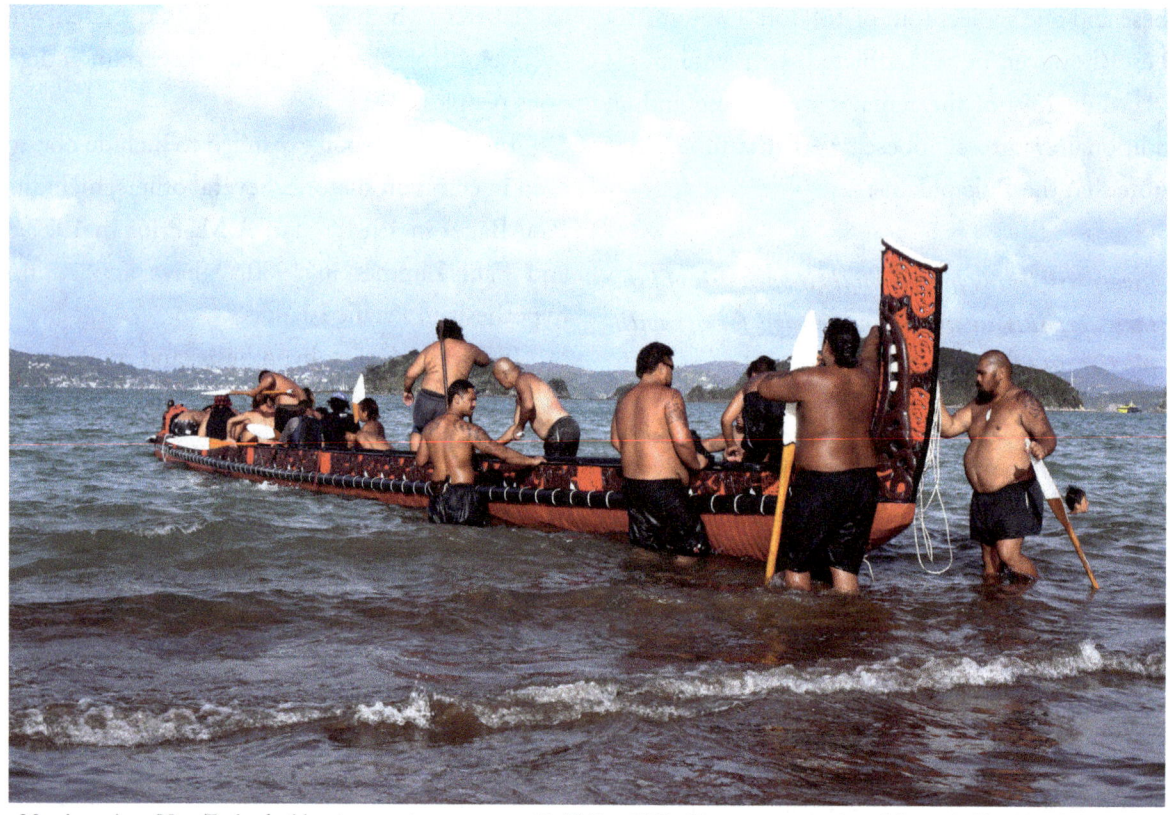

Maori warriors (New Zealand athletes), preparing war canoe, Te Ti Bay, 2009. Photo representative of the typical health of Maoris.

in 2003,[683] and finally, to 50% by 2017.[684] An additional 34% of adults were overweight in 2016-2017, indicating that 84% of adults were either overweight or obese (see 2009 photo of Māori athletes above). That same year, 69% of Pacific adults were obese, 29% of Pacific children were obese, and 18% of Māori children were obese.[684] In 2013-2014, an average of 5.6% of Māori over the age of 15 years also had diabetes, which is up more than 4-fold since 1962.[685]

As can be seen in the graph on New Zealand Māori p. 175 ("New Zealand/Māori: Obesity, Body Fat LA%, Veg Oils & Sugar, 1961-2019"), obesity increased from about 10% in 1977 to 50% in 2017. However, during the same period of interest, i.e., 1961 to 2019, sugar consumption was already high in 1961 at nearly 500 cal/day, and elevated only 17%, while vegetable oils increased 1,471%.

Clearly, the Māori on the island of Pukapuka developed obesity while consuming refined carbs and sugars, however, they remained quite healthy, whereas, when seed oils were introduced and elevated markedly in New Zealand, the Māori became severely overweight and diabetes elevated more than 4-fold, indicating they were much more metabolically ill. The prevalence of diabetes in the Western Pacific is among the highest in the world, including levels of 37.5% in Tokelau, 35% in the Federated States of Micronesia, 34.9% in Marshall Island, 28.8% in Kiribati, and 25.7% in the Cook Islands.[382]

It is well established that the Māori once enjoyed perhaps the most revered physiques in the world,

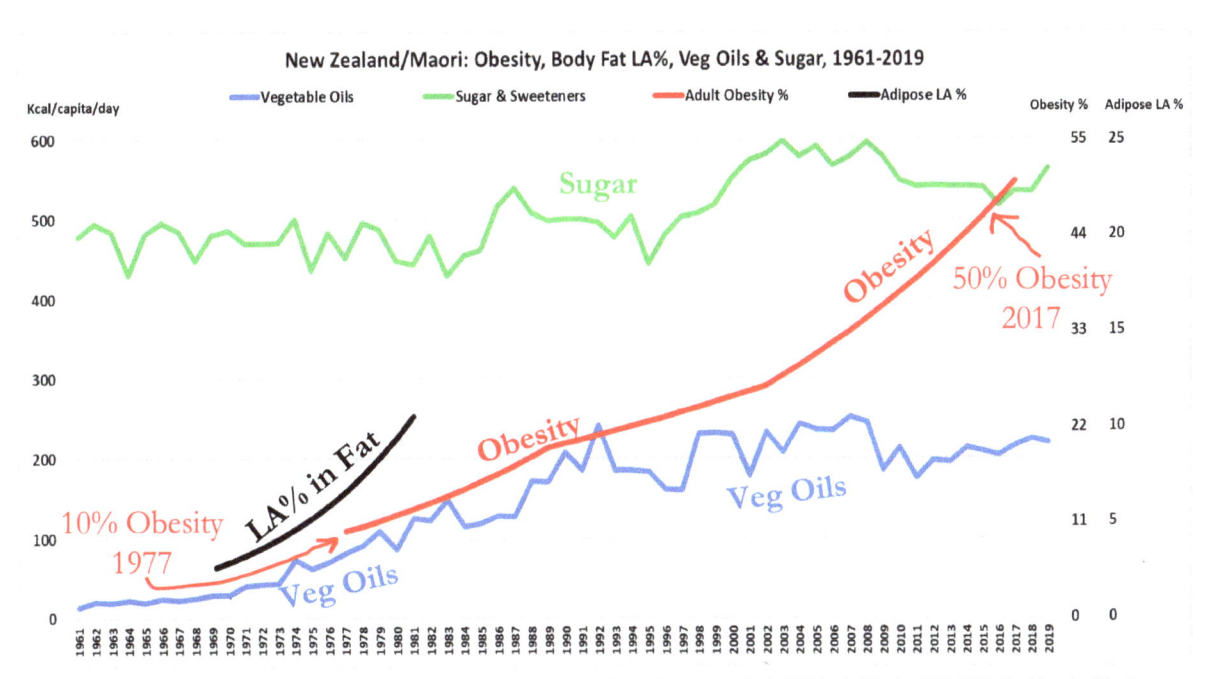

New Zealand/Maori: Obesity, Body Fat LA%, Veg Oils & Sugar, 1961-2019

References: 1) Obesity 1977: New Zealand Health Survey, Ministry of Health. Understanding Excess Body Weight. 2) Obesity 1989-2003: Tracking the Obesity Epidemic: New Zealand 1977-2003. 3) Obesity 2017: New Zealand Health Survey 2016/17. 4) LA% in Adipose, 1969: Shorland, FB. Amer J Clin Nutr. 1969;22(5):594-605. 5) Adipose LA%: Sutherland WHF. Metabolism Clinical & Experimental. 1981;30(9):839-844. 6) Vegetable oil and sugar consumption: FAO Food Balance Sheets, retrieved from Knoema.com. U.S. © C. Knobbe, 2022. Ancestral Health Foundation.

whereas today, they have one of the highest rates of obesity in the world. This has been driven by processed food and, in this case, sugars and seed oils together hold the enormous bulk of the responsibility. However, this is indeed a population study in which obesity elevated many-fold, over a period of just 40 years, with vegetable oils as the primary driver.

LA% IN BODY FAT (ADIPOSE) INCREASING OVER TIME – GLOBALLY – IN PARALLEL WITH INCREASING SEED OIL CONSUMPTION AND OBESITY

As reviewed previously, the lowest omega-6 linoleic acid (LA) adipose (body fat) levels in the world, as far as we are aware, were documented in the South Pacific Island countries, including the New Zealand Māoris at an average of 2.6%, *in 1969*.[674] The Europeans of New Zealand in the 1969 study had body fat LA which averaged 3.02%.[673]

The Pukapukans had average LA concentration in body fat of 3.22% for Pukapukans residing in Pukapuka, as well as an average of 2.6% for Pukapukans living on the island of Raratonga.[673] In the United Kingdom, a study completed in 1960 found body fat LA ranging from 2.5% to 6.5%, with an average of 4.5%.[686] Sweden had one study with body fat LA of 4.0% in 1958[694] [695] and one study in South Africa in 1963 found an average adipose LA of 5.9%.[687] Take notice that the lowest recorded body fat LA percentages were all either in the 1950s or 1960s.

In 1959, the U.S. adipose LA averaged 9.1%,[6] but, of course, the U.S. had and still has the highest seed oil consumption per capita in the world.

In 1962, as seed oils began to escalate on a

CHAPTER 4

global basis, body fat LA was found to be 5.5% in Columbia, 5.8% in Jamaica, 8.2% in Nigeria, 7.9% at one U.S. location (Boston, MA), and 9.4% in Japan.[688] Body fat LA climbed to 10.5% in 1981 in New Zealand men.

As edible seed oils continued their global ascent in consumption, in 1991 and 1992, body fat LA was 10.4% in Finland, 11.7% in Germany, 12.4% in Edinburgh, U.K., 12.9% in Coleraine, U.K., 13.1% in Norway, 13.4% in Switzerland, 14.1% in Malaga, Spain, 14.2% in Granada, Spain, 14.8% in Moscow, 15.3% in The Netherlands, and 24.6% in Jerusalem, Israel.[689]

In the 21st century, as seed oils continued to displace other fats and even carbohydrates, some of the body fat LA percentages were as follows: France, at 11% in 2014,[690] 12.5% in Prague, Czech Republic, in 2012,[691] 10.6% in Germany, in 2013,[692] 21.5% in the U.S. in 2008,[6] and an extraordinarily high 25.6% in Israel in 2002.

Thus, the body fat LA percentage in ancestrally living people in 1969 who did not consume seed oils averaged 2.86%. This included the Māoris of New Zealand, the Europeans of New Zealand, the Pukapukans of Pukapuka, and the Pukapukans of Raratonga, all reviewed previously.

This is what we will submit is an ancestral level of body fat LA – around 2.6 to 3.0%.

On the other hand, the westernized populations reviewed here since the year 1990, all of whom are confirmed to consume excessive seed oils, have an average adipose LA percentage of 14.2%. This includes only one averaged figure of 21.5% for the U.S. in 2008.

Any body fat LA percentage above approximately 4.0% is toxic – poisonous – and we'll review the biochemical reasons why subsequently.

Thus, not only does it appear quite evident that body fat LA percentage has risen markedly on a global scale, this is indeed in direct correlation with seed oil consumption (worldwide vegetable oil consumption to be presented subsequently). And while we believe that body fat LA percentage should be in the 2.5% to possibly 4.0% range in most cases,

Om-6 Adipose Linoleic Acid %: Ancestral vs Seed Oil Consuming Populations

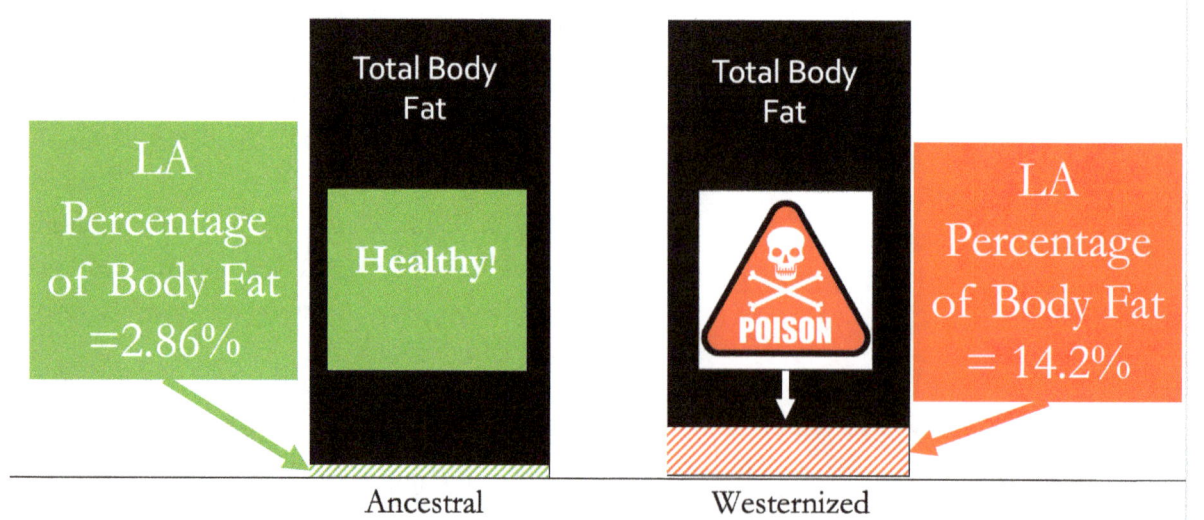

1) LA% Body Fat 1969 "Ancestral Data": Shorland FB, Czochanska Z, Prior IAM. Studies on Fatty Acid Composition of Adipose Tissue and Blood Lipids of Polynesians. Amer J Clin Nutr. 1969;22(5):594-605. 2) LA% Westernized Populations: see references cited herein. © C. Knobbe, Ancestral Health Foundation, 2021. All rights reserved.

in the past 40 years, we have not seen a single study that shows average body fat LA percentage anywhere even close to this range.

This enormous increase in body fat LA percentage, of course, reflects the profile and amounts of fatty acids – mostly omega-3, omega-6, and transfats – that we consume in our diets. We strongly suspect that accumulation of omega-6 LA beyond approximately 4.0% in the body fat sets the wheels in motion to develop a pro-oxidative, pro-inflammatory, toxic, and nutrient-deficient biological milieu, which drives a myriad of diseases, including CHD, cancer, metabolic syndrome, type 2 diabetes, and so much more.

And although the actual percentage of body fat as LA that is consistent with health and lack of chronic disease cannot be definitively known at this point based on many studies, the general concept and advice are the same. To achieve optimal health, we must reduce our body fat LA percentage and, in most cases, probably down to the 2.5% to 4.0% range. It is unlikely that humans can achieve substantially lower numbers and, in fact, that could be deleterious as well. Again, recall Paracelsus' dictum and the fact that there is an optimal range for all nutrients, including LA.

As previously reviewed, the mathematical formula which predicts body fat LA percentage, as a very rough approximation, is simply to take the last three years' average dietary LA consumption as a percentage of consumed energy and double it. We know that much of the world now consumes somewhere between 8% to 10%[180][173] and even ~12% of energy as LA,[6][3] with the U.S. and Israel consuming the greatest percentage per capita of LA; hence, the body fat LA% in the U.S. and Israel reflect that, at 21.5% and 24.6%, respectively.[6][689]

Therefore, even if we had no available data on seed oil consumption for an individual or a population, if we were to measure their average body fat (adipose) LA%, we would be able to have a pretty accurate estimate as to their seed oil consumption, at least as it relates to a percentage of their total fat consumption. The mathematical formula would literally allow us to approximate the average LA consumption for a given individual (or population in a larger study) over the past three years. That's pretty nifty.

If we were to observe only a single biomarker that will consistently both predict and track chronic disease, including overweight, obesity, CHD, diabetes, metabolic syndrome, diabetes, Alzheimer's disease, dementia, age-related macular degeneration (AMD), etc., it *wouldn't* be LDL or HDL cholesterol, triglycerides, glucose, hemoglobin A1c (HgbA1c), or any other typical biomarker, it would be *adipose LA%*. This is the one single biomarker that we believe might be the best predictor. Why? Because, in general, it is a biomarker that tracks the relative consumption of omega-6-rich seed oils.

Next, let's review the population study of Sweden before we get a little further into the deep molecular science, which, of course, we'll try to greatly simplify.

SWEDEN – LA RISES FROM 4% TO 7% IN BODY FAT, WITH PARALLEL RISE IN OBESITY

At this point, it should be mentioned that, outside of the U.S., where 37 studies of adipose (body fat) LA% were completed between 1959 and 2008 (Guyenet and Carlson),[6] there are far fewer adipose fatty acid analyses around the world. Perhaps most of them have been reviewed in this book, or at least we've presented a pretty fair sampling from around the world.

We believe it should also be appreciated that, before 1952, the presence of specific fatty acids in adipose (body fat) samples could be determined in *qualitative* analyses, but the *quantitative* analyses (percentages of fatty acids) could not be accurately determined. That all changed in 1952 when gas chromatography became available.[693] Thus, any attempts at quantitative analysis of body fat LA percentage prior to 1952 would undoubtedly have been quite imprecise, but perhaps not worthless. We are not aware of any such analyses worth mentioning.

In one of the few body fat LA analyses completed after 1952, but before the severe onslaught of westernized, seed oil-laden diets globally, is that of a study conducted in Sweden in 1958. Adipose (body fat) biopsies proved that body fat LA percentage was only 4.0% that year.[694] [695] In a subsequent study of body fat LA percentage completed in Sweden nearly five decades later, in 2006, body fat LA was 7%.[696] In both cases, adipose LA percentage was far lower than Americans, who averaged 9.1% in 1959 and 21.5% in 2008. With this knowledge, we should be curious as to the prevalence of obesity in Sweden.

Indeed, Sweden has far less obesity than most westernized countries. If we just look at the approximate time frame in which we have adipose LA percentage, obesity was only 0.9% in 1969 and gradually and steadily rose to 5.1% by 2000 in young men who were all 18 years of age.[697] For adults aged 25 to 64, in 1985 (the earliest available data) obesity was 6.8%, which elevated to 12.9% by 2002.[698]

Obesity in Sweden is obviously very low compared to the U.S. For vegetable oil data in Sweden, we limited the analysis to the high PUFA oils

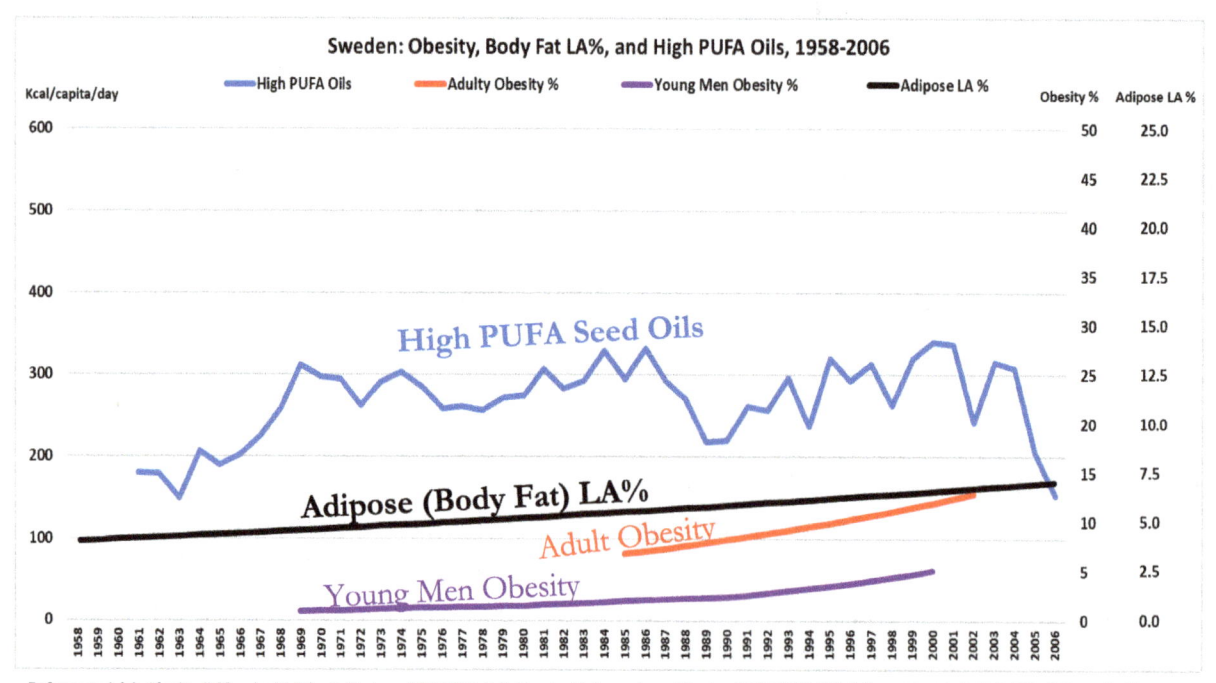

Sweden: Obesity, Body Fat LA%, and High PUFA Oils, 1958-2006

References: Adult Obesity: 1) Neovius M. Obesity Reviews. 2006;7(1):1-3. 2) Neovius M. Intern Journ Obesity. 2008;32:832-836. Adipose Linoleic Acid (LA)%: 1) Bergqvist U, Holmberg J. 4th International Conference on Biochemistry. Problems of Lipids, HM Sinclair, Ed., 1958, p. 60. 2) Gertow K. Eur J Clin Nutr. 2006;60:1406-1413. Vegetable Oils: FAO Food Balance Sheets, vegetable oils. Knoema.com. © C. Knobbe, 2022. Ancestral Health Foundation.

consumed (rapeseed, soybean, mustard, groundnut (peanut), sunflower, sesame, maize germ (corn), and cottonseed) since the country has significant consumption of far healthier oils, including coconut, palm, and olive oil (see the graph on page 178, "Sweden: Obesity, Body Fat LA%, and High PUFA Oils, 1958-2006").

Thus, in Sweden, we observe a strong correlation between high PUFA seed oil consumption, adipose (body fat) LA percentage, adult obesity, and obesity in young men. Furthermore, we observe that, while the consumption of seed oils is far less than in many westernized countries, this runs in parallel with their relatively low level of obesity.

U.K. – LIKE THE U.S., OBESITY & CHRONIC DISEASE RISING WITH SEED OILS, WHILE SUGAR CONSUMPTION FALLS!

Thomas A.B. Sanders, PhD, Emeritus Professor of Nutrition and Dietetics, King's College London, in 2016, reviewed that over the previous forty-year period in the U.K., total fat consumption had dropped from about 42% down to 35%, while saturated fat consumption fell from 12% down to 10%.[640] During the same time frame, polyunsaturated fat (PUFA) elevated from 4% to 6% of total consumed energy, while partially hydrogenated fats (trans fats) declined from about 2% of energy to well below 1% of energy.

If reducing fat and saturated fat were beneficial, then the U.K. ought to have improvements in health, right? However, we see anything but improvements. In fact, we see worsening trends in most every metric of health in the U.K. since the 1960s.

Obesity in the U.K. was about 7% in 1980,[699] which rose to 14.5% in 1993, and finally to 28% in 2019.[700] As reviewed in Chapter 2, coronary heart disease deaths in the U.K. elevated from 2.9/100,000 in 1921 to 550/100,000 in 1970.[269] [286] [287] [288] Adult diabetes in the U.K. was 2.5% in 1994, which rose three-fold to 7.5% by 2019.[701]

Chronic disease has riddled the U.K. just like most westernized populations. In 2005 approximately 38% of all deaths were due to cardiovascular disease, 25% due to cancer, 7% to chronic respiratory disease, 14% to other chronic diseases, and 1% to diabetes;[702] however, the latter number is artificially low since diabetes drives cardiovascular disease.

In 2015 and 2016, our colleague, Marija Stojanoska, MSc, of Macedonia, worked tirelessly to track down sugar consumption in the U.K back to the 18th century and vegetable oil consumption back to the early 20th century, all of which we published in the journal *Medical Hypotheses*, in 2017 (all data not shown).[4]

In Figure 4.1, we'll show a subset of that data beginning in the early 1940s, which reveals that sugar consumption in the U.K reached a peak of 142 grams/day (568 calories) in 1961 and then took a generally downward trend, reaching a low of 90 g/day (360 calories) in 2006, with the FAO data ending in 2011 with sugar consumption at 102 g/day (408 calories). Total vegetable oil consumption, on the other hand, was already at 20 g/day in 1942 and elevated to 50 g/day in 2019, which is the last available data (Knoema database).

Thus, during the same period of a 4-fold increase in obesity between 1980 and 2019, a tripling of diabetes prevalence between 1994 and 2019, and a presumed large increase in chronic disease deaths in the U.K. during the same approximate period, we observe that the total added sugar consumption declined 28% between 1961 and 2011. Vegetable oils,

CHAPTER 4

FIG. 4.1

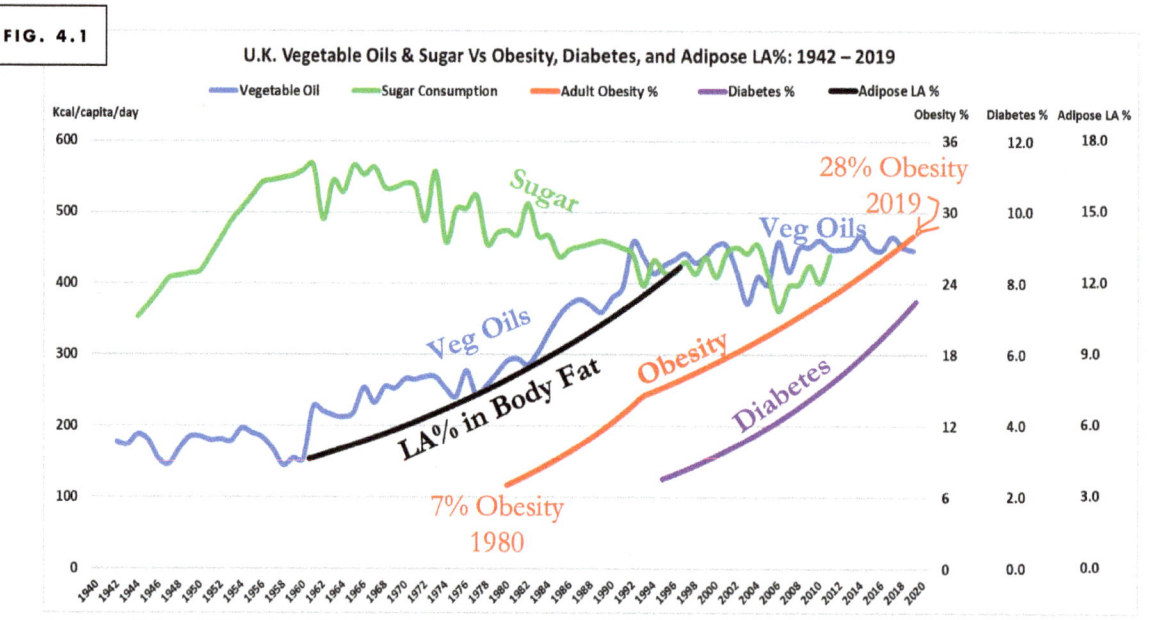

U.K. Vegetable Oils & Sugar Vs Obesity, Diabetes, and Adipose LA%: 1942 – 2019

References: 1) Obesity 1980: Lean M. ABC of obesity. Obesity—can we turn the tide? BMJ 2006;333(7581):1261-4. 2) Obesity 1993-2019: Moody, A. Health Survey for England 2019 – Overweight and obesity in adults and children. NHS Digital. 3) Diabetes: Fat, LN. Health Survey for England 2019 Adults Health. NHS Digital. 4) Adipose LA%: 1960: Kingsbury KJ. The Fatty Acid Composition of Human Depot Fat. Biochem J. 1961;78:541. 5) Adipose LA% 1997: Bakker N and the EURAMIC Study Group. Adipose Fatty Acids and Cancers of the Breast, Prostate and Colon: An Ecological Study. Int J Cancer. 1997;1997;72:587-91. 6) Vegetable oil and sugar consumption: FAO Food Balance Sheets, retrieved from Knoema.com. © Copyright C. Knobbe, Ancestral Health Foundation, 2022. All rights reserved.

FIG. 4.2

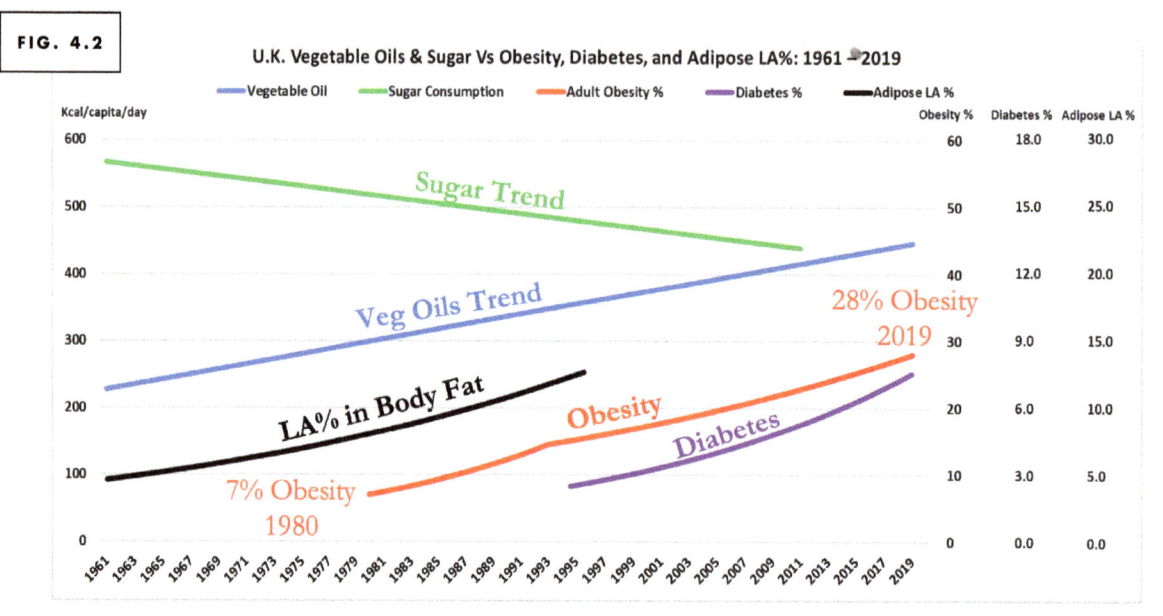

U.K. Vegetable Oils & Sugar Vs Obesity, Diabetes, and Adipose LA%: 1961 – 2019

References: 1) Obesity 1980: Lean M. ABC of obesity. Obesity—can we turn the tide? BMJ 2006;333(7581):1261-4. 2) Obesity 1993-2019: Moody, A. Health Survey for England 2019 – Overweight and obesity in adults and children. NHS Digital. 3) Diabetes: Fat, LN. Health Survey for England 2019 Adults Health. NHS Digital. 4) Adipose LA%: 1960: Kingsbury KJ. The Fatty Acid Composition of Human Depot Fat. Biochem J. 1961;78:541. 5) Adipose LA% 1997: Bakker N and the EURAMIC Study Group. Adipose Fatty Acids and Cancers of the Breast, Prostate and Colon: An Ecological Study. Int J Cancer. 1997;1997;72:587-91. 6) Vegetable oil and sugar consumption: FAO Food Balance Sheets, retrieved from Knoema.com. © Copyright C. Knobbe, Ancestral Health Foundation, 2022. All rights reserved.

on the other hand, doubled in consumption during the same approximate time-frame (1961 to 2019; see Figure 4.1, entitled "U.K. Vegetable Oils & Sugar Vs Obesity, Diabetes, and Adipose LA%: 1942- 2019").

Since Figure 4.1 regarding the U.K data makes it a bit difficult to observe the beginning and ending points for sugar and vegetable oils in relation to obesity, diabetes, and the LA% in body fat, we've produced a second graph which shows only the trend lines for sugars and seed oils versus the other conditions. This graph, entitled "U.K. Vegetable Oils & Sugar Vs Obesity, Diabetes, and Adipose LA%: 1961-2019," begins in 1961 and ends in 2019, as the title indicates (see Figure 4.2).

In this graph, one can observe the highly positive and linear correlation between vegetable oils, obesity, diabetes, and the LA% in body fat. However, here we clearly observe an inverse (negative) correlation between sugars and obesity, diabetes, and body fat LA%, that is, as sugar consumption substantially declines over a period of more than 50 years, obesity, diabetes, and LA% in body fat all climb remarkably. Furthermore, such evidence has been independently verified by other researchers.[703]

AUSTRALIA AND AUSTRALIAN ABORIGINALS: POPULATIONS WITH RISING SEED OILS, OBESITY AND CHRONIC DISEASE – WHILE BOTH SUGARS AND CARBS FALL

Prehistorians now believe that the Australian Aboriginal population, sometimes referred to as "Torres Strait Islanders," came to Australia from Southeast Asia at least 40—50,000 years ago.[704] They're undeniably the original people of Australia. For tens of thousands of years, the Aboriginals lived as hunter-gatherers under vastly differing conditions, in various climates, and as a result, with many varied diets based on available flora and fauna.[705]

The Aboriginal peoples were omnivorous, deriving their diet from a very wide variety of available plants and wild animals depending on geographic locale and season of the year. Virtually all animals were considered edible, including mammals, birds, reptiles, marine species, fish, shellfish, and even insects.

"Everything edible on an animal carcass was eaten, including muscle, fat depots, bone marrow and internal organs,"[705] wrote one anthropological nutrition researcher. Consumption of plants included, "tuberous roots, seeds, fruits, nuts, gums [plant gums] and nectar" as well as uncultivated plants such as "fruits, berries, seeds… beans" and honey.[705]

Numerous reports have described the Australian Aboriginals as being lean and physically fit, without having developed any of our westernized diseases, when they lived as hunter-gatherers. Following an analysis of the broad scientific literature on the subject, Professor of Nutrition, K. O'Dea, formerly of Deakin University, Geelong, Australia, published two tables that have been slightly modified and grouped together (page 182). This table indicates the health of the Aboriginals both before (left) and after (right) westernization of the diet.[705]

In his book, *Nutrition and Physical Degeneration* (1939), Weston A. Price, who had spent considerable time investigating the nutrition transition of the Aboriginals, wrote the following:

"Those individuals [Aborigines]… who had adopted the foods of the white man suffered extremely from tooth decay as did the white. Where they had no opportunity to get native food to combine with the white man's food their condition was desperate and

Health of Australian Aboriginals as hunter-gatherers, consuming native, traditional diet.	Chronic diseases in Australian Aboriginals after westernization of diet, with seed oils, sugars, refined flours, and processed foods.
Physically fit	Obesity of the android type (male-like)
Lean (BMI < 20 kg/m^2)	Hypertension
Low blood pressure	Body weight and blood pressure increase with age
No age-related increase in BMI or blood pressure	Type 2 diabetes mellitus
Low fasting glucose levels	Coronary heart disease
Low fasting cholesterol levels	Elevated triglycerides and low HDL-cholesterol levels
No evidence of diabetes	Hyperinsulinemia (high insulin, indicating insulin resistance, a precursor to or facet of diabetes)
No evidence of coronary heart disease	Insulin Resistance
No evidence of metabolic syndrome	Metabolic syndrome

Adapted from: O'Dea, K. Diabetes in Australian Aborigines: impact of the western diet and lifestyle. Journ Intern Med. 1992;232:103-117.
© Copyright C. Knobbe, Ancestral Health Foundation, 2022. All rights reserved.

extreme... *It is quite impossible to imagine the suffering that these people were compelled to endure due to abscessing teeth resulting from rampant tooth decay."*[706]

Like most of the populations that Price observed in the 1930s, the Aboriginals had no dentists.

In regard to Aborigines who had been provided government food subsidies, Price stated, "The rapid degeneration of the Australian Aborigines after the adoption of the government's modern foods provides a demonstration that should be infinitely more convincing than animal experimentation. It should be a matter not only of concern but deep alarm that human beings can degenerate physically so rapidly by the use of a certain type of nutrition, particularly the dietary products used so generally by modern civilization."[707]

One of Price's final statements on his analysis of the effects of westernized food on the Aborigines came in his final paragraph on the subject:

"While the Aborigines are credited with being the oldest race on the face of the earth today, they are dying out with great rapidity wherever they have changed their native nutrition to that of the modern white civilization."[708]

By many accounts, when Australian Aboriginals are exposed to westernized diets, a clear pattern of physical degeneration begins. The ultimate effects include the development of an android form of obesity (male-pattern with heavy trunk and abdomen), which emerges in both men and women, accompanied by insulin resistance that, in turn, leads to or is associated with, high blood sugars, high triglycerides, hypertension, and eventually, type 2 diabetes, and premature cardiovascular disease.[705] Indeed, by all accounts, Australian Aboriginals were healthy before European settlement and did not suffer from chronic disease.[709]

In 2016, the population of Australia was just over 24 million, and at that time, just under 800,000 of that population were represented as either Aboriginal or Torres Strait Islander, and these groups represented 3.3% of the population at that time.[710] And whereas we've already observed the devastating health effects of these people while consuming westernized diets, the remainder of data and analysis will regard Australia as a whole.

Like most of the world, the whole of Australia has westernized its diets with processed foods, seed oils, and refined flours and sugars, particularly since the mid-20th century. As Price discovered in the 1930s, only the most remote parts of the world – those that cannot be reached by roads or ports – are relatively immune to the commercialized "foods of the white man."[28]

In Australia, adult obesity has risen more than three-fold since the earliest available prevalence study. In 1980, adult obesity was about 9%,[711] which elevated to 20.3% in 1995, 20.4% in 2000, 25.9% in 2008, 29.1% in 2012, 29.0% in 2015,[712] and finally to 31.3% in 2018.[713]

Also, in 2018, the National Health Survey found that, in addition to 31.1% being obese, another 35.6% were overweight, with the total overweight and obesity resting at 67% that year.[713] Additionally, for men aged 65 to 74 years, 42.2% were obese.

In 2001, 3.3% of Australians reported being diabetic, and that number rose to 4.1% in 2007, 4.2% in 2011, 4.7% in 2014,[714] and a total of 4.9% in 2018.[713]

A total of 47% of Australians had one or more chronic disease conditions in 2018, which was up from 42.2% in 2008.[713] Hypertension (high blood pressure) affected 22.8%, arthritis affected 15.0%, asthma 11.2%, osteoporosis 3.8%, cancer 1.8%, and kidney disease 1.0%. Heart conditions, stroke, and vascular disease affected 4.8%, while mental and behavioral conditions affected 20.1% of people.[713] As of 2016, chronic, non-communicable diseases were estimated to account for 89% of all deaths in Australia.[715]

With regard to the dietary transition in Australia since the mid-20th century, we observe a fairly typical pattern – more processed foods accompanied by marked increases in seed oils – however, sugar consumption has been on a downward trend since 1961. Two different studies have verified these facts; the first of these two papers was published in 2011, by Alan W. Barclay and Professor Jennie Brand-Miller, at the University of Sydney, under the title, "The Australian Paradox: A Substantial Decline in Sugars Intake over the Same Timeframe that Overweight and Obesity Have Increased."[711]

The title tells the story, indeed. After reviewing the fact that obesity has increased three-fold in Australia, between the years of 1980 and the approximate date of the study (2011), the authors concluded the following:

"The findings confirm an 'Australian Paradox' – a substantial decline in refined sugars intake over the same timeframe that obesity has increased." [711]

To further substantiate or refute the data, which was initially based primarily on the FAO database, the researchers analyzed total sugars (both added and naturally occurring), as well as the consumption of confectionary, sugary products, and non-alcoholic sugar-sweetened beverages, including fruit juices, in the end concluding that the FAO data was verified and accurate.

There was no denying it – an inverse correlation between sugar consumption and obesity existed – as sugar consumption went down, obesity went up, at least in Australia. Barclay and Brand-Miller noted, however, that a similar situation existed in the U.K., i.e., obesity rising during the same timeframe that sugar consumption fell.

The second study on the so-called "Australian Paradox" was also published by Barclay and Brand-Miller, some six years later, in 2017.[716] The researchers again found that, over the period between 1980 and 2011, total sugar consumption had decreased from 152 g/day down to 127 g/day, which is a decrease of 16%. Once again, four different data sources all indicated the same phenomenon – obesity was still on the rise in Australia, despite substantial declines in sugar intake.

"This inverse relation between trends in the prevalence of overweight and obesity and changes in the consumption of added sugars has been termed the Australian Paradox. The rising prevalence of obesity in the face of apparently falling intake of added sugars challenges the widespread belief that energy from sugars is uniquely linked to changes in the incidence of obesity."[716]

These researchers, like most, did not mention or apparently consider seed oils as the culprit, which has been the norm in Nutrition.

Utilizing the FAO database as well, with more recent data accessed via Knoema, we've graphed the consumption of sugars and vegetable oils versus the trends of obesity, diabetes, and chronic disease prevalence (see graph below, "Australia: Vegetable Oils & Sugars Vs Obesity, Diabetes, and Chronic Disease, 1961-2019"). Measured in terms of energy, sugar consumption was 558 cal/day in 1961 and dropped

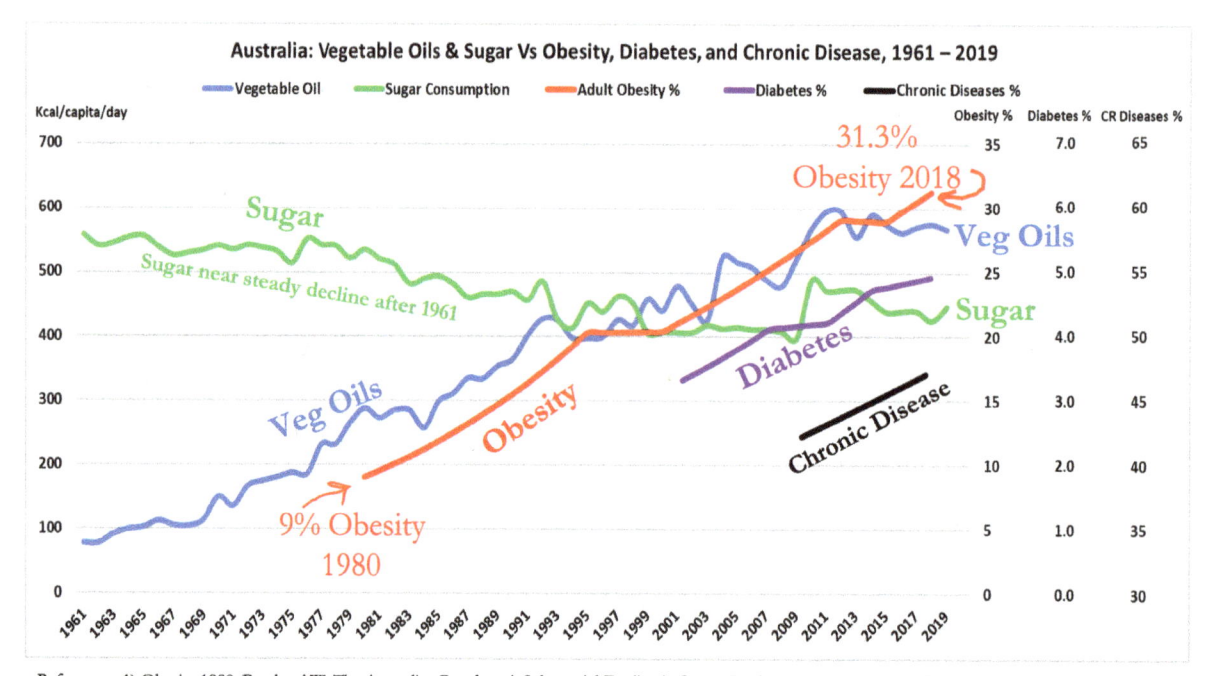

Australia: Vegetable Oils & Sugar Vs Obesity, Diabetes, and Chronic Disease, 1961 – 2019

References: 1) Obesity 1980: Barclay AW. The Australian Paradox: A Substantial Decline in Sugars Intake over the Same Timeframe that Overweight and Obesity Have Increased. Nutrients. 2011;3:491-504. 2) Obesity 1995-2015: Huse O. Obesity Research & Clinical Practice. 2018;12(1):29-39. 3) Obesity 2018: National Health Survey: First results. Australian Bureau of Statistics. 2017-18. 4) Diabetes, 2001-14: Diabetes. Australian Government, Australian Institute of Health and Welfare. 23 Jul 2020. 5) Diabetes 2018: National Health Survey (see number 3). Chronic Disease: National Health Survey (see number 3). 6) Vegetable oil and sugar consumption: FAO Food Balance Sheets, retrieved from Knoema.com. © Copyright C. Knobbe, Ancestral Health Foundation, 2022. All rights reserved.

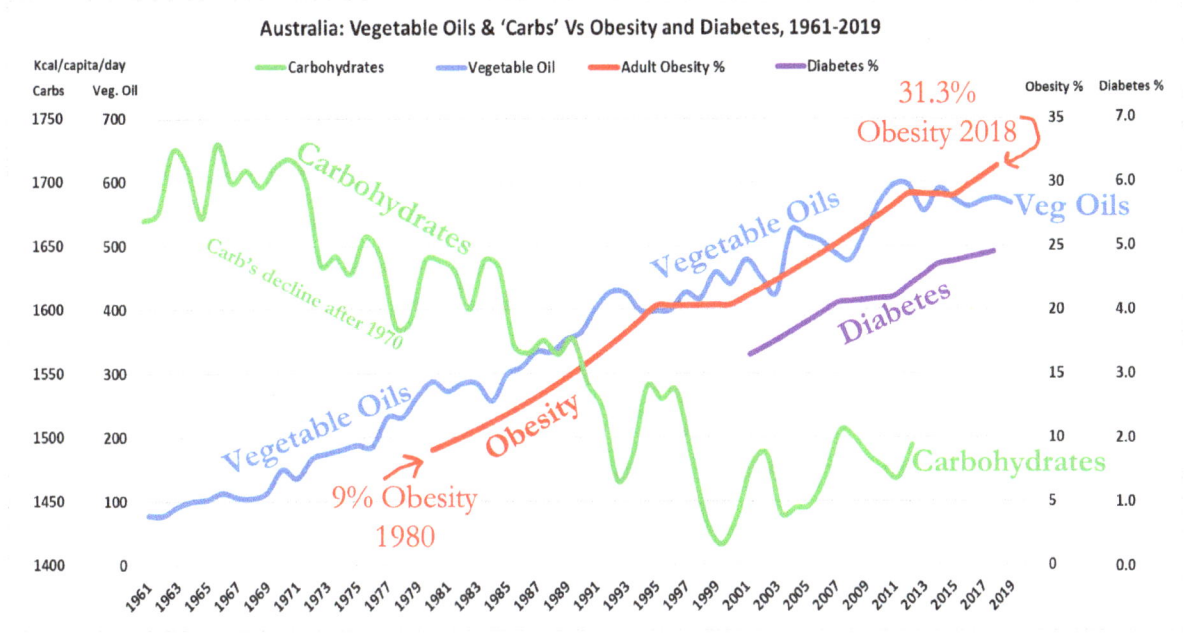

Australia: Vegetable Oils & 'Carbs' Vs Obesity and Diabetes, 1961-2019

[Graph showing carbohydrates declining from ~1669 kcal/capita/day in 1961 to lower values by 2019; vegetable oil consumption rising sharply; adult obesity rising from 9% in 1980 to 31.3% in 2018; diabetes rising from ~1% to ~5%.]

References: 1) Obesity 1980: Barclay AW. The Australian Paradox: A Substantial Decline in Sugars Intake over the Same Timeframe that Overweight and Obesity Have Increased. Nutrients. 2011;3:491-504. 2) Obesity 1995-2015: Huse O. Obesity Research & Clinical Practice. 2018;12(1):29-39. 3) Obesity 2018: National Health Survey: First results. Australian Bureau of Statistics. 2017-18. 4) Diabetes, 2001-14: Diabetes. Australian Government, Australian Institute of Health and Welfare. 23 Jul 2020. 5) Diabetes 2018: National Health Survey (see number 3). Carbohydrate Data: OurWorldInData.org. 3). 6) Vegetable oil and sugar consumption: FAO Food Balance Sheets, retrieved from Knoema.com. © Copyright C. Knobbe, Ancestral Health Foundation, 2022. All rights reserved.

to 447 cal/day by 2019 – a decrease of 20%. Total vegetable oils, on the other hand, elevated from 78 cal/day in 1961 to 567 cal/day in 2019, an increase of of 7.27-fold (627%) (reference in graph on page 184).

We've also examined carbohydrate consumption in Australia over the same time frame, finding a substantial decline in carbohydrates, again during the same period of time while obesity, diabetes, and chronic diseases all escalated. In 1961, total carbohydrate availability was 1,669 cal/day, and that decreased to 1,493 cal/day in 2013, which is a drop of 10.5%.[717] And again, this is during a period of a more than 3-fold increase in obesity, a marked rise in diabetes, and a substantial surge in the percentage of people afflicted with chronic diseases (see graph above, "Australia: Vegetable Oils & 'Carbs' Vs Obesity and Diabetes, 1961-2019").

Sugars are indeed problematic when consumed to excess, as they're nutrient-deficient food. They should be minimized, just as recommended by Weston A. Price in 1939 and 1945, and more recently by the WHO and many other authoritative institutions. Sugar-sweetened beverages, sweets, confectionary, and other added sugars should be minimized in favor of choosing more nutrient-rich foods, such as fruits, vegetables, and whole grains, when well tolerated.

Carbohydrates, per se, are not inherently problematic, except when they're processed (sugars and refined flours), and the evidence in the U.S., Australia, and Japan (to be reviewed) proves that obesity, diabetes, and chronic diseases have all escalated while carbohydrates are on the decline. Again, many have wrongly implicated both sugars and carbohydrates for one simple, unfounded reason: they tend to "run with" seed oils.

That's right. Great reductions of carbohydrates

often reduce seed oil consumption, and we'll review why in further detail subsequently, but for now, suffice it to say that the greatest sources of carbohydrates in westernized diets, for example, mixed chicken dishes, french fries, potato chips, tortilla chips, yeast breads, pasta dishes, pizza, rice containing dishes, muffins, donuts, candies, etc., are often enormous sources of seed oils.[718] The oils lie neatly hidden in these foods, fooling many into the belief that these foods are 'mostly carbohydrates.'

Thus, substantial carbohydrate restriction tends to reduce seed oil consumption, often leading to success, and voila – the "low-carb diet" works! But, when we understand why something works, now we're free to zero in on where the success comes from, which can be very liberating since many people do not prefer low carbohydrate diets. Furthermore, there are many beneficial nutrients in numerous whole food, higher carbohydrate food sources, including potatoes and other root vegetables, whole grains, fruits, etc.

PAPUA NEW GUINEANS OF TUKISENTA: EXTREME "HIGH CARB" BUT HEALTHY!

Yet another of the most fascinating ancestral diets in history is that of the Papua New Guineans that live at high altitudes, generally known as "Highlanders" because they reside at approximately 6,500 to 8,000 feet (~1800 – 2600 m) elevation. The primary population on which we'll focus is the people of Tukisenta, Papua New Guinea (PNG), who were the subjects of the largest and most comprehensive study of any ancestral population to date.

The Tukisenta, PNG population is incredibly unique because they exist on a subsistence economy based almost exclusively on the cultivation of sweet potatoes and pig herding, heavily in favor of sweet potato consumption.[720] Sweet potatoes originated in Central America and are believed to have been introduced to PNG about 1200 years ago.[719]

Dietary consumption of the Tukisenta, PNG population, on a caloric basis, consists of more than 90% sweet potatoes, with only small amounts of animal meats, the latter being mostly pork and small amounts of fowl. Yet, they've been found to be, at least by western standards, very healthy and largely free of chronic disease.[720]

Beginning in 1966, researchers Professor Peter F. Sinnett, senior research fellow, National Heart Foundation of Australia, and Professor H. Malcolm Whyte, The John Curtain School of Medical Research at The Australian National University, undertook the largest study of any ancestrally living population up to that time, to scientifically evaluate both the diet and health of the PNG Highlanders. Prior to initiating the study of the Tukisenta population, Sinnett and Whyte were aware that multiple hospital-based studies had already indicated that, in this population, cardiomyopathy, hypertension, and coronary heart disease were rare.[721] [722] [723] [724]

Remarkably, researchers Campbell and Arthur, in a study of 2000 admissions to the medical ward of the local Port Moresby General Hospital, between 1960 and 1962, found that only four patients (0.2%) had hypertension, and not a single case of admission was related to coronary heart disease or cardiomyopathy.[722]

Sinnett and Whyte assessed the entire population of Murapin, a tribal community located in the West Highlands, centered about Tukisenta. Some 1,489 people were studied, which included 779 people over 15 years of age. The on-location assessments took place over a period of about 3-and-a-

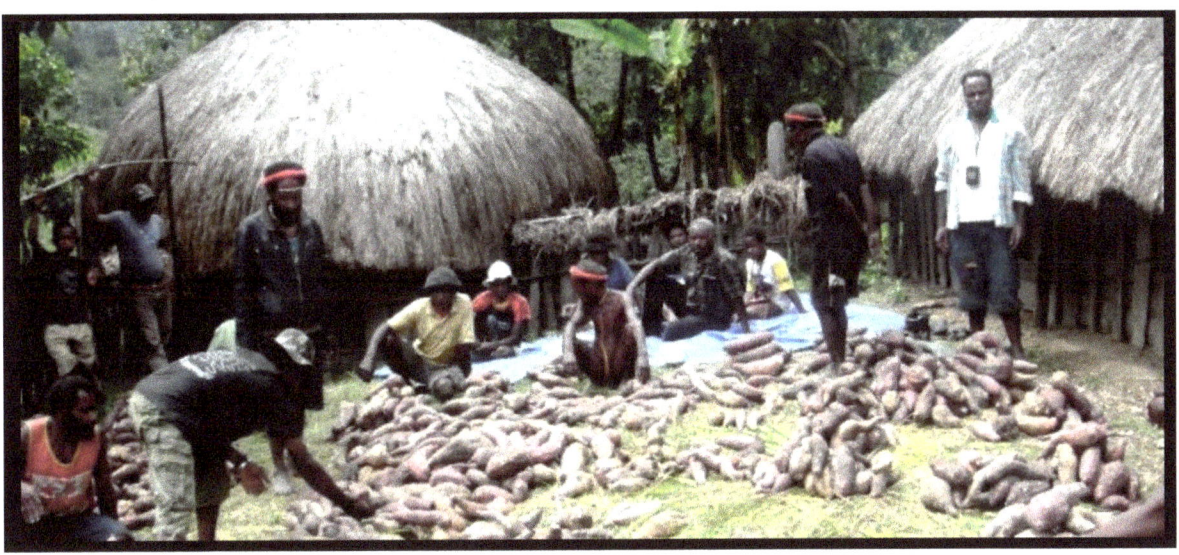

Papua New Guinean (PNG) Highlanders following a sweet potato harvest, the staple food of their ancestors for at least 1200 years. Residing at altitudes of 6,500 – 8,000 feet, the Highlanders had no access to seafoods, thus making more than 90% of their diet from sweet potatoes while occasionally feasting on pork and chicken.
© Copyright C. Knobbe, Ancestral Health Foundation, 2022.

half years, between October 1966 and early 1970. The research professors made some profound observations:

"The subjects were shorter and lighter than Europeans, muscular and mostly very lean…" and later reported, *"the population was lean, physically fit, and in good nutritional state… ischemic heart disease [CHD] is much less common than in Americans, and indeed, than in any other population which has been surveyed… No diabetes or gout was found…"* and finally, *"Ischemic heart disease was rare if not absent."*[720]

Furthermore, the Papua New Guineans' weight decreased with age, whereas the opposite effect had already been observed in European and American populations. They also were reported to have had no age-related macular degeneration (AMD).

Sinnett and Whyte's studies took almost two years to complete and were incredibly well detailed. Carbohydrates in the diet came almost exclusively from sweet potatoes and were confirmed to be greater than 90% of calories, with fat reported as an incredibly low 3% percent of calories.[720] They reported protein consumption to average 25 g per day.

In an extensively detailed previous paper on the PNG population, Sinnett and Whyte reviewed the dietary analysis, in which all foods consumed, during a period of one week, by a subset of 90 people from the population were weighed, recorded, and then analyzed subsequently. The types of potatoes consumed were biochemically analyzed for nutrient content.

They found that the average daily protein, fat, and carbohydrate, was 25.3 g, 6.2g, and 540 g for men, and 20.2g, 7.4g, and 410 g, for women, respectively.[725] Caloric consumption was 2,300 cal/day for men and 1,770 cal/day for women.

This indeed is only 2.4% fat for men and 3.8% in women (for an average of ~3%), which is by far the lowest fat and the highest carbohydrate diet of any ancestral diet of which we are aware. Undoubtedly, this diet appears to reach the upper threshold of possibility for high carbohydrate and low fat, at least of any naturally occurring diet where severe malnutrition does not occur.

Some might question the validity of Sinnett and Whyte's analysis and perhaps question whether the one-week analysis of their food consumption was long enough. However, the extensive duration of the investigation of the Highlanders over a period of more than three years, as well as the impeccable reputation of the research professors Sinnett and Whyte, strongly suggests that the data is valid and an appropriate representation of the long-term diets of the Highlanders.

Furthermore, similar findings were documented in two other PNG Highlander populations, one in 1947 and another in 1974, both of which independently verified extreme heavy dependence on a single vegetable staple.[726] [727]

In fact, in the 1974 PNG Highlander study, the population of Lufa had a diet extremely similar to the population of Tukisenta, with sweet potatoes being the staple crop and smaller amounts of yams, bananas, taro, pandanus, sugar cane, and leaves, with the animal source, again being small amounts of pork and other meats as very minor contributors.

In this population, total caloric consumption was 2,523 cal/day and the macronutrient ratios were 84% carbohydrate, 10% fat, and about 6% protein, yet the population was lean and apparently quite fit.[727] As we'll see subsequently, these are the approximate macronutrient ratios for the Okinawans around the year 1960, who were also once among the longest surviving people on the planet.

If we ended this review on the PNG Tukisenta Highlanders here, one might be left with the impression that this could be yet another near perfect diet, since it is indeed ancestral but did not cause any severe malnutrition. But there's more to the story.

There are some downfalls of such a diet, even though such a diet leads to remarkably better health outcomes than typical western diets. And this would only make sense if we view the Highlander's diet with appreciation for the principles laid out by Weston A. Price in the 1930s and 1940s. With so little animal fats in the diet, were the Highlanders getting enough of the fat-soluble vitamins A, D, and K2? If not, then we should expect to see some negative ramifications – and that is indeed what we see.

Sinnett and Whyte found and reported the following:

"The dental condition of this group was extremely poor. Of the adult population, 64% of males and 47% of females showed dental caries [cavities]. Periodontal disease was present in 96% of males and 87% of females."[725]

Vision declined precipitously with advancing age, apparently primarily because of cataracts, since the population had no cases of macular degeneration, and there was no mention of glaucoma (though ophthalmologists were not part of the team). Arthritis was quite common in the group, with 8.4% of adults having had complaints of joint pain, and, after the age of 60, 32% of males and 21% of females had complaints of severe joint pain.[725]

Without butter, milk, eggs, organ meats, cod liver oil, or beef tallow, the Tukisenta Highlander population was very likely deficient in vitamin K2, which drives calcium into teeth and bones.[728] As Price found, this would account for the very high degree of dental cavities and perhaps for the joint pains, though other causes might account for this as well, including iron deficiency.

The Highlanders also had almost no source of pre-formed vitamin A (retinol), which is present in substantial amounts in the animal sources listed above, but does not exist in sweet potatoes or any other plant sources. Plants provide "pro-vitamin A" carotenoids such as beta-carotene, which may be converted to the active form of vitamin A in the body, but conversion is typically only around 4% and may be negligible, which may have left at least some of this population deficient in vitamin A.[729] [730]

On yet another interesting note, tobacco was smoked by 73% of the males and 20% of the females, with 57% of males and 14% of females stating they were heavy smokers. Smoking declined with age in the population such that 46% of males and none of the females were still smoking beyond age 60.[720] The manner of smoking, however, was not traditional cigarettes, but rather, more akin to pipe smoking. The population was further exposed to almost constant smoke in their homes, due to the placement and near-continuous use of centrally placed open wood fires in the homes, which were entirely without chimneys and with very little ventilation.[720]

Perhaps as a result of the tobacco smoking and perpetual exposure to smoke in the homes, respiratory diseases were the most common cause of morbidity and mortality amongst the Papua New Guineans, with pneumonia accounting for 17% of hospital admissions. Acute bronchitis and pleurisy were also common, but there was no mention of emphysema or chronic obstructive pulmonary disease (COPD), key terms normally used in reference to cigarette smoking and lung disease.

And as far as reduced lung function with age, the authors reported the following:

"... the implied decrease in lung function in the subjects of the present study is not as great as was found for an agricultural population in South Wales..."[725]

In general, this evidence is consistent with the evidence in other cultures where tobacco smoking in populations without seed oil consumption appears to have dramatically reduced harmful effects.

In summary, the PNG Highlanders of Tukisenta had little or no obesity, were lean and physically fit, had little or no coronary heart disease despite a very high prevalence of tobacco smoking and smoke exposure, and had no diabetes or gout. However, they did have poor dental health, significant arthritis, and lung ailments, even if the latter was not emphysema. Their diet of more than 90% sweet potatoes and greater than 90% carbohydrate was tolerated well. If the population had also consumed just small amounts of either butter, eggs, whole milk, cod liver oil, organ meats, or even small amounts of beef, they would have achieved higher levels of fat-soluble vitamins and would have theoretically had far healthier teeth, bones, joints, and even lungs as well as greater immunity to pneumonia and other infectious diseases. Nevertheless, in the authors' own words, they summarized:

"...the [Tukisenta] subjects invariably were in good health."[725]

Just like all other ancestrally living populations who have had great resistance to chronic diseases, the Tukisenta Highlanders did not consume refined flours, sugars, seed oils, or artificially produced trans fats. In short, they consumed no processed foods.

Given that their diet was only 3% fat, and the bulk of that came from sweet potatoes and very small amounts of traditionally raised pork, **we have estimated their omega-6 LA consumption at about 0.6% of total calories**. Once again, we observe in a traditional living population that the ancestral diet provides less than 2.0% of calories as omega-6 LA. And again, contrast this to westernized diets that contain anywhere from about 6% to 12% omega-6 LA.

HIGH-PUFA DIETS: WHY THEY'RE DANGEROUS AND SATURATED FATS ARE HEALTHY

High-PUFA diets, as you have undoubtedly observed, potently promote every chronic disease that you can think of, including overweight, obesity, coronary heart disease (CHD), cancers, metabolic syndrome, type 2 diabetes, dementia, Alzheimer's disease, autoimmune diseases, age-related macular degeneration (AMD), and a myriad of other chronic diseases, both well-known and rare.

Beginning with the next section of this chapter as well as Chapter Five, we'll address why this happens at the metabolic, that is, molecular level. Besides seeing a correlation at the macro-level – for individuals or populations – we want to know what's happening at the molecular level.

Since cardiovascular disease is the world's number one killer, taking the lives of an estimated 17.9 million people each year – 32% of all deaths worldwide[731] – let's examine the biological (molecular) mechanisms which will indeed support the epidemiologic evidence that we've already reviewed.

HOW IS OMEGA-6 LA EXCESS DRIVING CORONARY HEART DISEASE?

In the classic medical textbook, *Western Diseases*, edited by Norman J. Temple, PhD, and Denis P. Burkitt, MD, contributing author Dr. Hans Diehl, clinical professor of Preventive Medicine at Loma Linda University, wrote the following:

"The failure of cholesterol reduction to reduce mortality from CHD [coronary heart disease] and from all causes in most human intervention trials has prompted considerable debate regarding the validity of the lipid hypothesis and the probable benefits of cholesterol reduction as a national health objective."[732]

If reducing cholesterol empirically and consistently, fails to resolve or reduce CHD, shouldn't this lead us to question the hypothesis? Again, the old adage comes to mind – If you can't prevent or reverse a condition, you probably don't understand it.

The "diet-heart hypothesis," first proffered by University of Minnesota's physiologist, Ancel Keys, PhD, nearly 70 years ago in the 1950s, holds that saturated fat drives cholesterol higher, cholesterol drives atherosclerosis, and that leads to CHD.[733] [734] The "lipid hypothesis" was born in 1913 by Nikolai N. Anitschkow, a young Russian pathologist, who reported that feeding pure cholesterol from eggs yolks dissolved in sunflower oil, produced atherosclerosis in rabbits.[735]

This hypothesis holds that low density lipoprotein (LDL) cholesterol, as it elevates, drives atherosclerosis.[736] There is just one problem with these hypotheses – neither has ever been proven. In fact, today there is at least as much evidence against these hypotheses as there is for them.[737] Let's examine just some of the contradictory evidence.

In 2009, William R. Ware, PhD, Emeritus Professor, University of Western Ontario, London, Ontario, Canada, reviewed 19 studies that, when evaluated collectively, appear to falsify the hypothesis that LDL cholesterol per se induces atherosclerosis, including another 10 studies which found no correlation between total cholesterol or LDL and the progression of atherosclerosis. These studies collectively found no correlation between total cholesterol levels and atherosclerosis at autopsy or coronary artery plaques on CT scans.[738] They also found only a trivial correlation between coronary artery calcium (CAC) scores and LDL levels.[738]

Danish physician, Uffe Ravnskov, MD, PhD, famous for questioning the lipid hypothesis, reviewed 19 studies that followed 30 cohorts and a total of 68,094 participants, finding that LDL cholesterol was inversely related to all-cause mortality for people aged 60 or above, that is, higher LDL was associated with a longer lifespan in 92% of people and, in the other 8%, no association was found.

Just since 2009, there have been nine independent meta-analyses (studies evaluating many studies), including studies by (lead authors only) Jakobsen (2009),[739] Mente)2009),[740] Skeaff (2009),[741] Siri-Tarino (2010),[742] Chowdury (2014),[743] Farvid (2014),[744] de Souza (2015),[745] Harcombe (2016),[746] and Zhu (2019),[747] every one of which found that saturated fat was not independently associated with heart disease.

Not to be deterred, the American Heart Association (AHA) subsequently released a Presidential Advisory on dietary fats, restating and re-establishing their nearly 6-decade-old dietary advice to reduce saturated fat and replace it with PUFA (omega-6 rich-oils), which will lower cholesterol.[748]

Indeed, the AHA continues to advise Americans to consume no more than 5% to 6% of their calories as saturated fats,[749] the 2015-2020 Dietary Guidelines for Americans recommends limiting saturated fat to less than 10% of calories,[750] and the World Health Organization also continues to recommend limiting saturated fat to less than 10% of calories.[751]

With each of these organizations, the recommendation to replace saturated fats with unsaturated fats – seed oils – remains deeply entrenched, while nations, countries, and the entire world becomes progressively more overweight, obese, and riddled with chronic diseases, including heart disease.

IT'S NOT NATIVE LDL, BUT RATHER, OXIDIZED LDL THAT IS THE PRIMARY DRIVER OF CHD

Low-density lipoprotein (LDL), or LDL-cholesterol, is not the problem in coronary heart disease, it's only when it becomes oxidized that it's a problem. In other words, LDL per se is not inherently atherogenic – causing CHD. It's only when it is oxidized that it causes CHD. That is the hypothesis which has its roots in research first published by Joseph Goldstein and Michael Brown, in 1979.[752]

Goldstein and Brown showed that LDL was not taken up into macrophages – which begins the atherosclerotic plaque in arteries – while in its native state, but rather, it must be chemically modified (acetylated) first.[753] Once chemically treated and modified from its original state (in an exacting way) macrophages would recognize and ingest the LDL and this, theoretically, might lead to atherosclerosis. Assuredly, once LDL was chemically modified from the native state, the macrophages would accumulate massive amounts of the modified LDL.

In 1979, Goldstein and Brown made it clear that they weren't certain of the implications of their findings, but suspected that modification of LDL in the body might lead to macrophages ingesting the LDL, which could lead to atherosclerosis and, therefore, CHD.[752]

CHAPTER 4

Over the next few years, the two researchers made many discoveries regarding cholesterol metabolism, particularly with regard to the regulation of serum cholesterol via the function of cell receptors that allow uptake of LDL.[754] Their discoveries were considered so valuable that in 1985, both researchers were awarded the Nobel Prize in Physiology or Medicine "for discoveries concerning the regulation of cholesterol metabolism."[754]

Many researchers noted that when macrophages had ingested enough LDL cholesterol, they became full of oily droplets and thus were termed "foam cells" due to their foamy appearance. This was not only the beginning of the development of atherosclerotic plaques, but was the mechanism for progression of disease as well. Goldstein and Brown reasoned that the macrophages would scavenge damaged LDL, in the process becoming foam cells, but that macrophages would not scavenge undamaged LDL.

They weren't sure what kind of damage was required for the LDL to be taken up, however, which would thereby initiate and perpetuate the development of arterial disease. The entire phenomenon was a mystery.

The breakthrough in this puzzle came in 1984, when three researchers, Urs Steinbrecher, Sampath Parthasarathy, and David Leake, who worked in conjunction with Daniel Steinberg and Joseph Witztum, all collectively discovered that the modification of LDL that would cause it to be taken up by macrophages was none other than lipid (fat) oxidation (technically called peroxidation). The oxidized LDL hypothesis was thus born.[755] The next question was, what factor or factors promote oxidation of the LDL particle?

Over the next 30 years, Steinberg and Witztum and affiliate colleagues collectively published more than 100 papers reviewing evidence that the oxidation of LDL occurs within the body which, in turn, drives atherosclerosis.[756] They also showed that oxidized LDL was both proinflammatory and immunogenic, which was further support for the hypothesis.[757]

Given the belief system that oxidation of LDL was indeed the initiating and propagating step for atherosclerosis, it was generally theorized that vitamin E, a good exogenous antioxidant, could be consumed and would reduce progression of disease. Could vitamin E alone be the silver bullet to reduce oxidation and prevent oxidized LDL?

Many large clinical trials were conducted with vitamin E, as well as beta-carotene and other antioxidants given orally, to determine if such supplementation could prevent atherosclerotic disease or progression. In 2010, these trials, meta-analyses, and immense data involving approximately 80,000 subjects had been completed. The outcomes? In the words of Steinberg and Witztum: "disappointingly negative."[757] In general, all such studies were a colossal failure. If oxidation of LDL is the inherent problem in atherosclerosis, then why did antioxidant supplements not prevent the disease?

The brilliant researchers, Steinberg and Witztum, gave every possible alternative consideration as to this abject failure:

"...vitamin E might be the wrong antioxidant in humans," "the dosage may have been too low," "treatment may have been started too late in life," and "antioxidant treatment may be beneficial only in some subset of patients..."[757]

At least in their latest review, no dietary advice was given.

Since the 1960s or even before, there has been intense vitriolic debate amongst the medical community regarding the diet-heart hypothesis, saturated fat, unsaturated fat (i.e., PUFA, or seed oils), cholesterol, and statin therapy (which lowers cholesterol at the expense of enormous potential side effects).[758]

However, one of the earliest studies to examine the relationship between LA (seed oil) versus oleic acid (e.g., olive oil) *enriched diets,* specifically with regard to LDL oxidation itself, was completed by Peter Reaven, MD, along with Steinberg and Witztum (1993).[759] Curiously, the group found that oxidation of LDL was worse with LA-rich diets given to people for eight weeks. In their own words, they wrote the following:

"Substitution of monounsaturated (rather than polyunsaturated) fatty acids for saturated fatty acids in the diet might be preferable for the prevention of atherosclerosis."[759]

Since approximately 1985, more than 9,000 papers have been published regarding oxidized LDL (PubMed search for "oxidized low density lipoprotein"). Without question, oxidized LDL has been accepted as a major mechanism for atherosclerosis leading to CHD. The question is, what causes LDL to become oxidized in the first place?

It has been shown that it is none other than linoleic acid (LA) itself that is the initial component to undergo oxidation when LDL becomes oxidized.[760] LA is also the most commonly oxidized fatty acid in LDL.[761] It has also been shown that once LA becomes oxidized in LDL, it is no longer recognized by the scavenger receptors in the liver, but the macrophages will take it up quickly leading to foam cells and atherosclerotic plaques.[177][178][179]

James J. DiNicolantonio, cardiovascular research scientist at St. Luke's Mid America Heart Institute, and James H. O'Keefe, published a paper in 2018 in which they reviewed 66 key papers all in support of an LA-rich diet causing atherosclerotic heart disease, summarizing as follows:

"Thus, expanding on the oxLDL [oxidized LDL] theory of heart disease, a more comprehensive theory, the 'oxidized linoleic acid theory of coronary heart disease,' is as follows: dietary linoleic acid, especially when consumed from refined omega-6 vegetable oils, gets incorporated into all blood lipoproteins (such as LDL, VLDL and HDL) increasing the susceptibility of all lipoproteins to oxidize and hence increases cardiovascular risk."[762]

There it is – the biological mechanism for seed oils as the primary driver of atherosclerosis – all explained in a single, logical, scientific, and unambiguous way. No such mechanistic sense has ever been given for saturated fat to cause atherosclerosis based on oxidized LDL. And it is impossible to do so because saturated fats, while indeed raising cholesterol mildly, protect LDL from oxidation.

Saturated fats, which are the least likely type of fat to oxidize,[763] not only do not cause heart disease, they protect us from heart disease. This is why, as reviewed previously, when we consume more carbohydrates than we can burn, our body converts those excess carbohydrates preferentially to saturated fat first and monounsaturated fats second.

In the conclusion of their paper, DiNicolantonio and O'Keefe wrote the following:

"In summary, numerous lines of evidence show that the omega-6 polyunsaturated fat linoleic acid promotes oxidative stress, oxidized LDL, chronic low-grade inflammation and atherosclerosis, and is likely a major dietary culprit for causing CHD, especially when consumed in the form of industrial seed oils commonly referred to as 'vegetable oils.'"[762]

So now all we need is evidence that ties together oxidized LDL to actual coronary heart disease, right? And we have that. The coronary artery calcium (CAC) score is a measure of the calcification within coronary arteries, taken by a CT scan utilizing sophisticated programs. Calcium shouldn't normally be in our coronary arteries, but rather, should be in our teeth and bones.

However, calcium tends to be deposited within our coronary arteries in the face of CHD, and the more calcium in the coronary arteries, generally the more atherosclerosis, and the greater the cardiac risk.[764] The most frequently used measure of this is called the Agatston score. According to University of Washington researchers, in review of expert consensus on CAC scanning outcomes,

"a zero calcium score makes the presence of atherosclerotic plaque very unlikely and may be consistent with a low risk of cardiovascular event in the subsequent 2 to 5 years. In contrast, a 'high' calcium score indicates greater likelihood of disease and may be consistent with moderate to high risk of a cardiovascular event during that time period."[764]

Oxidized LDL (Ox-LDL) has been correlated to coronary artery calcium (CAC) scores. In fact, whether CAC scores are zero, intermediate, or high, this has been correlated to increasingly higher circulating levels of Ox-LDL.[765] CAC scoring has been the subject of more than 2,500 published papers, and evidence now indicates that CAC scanning is strongly predictive of future coronary events, which includes myocardial infarction (heart attack) and CHD death.

CAC score and the predicted future of "cardiac events" is as follows: CAC score of 0, equals very low risk with event rate of 1.4% in 10 years; CAC score of 1-100, equals low risk with a 10 year event rate of 4.1%; CAC score of 101-400 indicates intermediate

Coronary Artery Calcium (CAC) Score	Risk Equivalent	10-Year Cardiac Event Rate (Average)
0	Very Low	1.4%
1-100	Low	4.1%
101-400	Intermediate	15%
> 400	High	26%
> 1,000	Very High	37%

Hecht HS. Coronary Artery Calcium Scanning – Past, Present, and Future. JACC Cardiovasc Imaging. 2015;8(5):579-596.
© C. Knobbe, 2022. Ancestral Health Foundation.

risk, with a 10-year event rate of 15%, CAC score greater than 400 indicates high risk, with a 10-year event rate of 26%; and finally, CAC score greater than 1,000 indicates very high risk, with a 10-year event rate of 37% (see table on page 194).[766]

Thus, a very substantial body of evidence, with roots going back more than 40 years, shows that Ox-LDL is the major culprit in the genesis and progression of atherosclerosis. Likewise, we also have a strong body of evidence, both theoretical and demonstrable, that Ox-LDL is driven by seed oil consumption high in omega-6 linoleic acid (LA), that LA and its metabolites actually define oxidation of LDL, and that higher Ox-LDL predicts higher CAC scores.

Seed oil consumption induces oxidized LDL, Ox-LDL predicts CAC scores, and CAC scores predict cardiac events. It's all very logical. And to end on a simple, practical plan to prevent progression of coronary heart disease and possibly reverse it as well? Get rid of the seed oils. Eat animal meats or fats, butter, eggs, and organ meats, instead.

WHY HIGH-FAT DIETS HAVE OFTEN BEEN 'PROVEN' DANGEROUS

To understand the vilification of saturated fats and deep lack of appreciation of excess LA as a primary culprit in the pandemic of chronic disease, it is important to understand how science operates, as this plays a large role in how we have reached this sad state of affairs. Most of the scientific investigations and literature from the past century has made little or no distinction between the types (or origin) of dietary fats, whether in observational studies or randomized trials.

Even the most distinguished researchers often make absolutely no distinction between fats in the diet that are derived from seed oils versus fats derived from 100% grass-fed, pasture-raised animals. In nearly all of such studies, therefore, there is no distinction between diets of 1 to 2% LA, which might well be considered ancestral, versus those of 8 to 12% LA, which are likely the most westernized. In our view, this may be the greatest, most consistent, and generalized systematic error in all of the scientific literature. The actual content of the LA in the diets being studied is seldom considered as a crucial variable in the outcomes.

Thus, numerous investigators have claimed that "high-fat diets" or "western diets," for example, produce obesity,[767] hypertension,[768] type 2 diabetes, and metabolic syndrome,[769] with claims that such diets may also promote heart disease[770] and cancers.[771] However, on deeper investigation, we often find that the investigators unknowingly and often unwittingly, used or observed diets very high in seed oils and, therefore, omega-6 LA.[769]

Many such diets in animal studies or in reference to human populations utilized (or observed) very high omega-6 seed oil diets, including soybean, corn, canola, cottonseed, rapeseed, sunflower, and safflower oils,[769] all of which push dietary LA percentage to very high levels. Yet many authors are entirely unaware, making no such distinction between these fats and naturally low LA fats such as those from butter, beef tallow, coconut oil, or palm kernel oil.

Once again, if we turn to existing population examples, we find that the Maasai tribe of Kenya and Tanzania,[257] the traditional Eskimos of Greenland,[772] the Tokelauans,[362] Kitavans,[773] various South Pacific Islanders,[774] the Aché of Paraguay,[775] and 19th century Americans,[776] all either consume or consumed, substantial amounts of fat and animal fats, yet generally remained exquisitely healthy and without overweight or chronic disease. But in all cases, dietary analysis proves that their omega-6 LA consumption was less than or equal to about 2% of the diet or at least that virtually none of their fats were derived from seed oils.

On the other hand, we have many examples of individuals and even populations on relatively low-fat diets, whose health has suffered markedly. Examples might include the Japanese of the past four decades (reviewed in Chapter 5), individuals on plant-based diets consuming substantial seed oils,[777] [778] and those on a macrobiotic (mostly grains) diet (when seed oils are included).[778] In all such cases, the omega-6 LA consumption is generally high, e.g., 6 to 8 percent of the diet or more.

It is our assertion, therefore, that it's neither the low-fat nor the high-fat diets which are inherently the issue. Rather, it's the type of fat that is infinitely more critical. So whether one consumes an average fat diet, a low-fat (high carb) diet, or a high-fat (low-carb) diet, it's not the percentage of fat that matters; it's the source of the fat, the LA content of that fat, and the presence of fat-soluble vitamins in that fat that matters the most.

In diets that are beneficial to health, the LA consumption is exceedingly low, that is, in the 1 to 2% range of the diet, and it doesn't matter if the diet is high-fat or low-fat. Achieving this level of LA in the diet, of course, can only be accomplished without seed oils. In fact, all natural diets without processed foods, seed oils, or substantial amounts of nuts and seeds (the latter of which is rare in ancestral diets), whether low in carbs or low in fat, will always be very low in omega-6 LA.

THE GREENLAND INUIT OR 'ESKIMOS' – CARNIVORES BUT HEALTHY AND HEART DISEASE FREE ON THEIR ANCESTRAL DIET

The headline of a Discover journal article reads, ***"The Inuit Paradox – How can people who gorge on fat and rarely see a vegetable be healthier than we are?"***[779] The headline is telling.

The historical discoveries of the traditional Inuit ('Eskimos') and their high animal fat diets, along with their purported lack of heart disease, must be told, as these are the scientific chronicles that catapulted omega-3 fatty acids into mainstream consciousness worldwide.[796] Interestingly, and more recently, the same science that established omega-3 fats as protective, as well as the assertion that the 'Eskimos' had little or no heart disease, have both been called into question.[797]

The term 'Eskimo' has been used for the groups of closely related Indigenous people that include the Inuit and the Yupik (or Yuit), collectively from Alaska, Northern Canada, Siberia, and Greenland. Today, the term 'Eskimo' may be considered unacceptable to some, and we'll refer to the population as Inuit, in keeping with preferred terminology across most of Alaska, Canada, and the Arctic.[780] However, any quotes in the literature will not be changed.

The story of the Inuit, who generally reside in the frozen tundra north of the Arctic Circle, represents the common theme that we observe over and over, and which has been presented as far back as the 1930s by Weston A. Price.[28] Native, traditional people enjoy tremendous health and great resistance to chronic disease of every type until they begin to westernize their diets.

Perhaps the first to recognize the health of the

Inuit was Hans Egede, missionary to Greenland in 1741, who wrote the following remark:

> "...*Greenlanders were strong and able bodied. You seldom see someone with a natural ailment, or disease, except for a weakness of the eyes caused by the keen winds of spring and the snow and ice, which hurt the eyes.*"[781]

In 1908, August Krogh and Marie Krogh, in a scientific expedition, completed a study of the diet and metabolism of the 'Eskimos' of Greenland.[782] In the brutally cold conditions of the Arctic, where temperatures may plunge to -50 °F (-45 °C), combined with the very brief summer, where temperatures generally do not rise above 50°F (10 °C), the geographic region presents few opportunities for plant foods.

The Krogh team wrote that the Inuit of Greenland consumed "a diet which is practically exclusively of animal origin" stating further that "The Eskimos are probably the most exquisitely carnivorous people on Earth, living, as most of them do, almost exclusively on meat and fish" surviving "for long periods... absolutely without vegetable food."[782] They noted that their only indigenous plant foods were whortleberries and a few seaweeds, mostly eaten in the summer or fall months.

The primary and favorite foods of the Inuit came from seals, which included the meat, liver, blood, and blubber, although they also consumed reindeer, walruses, whales, birds, bird eggs, and fish, with the latter primarily being Capelan (of the salmon family of fish).

The Krogh team carefully analyzed the Inuit diet, confirming that it was extremely rich in protein and fat, with trivial amounts of vegetable matter, and exceedingly low in carbohydrate. About half of the carbohydrates came from the glycogen stores in animal meats. They found that the Inuit consumed, on average, per day, an extraordinary 282 grams of protein, 135 grams of fat, and just 54 grams of carbohydrate, which worked out to be 2,559 calories, 44% protein, 47% fat, and about 8% carbohydrate.[782]

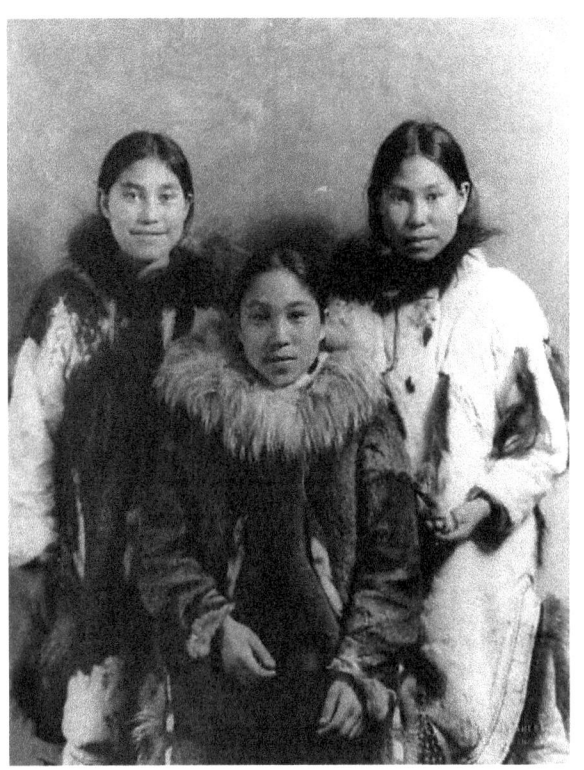

Studio portrait of three young Eskimo women, circa 1908-1915. Image in the public domain.

The Krogh team found that the Inuit were generally of short stature with a "distinct disposition to become fat," however, they confirmed that their health was "on the whole rather good."[782] Rheumatism was practically their only ailment but was quite common.

The team found that, despite consuming a diet that they described as being "like those of the carnivorous animals," the Inuit people had little or no uric acid diseases such as the painful condition of gout, the latter of which is a common concern in western medicine with 'high protein diets.'[783]

The Krogh investigators also made no mention of heart disease or cancer in the Eskimos, although, as we've reviewed, coronary heart disease was virtually unknown on a worldwide basis in 1908. The team concluded, "the diet does not appear to have any injurious effects whatever upon the people."[782]

The Inuit traditionally ate enormous amounts of seal oil, which is a marine omega-3-rich oil.[784] [779] In general, they would cut fist-sized chunks or narrow strips of seal blubber and place it into various containers that were made of skin, plastic, or glass. The oil would gradually separate from the solids in the blubber and float to the top.

They would then typically pour a few tablespoons of the oil on a plate and dip dried fish, dried meats, dried seal meat, or when occasionally available, even greens or bread into the oil before eating. In fact, in the 19th century, the trading of seal oil was common practice among the Inuit.[784]

In the 1930s, Weston A. Price evaluated both 'isolated and modernized Eskimos' and wrote extensively about his evaluations. In his words, Price wrote:

*"The Eskimo race has remained true to ancestral type to give us a living demonstration of what Nature can do in the building of a race competent to withstand for thousands of years the rigors of an Arctic climate. Like the Indian, the Eskimo thrived as long as he was not blighted by the touch of modern civilization, but with it, like all primitives, he withers and dies. **In his primitive state he has provided an example of physical excellence and dental perfection such as has seldom been excelled by any race in the past or present [emphasis added]**."*[785]

In the 1970s, Danish researchers Hans Olaf Bang, MD, PhD, and Jørn Dyerberg, MD, PhD, completed four primary expeditions to Greenland and produced multiple seminal scientific papers over that decade, which established that fish and omega-3 fats were ostensibly "heart healthy,"[786] [787] [788] [789] [790] a belief system that persists today.

With these multiple studies and publications, Bang and Dyerberg presented much evidence that, taken together, established that CHD in Greenland was still rare, at least up until that time. The curious and ironic finding, however, for a scientific community poised to vilify high-fat diets, was that the Greenland 'Eskimos' consumed a diet that was "extremely rich in animal fat," yet the population of northern Greenland was relatively free of heart disease and had virtual absence of myocardial infarction (heart attack).[787]

The following four pieces of evidence were presented in Bang and Dyerberg's papers:

First, between 1935 and 1943, the Chief Medical Officer for Greenland, Dr. Alfred Bertelsen, published four volumes of his and other physicians' collective experience in Greenland over the previous three decades, approximately,[791] but he did not even mention ischemic heart disease; nor did he use comparable terminology to indicate substantive CHD, although he did discuss atherosclerosis among Greenlanders.[792]

Second, based on the annual report of 1978 for the state of health of Greenlanders, between 1973 and 1976, death from ischemic heart disease accounted for an average of just 3.5% of all causes of death.[792]

Third, the same 1978 "state of health" report gave an annual average of 9.5 cases of myocardial infarction (MI, or heart attack), most of which were from the southern part of Greenland, which is the region known to be the most westernized in their diet.

Fourth, between the years 1968 and 1978, Bang and Dyerberg published the following evidence and excerpt:

"not a single death from ischemic heart disease or case of myocardial infarction [heart attack] was reported from the UmanaK district (population of about 2600) where the present investigations were carried out."[786]

Bang and Dyerberg also referenced that, Professor Bent Harvald, of Denmark, who was head of the medical department at Dronning Ingrids Hospital in Nuuk, the capital of Greenland, as well as a member of the Nordic Council for Arctic Medical Research,[793] published a paper in 1974 in which he wrote the following:

"MI [myocardial infarction, or heart attack] does not occur in the Eskimo population. On the other hand, ECG records in those older than 50 years of age show numerous abnormalities compatible with history of MI at least as frequent as in many Western populations. The same is true for frequent deaths caused by heart failure as a consequence of arteriosclerotic degenerative heart disease. It is therefore a mystery that there are no MIs [via translation from Danish]."[794]

At the time, Harvald had been at the Dronning Ingrids Hospital, now known as Queen Ingrid's Hospital, in Nuuk, since 1965, which was nine years.[793] Dronning Ingrids Hospital was and remains not only the largest hospital in all of Greenland, but also the central hospital for all of Greenland. If Harvald asserted that "MI does not occur in the Eskimo population," he was surely quite accurate, as he would have at least known of hospitalized cases during nine years of experience.

During the period of 1970 to 1978, Bang and Dyerberg made four expeditions to Greenland to complete dietary studies and numerous blood analyses of Greenlanders living in the UmanaK district. The latter is an area where ancestral diets were quite well maintained and the men were mostly employed in seal hunting and occasionally, whaling and fishing.

The scientific team also evaluated a similar number of Greenlanders residing in Denmark for comparison. They determined that, not only were the concentrations of cholesterol, triglycerides, LDL, and VLDL (very low density lipoprotein) lower in the Inuit of Greenland, but they also found, much to their surprise, that both the omega-6 LA and the omega-3 ALA were both much lower in the blood of the Inuit of Greenland as compared to their genetic cohorts in Denmark.

For example, the plasma LA in the Inuit of Greenland was only 40% the level of the Inuit in Denmark (20.3% vs 51.0%, respectively; specifically in the plasma cholesterol esters for the medically minded).[786]

Bang and Dyerberg also found that the Inuit of Greenland, whose dietary fat was dominated by seal meat and blubber, whale meat and blubber, and fish, had much higher long-chain omega-3 fatty acids, especially eicosapentaenoic acid (EPA) and docosahexaenoic acid (DHA).[786]

In fact, the EPA averaged more than 9 times as much in the diet of the Inuit of Greenland as compared to their genetic cohorts in Denmark (4.6% versus 0.5%, respectively) and EPA was also 17.5 times greater in the plasma of the Inuit of Greenland (15.8% versus 0.95% of total fats, respectively; again, in the plasma cholesterol esters).[786]

The Inuit of Greenland's diet was carefully evaluated and, roughly in order of descending calories for animal sources followed by plant sources, was seal meat and blubber, whale meat and blubber, fish, seal intestines, wildfowl, soup with seal meat, tinned food, bread, sugar, potatoes, milk (powder), and biscuits.

Note that there were no obvious sources of vegetable oils in this diet whatsoever, however, the tinned foods, bread, and biscuits were all likely sources of smaller amounts of oils. On the other hand, the diet of Denmark at that time already had very significant amounts of vegetable oil and sugar consumption, with 275 cal/day worth of edible oils and 525 cal/day worth of sugars in 1970.[795]

This is one of the few countries in which we've observed a downward trend in seed oil consumption in recent years. Unfortunately, no such data on sugar and seed oil consumption is currently available for Greenland, as the FAO has never tracked such data in Greenland.

Bang and Dyerberg repeatedly presented and discussed in their papers two seminal observations.[786][796] First, they made it abundantly clear that the levels of linoleic acid (LA) were far lower in the native, traditional living Inuit of Greenland, as compared to the Inuit of Denmark. This, they realized, was due to the low levels of LA in the diet of the Inuit in Greenland, who consumed little processed foods and very few vegetables (or vegetable oils), unlike their genetic cohorts in Denmark.

Second, they reasoned that the very high omega-3 EPA and DHA levels that they observed in the Inuit of Greenland were responsible for the lack of heart attacks and ischemic heart disease. This was a prescient theory that literally began the omega-3 revolution.

Whether or not the Greenlanders had CHD historically presents a contentious debate in the scientific literature,[797] as the evidence indeed is relatively scant and may be considered incomplete. However, historically this is nearly always the case when a disease or condition is rare. Try finding a study to prove malaria has a low prevalence in the U.S. currently. You won't find one. But you will find a slew of studies regarding the prevalence of malaria in Africa, where the disease is endemic.

In 2014, Bang and Dyerberg's extraordinary research and papers from the 1970s were the subjects of attack and controversy, with questions aimed at their assertion that heart disease was once rare in Greenland.[797] This, we suspect, was born out of the perpetual allopathic dogma that high animal fat diets produce coronary heart disease and, therefore, the evidence from the traditional living Inuit conflicts with such theory. However, so does the evidence from the Maasai, Tokelauans, and 19th century Americans (all reviewed previously).

J. Goerge Fodor and colleagues, who collectively argued that Bang and Dyerberg's papers were incorrect regarding the low incidence of heart disease in the Inuit of Greenland, cited much other evidence that CHD was 'as high or higher compared to non-Eskimo populations.'[797] However, nearly all of Fodor's evidence indicating that CHD was higher in the Inuit came from studies published after 1979.[797] This was independently verified by James DiNicolantonio as well.[798]

Detractors of theories and evidence that extreme high natural fat and saturated fat diets do not cause CHD may claim that such populations, for example, the Maasai or the Inuit, had atherosclerosis and, therefore, had "coronary heart disease." They may even conclude that 'their high fat and saturated fat diets are causing disease.' Indeed, there is no argument that atherosclerosis occurs in all populations, even young children.[799] But obviously, the general concern for all of us is not whether we have atherosclerosis, but whether we die of heart attacks, congestive heart failure, or any other preventable heart condition.

In 2003, Peter Bjerregaard of the Division for Research in Greenland, National Institute of Public Health, wrote, "The notion that the incidence of ischemic heart disease (IHD) is low among the Inuit subsisting on a traditional marine diet has attained axiomatic status. The scientific evidence for this is weak and rests on early clinical evidence and uncertain mortality statistics."[800]

And while Bjerregaard's statement is true, it is our collective opinion that Bang and Dyerberg's findings regarding the rarity of coronary heart disease among traditional living Inuit are indeed accurate. The historical evidence, ancestral diet, and everything we understand about the drivers of CHD and chronic disease applies in this population, just the same as in any other, all suggesting that CHD in the population was once rare.

Bang and Dyerberg apparently believed that the key factor in preventing atherosclerotic heart disease, which could end in heart attack, was substantially driven by the long-chain omega-3 fatty acid, EPA. In their 1978 paper, they wrote, "Indeed, enrichment of tissue lipids with E.P.A. whether by dietary change or by supplementation may reduce the development of thrombosis and atherosclerosis in the Western World."[790]

As chapter authors in the book *Advances in Nutritional Research* (1980), they attributed the low level of CHD in the Inuit of Greenland to the fact that their diet induced low levels of cholesterol, LDL, and VLDL, while producing high HDL. Furthermore, the diet resulted in high levels of omega-3 EPA and low levels of the omega-6 arachidonic acid (AA). Of all of these biomarkers, with regard to importance, they wrote, "Of the four factors influencing the tendency to thrombosis [e.g., a clot leading to heart attack] mentioned above, the [high EPA and low AA] seems the most important in explaining the rarity of ischemic heart disease in Greenlanders and is the only one with an experimental basis explaining the mechanisms of action. Our observations on the role of eicosapentaenoic acid [EPA] in reducing thrombosis in Greenlanders may turn out to be of importance in prophylaxis against ischemic heart disease both in Greenland and in other parts of the world."[786]

In other words, Bang and Dyerberg believed that the high EPA and the relatively low omega-6 AA fatty acids may have been key to preventing heart attacks..

With these papers and that final statement from Bang and Dyerberg, a great and ever-escalating interest in high levels of omega-3 fats was born, right along with supplementation of omega-3 fats. And while this may have merit to help prevent heart attacks, particularly when the diet has been too high in LA, let's return to the bigger issue, which is the consumption of LA.

In Bang and Dyerber's studies, just exactly as they reviewed, the omega-6 LA in the diet of the Inuit in Greenland averaged 5.0%, whereas it was 10% in the Inuit of Denmark.[786] LA consumption was exactly twice as high in Denmark at that time, and ischemic heart disease (~CHD) in Denmark was about 60 deaths/100,000 people per year, which was more than three times higher than Spain, nearly three times higher than France, about twice as high as Portugal, and substantially higher than Germany.[801]

If we compare CHD resulting in MI (heart attack) in Denmark at that time to that of the traditional living Inuit, as reviewed by Bertelsen, Bang, Dyerberg, and Harvald, it appears that CHD and heart attacks in Denmark were dramatically higher than in the traditional Inuit.

Unfortunately, body fat LA analysis in Bang and Dyerberg's research wasn't completed, but extensive fatty acid analyses of the blood were completed. In all three different studies of the blood, the LA% was markedly higher in the westernized Inuit of Denmark as compared to the Inuit of Greenland.[786]

For example (apologies for the technicality), the LA concentration in plasma cholesterol was 151% higher in Denmark than in Greenland (51% versus 20.3%, respectively), the LA concentration in plasma triglycerides and free fatty acids was 189% higher in Denmark than in Greenland (17.9% vs 6.2%), and the LA concentration in plasma phospholipids was 238% higher in Denmark than in Greenland (22.3% vs 6.6%).[786]

Now while this review has been quite technical, there is a simple take-home message. We now understand that all three of the above studies of LA concentration in the blood are reflective of the LA concentration in the diet and in the body fat.[802] [803] [804] In other words, with these serum studies of LA concentration, we can predict the body fat LA percentage, at least within a decent range of accuracy.

And with that knowledge, we can conclude that the low LA concentration in the relatively ancestral diet of the Inuit of Greenland led to low serum LA concentrations and would have most certainly led to low body fat LA concentrations.

Thus, once again, we can infer that the presumably very low level of vegetable oils and their derivatives (margarines and trans fats) in the diet of the traditional living Inuit protected them from much coronary heart disease and many other chronic diseases, while the higher LA diet in the Inuit in Denmark would not have.

Hence, the much higher prevalence of CHD in Denmark as compared to the extremely low prevalence of CHD in the ancestrally living population of Greenland. We cannot, however, conclude that there were no seed oils at all in the diet of the Inuit of Greenland in the 1970s, as the tinned foods, breads, and biscuits all were likely sources of oils and, furthermore, the 5% LA in the diet strongly suggests that edible oils were part of the dietary.

DIET AND DISEASE IN THE INUIT: OBESITY, DIABETES, AND CHD EMERGE WITH SEED OIL AND MARGARINE CONSUMPTION

For hundreds if not thousands of years, the traditional diet of the Inuit has been called *kalaalimernit*, and it consists mostly of marine mammals in the form of seal meat and blubber and whale meat and blubber, but also fish, with smaller amounts of wildfowl and terrestrial species, including caribou and muskox, and very little plant life, mostly seaweeds and berries during the very short summer. *Kalaalimernit* has gradually been replaced over the past two to three hundred years by westernized foods.[782 805 806 807]

According to Danish researchers who have studied the dietary transition in Greenland, "Since the 18th century, imported foods have been available like grain, rice, and sugar, but in 1900 *kalaalimernit* still made up 82% of the total energy intake (Bertelsen 1935). Roughly 50 years later, 21% of the diet was *kalaalimernit* in towns and 45% in villages (Uhl 1955). In 2018, the proportion was 14% in towns and 21% in villages, being caribou meat, fish, seal meat, whale skin and blubber (*muktuk*), the remaining being imported foods (Larsen et al, 2019). In larger towns, the same foods are available as in Europe although at higher prices."[808]

According to researcher Anders Koch, chronic disease conditions in Greenland are changing, which is occurring in parallel with the westernized foods:

> "The disease pattern [traditionally] was characterized by high rates of infectious disease and low rates of chronic diseases inclusive of diabetes. In 1940, the Danish physician and Chief Medical Officer for Northern Greenland, Alfred Bertelsen, wrote that, 'One case of diabetes is noted among the patients treated in 1910 at Julianahaab (Qaqortoq, South Greenland), and a few additional patients are known later to have been treated.'"[809]

Researchers found that, between 1962 and 1964, diabetes was found in less than 0.06% of the 4,249 Greenlanders examined at that time.[810] In three different surveys between the years of 1999 and 2014, among 4,520 people, diabetes was present in the range of 6.0 to 9.7%, which is nearly entirely type 2 diabetes.[809] Thus, between about 1962 and approximately 2010, diabetes prevalence elevated from 0.06% to an average of about 7.9%, which is an increase of 1,317-fold.

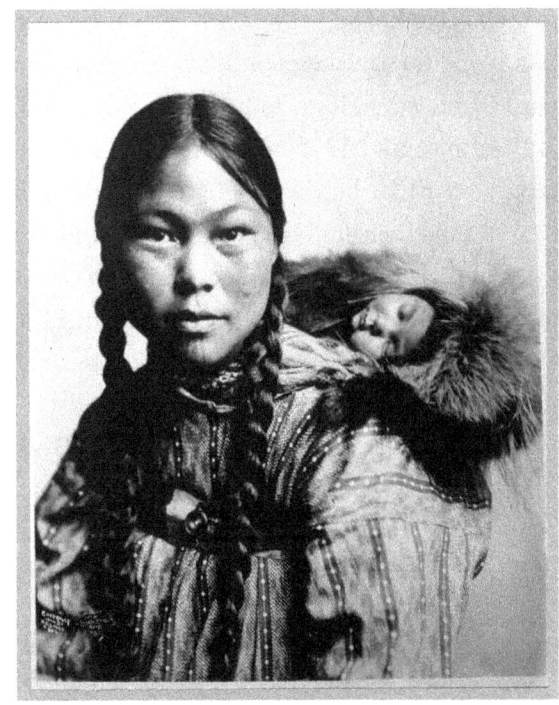

Eskimo mother with child. Photograph taken 1906. Photo courtesy U.S. Library of Congress.

Obesity in Greenland has also increased dramatically over the past 60 years. Obesity (BMI > 30 kg/m²) in Inuit men aged 50 to 69 years in Greenland was 2% in 1963, 10.8% in 1998, and 17.5% in 2008, while obesity in Inuit women of the same age groups was 8.3% in 1963, 23.0% in 1998, and 24.5% in 2008.[811] In 2018, adult obesity in Greenland reached 24% in men and 32% in women with an overall adult obesity prevalence of 28%.[812]

In regard to cancer prevalence, based chronologically on the works of Bertelsen in 1935, followed by the Chief Medical Officer of Greenland from 1951 to 1967, and finally, the Registry of Causes of Death at the National Institutes of Public Health, the approximate increase in cancer deaths in Greenland was three-fold between 1924 and 2009.[813]

Regarding CHD, in a study of 1,851 Inuit people around the year 1962, including 65% of the men aged 40 and above, only 1% had ischemic (poor blood flow) changes on EKG (electrocardiogram).[814] However, in a study completed in 2007, 12.2% of men and 13.4% of women had ischemic changes on EKG. Furthermore, in the 2007 study of 1,316 Inuit living in Greenland, the overall prevalence of CHD based on either chest pain consistent with CHD (angina), history of heart attack, or definite signs of heart attack on EKG, was 10.8% in men and 10.2% in women.[815]

The history strongly suggests that CHD was either extremely rare or nonexistent between 1908 and 1940 and perhaps began to rise after the 1970s. By any number of metrics, it appears plainly evident that CHD has increased remarkably just since the 1960s and even 1970s in Greenland, and may have increased almost infinitely since 1908. In the graph below ("Greenland: Obesity, Diabetes and Estimated CHD Vs High PUFA Oils & Margarines, 1908-2019"), we have estimated CHD as virtually non-existent in 1908 (0.1%), with an estimated trend indicated by the dotted line, ending in 2007 with the known data of an average of 10.5% CHD.

With regard to vegetable oils and their derivatives, like margarines and trans fats, although the FAO does not have consumption data, we were able to obtain data from OEC, which is an organization that tracks import and export data from many

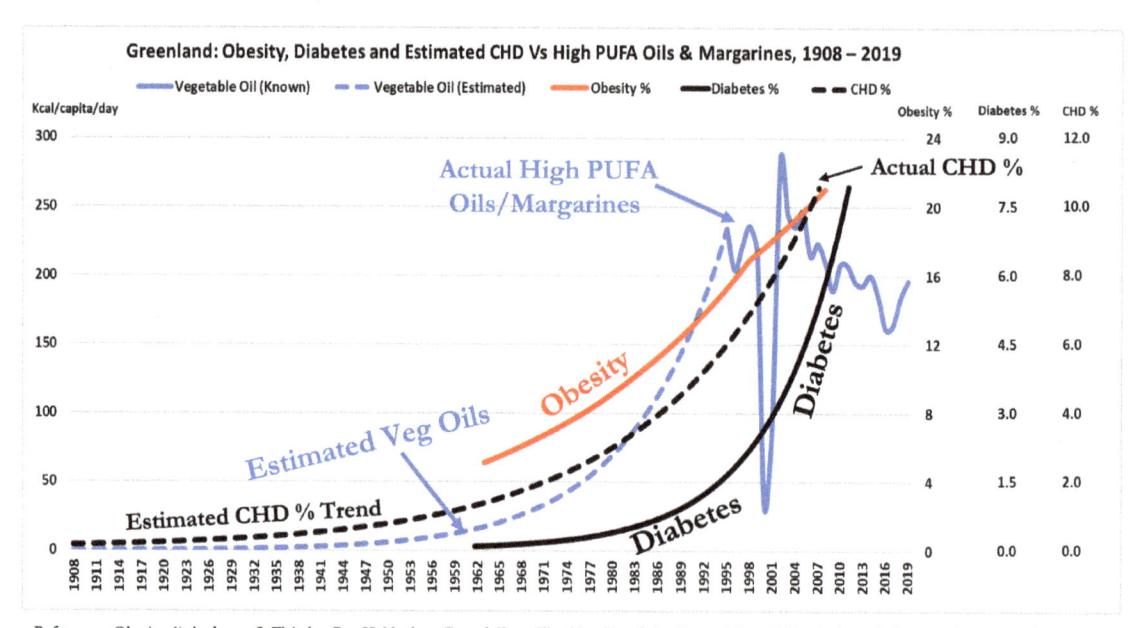

Greenland: Obesity, Diabetes and Estimated CHD Vs High PUFA Oils & Margarines, 1908 – 2019

References, Obesity: 1) Andersen S, Fleischer Rex K, Noahsen P, et al. Forty-Five Year Trends in Overweight and Obesity in an Indigenous Arctic Inuit Society in Transition and Spatiotemporal Trends. Am J Human Biology. 2014;26:511-517. 2) Greenland Obesity Prevalence. Global Obesity Observatory. Retrieved: https://data.worldobesity.org/country/greenland-81/#data_prevalence. Diabetes: 1) Sagild U, Littauer J, Jespersen CS, et al. Epidemiological studies in Greenland 1962-1964. Acta Med Scand. 2009;179(1):29-2. 2) Koch A. Diabetes in Greenland – how to deliver diabetes care in a country with a geographically dispersed population. Int J Circumpolar Health. 2019;2019;78(sup 1) CHD: 1) See Bertelsen A, 1940, herein. 2) Jørgensen ME. High prevalence of markers of coronary heart disease among Greenland Inuit. Atherosclerosis. 2008;196:722-778. Oils/Margarines: Imports and Exports, OEC. Animal and Vegetable By-Products. Retrieved: https://oec.world/en/profile/country/grl. © Copyright C. Knobbe, Ancestral Health Foundation, 2022.

countries and regions. The OEC data indicates that Greenland already had substantial consumption of margarines and seed oils by 1995, as indicated in the graph.[816] However, we know from the Krogh team studies that seed oils were nonexistent in 1908.

As such, in the graph on page 204, we've estimated seed oil consumption between 1908 and 1995, at which point the data becomes known and is presented here for the first time. There are large drops in the apparent consumption data provided by OEC for the years 2000 and 2001, however, we suspect this was failure on the part of the trade office to accurately track data for those years and is no fault on the part of OEC or ourselves.

HIGH LEVELS OF LONG-CHAIN OMEGA-3 FATS – LESS HEART ATTACKS BUT MORE STROKES?

From the landmark studies of Bang and Dyerberg on the 'Eskimos,' we learned that a very high consumption of the long-chain omega-3 fatty acids, EPA and DHA, appeared to have a protective effect against heart attack, but curiously, there would soon follow a concern that this might come at the expense of a greater risk of stroke. One paper regarding this possible effect in Greenland may be quoted as follows:

"a high incidence of stroke has been reported in Greenland as well as among Alaska Inuit and Alaska natives."[817] The paper continued, citing multiple references in support, "Similarly, a low mortality rate from ischemic heart disease and a high mortality from cerebrovascular disease have been reported among Greenlanders and in the Canadian Arctic population."[817]

In high doses, could the long-chain omega-3s lower the risk of atherosclerosis and heart attacks, and yet raise the risk of stroke?

There are two kinds of stroke: ischemic stroke and hemorrhagic stroke. Ischemic stroke is due to poor blood flow as a result of atherosclerosis, blood clots, or emboli, like plaques that break off and travel "downstream" until they occlude an artery, leading to compromised tissues served by that vessel. The latter is much like a heart attack, i.e., a blocked vessel with tissues dying of ischemia secondary to poor blood flow.

Hemorrhagic stroke occurs when a vessel in the brain leaks or ruptures, which might be due in part to high blood pressure, blood "thinning," weakened vessels such as aneurysms, and even ischemic strokes that then lead to hemorrhages. Logistically, given that fish oil – whether from consuming fish itself or from supplements – leads to reduced blood clotting, it seems reasonable to suspect that "thinning of the blood" in relation to high fish or marine life consumption might lead to hemorrhagic stroke.

Another breakthrough that came with Bang and Dyerberg's work was that, even without affecting cholesterol levels substantially, the relative amounts of different polyunsaturated fatty acids – omega-3s versus omega-6s primarily – could meaningfully influence cardiovascular pathways. This suggestion followed the fact that fish oils and their associated omega-3 fatty acids were deemed to have myriad effects such as preventing platelets from aggregating and inhibition of inflammation, which ultimately, appeared to suggest that fish oils could prevent cardiac related death. This was yet another revolutionary concept at that time.[796]

If we return briefly to the finale of Bang and Dyerberg's published research on the Greenland studies, published in 1980, they wrote the following:

"the Eskimo consumption of [omega-6] linoleic (18:2n6) and [omega-3] linolenic (18:3n3) acids is much lower than that of Danes. The intake of linoleic acid by Eskimos is less than half that of Danes, whereas that of linolenic acid is only one fifth."[786]

Indeed, this was true because seed oils are substantial sources of both omega-6 LA and omega-3 ALA, which is why the blood levels of both were far lower in the Inuit of Greenland who had little oils, than in the "Danes" in Denmark, who had much more. But what about the long-chain omega-3s? These are the ones thought to be so healthy.

Bang and Dyerberg reviewed that EPA, DHA, and one other long-chain omega-3 fat (docosapentaenoic acid) were dramatically higher in the Inuit people of Greenland, with the sum of those three fatty acids accounting for an *astonishing 13.1% of the diet compared to only 0.8% for the Inuit in Denmark.*[786]

As reviewed by the authors, the long-chain omega-3 fats, especially EPA and DHA, work synergistically to prevent clotting, which is how they prevent heart attacks and may also help to prevent atherosclerosis. The plaguing question, however, was whether or not this was too much of a 'good thing'?

Though we are not aware of any data on stroke in Greenland from the era of Bang and Dyerberg's studies, a 2011-2012 study in Greenland found that 156 strokes were registered.[817] Of these, 89.1% were ischemic strokes and the other 10.9%, hemorrhagic strokes. This is quite typical, that is, around 90% of strokes are of the ischemic type, not the hemorrhagic.

To compare stroke data between populations, we must understand that most stroke data is quoted as the number "per 100,000 person-years," which takes into account the number of people in the study as well as the term that they were in the study. So a study that followed 1,000 people for a total of 2 years would contain 2,000 person-years of data.

Thus, we need to compare the high omega-3 consuming Greenlanders to other populations for reference. If we just give each country a single number, all of which are "per 100,000 person-years," Greenland was (in "age-standardized" incidence rates) 149. Countries that had much lower average age-standardized incidence rates included Denmark at 93, France at 75, Germany at 85, and Italy at 97.5.[817]

If we only looked at these, we might begin to believe stroke rates are indeed much higher in Greenland. But then we see that (with the same definitions as before) the incidence rate for Norway was 154, Sweden 197.5, Portugal 189.5, Finland 254, and Japan topped the list at 317.5.[817] With this line-up, we begin to see that, by comparison, stroke incidence in Greenland might fall somewhere in the middle-range. Is the fear of fish consumption and stroke beginning to diminish?

An excellent review of the subject was completed at the Feinberg School of Medicine, Northwestern University in Chicago, Illinois, comparing people who never ate fish to those who ate fish up to 5 times per week. Using those who either never ate fish or ate fish less than once a month as the group for comparison, those who consumed fish 1 to 3 times per month had a 9% lower stroke risk, fish consumption once per week had an 18% lower risk, and fish consumption 5 times a week or more had a 31% lower risk of stroke.[818] With this data, there is a practically linear relationship – more fish, lower stroke risk. And the same study found no relationship between hemorrhagic stroke risk and fish consumption.

Numerous other studies have found either no association or an inverse association (more fish, lower stroke) between fish consumption and stroke.[819] Chinese researchers completed a meta-analysis, evaluating 33 separate, independent, cohort studies, summarizing as follows:

"Based on current evidence from prospective cohort studies, we concluded that fish consumption was associated with a decreased risk of stroke."[820]

From all available evidence, we would conclude that consuming fish, probably 2 to 3 times a week certainly, should not only reduce the risk of heart attack but also stroke. As always, the evidence is clear and strong that eating whole fish is what provides the benefit, while the evidence regarding the consumption of fish oil itself is less well addressed, at least in population studies.

Stroke, like all chronic diseases, is complicated, and many factors are involved besides fish or omega-3s. Stroke risk is increased by the presence of high blood pressure, diabetes, other cardiovascular disease, atrial fibrillation (abnormal heart rhythm), smoking, and alcohol consumption.[821] Clearly, every one of these conditions is preventable with ancestral diets and a choice not to smoke or drink heavily. As usual, prevention is key and it is not difficult.

THE TRADITIONAL INUIT DIET IS NOW WESTERNIZED – A LOOK BACK AT LA% IN THE TRADITIONAL DIET

The traditional Inuit diet falls at the extreme other end of the spectrum of macronutrient ratios as compared to the Papua New Guineans of Tukisenta. Whereas the Papua New Guineans of Tukisenta were shown to consume 94.6% carbohydrate, 3% fat, and about 2.4% protein in their traditional diet, the Inuit reviewed by the Krogh team in 1908 were confirmed to consume only 8% carbohydrate, 47% fat, and 44% protein.

Thus, the Inuit were among the highest animal fat consumers in the world, while the Papua New Guineans of Tukisenta had only trivial amounts of animal fats in their diet. And despite the fact that these two diets are polar opposites in terms of macronutrient ratios and derivation of calories, both diets have been shown to succeed very well in preventing chronic disease. It is obvious that both diets, if followed traditionally, are far more successful at preventing chronic disease than any westernized diet.

In the traditional diet of the Inuit, most of the fat came from seal blubber, and given the concern about omega-6 in the diet, the LA content in seal blubber should be of interest, right?

In a very large study of the fatty acid profiles of a total of 760 Alaskan harbor seals, which are the most abundant seals globally, the average LA as a percent of body fat in four different species was an incredibly low 0.67 to 1.21%.[822] Whale blubber, as a percent of body fat, has been shown to average just 1.64% LA.[823] This indicates that both seal blubber and whale blubber are even lower in LA than 100% grass-fed beef, which is often only about 2.0 – 2.6%!

If we make the assumption that the great majority of the fat in the diet of the 1908 Inuit was from seal meat blubber, which is a very close approximation, even at the upper limit of 1.21% LA of total fatty acids (total fat), this calculates to just 1.62 grams of LA per day, which is only 14.6 calories, or 0.6% of total calories!

Once again, as we observe in all native, traditional diets, the LA ranges between about 0.6% and 2.0% of total fats. Even in the mostly traditional diet of the contemporary Inuit of Greenland who were studied by Bang and Dyerberg, the LA content of the diet was 5.0%, which strongly suggests that there were seed oils in their tinned foods and very likely in their large portions of breads and biscuits (14.6 servings/week).[786] None of these three foods were part of their traditional diet, of course. Most processed breads and biscuits contain seed oils, which would have quickly raised their omega-6 consumption to these approximate levels.

More importantly, as in every ancestrally living population, the **traditional Inuit consumed neither refined flours, added sugars, or seed oils** whatsoever, and given that their diet came almost exclusively from wild-caught animals, seaweed, and a few berries, the *LA consumption would indeed have been exceedingly low, in this case, under 1.0% of total calories.*

It seems clear from much epidemiologic evidence, that wild-caught fish and seafood, while very healthy food sources, are not required in order to prevent CHD or other chronic disease. This is proven by the studies of the Maasai, the Papua New Guineans of Tukisenta, and perhaps the greater percentage of 19th century Americans, none of whom had significant sources of fish or seafood, yet remained virtually free of most chronic disease.

In conclusion, the traditional ancestral diet of the Inuit of Greenland contained the following:

- All nutrient-dense, non-processed foods
- Food choices loaded with fat-soluble and water-soluble vitamins (e.g., liver, fish, and seafoods)
- Excellent sources of minerals
- An LA content under 1.0% of calories

Quite frankly, it's no wonder the traditionally living Inuit were robust, healthy, and free of chronic disease.

IS ISRAEL A 'PARADOX'? THE QUINTESSENTIAL NATION FOLLOWING THE AHA'S 'HEART HEALTHY DIET' REPLETE WITH VEGETABLE OILS – BUT IS IT WORKING?

The high-PUFA seed oils have long been shown to reduce total cholesterol levels and with that, and that alone, these oils have been widely recommended in allopathic medicine for both prevention and management of coronary heart disease. As previously reviewed, the American Heart Association (AHA) has recommended for decades very low consumption of saturated fat and continues to advise that all Americans should be substituting unsaturated fats – 'vegetable oils' – in place of saturated fats.

The AHA recommends consumption of 5 to 10% of calories in the form of omega-6 PUFA, including soybean oil, corn oil, and sunflower oil, which are ~56% LA, ~59% LA, and ~68% LA, respectively (see tables in Chapter 6).[824][825]

Since the mid-1990s, Israel appears to have had the greatest compliance with such established recommendations, as their diets have been somewhat low in calories, low in total fat, exceedingly low in saturated fat,[826][827] and simultaneously 'boast' an estimated 12% of calories as LA, which is the highest relative omega-6 consumption of any large population worldwide.[827]

For comparison, recall that Americans averaged approximately 11.8% of calories as LA in 2008.[6] A study in Jerusalem found that omega-6 consumption averaged 10.1% of total calories, with 90% of subjects consuming more than 6% PUFA, and a quarter of the studied group consuming more than 12% PUFA, all as a percentage of total calories consumed.[828]

About as far back as evidence allows, the Jewish population has had an extraordinary consumption of vegetable oils and trivial amounts of added animal fats in the diet. Following the establishment of the State of Israel in 1948 and with the arrival of many groups of immigrants, oil and fat consumption rose from 15 kg/capita/year (33 lbs/yr) in 1950 to 21 kg/capita/yr (46.2 lbs/yr) in 1970.[829] During the same time frame, fish intake dropped from 17 kg/capita/yr (37.4 lbs/yr) in 1950 to 10 kg/capita/yr (22 lbs/yr) in 1973.

Between the years of 1961 and 2019, total vegetable oils consumption began at a low of 317 cal/day in 1961, peaked at a high of 695 cal/day in 2017, and ended in 2019 at 601 cal/day.[830] During the same time frame, butter and ghee (clarified butter) consumption together ranged from as low as 11 cal/day (about one gram or a fifth of a teaspoon) and never rose above 31 cal/day (just over 3 grams, or a little over a half teaspoon), while added animal fats (e.g., tallow, suet, lard, etc.) ranged anywhere from 3 to 31 cal/day (i.e., one-third of a gram to about 3 grams).

In terms of total fats, in 1990, vegetable oils accounted for a staggering 71.4% of the fats, margarine 26.2%, and butter 2.4%. By 1999, these figures were 75.8% vegetable oils, 21.4% margarine, and 2.7% butter.[828] In 2019, total added fats in the diet of the population of Israel included 601 calories of vegetable oils, 26 calories of butter, and 14 calories worth of animal fats.[830]

Thus, for that year, vegetable oils accounted for 94% of added fats, butter 4%, and animal fats 2%. Proportionally, this is the largest consumption of vegetable oils and the lowest consumption of added animal fats of any population that we are aware of. Macronutrient ratios in Israel for year 2013 were 14% protein, 48% carbohydrate, and 38% fat, which is very typical of western countries.[831] Nothing unique there.

Given that seed oils high in PUFA drive LA (and ALA) high in the adipose, the Israeli diet ought to produce very high levels of adipose LA concentration. Indeed, the average values of body fat LA as a percent of total fatty acids (the standard method of presenting these values) was already a staggering 23.94% by 1976,[832] exceeding most all other absolute values in the world by a full 10% and, obviously, exceeding the ancestral values of the Tokelauans at 3.8%,[17] the traditional New Zealand Maoris at 2.6%,[674] and the Pukapukans of Raratonga at 2.6%,[674] all by more than 20%!

The more recent adipose LA levels of the Israelis has remained about the same as the 1976 level, measuring 23.9% in 1995,[833] 24.6% total omega-6 in 1997,[689] and finally, 25.6% adipose LA in 2002.[834] This correlates well with the fact that their seed oil consumption was already known to be very high in 1950 and has only increased. In general, this extreme high percentage of body fat LA is likely the upper limit, at least for a population at large, although individual levels may rise even further in some people.

If we view the Israeli diet through the lens of the AHA and the "ivory tower" diet dictocrats, whose 60-year-old belief system maintains that animal fats are detrimental and vegetable oils are beneficial, the Israeli diet ought to be the perfect diet. At least from a health standpoint, if allopathic medicine is correct, they should be living in a utopian society, right? So, let's examine the effect of this diet on the Israelis.

In regards to obesity prevalence, the first available study in Israel was completed in 2000, which was many decades after their seed oil consumption became very high. Adult obesity (BMI >30) in Israel was 22.9% in 2000,[835] 22.8% in 2013, and 24.1% in 2019.[836] Overweight for those same years was 39.3%, 34.1%, and 34.47%, respectively. Thus, total overweight and obesity was 62.2% in 2000, 56.9% in 2013, and 58.57% in 2019.[835,836] Well over half of the nation has been either overweight or obese for more than 20 years.

The prevalence of diabetes in Israeli Jews in the year 1996 was 3.4%,[837] which rose to 9.6% in 2013 and 9.71% in 2019.[836] In other studies from the Hadera District in Israel, in 2011 the prevalence of adult-onset diabetes was 21% among the Arab population and 12% among Jews; Arabs and Jews represent 21% and 74% of Israelis, respectively.[838]

Using a weighted average for the entire country, this indicates that about 13.9% of adult Israelis had type 2 diabetes mellitus (T2DM) by 2011. In this same study, the prevalence of T2DM had risen to 25% of Arabs by age 57 and 25% of Jews by age 68.[838] In 1996, Israel had the highest death rate from diabetes in the world.[839] Israel's Health Ministry report of 2008 found that, compared to the U.S. and Europe, Israel ranked number one in mortality rates for diabetes, kidney disease, and sepsis (severe infections that involve dissemination of bacteria in the blood, which is life-threatening).

Israel also has a very high rate of deaths from hypertension, reporting 9 deaths per 100,000 in 2008, compared to 5.8 in the U.S., 5.7 in Germany, 4 in France, and 1.5 in the U.K.[840] Deaths due to kidney disease were very high as well at 18.3 deaths per 100,000, compared to 11.7 in the U.S., 7.1 in Germany, 5.165 in France, and 3.5 in the U.K.

If we look back at CHD prevalence in Israel during the 1970s, we make some interesting observations. CHD in the U.S was one of the highest in the world, being about ten-fold greater than Japan.[832] In Israel at that time, the CHD mortality rate was about three-fourths as high as the U.S. and six times higher than Japan.[841]

In the 1990s, the prevalence of CHD, diabetes, and cancer in Israel was quite comparable to other western countries. In 1995, the standardized mortality rate from CHD in Israel was 235 for men and 168 for women, compared with 246 for men and 131 for women in the U.S. and Europe.[842] Thus, the death rate from CHD was approximately the same in men in the U.S. and most of Europe, but was substantially higher in women.

In a study of myocardial infarction (MI, or heart attack) rate among the 25 to 64 year old residents of Jerusalem between 1995 and 1997, the age-adjusted incidence of CHD events, which was defined as either acute MI or CHD death, ranked high.[843] As compared to 21 countries (in the MONICA populations), the incidence of CHD events in Israel was third highest in men and eighth highest in women. However, the one glimmer of good news for Israelis was that the fatality rate from heart attacks was remarkably low.

Cancer is the leading cause of death in Israel, followed in decreasing order by heart disease, diabetes, cerebrovascular disease (stroke), septicemia (sepsis), dementia, kidney disease, chronic lung diseases (primarily chronic obstructive pulmonary disease, COPD), pneumonia and influenza, and accidents.[844]

The Israel National Cancer Registry, within the Israeli Ministry of Health, reported in 2016 that over the past 50 years, the number of patients diagnosed with cancers in Israel had risen five-fold, while the population increased about 3.4-fold, indicating a substantial increase in cancer cases.[845] Between 1970 and 2001, colon cancer incidence in Israel increased 270% in males and 185% in females.[846]

The 2008 Health Ministry Report for Israel also found that, compared to the U.S. and all of Europe, Israel had more deaths due to sepsis, which is an overwhelming whole-body infection and inflammation that most often follows lung (pneumonia), kidney, or bladder infection. In April of that year, the Ministry of Health reported that 3,700 patients were diagnosed with sepsis, which were related to "antibiotic-resistant blood infections," and 1,500 of those afflicted died.[840]

While sepsis accounted for 19.7% of deaths worldwide in 2017, those who both develop and succumb to the condition are overwhelmingly those living in the lower socio-economic regions such as Sub-Saharan Africa, Oceania, South Asia, East Asia, and Southeast Asia.[847] These are mostly regions made up of countries unified as being low or middle-income countries, linked by nutrient-deficiency. Israel, however, is considered a high-income country, ranking 19th out of 189 countries on the 2019 UN Human Development Index, with a "very high" standard of living.[848]

However, in Israel, the lack of animal fats and the extraordinary supply of vegetable oils would leave much of the country on the brink of fat-soluble vitamin deficiencies since vegetable oils contain neither pre-formed vitamin A, D, or K2,[163][164][165][166] all of which are critical to immune function.[849] Lack of animal meats and fats, which are the critical sources of these fat-soluble vitamins, particularly vitamin A, have been considered to be essential factors in enhancing immunity against infectious diseases, including COVID-19.[849]

The World Health Organization (WHO) recommends protein-rich animal sources daily to protect immune function, especially eggs and fish.[850] In 1992, the WHO and the Food and Agriculture Organization of the United Nations (FAO) both concurred, making the following statement:

"Regular consumption of vitamin A-rich foods such as animal products, orange and yellow fruits and vegetables, dark green edible leaves, and palm oil could prevent VAD [vitamin A deficiency]."[851]

However, palm oil, like all oils that are not of animal origin, only contains carotenoids, and no pre-formed vitamin A (see reviews above and elsewhere herein). At about 10% LA, palm oil, which is a tropical oil, is a much safer oil to consume than all of the high-PUFA seed oils; however, it will not have the safety of being very low in LA and also containing fat-soluble vitamin content, like butter and beef tallow, for example.

In the graph on page 212 ("Israel: Vegetable Oil, Sugar, Butter, and Animal Fats Vs Obesity and Diabetes, 1961-2019"), we observe the near tripling of diabetes in Israel during the period of 1996 to 2019, when diabetes elevated from 3.4% to 9.71%. We also observe a slight increase in obesity during this approximate period, from 22.9% in 2000 to 24.1% in 2019.

However, during this same period of time, sugar consumption dropped from 482 cal/day in 1996 down to 341 cal/day in 2019, which is a decrease of 29%. Sugar consumption dropped after 2000, precisely as diabetes elevated geometrically.

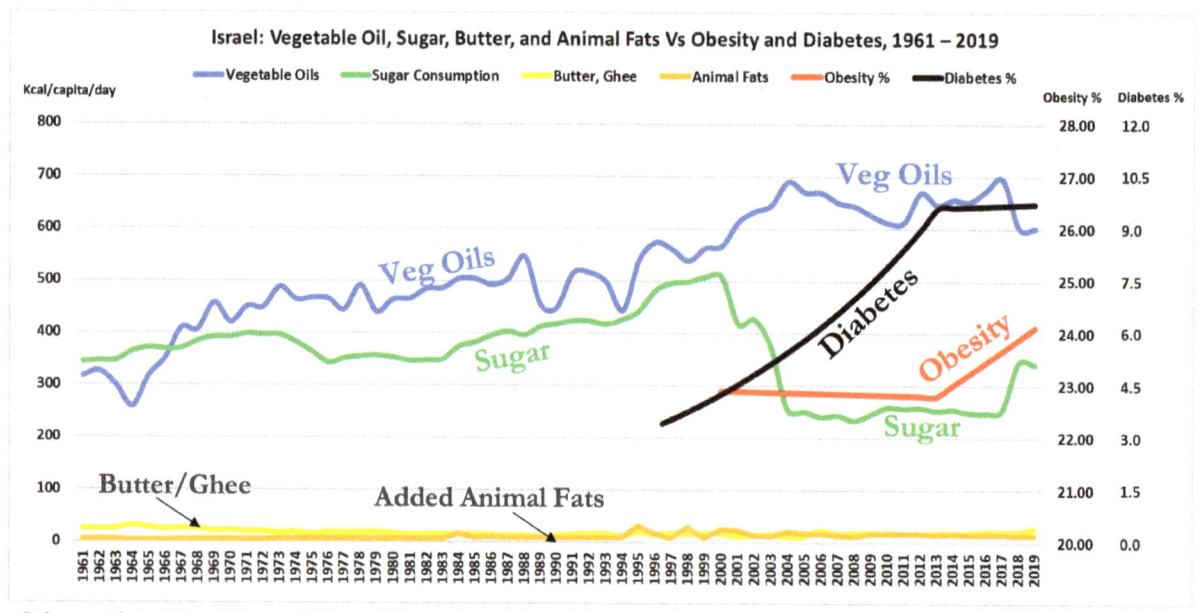

Israel: Vegetable Oil, Sugar, Butter, and Animal Fats Vs Obesity and Diabetes, 1961 – 2019

References: Obesity 1) Yr 2000: Kaluski D N, Berry EM. Prevalence of obesity in Israel. Obes. Rev. 2005:6(2):115-6. 2) Obes Yrs 2013-2019 2) "Results Summary, Prevalence of obesity among adults (ages 20-64)." Israel National Program for Quality Indicators in Community Healthcare." Years 2013-2019. Diabetes: 1) 1996: Health Information Svcs. Israel Ministry of Health: http://www.health.gov/il/units/healthisrael/63.htm. 2) See ref. #2 for obesity. Data for vegetable oils, sugar, diabetes, and sugar: https://knoema.com/FAOFBS2017/food-balance-sheets. © Copyright C. Knobbe, Ancestral Health Foundation, 2022.

During the same timespan, total vegetable oil consumption increased from 574 calories per day in 1996 to a high of 695 calories in 2017, before dropping to 601 cal/day in 2019. As reviewed previously, consumption of butter/ghee and added animal fats remained almost trivial.

Thus, we clearly observe that Israel, the quintessential nation following the American Heart Association's advice, has health concerns that rival the U.S., Western Europe, and, indeed, the most westernized countries worldwide. The population is clearly riddled with overweight, obesity, and chronic disease. From a health standpoint, the Israelis are the polar opposite of ancestrally living populations.

Furthermore, the correlation between chronic disease and seed oil consumption has never been more clear. We observe a marked increase in diabetes between 2000 and 2019, which also indicates much more metabolic syndrome, at the same time that sugar consumption fell by about one-third. Israel, in fact, now joins the United States, United Kingdom, and Australia as the fourth country where we have observed overweight, obesity, diabetes, and metabolic disease all increasing while sugar consumption was precisely on the decline. In each case, however, seed oil consumption has continued to rise.

CHAPTER 4: SUMMARY

All known ancestral diets are low in omega-6 LA because they contain no seed oils and are also low in nuts and seeds, which are the only other substantial sources of omega-6 in the diet. It is our conclusion that ancestral diets generally contain no more than about 2% LA. On the other hand, all westernized diets are generally replete with seed oils, leading to marked accumulations of omega-6 within the tissues of the body. Westernized diets today contain about 8 to 12% LA, which is at least 4 to 6 times too much LA on a percentage basis, and approximately 8 to 12 times too much LA by mass (weight).

Omega-6 LA and omega-3 ALA are essential fatty acids in the diet and must be consumed with a minimum of about 0.5% of calories. These levels are easy to achieve if one eats any kind of food by mouth. There are questionable benefits of getting much more than the required amounts and, by all accounts, levels of LA higher than about 2% of calories will likely begin to promote chronic disease, such as CHD, cancers, diabetes, and overweight.

It has been understood for around 60 years that the PUFA fats – such as LA and ALA – accumulate in body fat and reflect the proportions consumed in the diet. We've observed four populations consuming ancestral diets in 1969 that had adipose LA levels averaging 2.86%, whereas, in the past 20 years approximately, adipose LA levels average about 14.2% in westernized populations. These are staggering differences and reflect that virtually the entire world (with the exception of a very few ancestrally living populations) is consuming extraordinary levels of omega-6 fats.

In population studies, we've observed that the New Zealand Maori and the Pacific Islanders, in general, once had the most revered physiques in the world and were apparently supremely healthy. As is the typical scenario with the westernized food transition, the New Zealand Maori and Pacific Islanders, in general, have all suffered severely.

The New Zealand Maori, who undoubtedly had little or no obesity in the 19th century, now join other Pacific Island populations as being among the most obese in the world. As of 2017, 84% of the Maori are either obese or overweight. As we've seen, sugar consumption since the 1960s has changed little in New Zealand, but seed oil consumption has continued to climb steadily.

Sweden had body fat LA percentage of just 4.0% in 1958, which elevated to 7% by 2006, which still compares very favorably to other westernized nations. Accordingly, their level of obesity, which was only 6.8% in 1985, has risen 'only' to 12.9%. This was paralleled by substantial increases in seed oils.

The United Kingdom has seen a 4-fold increase in obesity and an even more recent 3-fold increase in diabetes, right along with increasing levels of LA in the body fat. Interestingly, sugar consumption steadily dropped by a total of 28% over a 50-year period, while obesity and diabetes rates steadily and dramatically increased.

Obesity in Australia was 9% in 1980 and climbed to 31.3% by 2018, which is a more than 3-fold increase, with modest increases in diabetes recently. During the same timeframe there has been a marked decline in sugar consumption and carbohydrate consumption.

The Papua New Guineans of Tukisenta have one of the most unusual diets of all – more than 90% sweet potatoes – with 94.6% of calories as carbohydrate, 3% fat, and only about 2.4% protein, but they are not vegan as they occasionally consume large amounts of pork and sometimes fowl. In the late 1960s to early 1970s, researchers Sinnett and Whyte found them to be lean, healthy, and virtually free of diabetes, gout, and coronary heart disease. We have calculated that the Papua New Guinean "Highlanders" of Tukisenta consumed a diet that was only about 0.6% LA.

The Inuit, often called 'Eskimos' in the past, were known as the "the most exquisitely carnivorous people on Earth," and although they were not as lean as many other populations while consuming their traditional ancestral diet, they were indeed healthy. They are believed to have had little if any heart disease, and diabetes was virtually non-existent up until about 1960. Since the 1970s, obesity and diabetes have markedly increased while it appears clear that seed oils have elevated to occupy around 10% of calories by 2000. The traditional diet of the Inuit consisted of seal meat and blubber, whale meat and blubber, some fish, walruses, caribou, reindeer, birds, bird eggs, and a very few seaweeds and berries. While consuming their ancestral diet, we've calculated that their omega-6 LA was only about 0.6%.

Israel has been called 'paradoxical' since they have so carefully followed both the American Heart Association and conventional medicine's admonishment to avoid saturated fats and consume more 'heart healthy' seed oils and less meat, yet have high rates of CHD and chronic disease. The Israelis consume precious few animal fats and an extraordinary degree of vegetable oils, which has pushed their body fat LA% to approximately 25%, which is higher than any country in the world that has been measured.

However, the Israelis have experienced levels of CHD, cancers, obesity, diabetes, kidney disease, high blood pressure, and other chronic diseases that rival the worst of the westernized populations. Total obesity and overweight was 58.57% in 2019. Seed oils have been very high since the early 1960s but have elevated to rival the greatest consumers of seed oils in the world, which is the United States. The main difference between the U.S. and Israel is that the U.S. consumes much more meat, which is beneficial, but also substantially more sugar. Sugar consumption has fallen sharply in Israel since 1996, while seed oil consumption continues to rise, and the Israelis have experienced a tripling of diabetes since then.

Coronary heart disease (CHD) has been shown to be causally linked not to LDL, but rather to oxidized LDL. Oxidized LDL (Ox-LDL) is driven primarily by seed oil consumption and, in fact, we measure oxidized LDL based on the presence of oxidized linoleic acid metabolites in the LDL.

Ox-LDL is rapidly removed from the blood and taken up by macrophages, which become "foam cells," and this drives atherosclerosis. Ox-LDL is strongly correlated with progression of the coronary artery calcium (CAC) score, which closely represents the degree of atherosclerosis in the arteries. Thus, Ox-LDL is predictive of the CAC score and the CAC score, in turn, is predictive of coronary "events," such as heart attacks and cardiac death. So how do we reduce our oxidized

LDL? Simple. Stop consuming seed oils and keep omega-6 consumption low.

And how do you keep LA low in your diet? Simply remove soybean, corn, canola, cottonseed, rapeseed, grapeseed, sunflower, safflower, rice bran, and most other oils. Most of these oils are from 20% up to 75% LA. Olive oil may range from about 3 to 27 % LA, with an average of around 10% LA, thus making it a potential contributor to higher LA body fat concentrations if body fat LA is already elevated.

High-quality extra virgin olive oil is certainly dramatically better than all of the seed oils and likely can be part of a healthy diet if one is already healthy. In contrast to seed oils, the traditionally raised animal fats of butter, lard, and beef tallow, for example, will be very low in LA, generally less than about 2% to 3%. These, we will submit, are the safest, healthiest, and most nutritious fats of all, and for most people, should be considered staples of the diet. These fats are the traditional fats of most populations, and they should remain that way.

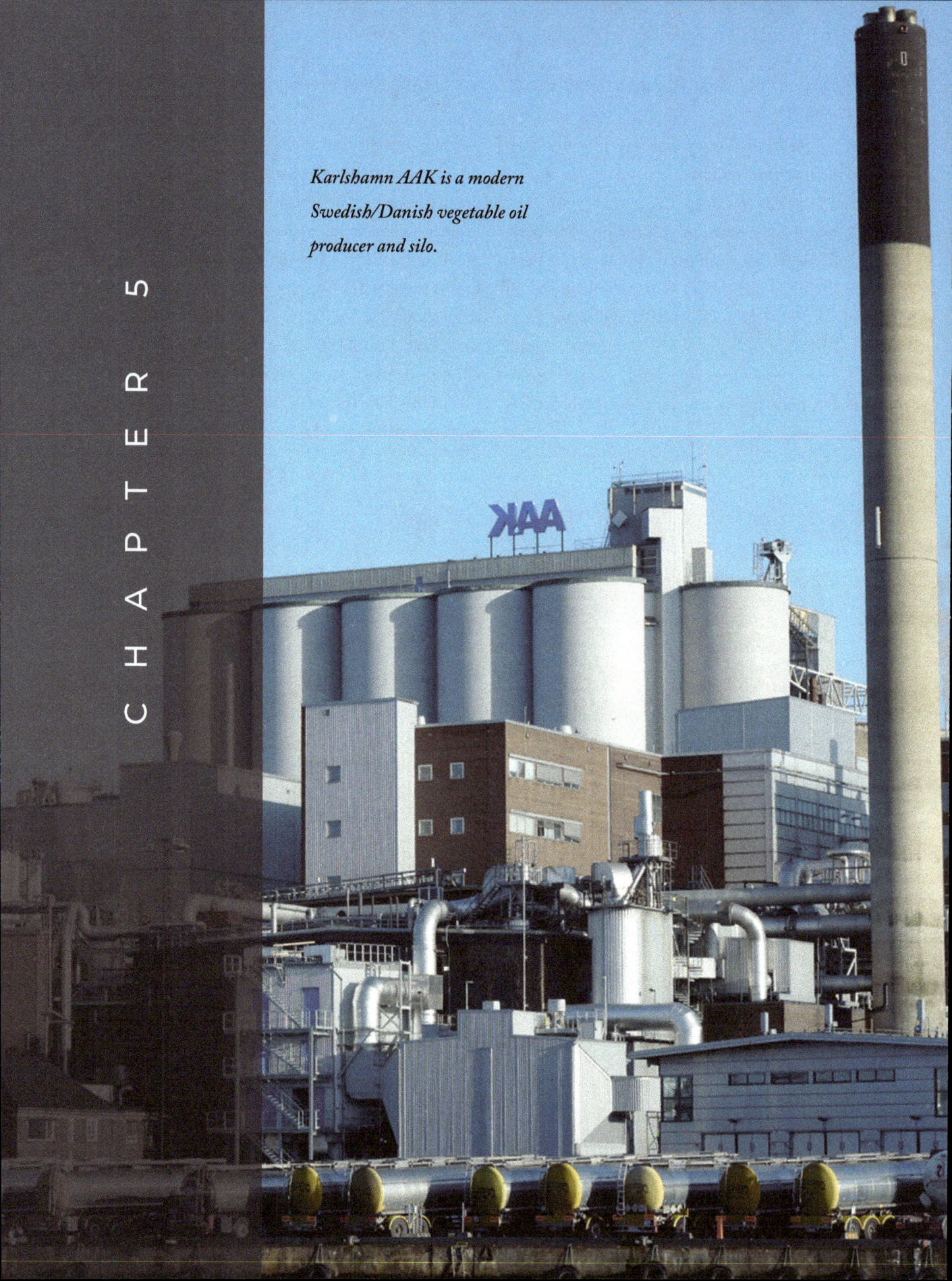

CHAPTER 5

Karlshamn AAK is a modern Swedish/Danish vegetable oil producer and silo.

CHAPTER 5

WHAT THE DEEPER SCIENCE SAYS

"All that man needs for health and healing has been provided by God in nature, the challenge of science is to find it."

– PARACELSUS

WHY YOUR LA MUST BE LOW!

In Chapter 3, we reviewed that the one single characteristic of ancestral diets, which is true regardless of whether they are high in fat (i.e., low-carb), low in fat (i.e., high carb), or even low in protein, is that they're low in omega-6 LA fats. Whether they're made up mostly of animal meats and fats, such as the traditional Inuit, Eskimos, or the Maasai, or they're very high in carbohydrates and are made up mostly of rice or sweet potatoes, such as the traditional Japanese, Okinawans, and Papua New Guineans of Tukisenta, **all ancestral diets are low in LA. All of them!**

And they're also fantastically healthy, providing for healthy children and healthy adults, all resistant to overweight and chronic disease. They're all also approximately 2% or less LA in the diet as a percentage of total calories. And why is this? The most parsimonious explanation is because none of them contain seed oils.

We have reviewed that there has been a pervasive, systematic, and nearly inexplicable belief system of treating all fats the same within the scientific literature. Literally in tens of thousands of scientific investigations (or more), whether the fats are from seed oils and contain 50% LA, or from animal fats such as butter, lard, or beef tallow, and contain only 2% LA, they're most often treated the same from the investigators' standpoint. This is also the case for animal fats that vary markedly in LA.

For example, lard from swine (pigs) that are fed an ancestral diet, have been shown to have LA of 2%, whereas conventionally raised swine from concentrated animal feeding operations (CAFOs), where pigs are fed a standard diet of GMO corn and soy, typically have a body fat LA of 20% (review and references in Chapter Six).

Yet, when investigators use CAFO pork fat (lard) in a study, negative (harmful) results attributed to the animal fat are not recognized as being related to the very high omega-6 content of the lard (up to 20 to 25%) which can even be higher than some edible oils, such as olive oil (~10% LA), palm oil (~10% LA) and canola oil (~21% LA) (see Chapter Six for references).

This systemic failure in Medicine and Nutrition may be the result of two most certain facts: First, seed oils have currently been in the food supply for about 155 years, making them appear to many investigators as normal "fodder" for the human race. Of course, these are investigators who simply are not aware of either the history of edible oils or the deep science and stark contrasts between high- and low-PUFA diets.

Second, seed oils have been promulgated as 'heart healthy' since at least 1961, soon after the American Heart Association (AHA) was influenced by American physiologist, Ancel Keys, who held a prominent position on the board of the AHA at that time.[303]

Thus, many investigators believe seed oils are indeed 'heart healthy' since they lower cholesterol. Therefore, "high-fat diets" used in animal studies and even in human subjects have most often ignored the single most important consideration of the entire diet, which is the source of the fat and, therefore, the omega-6 LA content.

SIMPLIFIED MOLECULAR BIOLOGY OF HOW AND WHY EXCESS LA DRIVES OBESITY AND CHRONIC DISEASE

Omega-6 LA in excess drives overweight and obesity through a number of pathways. First, when LA is consumed to excess, cellular pathways become dysregulated, leading to both proliferation of fat cells and increased fat deposition in fat cells.[852][853] The second major effect of excess LA is that it cripples the burning of fat for fuel (β-oxidation),[854][855] which likely induces a form of "fat partitioning," that is, a preferential storing of fat within the cell because the cellular machinery to burn fat for fuel is damaged.[855]

This is known as mitochondrial dysfunction, and it is unquestionably induced by excess LA, which is characterized by cellular accumulation of fat.[856][65] When this occurs in the liver it leads to hepatic steatosis, also known as "fatty liver disease" or non-alcoholic fatty liver disease.[856] When this occurs systemically, excess body fat accumulates, commonly to the state of obesity and morbid obesity.[857]

A third pathway for LA excess to induce overweight is that it increases the brain's resistance to the effects of leptin, a condition known as leptin resistance.[858][859] Leptin is a hormone produced by fat cells which normally sends a signal to the brain to communicate that cells are energy replete, i.e., "I'm full." But when omega-6 is high, this leptin signal in the brain is impeded while appetite is stimulated.

A fourth pathway for excess LA to induce undesirable weight gain is through inflammation, which is a hallmark of obesity.[860][861] The fifth and perhaps final major pathway by which over-abundance of LA induces overweight is via dysregulation of the cannabinoid system, which has a role in regulating satiety and energy homeostasis. The endocannabinoid system (ECS) is well recognized for its appetite-promoting effects and this has been exploited in *Cannabis* medical applications for terminally ill patients with cancers, for example. The ECS, however, is stimulated by circulating endocannabinoids derived from LA and its metabolite, arachidonic acid (AA), which itself produces overeating.[862][863][864]

We've reviewed the oxidized LDL pathway as the primary mechanism to induce atherosclerosis and CHD, in Chapter Four. Omega-6 LA in excess, in general, induces chronic disease via four major pathways: 1) Oxidation, 2) Inflammation, 3) Toxicity, and 4) Nutrient-deficiency. Each of these will be considered next.

SEED OILS AND HIGH LA DIETS ARE HIGHLY PRO-OXIDATIVE

There has been a pervasive belief system in medicine that inflammation is perhaps the key central player of most all chronic disease, ranging broadly from coronary heart disease, to metabolic disease and diabetes, to Alzheimer's disease, and macular degeneration.[865][866] However, many decades of research and investigation lead us to believe that oxidation, and not inflammation, is by far the greater contributor to the root cause of chronic disease.[867] However, increasing oxidation does, indeed, also lead to increased inflammation.[868]

Oxidation of fats, proteins, and DNA, we believe, is the key central component of overweight, aging, and nearly all chronic disease. Unfortunately, this concept is, in many regards, vastly more complex, elusive, and difficult to grasp and comprehend than is the concept of inflammation.

Oxidation is a process defined at the molecular level by what are called "redox reactions," which stands for oxidation-reduction, because the two processes always occur together. Oxidation of any molecular species is the loss of electrons, while reduction of a molecular species indicates a gain of electrons.

When one molecule is oxidized, the reacting molecule must simultaneously be reduced. Hence, the term "Redox" in relation. An easier way to think of oxidation is the concept of the "rusting" of metal. When bare metal becomes wet, it undergoes oxidation. That is rust.

When we have excessive oxidation in our bodies, it's like we're rusting inside, and this is exceedingly dangerous.[867] However, this process doesn't necessarily require oxygen.[867] When it comes to all of the proteins, lipids (fats), and DNA (e.g., chromosomes) that can be oxidized, as well as the three basic kinds of fatty acids (saturated, monounsaturated, and polyunsaturated), it is the polyunsaturated fatty acids (PUFA) that are by far the most likely to undergo oxidation.[869] The PUFA, once again, are made up of both omega-6 and omega-3 fatty acids.

For the moment, we should recall that the concentration of PUFA in our diet reflects the PUFA in our bodies. And again, we've seen that the LA body fat concentration in ancestrally living people in the Pacific Islands averaged 2.86%, but that LA since the 1990s in the Western World averages about 14.2%. In the histogram graph below ("Vegetable Oil Fats are Dangerous Because They Oxidize"), we observe the fat type along with its respective LA%, plotted against its specific peroxidation index (PI).

The PI is an exceedingly complicated measure of a fat's ability to undergo oxidation (peroxidation) and become rancid. Think of a rotting fish – that is rancidity. Same with rotting beef or any other

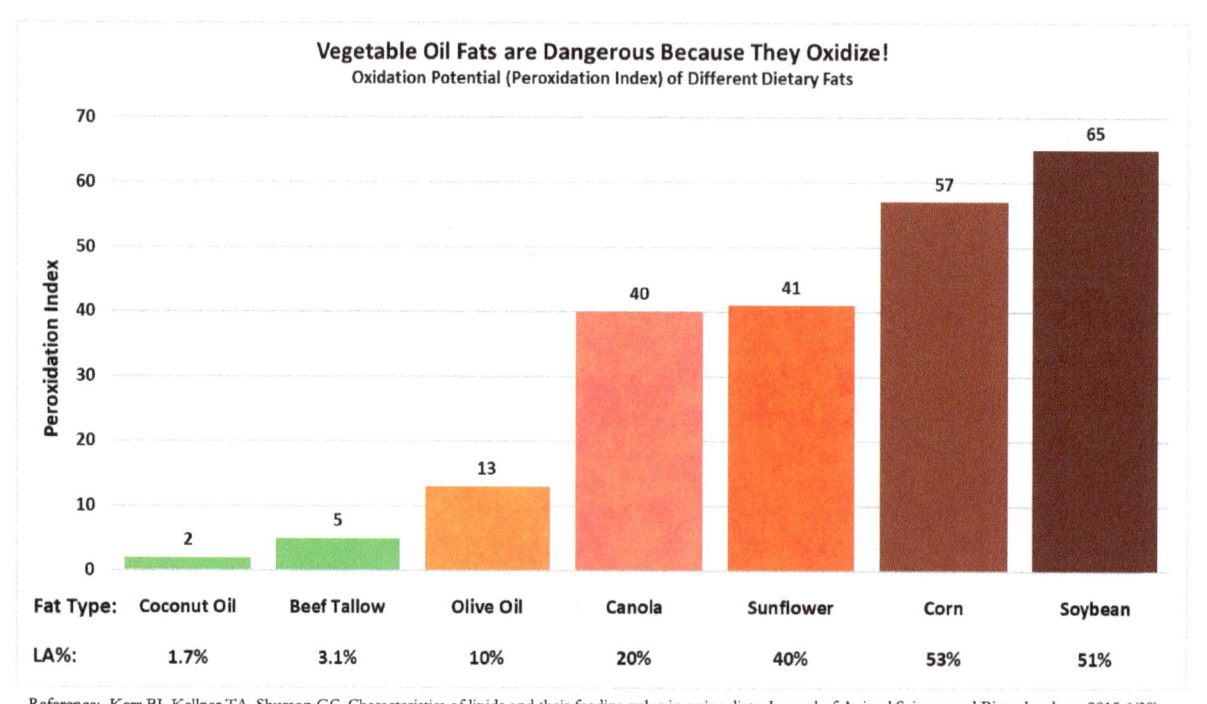

Vegetable Oil Fats are Dangerous Because They Oxidize!
Oxidation Potential (Peroxidation Index) of Different Dietary Fats

Fat Type:	Coconut Oil	Beef Tallow	Olive Oil	Canola	Sunflower	Corn	Soybean
Peroxidation Index	2	5	13	40	41	57	65
LA%:	1.7%	3.1%	10%	20%	40%	53%	51%

Reference: Kerr BJ, Kellner TA, Shurson GC. Characteristics of lipids and their feeding value in swine diets. Journal of Animal Science and Biotechnology. 2015;6(30). DOI: 10.1186/s40104-015-0028-x. © Copyright C. Knobbe, Ancestral Health Foundation, 2022.

kind of meat. The reason they emit a malodorous air is because the PUFA fats are in some stage of oxidation (peroxidation). It's the PUFAs that are oxidizing and far lesser amounts of the monounsaturated and saturated fats, because the PUFAs have the most double bonds.

In revisiting the graph on page 220 ("Vegetable Oil Fats are Dangerous Because They Oxidize!"), we observe that coconut oil has the lowest peroxidation index (PI) of 2 and it only has 1.7% LA, beef tallow (fat) is next lowest and it has a PI of 5 and only 3.1% LA, followed by olive oil with a PI of 13 and 10% LA, canola with a PI of 40 and 20% LA, sunflower oil with a PI of 41 and 40% LA, corn oil with a PI of 57 and 53% LA, and soybean oil with a PI of 65 and an LA of 51%.

When we eat fats, these exact same fats gradually contribute to our cellular membranes and reflect whichever fats we've been eating. The old adage that states, 'We are what we eat," is true when it comes to the amounts and types of PUFA fats we consume; however, recall that it is not true when it comes to the carbohydrates we consume.

The latter is true, as we've reviewed previously, because the ultimate fate of carbohydrates is either to be burned for energy, stored as glycogen (which is still carbohydrate), or when these conditions are met, we then convert excess carbohydrates into saturated fats and monounsaturated fats, in that order of preference.

Therefore, because we don't want to be a set-up for our bodies to oxidize, which leads to untold destruction and disease, we want to consume fats with a very low peroxidation (which, for simplicity, will be referred to as oxidation) index and very low LA. Notice that they go hand-in-hand.

There are several further observations here, however. First, from the graph on page 220, one might conclude that we should be eating all coconut oil, instead of beef fat. This would be an incorrect conclusion and an extraordinary mistake.

Remember, this is oxidation measured in a lab, not in a body, so there are some very critical differences. The beef fat comes with vitamins A, D, and K2, whereas the coconut oil has none of these. A diet with 100% coconut oil as the only source of fat would ultimately be lethal, because no vitamins A, D, or K2 would be present.[148] The same goes for all the other vegetable oils, just as E.V. McCollum showed in the many animal studies completed before 1918.[148][149]

Beef fat (and the fat of other traditionally raised animals) as the primary source of fat not only sustains health as we've seen in many traditional population studies, but it does it phenomenally well. Nineteenth century Americans were the perfect examples. Coconut oil also sustains health remarkably well because it is exquisitely unlikely to oxidize, just as we observed in the Tokelauans.

However, the traditional populations who consumed coconut oil in enormous amounts – such as the Tokelauans – also consumed a great deal of fish, which provided their fat-soluble vitamins. Yet another caveat from this study and the graph on p. 220, is that the beef fat peroxidation index might well have been even lower had the beef tallow come from 100% grass-fed, pastured cattle, however, in this case the source of the tallow was not cited.

Nevertheless, even concentrated animal feeding operation (CAFO) cattle would have very low LA, but would also have lower nutrient densities in the meat. With that said, even grocery store CAFO-raised beef would be far superior to the high-PUFA oils because the LA is very low (around 3% or less, typically), the oxidation index is very low, and beef fat supplies significant amounts of vitamins A, D, and K2 (see Chapter Six).

From the same graph regarding the oxidation potential of different dietary fats, it should be clear that we don't want to fill up our fat stores and cellular membranes with high-PUFA oils, like canola, sunflower, corn, and soybean, which all have oxidation indexes that are orders of magnitude higher than coconut oil and beef tallow. By logical extrapolation, all vegetable oil sources should be avoided.

Olive oil has a substantially higher oxidation index than coconut oil or beef fat, but a relatively low LA (~10%), which is why it has (in part) a far better track record (e.g., Mediterranean diet) in sustaining health when compared to westernized populations that consume substantial amounts of seed oils. Nevertheless, even olive oil does not have the very low oxidation index of coconut oil or traditional animal fats, it is generally about 4 to 5 times higher in LA, and it contains none of the fat-soluble vitamins required for life.

Indeed, our cells must have small amounts of PUFA, including LA, in very specific places including cell membranes, the membranes of mitochondria (the powerhouses of the cell), and for the production of signaling molecules called prostaglandins and eicosanoids. So while LA is an essential fat, it is nearly impossible to become deficient in this fat if one is eating food (as it is contained in all common foods, as reviewed previously).

The problem of excess omega-6 LA in the body is that it is highly subject to oxidation, or what lipid scientists call peroxidation, which is a damaging attack on the double bonds of lipids.[870] When LA (and other unsaturated fats) are attacked by free radicals (e.g., hydroxyl radicals, superoxide radicals, hydrogen peroxide, and singlet oxygen), they develop a degenerated and dangerous kind of fat called a lipid hydroperoxide, which can then further degenerate into other downstream products that are even far more dangerous (reviewed below).[871]

Saturated fats are extremely resistant to oxidation because they contain no double bonds, whereas monounsaturated fats are more subject to peroxidative attack because they contain a single double bond, and polyunsaturated fats (PUFA) are by far the most subject to oxidation because they contain two or more double bonds.[872] In one study, lipid chemists confirmed that, as compared to saturated fatty acids, monounsaturated fatty acids (MUFA) were 12-fold more likely to oxidize, and PUFA were found to be 25-fold more likely to oxidize.[872]

Brian J. Kerr, research scientist at the USDA-ARS-National Laboratory for Agriculture and the Environment, and colleagues, have shown that saturated fats with zero double bonds have a peroxidation index (PI, or proneness to oxidation) of zero, whereas monounsaturated fats, like oleic acid, which makes up the bulk of olive oil and has one double bond, has a PI of 0.1, omega-6 linoleic acid (LA) has two double bonds and a PI of 1.0, and omega-3 ALA (alpha-linolenic acid) has three double bonds and a PI of 2.0 (see graph on page 223, "Vegetable Oil Fats Have High Potential to Oxidize").[873] This, in essence, is why we don't want to be filling up our bodily fat stores and cellular membranes with an over-abundance of PUFA, which are extraordinarily more likely to oxidize!

The point of all of this is that saturated fats and monounsaturated fats, unlike polyunsaturated fats (omega-6 and omega-3), are very unlikely to undergo this type of damaging oxidation because they're biologically stable. The saturated and mono-

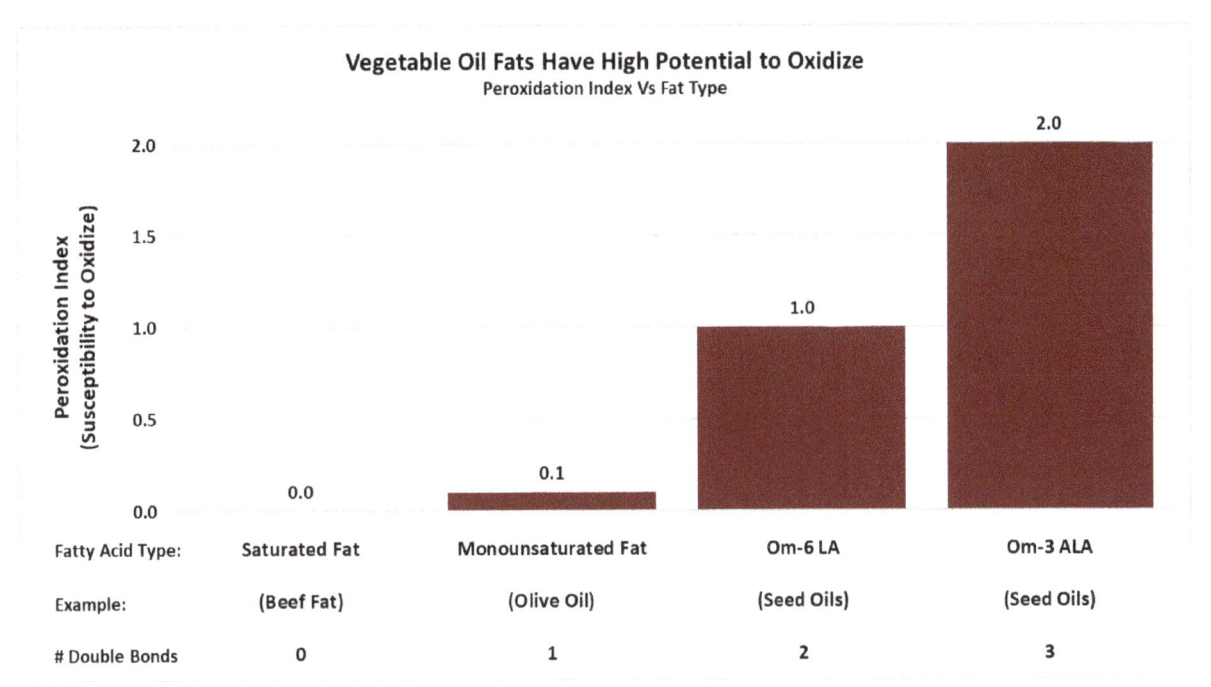

Vegetable Oil Fats Have High Potential to Oxidize
Peroxidation Index Vs Fat Type

Fatty Acid Type:	Saturated Fat	Monounsaturated Fat	Om-6 LA	Om-3 ALA
Peroxidation Index	0.0	0.1	1.0	2.0
Example:	(Beef Fat)	(Olive Oil)	(Seed Oils)	(Seed Oils)
# Double Bonds	0	1	2	3

Reference: Kerr BJ, Kellner TA, Shurson GC. Characteristics of lipids and their feeding value in swine diets. Journal of Animal Science and Biotechnology. 2015;6(30). DOI: 10.1186/s40104-015-0028-x. © Copyright C. Knobbe, Ancestral Health Foundation, 2022.

unsaturated fatty acids are the fats that our bodies choose to store for surplus energy needs, as they're biologically stable, yet they also serve as the perfect fuel to be burned for energy, which lipid scientists call beta-oxidation.

Thus, contrary to popular belief, saturated (and monounsaturated) fats are a far healthier alternative even if consumed to excess, whereas an excess of the polyunsaturated fat LA – anything above about 2% of calories – progressively becomes more harmful.[65][208][218][266][267] This is a major reason why the healthy natural meats of grass-fed, pasture-raised, and naturally fed animals, as well as wild-caught fish and seafood, which all have exceedingly small amounts of LA, are supremely healthy (data presented in Chapter Six).

Next, we must consider once again that the half-life of the polyunsaturated fatty acids in our bodies is about 600 to 680 days, reflecting the diet over the past two to three years, and that the total body fat turnover may occur over a period of 800 to 900 days.[664][6] Thus, the french fries eaten today, or the onion rings, chips, potato chips, chicken "tenders," fried fish, fish and chips, fried chicken, or any other foods cooked in or made with vegetable oils, even after a single serving, will take up residence within our cellular membranes and fat stores, negatively impacting our physiology for about three years!

Now, let's contrast that, for the moment, with tobacco smoking. Cigarette smoking exacts its bodily harm not just in the lungs, but throughout the body, primarily because the inhaled smoke induces a pro-oxidative state throughout the body, very similarly to vegetable oils.[874] However, with cigarette smoking, the increased oxidative effect is driven by inhaled toxicants that gain access to the blood via the lungs.

After cessation of smoking, one study showed that multiple biomarkers of oxidative stress in the

Poisoned for 6 Months to 1 Year After Quitting

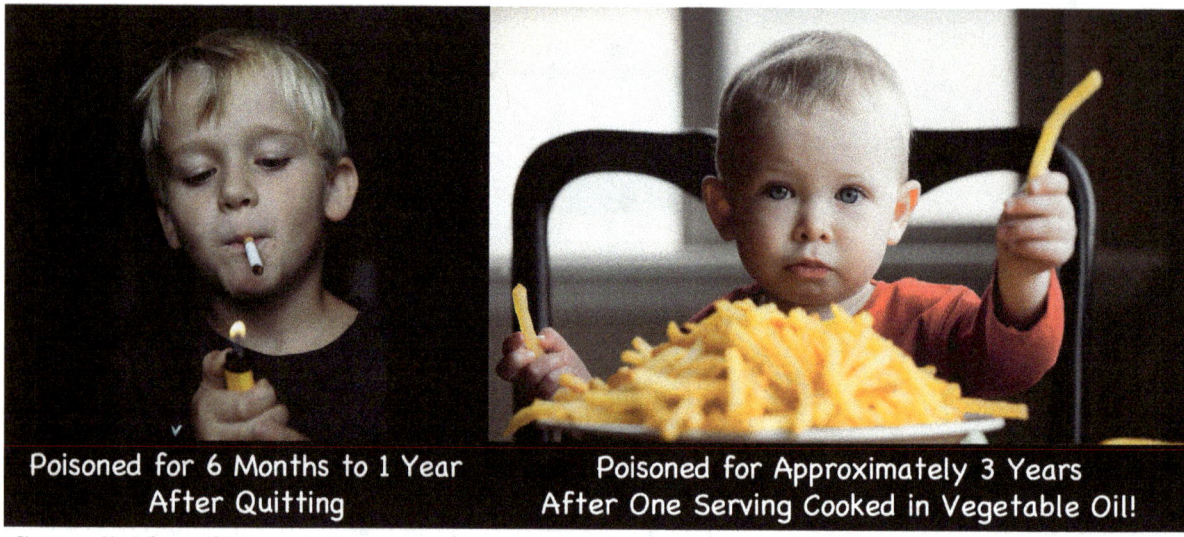

Poisoned for Approximately 3 Years After One Serving Cooked in Vegetable Oil!

Cigarette smoking induces verifiably increased oxidative stress persisting up to one year after discontinuation. Reference: 1) Zhou JF, et al. Effects of cigarette smoking and smoking cessation on plasma constituents and enzyme activities related to oxidative stress. Biomedical and Environmental Sciences. 2000;13(1):44-55. 2) Fatty acid accumulation and content in adipose has a half-life of approximately 600 days and represents fatty acid consumption for the past 2 to 3 years. Reference: Beynen AC, et al. A mathematical relationship between the fatty acid composition of the diet and that of the adipose tissue in man. © Copyright C. Knobbe, Ancestral Health Foundation, 2022.

blood (lipoperoxides, nitric oxide) were increased while other biomarkers of stress (vitamin C, vitamin E, superoxide dismutase [SOD], catalase, and glutathione peroxidase) were decreased.[874] These biomarkers remained increased and decreased, respectively, at six months after cessation of smoking but were normalized in comparison to the nonsmoking control group at one year.

Thus, the pro-oxidative effects of long-term smoking continue for no more than about one year after discontinuation of smoking whereas seed oils' pro-oxidative effects last for about three years after discontinuation of consumption.

In the side-by-side photos above, we see a young boy smoking a cigarette – an action most any of us would find deplorable. In the adjacent photo, we observe a much younger boy consuming french fries – a behavior that most parents readily accept. However, in our scientific view, the french fries are tremendously more harmful than cigarette smoking, as the heated oils and high omega-6 fats will induce a pro-oxidative state in the young boy that will last approximately three years, whereas the pro-oxidative state of cigarette smoking will abate within one year.

When one consumes LA in the diet, it must be transported within lipoproteins in the blood (HDL, LDL, VLDL, and chylomicrons), and it then has a marked tendency to accumulate in fat cells, within the lipid droplets inside many cell types, and in your cellular membranes.[6][870]

In this scenario, your body is a "sitting duck," set up for destructive oxidation reactions, because the LA is exposed to "free radicals," which are constantly generated during normal metabolism and production of cellular energy.[870]

In fact, our bodies make large amounts of free radicals every second of our lives. Perhaps the most common and important of these are hydroxyl radicals. A typical cell produces around 50 hydroxyl radicals per second, which is around 4 million per day.[875] Based on the most recent and highly sophisticated estimates, the average 70 kg (154 lb) "reference man" has 30 trillion (3.0×10^{13}) cells.[876] At

4 million hydroxyl radicals per day, that computes to be 120,000,000,000,000,000,000 (1.2 x 10[20] free hydroxyl radicals per day! And this is only of the hydroxyl radical type – there are many other types of radicals.

However, free radicals are not just intrinsically dangerous – each one acting like the proverbial "bull in a China shop" -- but, remarkably, free radicals are important biological signaling molecules that are needed in normal metabolism.[877] The problem arises primarily when there is an excess of unsaturated lipids (omega-6 LA) in our bodies because the free radicals react with these, beginning a vicious chain reaction. This is the simplified version…

Free radicals, like the hydroxyl radical, have the potential to attack any biomolecules, which includes proteins, lipids, carbohydrates, nucleic acids, DNA, hormones, enzymes, and many other biological molecules.[878] [879] But of all the biological molecules around, it is the unsaturated lipids (omega-6 and omega-3) that are the most likely to be the subject of oxidative attack.[880] Then, if these unsaturated lipids are prominent in our cellular membranes because we've eaten far too many of them for far too long, when one of these is attacked, it begins a vicious cycle of attack. Here's why.

When we consume vegetable oils laden with very high amounts of omega-6, LA, both LA and the downstream fatty acids (e.g., arachidonic acid) that are derived from it accumulate in your cells. These then become the subject of oxidative attack by, for example, a hydroxyl radical. This ultimately produces degenerated products called lipid hydroperoxides, but these are short-lived and rapidly give rise to further end-products known as advanced lipid oxidation end products, often abbreviated as ALEs.[881]

However, when one molecule of LA undergoes oxidation, there is an intermediate molecule produced called a peroxyl radical, which will react with an unsaturated fatty acid (e.g., another LA molecule) sitting next to it, which produces another lipid radical. This phase is called propagation and it is a chain reaction mechanism that perpetuates a severely destructive "vicious cycle." The process is amplified dramatically based on an overabundance of unsaturated fats being present in cell membranes, which is precisely the situation with high LA-containing diets.

Filling up our cells and cell membranes with LA molecules is dangerous indeed. Perhaps the best analogy is that it's akin to using a welder. Welding produces huge numbers of sparks. In the usual scenario, however, the sparks fly off the welding tip and land safely on dry ground, concrete, or another hard surface. There's nothing there to catch on fire. We remain safe, and there's no fire. This metaphor holds true in low LA diets, which are the key component of ancestral diets (as they never contain seed oils).

Now suppose you're welding, but you've surrounded yourself with thin, dry tissue papers, one foot deep. They're going to catch fire. This is exactly what it is like to fill up our cells with LA. The body in this scenario is like a house afire. We refer to this entire process which begins with an overabundance of omega-6 LA as a *"catastrophic lipid peroxidation cascade,"* or *"CLIPS."* However, the pro-oxidative phase that we've just discussed is only the beginning. This cascade, which begins with overconsumption of LA, is also pro-inflammatory, toxic (secondary to the advanced lipid oxidation end products), and finally, nutrient-deficient.

SEED OILS ARE PRO-INFLAMMATORY

The oldest, most well-known, and most highly accepted effect of high omega-6 diets is that they're pro-inflammatory.[882] As with almost any science, not all the evidence is supportive. However, we'll briefly review the highlights, which are theoretical, observed, and logical, but not always proven.

High omega-6 LA-containing diets have been linked to increased inflammation, mainly because LA gives rise to the production of the longer omega-6 fatty acid called arachidonic acid (AA), and AA is the precursor to pro-inflammatory mediators, including prostaglandins and leukotrienes.[882]

For example, LA stimulates a marked proinflammatory state in the vascular endothelium,[883] and the prostaglandin-2 series (PGE-2) of molecules have potent inflammatory and cell proliferation effects.[884] In short, LA gives rise to AA, which produces mediators that are inflammatory, atherogenic (atherosclerosis-inducing), and prothrombotic (clot-inducing), which may collectively play a substantial role in heart attacks and strokes.[885]

The omega-3 fatty acids, which can be derived from ALA, include inflammation-resolving mediators, such as resolvins, protectins, and maresins, all of which come from the long-chain omega-3 fatty acids, EPA and DHA.[882] [885]

TOXICITY FROM SEED OILS: OXLAMS & ALES ADD EVEN MORE HARM

As previously reviewed, when LA is attacked by a hydroxyl radical (or other radical), it will give rise to lipid hydroperoxides. These are highly labile

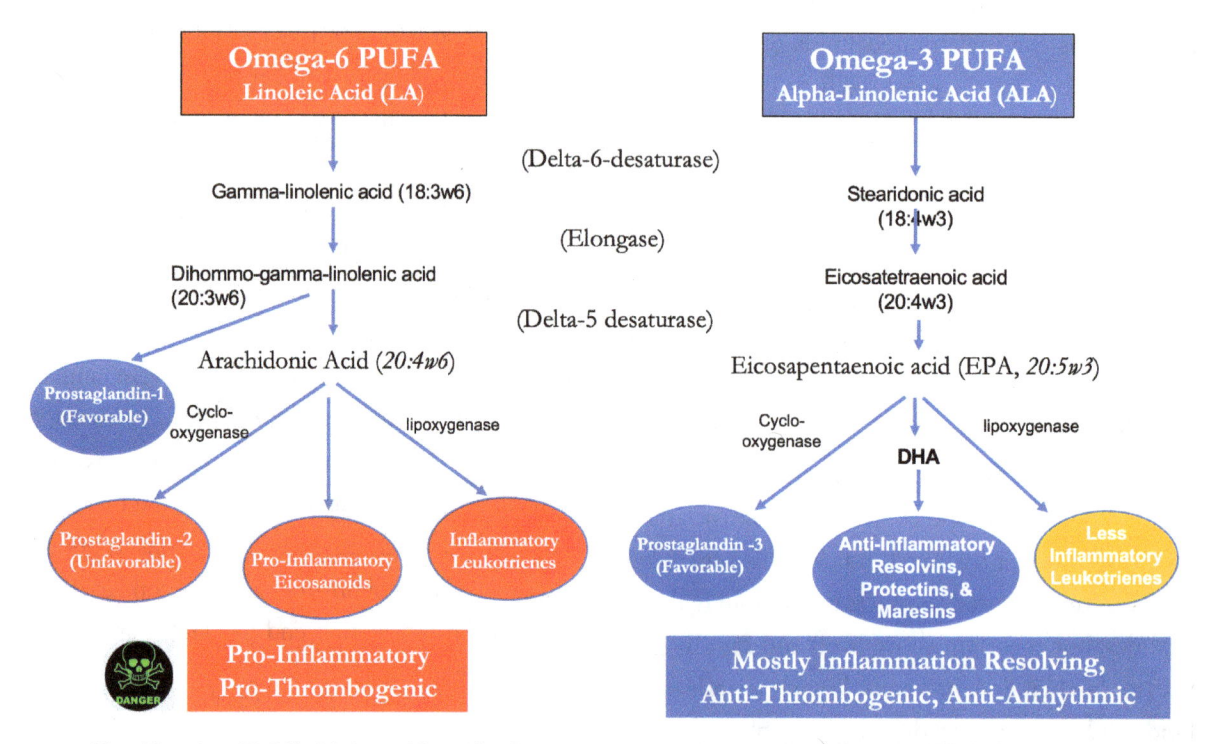

Adapted from: Innes JK, Calder PC. Omega-6 fatty acids and inflammation. Prostaglandins Leukot Essent Fatty Acids. 2018;132:41-48.
© Copyright C. Knobbe, Ancestral Health Foundation, 2022.

products and may be quickly converted to two other primary oxidized lipid products, referred to as 9- and 13-HODE (hydroxy-octadecadienoic acid).[886] These two constituents are sometimes referred to as **oxidized linoleic acid metabolites**, or **OxLAMs**. The two OxLAMs, 9- and 13-HODE, are the major oxidative constituents of Ox-LDL, and these are known to contribute to the atherogenicity of Ox-LDL, that is, these molecules are very important constituents in the cause of atherosclerosis and coronary heart disease.[886 887 888]

The LA-derived lipid hydroperoxides are highly unstable and rapidly decompose into a series of other dangerous compounds called **advanced lipid oxidation end products (ALEs**, also referred to as advanced lipoxidation end products). These include 4-hydroxy-nonenal (HNE), malondialdehyde (MDA),[889] acrolein,[890] and carboxyethylpyrrole.[891]

These four ALEs are ultimately derived from omega-6 LA and/or omega-6 AA and, unlike free radicals which have extremely short "lives," these ALEs are relatively stable and they freely roam around our tissues exacting destruction against many biomolecules, such as DNA, proteins, and lipids, permanently altering the structure and function of such molecules, resulting in widespread damaging effects.[892]

One might initially think that the ALEs consist only of HNE, MDA, acrolein, and carboxyethylpyrrole, but such would be an extreme underestimate. In fact, lipid scientists have determined that there are literally hundreds of such ALEs, all of which may be highly toxic in our bodies.[893]

In the graph below, "Heating Vegetable Oils Increases Toxicity," as shown by Bente Halvorsen and colleagues at the University of Oslo, in

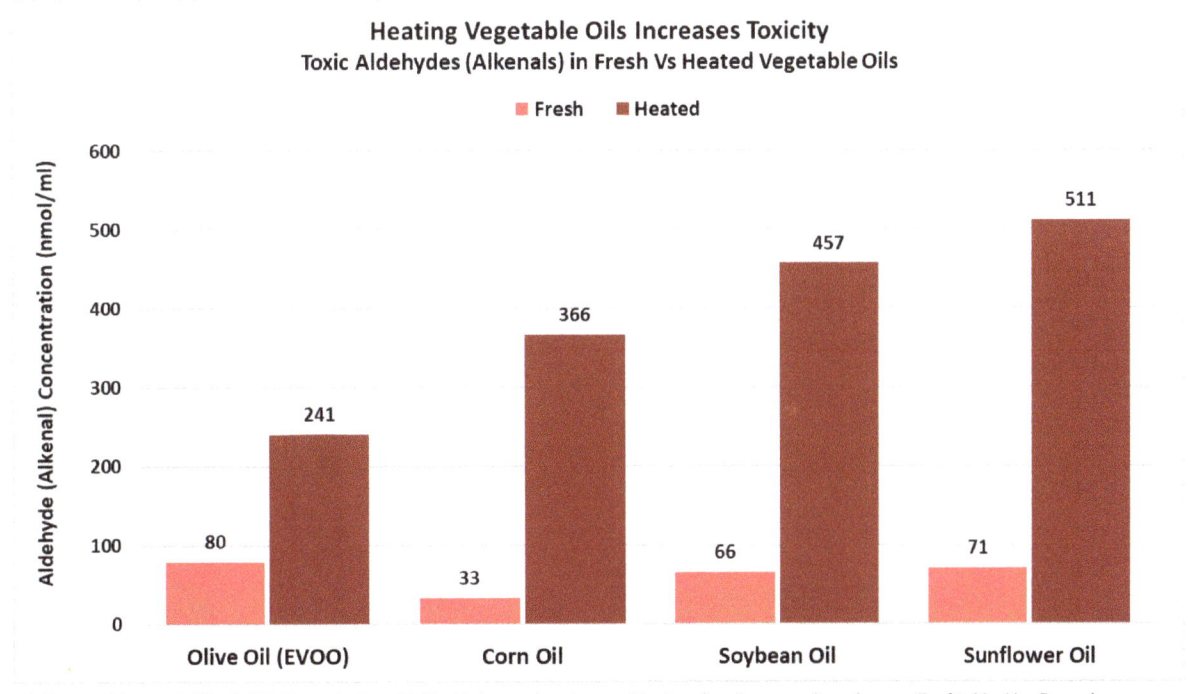

Heating Vegetable Oils Increases Toxicity
Toxic Aldehydes (Alkenals) in Fresh Vs Heated Vegetable Oils

Oil	Fresh	Heated
Olive Oil (EVOO)	80	241
Corn Oil	33	366
Soybean Oil	66	457
Sunflower Oil	71	511

Aldehyde (Alkenal) Concentration (nmol/ml)

Reference: Halvorsen L, Blomhoff R. Determination of lipid oxidation products in vegetable oils and marine omega-3 supplements. Food & Nutrition Research. 2011;55:5792. Each measurement made before and after heating of oil and each oil heated at 225 °C (437 °F) for 25 minutes. © Copyright C. Knobbe, Ancestral Health Foundation, 2022.

Norway, we also see that the ALEs (also referred to as (toxic) aldehydes or alkenals) increase markedly when oils are heated.

Notice the enormous increase in these toxic ALEs in four commonly used oils (olive, corn, soybean, and sunflower) when the oils are heated to 225 °C (437 °F) for just 25 minutes, which simulates oven roasting/baking.[894] Soybean oil, the second most commonly consumed edible oil worldwide (behind palm oil),[895] showed increased toxic aldehyde content secondary to typical oven baking, which was 7-fold greater than baseline.[894]

Halvorsen and colleagues also ran one of the single most comprehensive studies comparing ALEs (alkenals) in a very large series of vegetable oils versus marine omega-3 supplements. In the study, they evaluated total ALEs content in 22 different vegetable oils and 33 different marine omega-3 supplements, all of which were available in Oslo, Norway, at the time.

The vegetable oils included the oils of olive, corn, sunflower, soybean, and rapeseed. The marine omega-3 supplements included fish oil, krill oil, seal oil, and cod liver oils. Given that the peroxidation index (PI) progressively increases based on the number of double bonds, we should expect the marine omega-3 supplements to oxidize easily, producing higher levels of ALEs on a per weight (mass) basis, and that is exactly what Halvorsen's group found.

As seen in the graph below, "We Should Avoid Vegetable Oils and Eat Fish," the ALEs in the marine oil supplements ranged from 158 to 932 nmol/mL, with an average of 492 nmol/mL.[894] The vegetable oils had a range of 33 to 119 nmol/mL, with an average of 69 nmol/mL. If you have been consuming marine omega-3 supplements, you might find such evidence quite alarming, however,

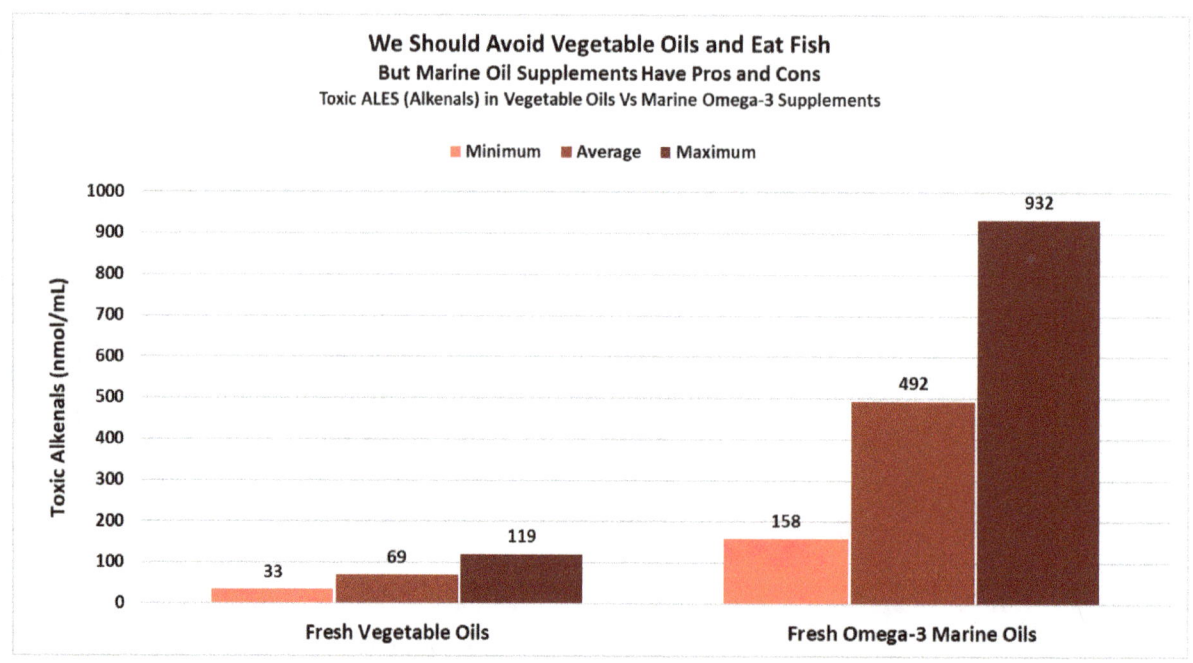

We Should Avoid Vegetable Oils and Eat Fish
But Marine Oil Supplements Have Pros and Cons
Toxic ALES (Alkenals) in Vegetable Oils Vs Marine Omega-3 Supplements

	Minimum	Average	Maximum
Fresh Vegetable Oils	33	69	119
Fresh Omega-3 Marine Oils	158	492	932

Toxic ALES (Alkenals) in a selection of 22 vegetable oils, including olive, corn, sunflower, soybean, and rapeseed and 33 omega-3 marine oils, including fish oil, krill oil, seal oil, and cod liver oils. Reference: Halvorsen BL, Blomhoff R. Determination of lipid oxidation products in vegetable oils and marine omega-3 supplements. Food & Nutrition Research. 2011;55. Doi.10.3402/fnr.v55i0.5792. © Copyright C. Knobbe, Ancestral Health Foundation, 2022.

there are some further considerations and caveats.

In terms of their ALEs content, the marine omega-3 supplements appear, at first glance, to be very dangerous indeed, with far higher concentrations of ALEs per gram (or mL) as compared to the fresh, unheated vegetable oils. However, the typical "dose" of marine oils (e.g., fish oil, cod liver oil) is generally very low, on the order of 0.5 g to perhaps 3.0 g/day. In contrast, many westernized populations are routinely consuming 20 to 80 g of vegetable oils per day.

Furthermore, "culinary oils" generally do not include fish oils, whereas the high-PUFA oils are commonly used for cooking. Therefore, not only does the dose of ALEs in vegetable oils far exceed that in virtually any marine oil supplement, but the vegetable oils are often heated, whereas the fish oils and cod liver oils are not. Finally, cold-pressed cod liver oils will supply vitamins A and D3 in substantial amounts[896] and, for those who are not acquiring these vitamins from other sources, we would submit that the benefits far outweigh the risks.

The consumption of fish oils for the sake of omega-3 (e.g., in capsules or glass bottle containers) is somewhat controversial in the scientific literature,[897] whereas the consumption of fish has been shown to be beneficial in nearly all studies, including meta-analyses.[897][898] When we consume a fillet of fish, the preservation of the flesh, as well as the oils (fats) that are naturally present in the fish, is rather "guaranteed by the antioxidant[s] and antimicrobial properties" of the fish fillet as a whole, at least when properly refrigerated or frozen.[899] Such is not the case when we remove fat from the fish (or other marine life) and put it into a capsule or bottle.

Another major caveat to consider with respect to the relatively high content of ALEs in marine omega-3-rich oils is the historical fact that the Inuit (often referred to formerly as 'Eskimos') consumed enormous amounts of seal fat as their major source of fat,[784] yet they remained very healthy (see previous review, Chapter Four). Obviously, seal oil was extracted from the animal and had the potential for oxidation with the production of significant ALEs; however, the oil was typically stored with the solid fat (blubber) and the conditions were frigid, so this would be expected to help deter ALEs development.

Furthermore, if we contrast seal oil to cod liver oil, seal oil can similarly be an excellent source of vitamin A and may also provide small amounts of vitamin D generally (see Canadian Nutrient File 2015 for types, data, and resources).[900] There are pros and cons to consuming fish oils in supplement form or even cod liver oils. However, both may have benefits and all points should be considered. In short, much depends on the remainder of the diet in a given individual.

With regard to other studies involving seed oils and ALEs, Andrew W.D. Claxson and colleagues, of the Inflammation Research Group at the London Hospital Medical College, also thermally stressed various culinary oils and fats by heating them for 30 to 90 minutes at 180 °C (356 °F), followed by assessment for ALEs presence.

The group found that the high PUFA edible oils, including the oils of corn, sunflower, soybean, rapeseed, groundnut (peanut), and grapeseed, all "generated high levels" of the toxic ALEs, whereas commercially available olive oil, coconut oil, lard, and beef fat (drippings) all "generated only very low levels" of the toxic ALEs.[901]

Martin Grootveld, PhD, Professor of Bioanalytical Chemistry and Chemical Pathology, De

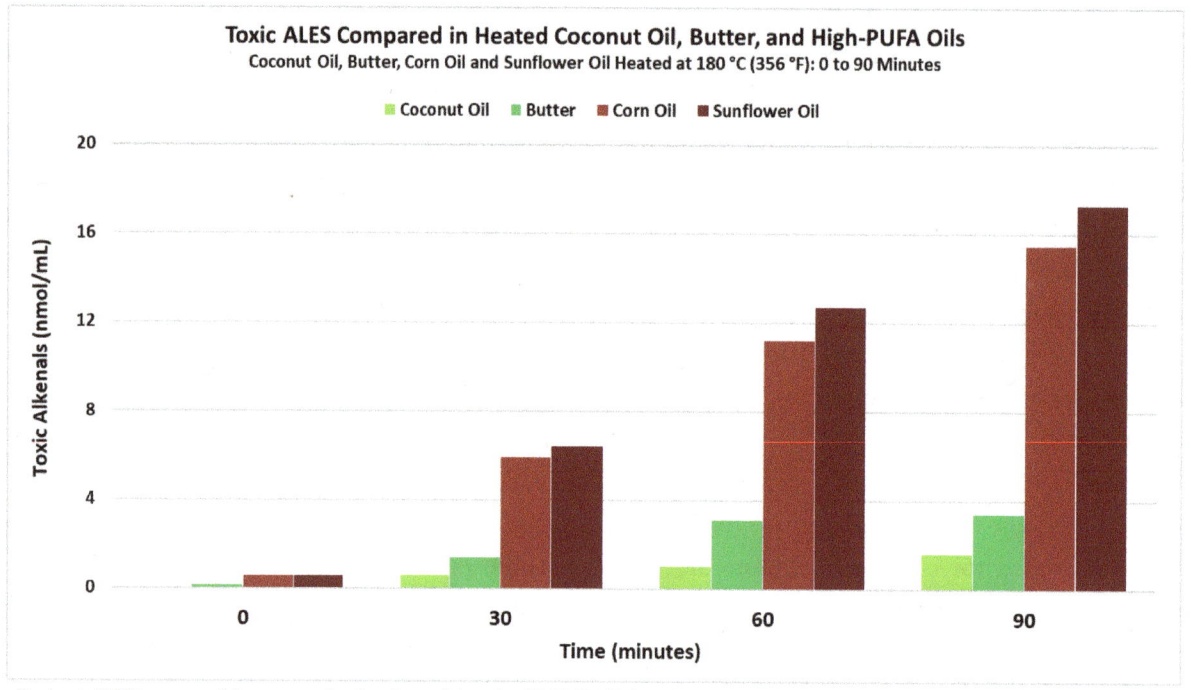

Toxic ALES Compared in Heated Coconut Oil, Butter, and High-PUFA Oils
Coconut Oil, Butter, Corn Oil and Sunflower Oil Heated at 180 °C (356 °F): 0 to 90 Minutes

Total toxic ALES in coconut oil, butter, corn oil, and sunflower oil, heated at 180 °C (356 °F) for 0, 30, 60, and 90 minutes. Reference: Grootveld M, Percival BC, Grootveld KL. Chronic non-communicable disease risks presented by lipid oxidation products in fried foods. Hepatobil Surg Nutr. 2018;7(4):305-12. © Copyright C. Knobbe, Ancestral Health Foundation, 2022.

Montfort University, Leicester, England, has contributed perhaps the largest body of research that confirms seed oils, particularly when heated, produce large quantities of ALEs.[902][903][904][905][906][907]

Grootveld and colleagues, over a period of more than two decades, have shown in many studies that seed oils develop very large quantities of toxic ALEs when they're heated. They've also demonstrated that these dangerous compounds are "readily absorbed from the gut into the systemic circulation,"[902] thus leaving no doubt that the presence of ALEs in vegetable oils and foods fried in vegetable oils are credible biological threats.

Grootveld has drawn causative connections between ALEs and cardiovascular disease,[902] atherosclerosis, inflammatory joint disease, rheumatoid arthritis, and digestive tract disorders.[903] Furthermore, the Grootveld team of researchers has found the toxic ALEs to be causative of mutagenicity and genotoxicity, "properties that often signal carcinogenesis; and teratogenicity, the property of chemicals that leads to the development of birth defects."[903] More recently, Grootveld and colleagues have additionally linked ALEs as significant contributors to cancers and neurological diseases.[907]

In the graph above, "Toxic ALEs Compared in Heated Coconut Oil, Butter, and High PUFA Oils," which is drawn on the data provided by Grootveld and colleagues, we observe the increase in ALEs when four different fats (coconut oil, butter, corn oil, and sunflower oil) are heated to 180 °C (356 °F) for 30, 60, and 90 minutes. Notice that, for each point in time, coconut oil has the lowest levels of ALEs, followed by butter, corn oil, and sunflower oil.[905] One should also notice that at all time points, coconut oil (2% LA) and butter

(~2-3% LA), maintain very low levels of ALEs, even up to 90 minutes of heating.

In an article published in *The Telegraph* (London, England), in which Grootveld's research was reviewed, the author wrote as follows:

> *"Scientists found that heating up vegetable oils led to the release of high concentrations of chemicals called aldehydes [one type of the ALEs group], which have been linked to illnesses including cancer, heart disease, and dementia."*[908]
>
> *Grootveld was quoted as saying, "A typical meal of fish and chips," fried in vegetable oil, was shown to contain "100 to 200 times more toxic aldehydes than the safe daily limit set by the World Health Organization." "In contrast," they wrote, "heating up butter, olive oil, and lard in tests produced much lower levels of aldehydes. Coconut oil produced the lowest levels of harmful chemicals."*[908]

Professor Grootveld, whose scientific papers are daunting except to other lipid chemists, made clear and simple points in the interview:

> *"For decades, the authorities have been warning us how bad butter and lard was. But we have found butter is very, very good for frying purposes and so is lard," he said. "People have been telling us, " he continued, "how healthy polyunsaturates are in corn oil and sunflower oil. But when you start messing around with them, subjecting them to high amounts of energy in the frying pan or the oven, they undergo a complex series of chemical reactions which results in the accumulation of large amounts of toxic compounds."*[908]

One final consideration that should be mentioned before reviewing the different destructive effects of some of the individual **ALEs is that they are not just produced exogenously – outside the body – but** they are also produced endogenously **– within the body.**[909] Thus, even if ALEs are present only in low amounts in unheated vegetable oils, consuming a high omega-6 LA diet will increase the concentration of LA within our cells, beginning the catastrophic lipid peroxidation cascade (CLIPS) within our bodies to produce ALEs endogenously.[910] [911] [912]

HNE, THE CLASSIC AND MOST TOXIC ALE, INCREASES WITH COOKING OF VEGETABLE OILS

The advanced lipid oxidation end product (ALE) known as 4-hydroxy-2-nonenal (HNE) is one of the most well-known ALEs produced from the oxidative degradation of LA. HNE, like almost any compound one would find in the human body, has what is known as a hormetic effect, that is, it is beneficial in small amounts but toxic at high amounts.[913] HNE at normal physiologic levels promotes cell survival, acts as an important signaling molecule, stimulates gene expression, enhances cellular antioxidant capacity, and results in cellular adaptive responses.[914]

At high levels, HNE promotes damage to various proteins and other biomolecules and induces programmed cell death (apoptosis) or destructive cell death (necrosis).[913] [914] This explains why natural animal fats, such as beef fat, butter, and coconut oil, all produce small amounts of HNE, which are beneficial. However, it is the unnaturally derived "factory fats," such as soybean, corn, canola, sunflower, safflower, cottonseed, rapeseed, and other high-PUFA oils that produce large amounts of ALEs, including HNE. Perhaps this is a good time to remind ourselves of Paracelsus' dictum (paraphrased), "The dose makes the poison."

HNE has not only been implicated, but has also generally been found in higher concentrations in association with atherosclerosis,[915][916][917] neurodegenerative diseases like Parkinson's disease and Alzheimer's disease,[918][919][921] cancer,[920][914] obesity, type 2 diabetes, metabolic syndrome,[921][914] age-related macular degeneration (AMD),[922] chronic kidney disease,[923] chronic obstructive pulmonary disease (COPD, e.g., emphysema or chronic bronchitis),[924] liver disease,[914] neuropsychiatric disorders including major depression, bipolar disorder, schizophrenia,[925] and chronic disease in general.[914]

We should also recall, HNE is just one of hundreds of ALEs that are produced in higher amounts in seed oils, particularly when they're heated. One of the major factors which determines the "exposure" (dose) of HNE is, of course, the heating of high-PUFA seed oils.

Neurosurgeon, Dr. Tetsumori Yamashima, Kanazawa University Graduate School of Medical Science, in Kanazawa, Japan, published a paper in the *Journal of Alzheimer's Disease & Parkinsonism*, entitled, ***"The Scourge of Vegetable Oil—Destroyer of Nations.***"[926] In the opening of this paper, Dr. Yamashima wrote the following:

> *"If you think vegetable oil such as soybean, canola and sunflower is healthy, your brain and body will be harmed without you knowing it! If you take linoleic acid, an omega-6 fatty acid which is easily oxidized in delicatessen fried foods, fast foods and processed foods, it rusts your cells, so brain function declines, your mood becomes unstable, and thinking ability decreases."*[926]

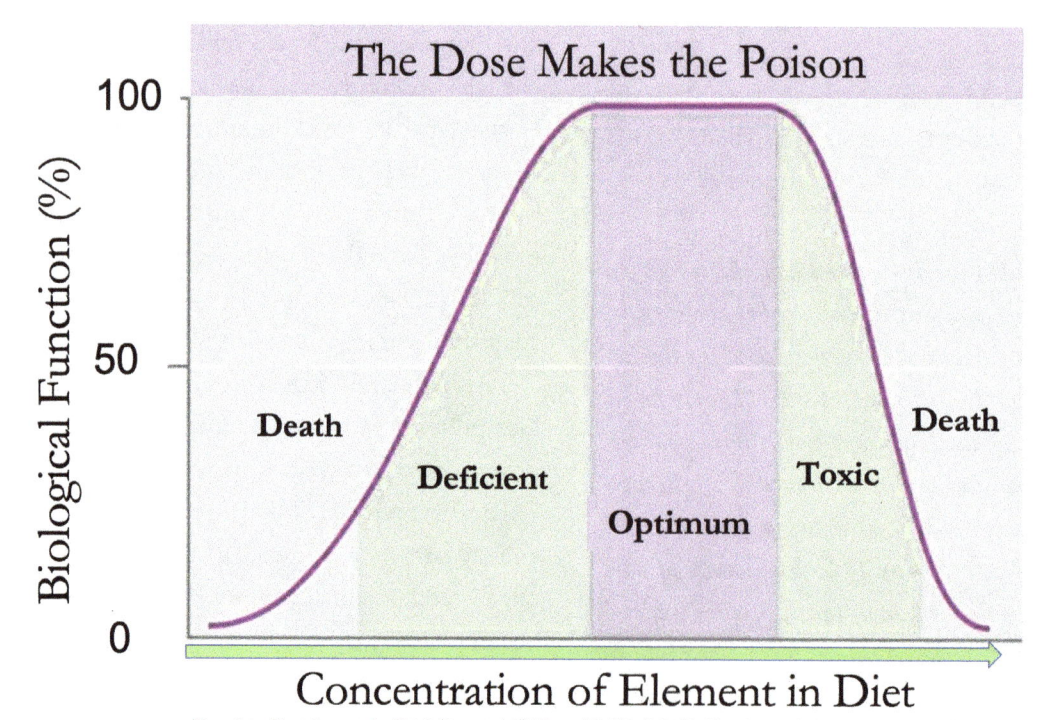

The Dose Makes the Poison

Biological Function (%) vs *Concentration of Element in Diet*

Regions: Death — Deficient — Optimum — Toxic — Death

Theophrast Paracelsus: works. Vol. 2, Darmstadt 1965, pp. 508-513. © C. Knobbe, Ancestral Health Foundation, 2021.

HNE in Plasma by Age

Hydroxynonenal (HNE) plasma concentration by age, 5-90 years. Yamashima Y. The Scourge of Vegetable Oil—Destroyer of Nations. J Alzheimer's Dis Parkinsonism. 2018;8:446. doi: 10.4172/2161-0460.1000446. Graph title and labels modified. Creative Commons Attribution 4.0 License.

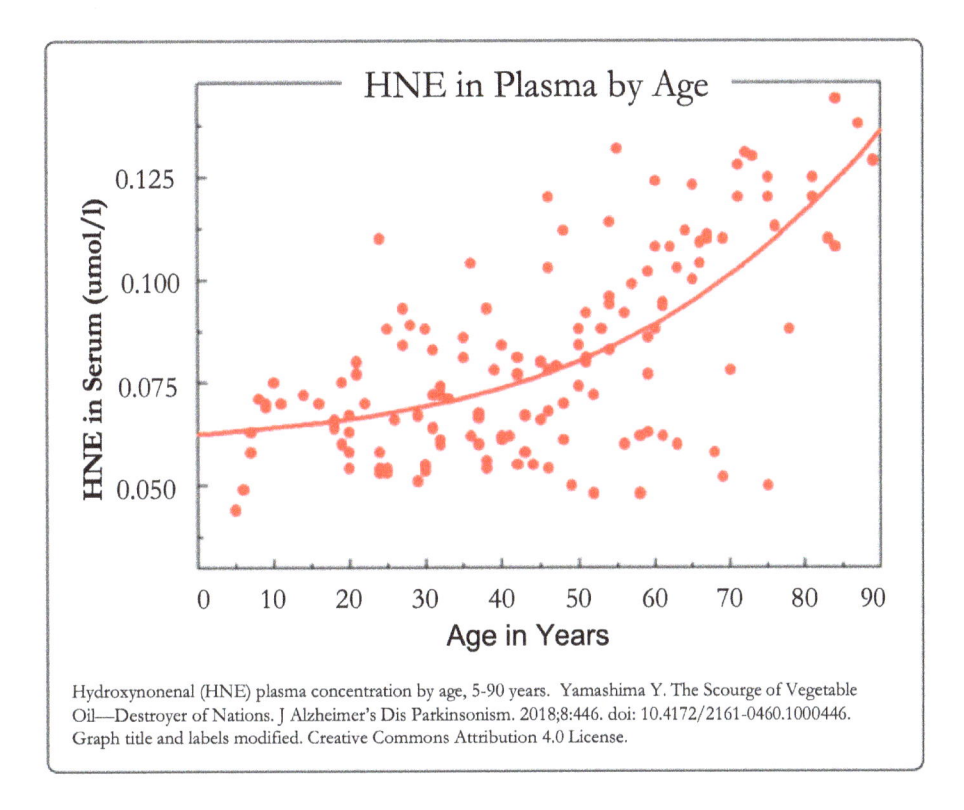

Yamashima showed that HNE may accumulate in the body progressively over a lifetime, somewhat predictably, with average levels more than twice as high at age 90 as at age 10 (see graph "HNE in Plasma by Age" above). Encouragingly, Yamashima's data, also shows that many people in their 60s and 70s have levels lower than the average 5 year-old, and many people in their 60s and 70s have HNE that is around one-third the level of cohorts their age, which suggests that these are the people consuming very low levels of seed oils, whether heated or not (see graph above).

Dr. Yamashima addressed the fact that HNE is produced primarily by the heating of high-PUFA vegetable oil, which is absorbed and accumulates in our bodies and in our brains. He wrote:

"Since hydroxynonenal is fat-soluble, it easily permeates blood vessels and cell membranes, and diffuses in the body just like poison gas. My own research with Japanese monkeys showed that the toxic substance that kills neurons in a brain with Alzheimer's disease was not amyloid beta which was suspected for more than half a century, but in fact was hydroxynonenal which is generated when vegetable oil is heated."[926]

Brian J. Kerr and colleagues, at the USDA Animal Research Service (ARS), National Laboratory for Agriculture and the Environment, thermally stressed corn oil (~53% LA) by heating the oil to 374 °F (190 °C) for up to 12 hours.[873] In the graph on page 234 ("Heating Vegetable Oils Increases Toxicity Over Time"), we can see that the dangerous toxicant, HNE, was only 2 ug/g before heating but increased to 45.1 ug/g within five hours of heating and remained at approximately that level through 8 hours of heating.

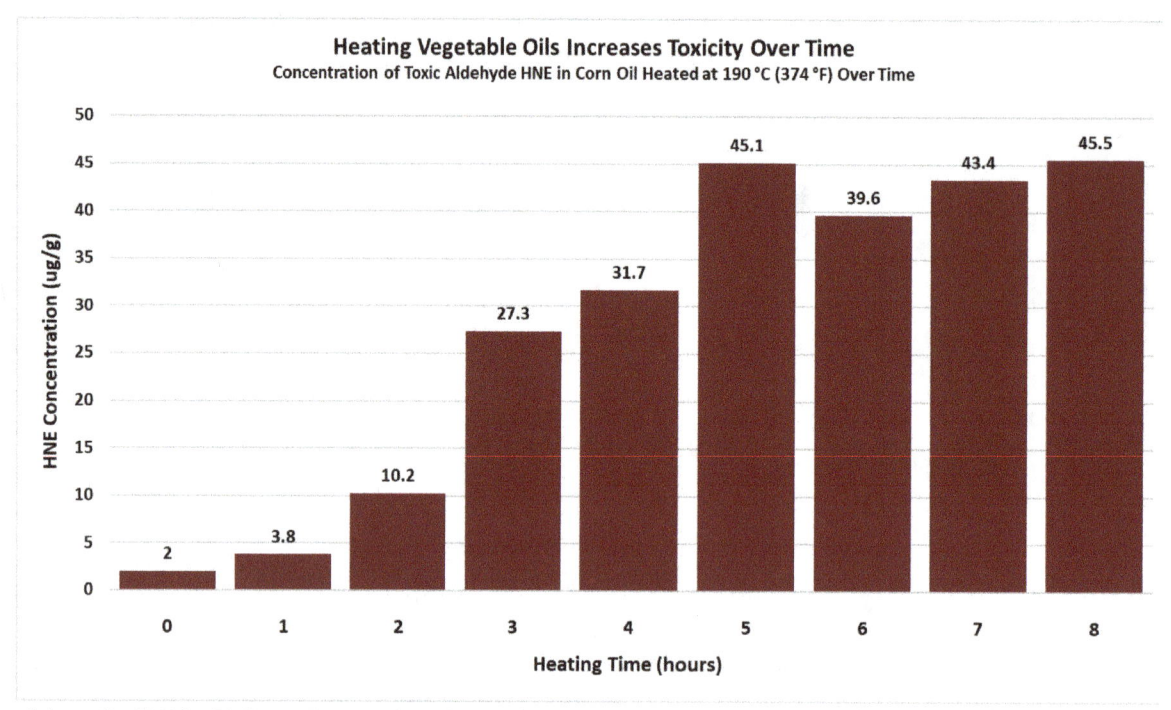

Heating Vegetable Oils Increases Toxicity Over Time
Concentration of Toxic Aldehyde HNE in Corn Oil Heated at 190 °C (374 °F) Over Time

Heating Time (hours)	HNE Concentration (µg/g)
0	2
1	3.8
2	10.2
3	27.3
4	31.7
5	45.1
6	39.6
7	43.4
8	45.5

Reference: Kerr BJ, Kellner TA, Shurson GC. Characteristics of lipids and their feeding value in swine diets. Journal of Animal Science and Biotechnology. 2015;6(30). DOI: 10.1186/s40104-015-0028-x. © Copyright C. Knobbe, Ancestral Health Foundation, 2022.

MALONDIALDEHYDE (MDA): ANOTHER DESTRUCTIVE ALE FROM SEED OILS

Malondialdehyde (MDA) is another of the ALEs that is a widely used biomarker of oxidative stress and, once again, it is derived almost exclusively from PUFA fats (vegetable oils), making overconsumption of LA the greatest driver.[927] MDA has been claimed to be the single most important end-product of lipid oxidation.[928] [929] MDA has been extensively purported to induce genotoxicity, which is the ability of a toxin to chemically alter DNA, leading to altered cell function and possibly mutations.[930]

MDA is also known to be mutagenic, which is the capability of a toxin to induce mutations in cells that may well lead to cancer.[930] With extensive investigations supporting this evidence, the National Institute for Occupational Safety and Health (NIOSH) of the USA has listed MDA as both a carcinogen and mutagen.[927] In 2015, the Belgian Superior Health Council deemed MDA to be a major concern for human health.[931]

Both HNE and MDA,[932] [177] along with 9- and 13-HODE,[887] [888] are all known to collectively alter the LDL particle into the oxidized state, that is, producing Ox-LDL, which is the atherogenic molecule that induces coronary heart disease. And, of course, as we've reviewed previously, it is the oxidation cascade of LA that ends in the production of 9- and 13-HODE, HNE, and MDA.

In a large sampling of foods, MDA was found to be above detection limits in 84% of analyzed foods, with dry nuts, fried snacks, french fries, and cured minced meat products contributing the most to the intake of both MDA and HNE.[933] Infants may be the most at risk when it comes to toxic exposure from foods, due to the extreme nature of processing with infant formulas.[934]

Infant milk formulas are particularly vulnerable because manufacturers remove butter from those containing bovine milk and replace the fat with vegetable oils, under the advice that such oils are 'heart healthy.'[934] With seed oils in the infant 'milks,' MDA has been detected at levels ranging from 200 to 1200 parts per billion (PPB), which is almost solely because the majority of fats in the formulae are primarily from high-PUFA oils.[935] And just like HNE, MDA is readily absorbed from the gut.[936] Thus, infants consuming such seed oil-laden formulae are placed at great risk of harm, particularly at the start of their young fragile lives.

Researchers from South China University of Technology have shown that the MDA levels of various oils are roughly proportional to the PUFA content of the oil and rise markedly over time. For example, the MDA content elevated markedly in all oils tested over a 30 day period of storage at 140 °F (60 °C).[927] However, while all oils tested were under 1 ug/g when fresh, over the 30-day period, the high-PUFA oils (linseed, corn, and rapeseed) produced much higher levels of MDA than did the low PUFA oils (palm and camellia).

In scientific analyses, MDA is the most widely used biomarker of oxidative stress in the body. Not surprisingly, MDA levels are also used to assess the oxidation status of foods. In keeping with the theory that ALEs from seed oils are drivers of chronic disease, it should also come as no surprise that MDA levels are strongly tied to hypertension, diabetes, atherosclerosis, heart failure, and cancer, and that higher levels of MDA have been shown in patients with breast, lung, oral, ovarian, and endometrial cancers, as well as complex regional pain syndromes, and even glaucoma.[937]

Other research has drawn strong correlations to increasing MDA and type 1 and type 2 diabetes, increasing BMI, and obesity.[938] This, of course, is linked to the fact that high omega-6 LA consumption drives whole body oxidative stress.

ACROLEIN, THE MAJOR TOXICANT IN CIGARETTE SMOKE: HIGHER IN VEGETABLE OILS!

Acrolein is yet another of the major types of ALEs (aldehydes) produced by the oxidative degradation of vegetable oils and LA. It should immediately pique our interest that acrolein is considered such a potent toxicant that the EPA has published a 106-page document entitled the "Toxicological Review of Acrolein."[939]

Acrolein is a ubiquitous environmental pollutant to which we may be exposed as a result of food and water consumption, cigarette smoke, automobile exhaust, and biocides (herbicides and pesticides), but also may be produced endogenously (within the body), the latter of which comes mainly from – you guessed it – the oxidation of unsaturated lipids, like LA.[940]

According to Department of Pharmacology and Toxicology researchers at the University of Louisville, Kentucky, "Acrolein has been suggested to play a role in several disease states including spinal cord injury, multiple sclerosis, Alzheimer's disease, cardiovascular disease, diabetes mellitus, and neuro-, hepato- [liver], and nephro-[kidney]toxicity."[940] The researchers explain that acrolein has diverse toxic effects, damaging DNA, proteins in our bodies, mitochondria (the powerhouses of our cells), cellular membranes, immune systems, and more.

Given that there are numerous sources of acrolein, we should focus on the most modifiable sources, which would include fried food, cigarette smoke, alcoholic beverages, charred meats, and, of course, the endogenously produced source of acrolein, which is the oxidation of unsaturated fats within our bodies.[940] Very simply, when it comes to fried foods, the problem is not animal meats and traditionally raised animal fats, which are low in PUFA, but rather cooking with vegetable oils (once again).

Researchers from the Department of Pharmaceutical Sciences, Oregon State University, published in 2008 a paper that would still be considered one of the most comprehensive reviews on both the dangers and sources of acrolein. In that paper, the authors stated, "Smoking of tobacco products equals or exceeds the total human exposure to acrolein from all other sources."[941]

Curiously, the research provided by Professor Martin Grootveld and other lipid scientists may challenge that statement, given the enormous production of acrolein in high-PUFA vegetable oils with lengthy heating as is utilized in fast-food restaurant cooking.[905 906 907]

In 2018, for example, Dr. Grootveld and colleagues found that a typical 154 g serving of "potato chips purchased from fast-food restaurants, including ubiquitous large chain global ones," were found to contain anywhere from about 1.0 to 1.5 mg of acrolein per serving.[905] Grootveld and colleagues are British, and it should be pointed out that what are referred to as "chips" in the U.K. would generally be called "french fries" in the U.S., "frites" or "pommes frites" in French-speaking countries, "finger chips" in Indian English, and "frieten" in Dutch speaking countries.

Let's put the 1.0 to 1.5 mg acrolein in a typical serving of french fries into perspective, because acrolein is not only toxic, it is the "major cigarette-related lung cancer agent." The 'famous' McDonald's french fries, in a large size, is 154 grams (the same mass that Dr. Grootveld used for reference).[942]

The World Health Organization (WHO) recommends that the "Maximum Human Daily Intake" (MHDI) for acrolein should be no more that 525 ug (0.525 mg)[943] whereas the Australian Government Department of Health (AGDH) recommends that the maximum "no-observed-adverse-effect level (NOAEL)" for acrolein should be no more than 35 ug (.035 mg).[944] Therefore, the single serving of McDonald's large french fries exceeds the WHO MHDI by about two- to three-fold and exceeds the AGDH's NOAEL level by about 28 to 43-fold!

Now let's contrast the fast-food french fries cooked in vegetable oils, again using the McDonald's large (154 g) serving size, in comparison to the acrolein in cigarette smoke. As Grootveld reviewed, the acrolein in typical fast-food restaurants' large size french fries is about 1.0 to 1.5mg (1000 to 1500 ug).

Researchers at Phillip Morris Research Laboratories scientifically evaluated 12 different representative cigarettes to assess the yield of smoke constituents under FTC/ISO (strict laboratory) conditions, and found that the production of acrolein ranged from a low of 15.5 ug to a high of 98.2 ug per cigarette with an average of about 53.9 ug.[945] This indicates that the acrolein in a typical large size fast-food french fries is equivalent to smoking 18 to 28 average cigarettes or up to 97 cigarettes lowest in acrolein! Need we wonder what is wrong with fast food?

Given that acrolein is considered a "major cigarette-related lung cancer agent,"[946] and it is greatly derived from the oxidation of seed oils, perhaps we should not be surprised to find that in rural China, frequent wok cooking (15 to more than 30 times per month) with seed oils (rapeseed or linseed oil) has been associated with an approximate doubling of lung cancer risk.[947] Perhaps the most surprising statistic in this regard is that 88.4% of the women with lung cancer in this study did not smoke cigarettes.

Acrolein is considered a cause or contributor to cardiovascular disease[948] [949] lung cancer,[947] Alzheimer's disease,[950] urinary tract cancers,[951] ischemic stroke,[952] and age-related macular degeneration (AMD),[953] among other chronic diseases. It behooves us to avoid the major sources that we can modify, particularly seed oils and cigarette smoking.

CARBOXYETHYLPYRROLE (CEP) – MORE FALLOUT FROM SEED OIL EXCESSES

Carboxyethylpyrrole, abbreviated CEP, is the final ALE that we will review in any detail, however, keep in mind that the oxidation of seed oils produces hundreds of ALEs. CEP is produced just like the other ALEs, from the oxidation of LA, primarily. The curious situation with CEP, however, is that it has the capacity to bind with proteins in our bodies, making them antigenic to our immune system, and this may be followed by what may be considered an autoimmune response.[954] Through this and other mechanisms, CEP has been implicated as important in the potentially blinding disease age-related macular degeneration (AMD), but also in autism, cancers, and wound healing problems and failures.[954]

CEP is well-known in the field of ophthalmology as playing a very critical role in the development of AMD with central vision loss because CEP accumulates both in the retina and in the layer of cells that supports the retina, known as the retinal pigment epithelium (RPE).[955] And in both cases, the CEPs are known to be produced endogenously (within the body) and in the case of AMD, may lead to what are known as "anti-CEP antibodies."

These are antibodies that attack whatever the CEP is bound to, which, in this case, could be structures in the retina and retinal pigment epithelium. This is yet another mechanism by which ALEs can produce destruction, in this case potentially leading to central vision loss, i.e., even blindness. In fact, researchers have found that CEP bound to proteins (called CEP-adducts) are massively accumulated in

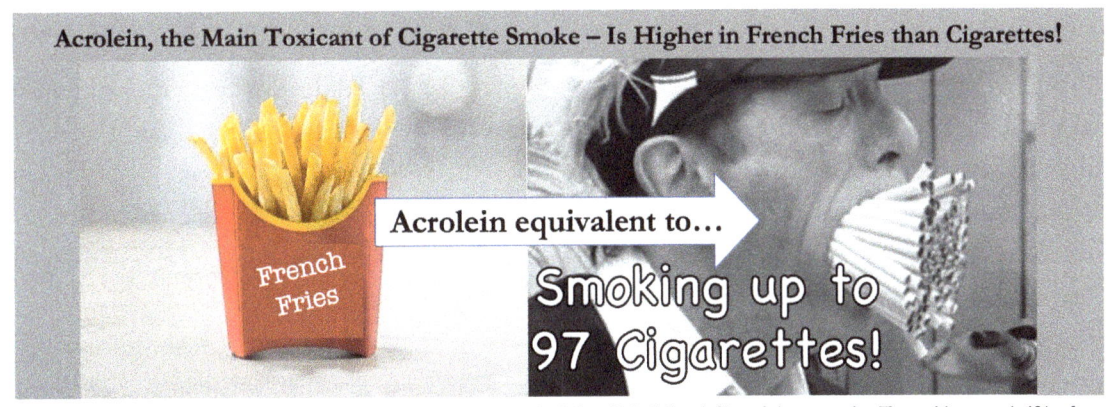

Acrolein, the Main Toxicant of Cigarette Smoke – Is Higher in French Fries than Cigarettes!

French Fries — Acrolein equivalent to... Smoking up to 97 Cigarettes!

Acrolein, the primary aldehyde (advanced oxidation end product) in cigarette smoke, is found in both French fries and cigarette smoke. The acrolein content in 154g of French fries (typical large fries) cooked in vegetable oils in typical fast food restaurants is equivalent to smoking 18-28 average cigarettes, or 97 cigarettes lowest in acrolein. References: 1) Grootveld M, et al. Chronic non-communicable disease risks presented by lipid oxidation products in fried foods. Hepatobiliary Surg Nutr. 2018;7(4):305-312. 2) Roemer E, et al. Chemical composition, cytotoxicity and mutagenicity of smoke from US commercial and reference cigarettes smoked under two sets of machine smoking conditions. Toxicology. 2004;195:31-52. © Copyright C. Knobbe, Ancestral Health Foundation, 2022.

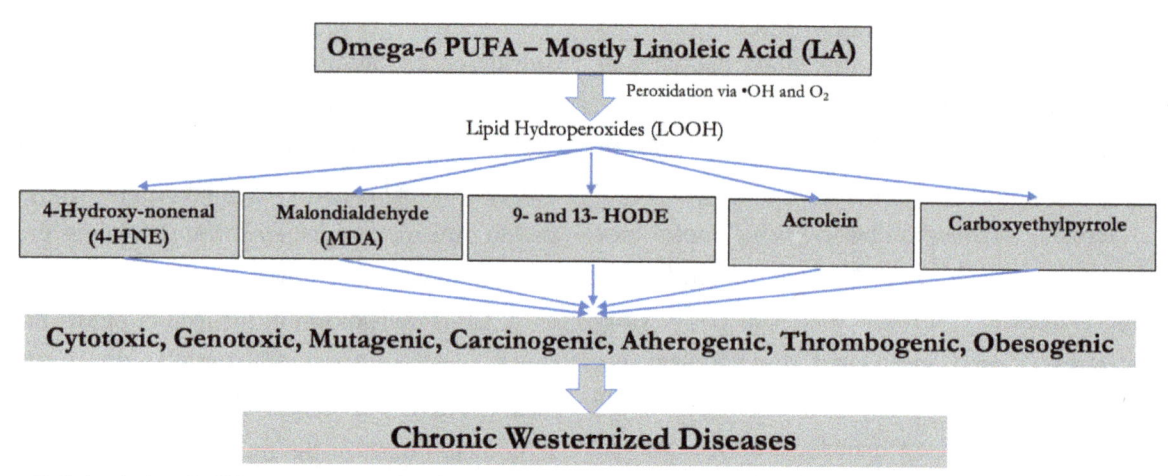

```
          Omega-6 PUFA – Mostly Linoleic Acid (LA)
                            │
                            │ Peroxidation via •OH and O₂
                            ▼
                 Lipid Hydroperoxides (LOOH)
         ┌──────────┬──────────┼──────────┬──────────┐
         ▼          ▼          ▼          ▼          ▼
   4-Hydroxy-   Malondi-    9- and 13-  Acrolein  Carboxyethyl-
   nonenal      aldehyde     HODE                  pyrrole
   (4-HNE)      (MDA)
         └──────────┴──────────┼──────────┴──────────┘
                               ▼
   Cytotoxic, Genotoxic, Mutagenic, Carcinogenic, Atherogenic, Thrombogenic, Obesogenic
                               ▼
                  Chronic Westernized Diseases
```

Verified mechanisms via which omega-6 excess, mostly linoleic acid (LA), lead to primary and advanced lipid oxidation end products (ALES), with associated and linked pathological developments. References herein. © Copyright C. Knobbe, Ancestral Health Foundation, 2022.

the retinas from individuals with AMD, but not in those without the disease.[954] And CEP bound proteins in the plasma of subjects with AMD have also been found to be about 60% higher than those without AMD.[955][956] CEPs also promote wet AMD, which is the type of AMD that is by far most likely to end in central blindness.[957]

OMEGA-6 LA EXCESS, MITOCHONDRIAL DYSFUNCTION, OVERWEIGHT AND CHRONIC DISEASE

Warning: Deep Science Ahead!

In the mitochondria, which are the powerhouses of the cell, excess LA may have the greatest impact and the most dreaded consequences. This is the case because when a person consumes seed oils and LA to excess, which is in fact, almost any amount, the LA accumulates within their cells and causes oxidative destruction on a massive scale.[6][180][958]

One of the key molecules that is oxidized and, therefore, damaged, in this scenario, is a molecule called cardiolipin.[854] Cardiolipin is the "lynchpin" upon which the mitochondria depend. It is critical because your mitochondria produce power like a generator for your body, by first accumulating what is known as a proton gradient within the mitochondrial membranes before using that stored energy from the proton gradient to create ATP, which is the energy currency of the cell. Let's examine how this works in a healthy low LA diet.

IN A LOW LA DIET, OXIDATION IS LOW AND MITOCHONDRIA WORK LIKE A MARVEL OF ENGINEERING

When we eat food, whether carbohydrate or fat, most of it (~whatever is not stored) will be used to create large amounts of a molecule called acetyl CoA, which enters the Krebs cycle to finally produce two high-energy carriers of electrons called NADH and FADH2.[959]

Just think of these high-energy electron carriers as electricity that will be used to power an engine. Inside the mitochondria, the NADH and FADH2 molecules transfer the energy-dense electrons to the electron transport chain (ETC), which uses the energy of the electrons to pump hydrogen ions – called protons – from the inner mitochondrial matrix into the intermembrane space to produce a proton gradient (see the image on page 240, "Normal Mitochondrial Energy Production in Low LA Diet").

This proton gradient is an enormous source of potential energy, which, just like a battery, has the capability to produce energy! How does it accomplish this? The protons (H+ in the diagram), because of the gradient, pass through an ETC complex (a protein) called ATP synthase, which adds a phosphate group to ADP (adenosine diphosphate) to create ATP (adenosine triphosphate).[959] ATP is the ultimate energy currency of the cell. This, in perhaps its simplest form, is the process by which the enormous majority of our energy is made, and this fuels the functions of cells. And keep in mind, our cells are really a microcosm of the whole body. If they're healthy, we're usually healthy.

The key "lynchpin" of producing energy, as one can see, is the production of the proton gradient. Without that, the energy production begins to fail. The proton gradient can only be held in place when the phospholipid membrane, which acts like a dam holding water, is able to hold the stored energy of the proton gradient.[960] [961] It must be secure and without leaks! And the key to maintaining that, as scientists have now unraveled, is a molecule called cardiolipin.[854]

Cardiolipin associates with proteins inside the mitochondrial membrane,[977] and when all is well and the cardiolipin molecules are in their natural state, the molecules all fit together in the membrane (phospholipid membrane) of the mitochondria, they function as they should, and they hold the proton gradient.[977] [962]

In the classic model of cardiolipin that was discovered in the heart – hence the name -- is a glycerol backbone and four acyl "tails," which are generally made up of – ironically – four linoleic acid (LA) molecules.[963] When the four LA molecules are in their normal state (unoxidized), the "tails" of the cardiolipin molecules all fit together neatly and they rather "insulate" the intermembrane space to hold the proton gradient. With a secure membrane, the electron transport chain (ETC) can build the proton gradient, and the protons can be used to make ATP. Everything runs smoothly, and energy (ATP) is produced in this marvel of engineering (see the over-simplified model on page 240).

The above scenario applies when LA in the diet is low, and the mitochondrial membranes are competent because the unoxidized tails of LA in cardiolipin fit together nicely. In this scenario, the membrane remains secure, the electron transport chain and proton gradients function as intended, and energy in the form of ATP is abundantly produced. However, now let's examine what happens when the diet is rich in LA, causing oxidation throughout the body.

IN AN OMEGA-6 LA RICH DIET, OXIDATION IS HIGH AND MITOCHONDRIA BEGIN TO FAIL

It is clear that increasing LA consumption in the diet increases the LA in cardiolipin proportionately.[964] [965] This may increase oxidative stress locally within the mitochondria, leading to oxidation of the LA within the cardiolipin.[966] Thus, even though LA is such a critical component of cardiolipin, it becomes damaged in a high LA diet through oxidation, and either A) undergoes a conformational ("shape") change, or B) is replaced by another fatty acid (usually the longer chain DHA or AA).[963]

Normal Mitochondrial Energy Production in Low LA Diet!

Over-simplified proposed mechanism of normal mitochondrial energy production in low LA diet with healthy cardiolipin. © Copyright C. Knobbe, Ancestral Health Foundation, 2022.

Either of these outcomes may devastate the form and function of the inner mitochondrial membrane, the electron transport chain, and the proton gradient, leading to mitochondrial dysfunction (see figure on page 241).[966]

Why? Because when the LA is damaged through oxidation and undergoes a shape change or is replaced by another fatty acid molecule, the 3-D conformational change causes the membrane to become "leaky" (see the diagram on page 241, "Mitochondrial Energy Failure in High LA Diet!"). In this case, the protons may leak through the membrane, resulting in energy failure, rather than passing through the ATP Synthase to create ATP (energy). An immediate and secondary "fallout" from this is increased reactive oxygen species (ROS), which fuels even worse oxidation of lipids – leading to a vicious cycle.[963][966]

There is an alternative explanation for this loss of power in the mitochondria in a diet that is excessive in LA. The natural shape of the cardiolipin is critical to transferring electrons in the mitochondrial electron transport chain (ETC). In this alternative model, it is known that the ETC typically forms a "respiratory supercomplex" with proteins (complexes) in the ETC, which supports the transfer of electrons and protons.[966]

Cardiolipin normally localizes to the hairpin turn of mitochondrial cristae, which are the folding structures within the inner mitochondrial membrane, and it is here that cardiolipin functions as a "glue" to stabilize the proteins of the electron transport chain to enhance electron transfer and reduce reactive oxygen species (ROS) production.[967][968][969]

However, when cardiolipin is oxidized, it is no longer able to easily form the "supercomplexes." The hairpin curvature of the cristae is lost resulting in disruption of the ETC functionality.[969] This leads to reduced transfer of electrons in the ETC, and production of ATP is radically diminished.[966] A second-

Mitochondrial Energy Failure in High LA Diet!

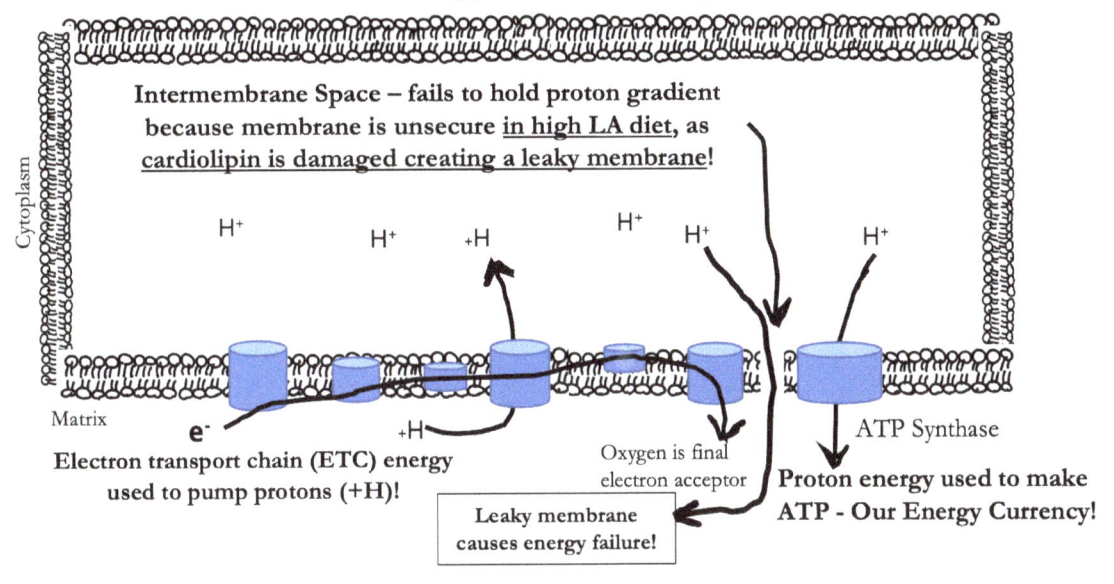

Intermembrane Space – fails to hold proton gradient because membrane is unsecure <u>in high LA diet, as cardiolipin is damaged creating a leaky membrane!</u>

H⁺   H⁺   +H   H⁺   H⁺   H⁺

Cytoplasm

Matrix   e⁻   +H   Oxygen is final electron acceptor   ATP Synthase

Electron transport chain (ETC) energy used to pump protons (+H)!

Leaky membrane causes energy failure!

Proton energy used to make ATP - Our Energy Currency!

Over-simplified proposed mechanism of partial mitochondrial energy failure in high omega-6 LA diet due to damaged (remodeled) cardiolipin, creating leaky inner mitochondrial membrane. © Copyright C. Knobbe, Ancestral Health Foundation, 2022.

---

ary result is increased reactive oxygen species (ROS), just as in the first proposed mechanism.[961][970][971][972] In either case, the end result is that the affected mitochondria are ineffective at producing power. And regardless of the ultimate molecular mechanism, the end result is the same – devastation of cellular energy production.

With either mechanism, this loss of mitochondrial power generation is profoundly dangerous to cells, as energy failure leads to increased oxidative stress, which, in turn, leads to increased inflammation and a whole host of sequelae.

The key point of this entire discussion is that high LA diets lead to higher oxidative stress, oxidation of cardiolipin, electron transport chain malfunction, and increased reactive oxygen species, which collectively leads directly to insulin resistance,[973][974][975] obesity,[973] and non-alcoholic fatty liver disease.[976] This is not related to any excess consumption of sugar, carbohydrate, or even fat. It is explicitly related to excess LA in the diet, which comes largely from seed oils (in westernized diets).

Researchers confirm that this associated loss of cellular energy production (mitochondrial dysfunction) secondary to cardiolipin remodeling will impair the reparative processes of injured cells and result in disorders of neurological signal transduction, muscle contraction, and circulation of blood, as well as cardiovascular diseases, heart failure, inflammation, ischemia (poor blood flow), premature aging, and many other diseases that may lead to premature death.[977]

Mitochondrial dysfunction is strongly related to DNA mutations and cancers.[978] Such energy failure can also lead to an increase in cell death (known as apoptosis), which may lead to disorders like Alzheimer's disease,[985] Parkinson's disease, amyotrophic lateral sclerosis (ALS),[979] age-related macular degeneration (AMD),[980] and many other neurologic disorders.

Finally, energy failure as a result of mitochondrial dysfunction will induce fatigue.[981] All the while, affected cells fail to properly burn energy for fuel, so instead, they store it as fat, which greatly contributes to being overweight. Overweight cells are a microcosm of how we become overweight. Just envision this process going on in all of your cells (see the graphic on page 243, "Omega-6 LA Excess +Westernized Diet +Nutrient Deficiencies").

One of the key and unifying identifiers of all so-called westernized chronic diseases is mitochondrial dysfunction (see graphic on page 243).[982] But why would they all share this pathological feature? Peroxidative damage to cardiolipin is the integral step leading to mitochondrial dysfunction, which has been shown to be critically important in all of the following: Many conditions of the heart and central nervous system (brain and spinal cord),[983] cardiomyopathies,[984] cardiovascular diseases, neurodegenerative diseases, Alzheimer's disease,[985] obesity, insulin resistance, type 2 diabetes, cancers, and more.[982]

Conventional medicine fails to connect the dots on all of this, viewing each of these diseases as if they're mostly unrelated. But in reality, probably 99.5% of the world's population is now consuming some amount of seed oils. The presence of this biological poison – seed oils – is now pervasive and ubiquitous. But commonality and a long history of use does not mitigate the fact that the seed oils are extremely dangerous.

SEED OILS DISPLACE ANIMAL FATS AND VITAMINS A, D, AND K2: THE COUP DE GRÂCE OF SEED OIL DEVASTATION

In the early 20th century, E.V. McCollum and other researchers all collectively found that animal growth rapidly came to a halt if seed oils were the only fat provided in the animals' diets, whereas growth could proceed normally when small amounts of butter, whole milk, egg yolks, or cod liver oil were given.[148] [149] It was also discovered that adult animals, if given provisions of food that contained seed oils as their only source of fat, soon began to develop rough coats, severely dry and inflamed eyes, dental decay, and eventually, weight loss. In both scenarios, whether young or adult, if the experimental diets containing only seed oils were continued, the animals would succumb to early deaths.[149] [151] [152]

What was discovered over many succeeding decades was that butter, whole raw milk, egg yolks, offal, and cod liver oil were all excellent sources of the fat-soluble vitamins A, D, and K2 (cod liver oil may be deficient in K2) but not a single edible oil of any type, including all the high-PUFA seed oils, olive oil, nut oils, or even the tropical oils (coconut, palm, and palm kernel) contain any of these vitamins (see Chapter One). Beef tallow (fat) as the sole source of fat was slightly less efficient in supplying all of the fat soluble vitamins as compared to butter, whole milk, egg yolks, offal, and cod liver oil, but was still very good.

By 1939, Weston A. Price had discovered that the modernized "foods of commerce," such as refined flours, sugars, and seed oils, caused a great displacement of the natural foods which are rich in the fat-soluble vitamins.[28] Remarkably, Price showed that the diets of traditional living people contained ten times more of the fat-soluble vitamins A, D, and K2, as compared to Americans at that time, and that deficiencies of these vitamins occurred in westernized diets leading to a great multitude of degenerative conditions, includ-

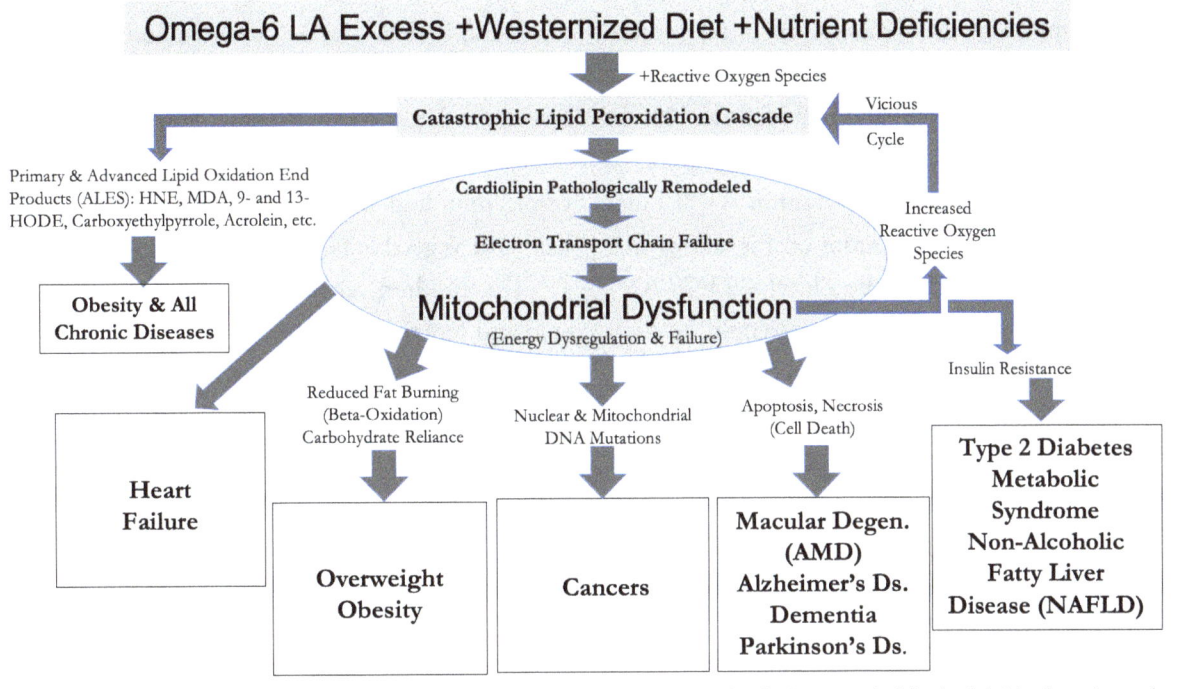

Omega-6 LA Excess + Westernized Diet + Nutrient Deficiencies

```
                        +Reactive Oxygen Species
                                 ↓
                Catastrophic Lipid Peroxidation Cascade  ← Vicious Cycle
                                 ↓
Primary & Advanced Lipid Oxidation End    Cardiolipin Pathologically Remodeled    Increased
Products (ALES): HNE, MDA, 9- and 13-              ↓                              Reactive Oxygen
HODE, Carboxyethylpyrrole, Acrolein, etc.  Electron Transport Chain Failure       Species
            ↓                                      ↓                                ↑
    Obesity & All                         Mitochondrial Dysfunction
    Chronic Diseases                    (Energy Dysregulation & Failure)
                                                                        Insulin Resistance
         Reduced Fat Burning      Nuclear & Mitochondrial   Apoptosis, Necrosis
         (Beta-Oxidation)              DNA Mutations         (Cell Death)        Type 2 Diabetes
    Heart  Carbohydrate Reliance                                                 Metabolic
    Failure                                                                      Syndrome
                                                               Macular Degen.    Non-Alcoholic
                 Overweight              Cancers               (AMD)             Fatty Liver
                 Obesity                                       Alzheimer's Ds.   Disease (NAFLD)
                                                               Dementia
                                                               Parkinson's Ds.
```

Proposed mechanisms via which omega-6 excess, mostly linoleic acid (LA), especially when combined with a westernized diet that is deficient in nutrients and antioxidants, induces a "catastrophic lipid peroxidation cascade," leading to mitochondrial dysfunction. All listed conditions are linked by these biological mechanisms and mitochondrial dysfunction. © Copyright C. Knobbe, Ancestral Health Foundation, 2022.

ing dental decay, arthritis, cancers, and a marked reduction in resistance to infectious diseases such as tuberculosis (see Chapter One).[28]

The fat-soluble vitamins, as shown by Price[28] and more recent researchers such as our friend and colleague, Chris Masterjohn, PhD,[986][987] work in synergy to provide not only optimal growth in infants and children, but also to preserve excellent health in adulthood. Modern science fails to recognize this and, instead, has greatly exaggerated the potential negative effects of aging[988] and genetics,[989][990] while fantastically underestimating the impacts of nutrient-deficiencies and toxic foods (mostly seed oils and industrially produced trans fats).

VITAMIN A DEFICIENCY: A RAMPANT CONDITION

Though each and every one of the 13 vitamins are necessary for both proper growth and development as well as maintenance of health in adulthood, it is clear from the anthropologic studies by Weston A. Price conducted in the 1930s that deficiencies of the fat-soluble vitamins – A, D, and K2 – were severe in populations on five continents if they were consuming the "displacing foods of modern commerce," and *only* if they were consuming the "displacing foods."

And while deficiency or absence of any vitamin may ultimately prove lethal, Price found that it was deficiencies of the fat-soluble vitamins that were by far the most common in the processed food laden diets. It is these three vitamins that will be reviewed briefly.

CHAPTER 5

One of the oldest diseases known to man, which stems from the deficiency of a fat-soluble vitamin, is night blindness. Descriptions date back to ancient medical papyri and included the correct prescription for its cure, which was consumption of liver (a tremendous source of vitamin A).[991] Hippocrates (460 – 375 BC) wrote on the use of fish oils as medicine and Pliny the Elder(~ 23-79 AD) wrote that the oil of dolphin livers could be used internally for chronic skin eruptions.[992]

At the end of the 18th century, Thomas Percival had introduced cod liver oil – a potent source of vitamins A and D – into the British Pharmacopoeia and he wrote, "…I believe no medicine in the materia medica is likely to be of more service."[993] In much of the world, during the 19th and 20th centuries, cod-liver oil was considered to be both food and medicine.

In fact, when not being regularly consumed, cod-liver oil was prescribed by physicians to treat numerous diseases and ailments, including night blindness, rickets, anemia, "consumption" (tuberculosis), scrofula (lymphatic tuberculosis), rheumatism, gout, lupus, palsy, constipation, impaired digestion, and "impaired nutrition."[994][995][996][997] In the U.S., cod liver oil was introduced into medical practice around 1845, when it was listed as a non-officinal drug in the *United States Dispensatory* in 1836 and remained listed there until 1960.[997]

In 1919, just shortly after E.V. McCollum began to publish works on the "fat-soluble A" (vitamin A) and the "water-soluble B" (the different types of B vitamins had not yet been elucidated [Chapter One]), physician Carl E. Bloch (1872-1952) completed studies on Danish children, aged one to four years, who presented with night blindness and severe dryness of the corneas of the eyes.[998]

Bloch suspected nutritional deficiencies in these children who were subsisting on fat-free milk, oatmeal, and barley soup – a dreaded consequence of World War I. Bloch prospectively studied 32 of the institutionalized toddlers, providing half of them with meals containing animal fats in the form of whole milk and butter, while providing the other half with 'vegetable fats' in the form of margarine.

The children receiving the animal fats recovered and remained healthy, while 50% of the group receiving the vegetable oil-laden diets developed corneal xerosis – a condition of severely dry, hazy corneas. Bloch rapidly cured all of the ailing children consuming the vegetable oil-laden diets by treating them with cod liver oil, concluding that the whole milk and butter, as well as the cod liver oil, all contained a fat-soluble nutrient that protected against night blindness and the severe dry eye conditions.[998][999]

In 1924, Danish physician Olaf Blegvad, M.D., published his analysis and treatment of nearly 450 cases of keratomalacia (severe and decompensating dry eye) due to diets deficient in vitamin A.[1000] Blegvad confirmed that deficiency was largely attributed to "the use of skimmed milk or of vegetable fats as a substitute for butter" concluding, "The treatment includes a corrected diet including large amounts of the vitamin [via milk, butter, eggs, liver, etc.]."[1000]

Additionally, a series of trials were conducted in the 1920s and 1930s providing foods rich in vitamin A (there were no supplements of any kind at that time), which found vitamin A greatly beneficial as a treatment for a wide variety of infections.[1001][1002][1003][1004] Vitamin A rich foods had also been shown in some cases to prevent infections. By 1928, researchers H.N. Green and Sir Edward Mellanby, at the University of Sheffield, England, reviewed that vitamin A was commonly being referred to at that

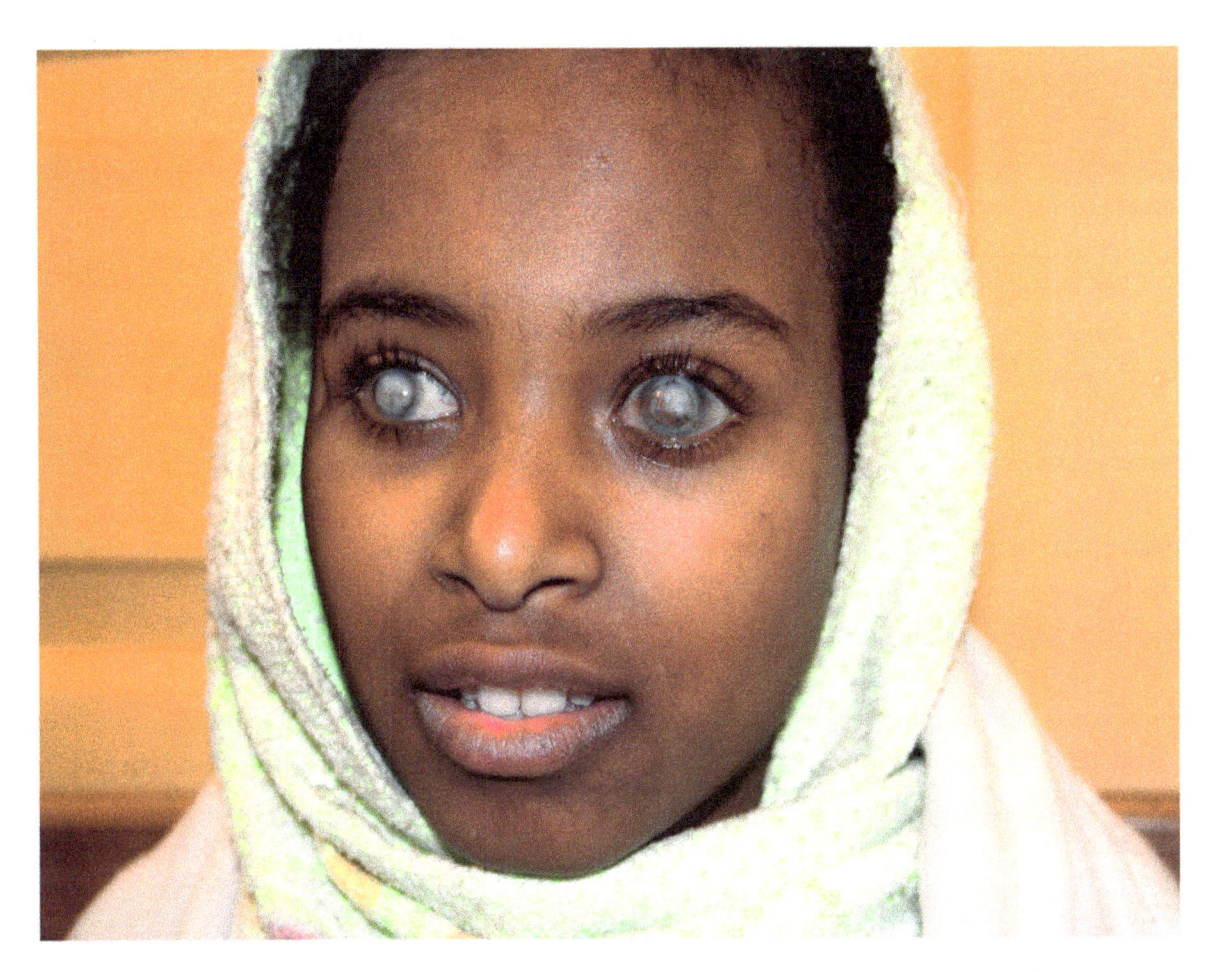

Vitamin A deficiency resulting in bilateral blindness in this 12-year-old girl, Ethiopia, 2009. She has undergone a corneal transplant, left eye, which failed. Image courtesy of Community Eye Health Journal, Dec 2009;22(71):33-35. Image license under CC BY 2.0.

time as the "growth promoting vitamin" while they referred to it as an "anti-infective agent."[1005]

Thus, by the early 1930s, it had clearly been established that very low animal fat diets and diets in which vegetable oils displaced animal fats led to deficiencies of vitamin A. Through about 1940, this had been remedied by the use and prescription of cod liver oil by both the lay public and physicians.[1006] However, with the advent of antibiotics – and after World War II – cod liver oil prescriptions, recommendations, and general consumption all rapidly declined.[997]

While vitamin A levels in the blood (serum retinol) may be established in routine analyses, the values may have little relation to whole-body stores of vitamin A (about 90% of stores are in the liver), since the vitamin is so critical that the body homeostatically maintains blood levels until stores are dangerously low.[1007] A liver biopsy would indeed be the only methodology to establish whole body stores, however, the risk and invasiveness of the procedure abrogates use for routine vitamin testing.[1008] By the late 1930s, the question of how to suitably establish vitamin A levels was already a consideration.

Researchers began to take advantage of the fact that vitamin A is the critical nutrient in night blindness through a clinical exam called "dark adaptation testing."[1009] Dark adaptation testing is a measure of the rate at which one develops sensitivity to see in darkness, for example, when entering a dark room after coming out of bright light. In studies completed in 1938,[1009] 1939,[1010] and 1941,[1011] researchers established that dark adaptation testing was the single most suitable index for detecting vitamin A deficiency.

In 2006, vision scientist Cynthia Owsley, PhD, along with colleagues at the University of Alabama at Birmingham, completed studies of dark adaptation and vitamin A treatment in 104 subjects, all over 50 years of age, both with and without age-related macular degeneration (AMD).[1012] The group was randomly and equally divided into control and experimental groups and both groups underwent baseline dark adaptation testing. The experimental group then received very large doses of vitamin A (50,000 IU/day) for 30 days, while the control group received a placebo.

Thirty days later, both groups underwent repeat dark adaptation testing. In the experimental group, which was given the large doses of vitamin A, both AMD and non-AMD subjects all experienced improvements in their dark adaptation times. Given that all subjects in the experimental group, whether their retinas were normal or not, had improvements in dark adaptation, is a strong suggestion that vitamin A deficiency is a rampant condition in the U.S., at least in those over age 50. Had vitamin A status been normal in these subjects, dark adaptation times should not have improved.

In 1949, after evaluating years' worth of studies and evidence, the U.K.'s Medical Research Council (MRC), under the direction of Sir Edward Mellanby, advocated that adults should consume 2,500 IU per day of vitamin A, or 7,500 IU carotenoids per day if depending on carotenoids from plant sources for vitamin A (carotenoids may convert to vitamin A, but conversion is relatively poor, e.g., about 4% on average from vegetables).[1013] [1014]

In 1975, Sauberlich and colleagues established the recommendation that 4,000 IU of vitamin A or ß-carotene per day should be consumed.[1015] In 2020, the U.S. Recommended Dietary Allowance (RDA) for vitamin A for those 14 years of age or older was set at about 3,000 IU for males and 2,330 for females.[1016] Yet, the 2007-2008 NHANES study found that adult men in the U.S. consumed an average of 2,161 IU and adult women consumed 1,931 IU.[1016] This represents a chronic under-consumption averaging about 840 IU/day for men and 400 IU/day for women, which represents a near mathematical certainty for population-wide vitamin A deficiency.

It is, therefore, a foregone conclusion that the enormous majority of Americans are falling markedly short of the recommendations made by all authorities regarding vitamin A consumption. This will assuredly contribute to many chronic diseases, including cardiovascular disease,[1017] cancers,[1018] and very likely, age-related macular degeneration,[1012] while it will assuredly negatively impact health, survival, and vision.[1019]

Today, vitamin A is arguably considered the most multifunctional vitamin in all of animal physiology, being critically important for its role in vision, immunity, reproduction, embryonic development, cellular differentiation, mucus membrane maintenance, epithelial cell function (e.g., the skin and gut), antioxidant functionality, redox signaling, and even energy balance.[1020] In fact, studies have concluded that vitamin A is involved in regulating at least 500 human genes.[1020] It is even proven to have direct involvement in insulin resistance and lipid metabolism, while also having a role as an electron carrier, indicating that vitamin A is critical to mitochondrial function.[1021] [1022]

Cod liver oil, a great source of vitamins A and D, benefitted millions of people historically, and likely saved countless lives. It remained in the *U.S. Dispensatory* for over 120 years and had a nearly 200-year history of use for prophylaxis of infections, prevention of disease, and treatment of a myriad of conditions. However, for nearly all physicians today, it is a relic of the past. Allopathic physicians today will rarely make recommendations for food sources of vitamins A and D, and recommendations for liver, cod liver oil, or fish roe (eggs), whether for night vision complaints, dry eyes, dry skin, infectious disease, allergies, or any other systemic condition, is practically unheard of.[1023] This is both a tragedy and a travesty.

WE NOW FACE A PANDEMIC OF VITAMIN D DEFICIENCY, DESPITE SUPPLEMENTS

Rickets is a disease characterized by poor calcification of the bones with consequent softening and distortion, often resulting in bowlegs. The disease was first described by physicians in the 1600s, however, it seemed to still be rare.[1024] It appears to be unknown if the condition existed before then. The Industrial Revolution in Great Britain in the late 1700s seems to have brought with it the scourge of rickets. Factory work, working indoors, and the smoggy air of industrialized cities, in retrospect, appears to have been associated with a plague of this disease that affected much of Europe.

Children affected with rickets in infancy have persistently soft bones – much like cartilage – and afflicted babies and toddlers are delayed in their ability to sit, crawl, and walk.[1024] As they do begin to stand or walk, their soft and weakened bones bend under their weight, leaving them with the characteristic signs of bowed legs or knock knees, but also distorted ribs, i.e., "pigeon breast." The scourge of rickets also frequently causes tetany – painful spasms of the hands, feet, and larynx – sometimes precipitating difficulty breathing, nausea, convulsions, and even death.

In about 1919, Sir Edward Mellanby of Great Britain, an acolyte of nutrition researcher, E.V McCollum, became deeply disturbed by the high incidence of rickets, which was especially severe in Scotland.[1025] Mellanby suspected the disease might be due to a vitamin deficiency. He took the diet most commonly consumed by the Scottish people, which was oatmeal, and fed it to dogs that he also unintentionally kept indoors, away from sunlight.

The dogs developed rickets just like humans.[1026] Just as McCollum had treated and reversed growth failure and xerophthalmia (a severe dry eye condition) with cod liver oil, Mellanby likewise treated the dogs with cod liver oil, which resulted in cures. With that, Mellanby suspected that rickets must have been a vitamin A deficiency.[1026]

McCollum was apprised of Mellanby's findings and set out to test the hypothesis that vitamin A was the missing nutrient in the development of rickets. He heated and aerated the cod liver oil, which he knew could destroy vitamin A, yet he found it could still cure rickets.[1027] In 1922, McCollum and colleagues concluded that a fourth vitamin (after vitamins A, B, and C had been discovered) was responsible, which they called "vitamin D."

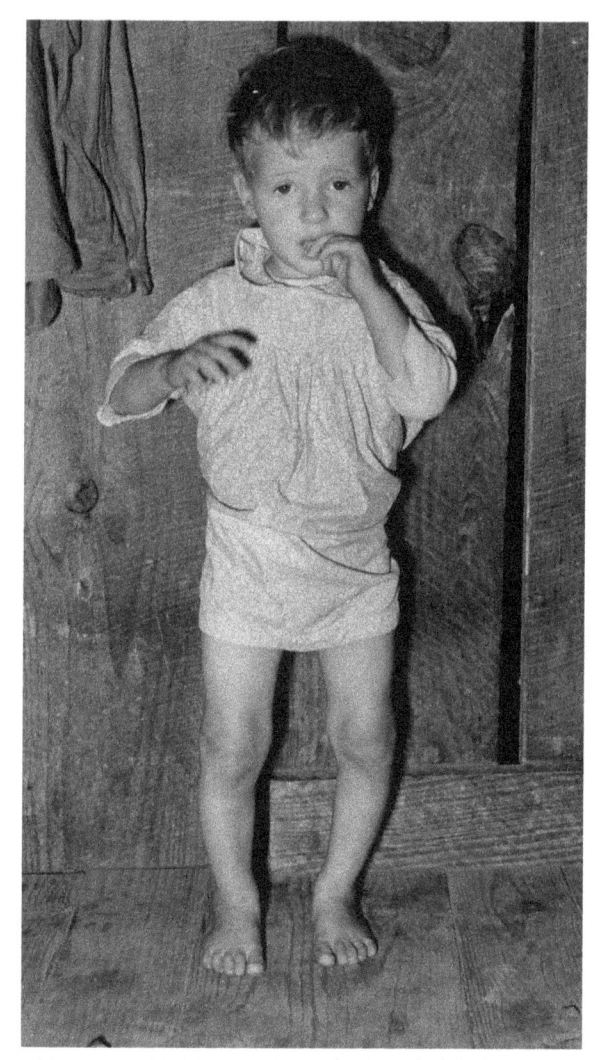

Two-year-old child with rickets, 1939. The child had never spoken, nor received any medical attention. Image in the public domain, courtesy of the U.S. Library of Congress.

During the same time that McCollum was completing investigations in the U.S., K. Huldschinsky, a physician in Vienna, and Harriette Chick, a determined researcher of the Medical Research Council (MRC) in England, both independently found that children suffering with rickets could be cured by either sunlight exposure or even artificially produced UV light.[1028][1029] It was soon concluded that sunlight or UV light could produce vitamin D from a lipid fraction in the skin, even if it wasn't provided in the diet.[1025] This was the first time that a vitamin was recognized that could be produced endogenously, rather than strictly provided in the diet, like vitamins A, B, and C.

Eventually, in studies completed in the late 1930s and early 1950s, R. Nicolaysen and colleagues showed that vitamin D increased the absorption of calcium from the intestine.[1030][1031] This helped pave the way to a better understanding of how vitamin D influenced calcium metabolism, but the research regarding the complexities of vitamin D was still in its infancy.

By 1971, research groups had worked out the complicated metabolic pathways from sun exposure or UV light to the development of an active form of vitamin D. When a cholesterol precursor in the skin, called 7-dehydrocholesterol, is "irradiated" by sunlight (UV), it converts to a pre-vitamin D3, which then circulates in the blood to the liver where it is converted to 25-hydroxyvitamin D3; that metabolic component circulates to the kidney where it is converted into the active form of vitamin D, which is 1,25-dihydroxyvitamin D3.[1024] Thus, sunlight is an extraordinarily important source of vitamin D, especially when dietary sources are minimal.

In 2000, National Academy of Sciences authors reviewed that vitamin D had already been found in the nucleus of cells that had nothing to do with bones, teeth, or calcium balance, such as the brain, lymphocytes (infection-fighting white blood cells), and skin.[1024] As of 2015, vitamin D has now been shown to control more than 900 genes.[1032] By another estimate, as many as 2,000 genes are currently considered to have vitamin D response elements, indicating that vitamin D plays a role in the functionality of thousands of proteins representing incalculable effects.[1033] Deficiency is now known to adversely affect up to 80 different metabolic pathways.

The Institute of Medicine (IOM) has defined vitamin D deficiency based on 25(OH)D3 – the usual target for assessing vitamin D status – as serum concentrations less than 20 ng/ml.[1034] The current guidelines for Americans suggest that optimal vitamin D status be greater than 30 ng/ml.[1033] In the U.S., currently, approximately 70% of adults and 67% of children aged 6 to 11 years have inadequate levels of vitamin D, and these statistics remain true even if fortification and supplemental vitamin D are considered.[1035][1036][1037]

Globally, vitamin D deficiency is now recognized as a pandemic, which is associated with at least 17 different cancers, many autoimmune diseases, heart disease, hypertension, stroke, obesity, depression, fibromyalgia, chronic fatigue syndrome, osteopenia, osteoporosis, periodontal disease, fractures in adults, rickets in children, and birth defects.[1038][1039]

But why is there such a pandemic of deficiency? First, there are very few foods that naturally are excellent sources of vitamin D,[1038] and some of those that are, such as fatty fish, fish livers, cold-extracted cod liver oil, some offal (organ meats), and egg yolks, are not widely consumed in westernized populations.[1039][1040]

Perhaps even far more problematic in the pandemic of vitamin D deficiency is the fact that sun exposure has been vilified for risk of skin cancers. The American Academy of Dermatology broadly and strongly advocates for intense sun avoidance and sunscreen use.[1041] Allopathic medical authorities, in general, have made strong recommendations to avoid all sun exposure, placing the entire world's population at much higher risk of vitamin D deficiency.[1042]

Even worse, the broad recommendations for use of topically applied sunscreens, which block more than 99% of incident UVB radiation (at "sun protection factor" [SPF] of 15), reduces the synthesis of vitamin D in the skin by 99%.[1043] One study estimated that an approximate 12% of deaths in the U.S. each year – about 340,000 deaths per year – are linked to reduced and inadequate sun exposure.[1044] Yet another study determined that sun exposure avoidance as a risk factor for death is comparable to cigarette smoking.[1045] Hundreds of studies, quite frankly, have repeatedly proven the link between vitamin D deficiency and a myriad of chronic, degenerative conditions.[1033]

An extraordinary finding is that approximately 90% of vitamin D is formed within the skin secondary to sunlight exposure.[1046] In other words, only around 10% of vitamin D is originating from the diet, which of course, would require, primarily, the consumption of fatty fish, fish liver (e.g., smoked cod liver), or cod liver oil, with much lesser amounts coming from numerous other animal sources.

Thus, for those who neither consume these natural sources or get regular sun exposure of 'unprotected' skin, the risk of vitamin D deficiency is tremendously high.

Educator, Marc B. Sorenson, Ed.D, and physicist, William B. Grant, PhD, in their scientific book, *Embrace the Sun*, completed analyses of approximately 1,300 studies, concluding as follows:

> *"There are 324 deaths associated with diseases of low sun exposure for every 1 death related to diseases of high sun exposure."*[1047]

Curiously, they've shown that melanoma – the only skin cancer that generally could threaten life

– affected only 1 person in 1,500 in the year 1935, whereas in 2014, it affected 1 in 50, an increase of 3,000%.[1048] However, they showed that in 1910, 33% of the U.S. population was employed in farming (obviously, with extensive sunlight exposure), whereas by 2000 only 1.2% of the population was employed in farming, which is a decrease of 96%. Citing eleven scientific papers in support, Sorenson and Grant wrote as follows:

"Many other papers in the scientific literature show that both incidence and death rate from melanoma are reduced with increasing exposure to sun."[1049]

Interestingly, they've also reviewed that 75% of melanomas occur on skin that is relatively unexposed to sunlight, for example, on the back or the upper legs, whereas they much less commonly present on areas of high sun exposure, such as the face and arms.[1050] Even for melanoma, the best prevention of a potentially lethal cancer is sunlight exposure. So while no authorities, including Sorenson, Grant, or ourselves, recommend sunlight exposure to the point of burning, regular sunlight exposure of unprotected skin provides extraordinary health benefits.

Given the remarkable synergistic effects of vitamins A and D, it should also be noted that exposure of the skin to the sun, surprisingly, "has opposite effects on vitamins A and D, catabolizing vitamin A but increasing the concentration of vitamin D."[1051] Furthermore, it has been hypothesized that lack of sunlight exposure and/or vitamin D deficiency may increase the accumulation of some of the active forms of vitamin A known as retinoids, and this may also increase susceptibility to infection.[1051] Thus, an important and delicate balance exists between these vitamins, which can best be remedied via consumption of appropriate amounts of vitamin A-rich foods while also receiving adequate sunlight exposure.

SUNLIGHT, MELATONIN PRODUCTION, AND MITOCHONDRIAL HEALTH: BEYOND VITAMIN D

The health of our mitochondria and hence, our body, is critically affected by the exposure of our skin to sunlight. Furthermore, the benefits of sunlight reach far beyond the production of vitamin D. Indeed, the effects of natural sunlight on our skin are so far-reaching and complex that we will likely never fully appreciate the countless benefits.[1047] Only a brief synopsis of yet another of the most important effects of sunlight exposure will be reviewed here.

The spectrum of light from the sun is 7% ultraviolet (UV), 39% visible (VIS), and 54% infrared radiation (IR).[1052] The latter term "radiation," while often thought of as dangerous, scientifically refers to the emission of energy as electromagnetic waves. Thus, we could call the sun's rays UV radiation, visible radiation, and IR, with none of these necessarily being dangerous, such as x-ray radiation.

Both the visible and the infrared light, in proper "doses," have been known for more than 50 years to produce health benefits "via the promotion of healing processes."[1051] IR can be divided up into near, mid, and far. Near IR (NIR) appears to be the most biologically active. NIR provides the warmth we feel from the sun, is healing and restorative, has often been referred to as low-level light therapy (LLLT) or photobiomodulation (PBM), and has been reported to be beneficial in thousands of studies dating back to 1968.[1051]

Melatonin, an extraordinary hormonal regulator of sleep, has also been shown to be a profoundly important and powerful subcellular antioxidant. In 2013, Professor Russel J. Reiter, PhD, and Du-Xian Tan, MD, PhD, first hypothesized that the mitochondria were the original sites of melatonin synthesis, which would suggest that melatonin could be produced in many, if not all, cell types.[1053]

Classically, melatonin is produced in the pineal gland (located in the center of the brain) and is produced in response to absence of light, thereby inducing sleep at nighttime.[1054] This was long believed to be the sole source of melatonin production. But thanks to Reiter's research, we now understand that 95% of the melatonin produced in the human body is in the mitochondria in response to NIR on the skin.[1055]

A number of researchers then demonstrated that melatonin was produced in many species and in many different cell types.[1056][1057][1058] In late 2017, researchers Denis Odinokov and Michael Hamblin proposed that photons of light from NIR could stimulate melatonin synthesis in the mitochondria.[1059]

Then, in 2019, Russel Reiter and Scott Zimmerman delved more deeply into the theory and expanded upon Odinokov and Hamblin's hypothesis, further postulating that natural sunlight, via NIR, not only would stimulate melatonin within the mitochondria, but that mitochondrial melatonin might act as a powerful antioxidant locally, quelling the ROS that develop there.[1060] This is a deeply fascinating and compelling theory, which is supported by tremendous evidence.

NIR penetrates several centimeters deep within the body and is able to pass through clothing, epidermis, dermis, and ultimately may reach the subcutaneous tissues.[1060][1059] At all levels, however, NIR induces the production of melatonin within the mitochondria, which reduces ROS such as hydroxyl radicals, superoxide, and hydrogen peroxide.[1060] Thus, mitochondrial melatonin is now known to improve the efficiency of the electron transport chain (ETC),[1061] enhance ATP production,[1062] and reduce mitochondrial damage from ROS.[1063] It is indeed one of the single most effective antioxidants known.

Throughout nearly all of history, mankind and all living creatures, while outdoors in the daytime, were exposed to sunlight which produced extraordinary amounts of mitochondrial melatonin, all due primarily to NIR exposure from the sun. In natural sunlight, 70% of the photons hitting the body are from NIR, with the remainder being those from UV or visible light.[1060]

Today, however, the enormous majority of people work and reside primarily indoors, being exposed almost exclusively to light-emitting diode (LED), organic light-emitting diode (OLED), fluorescent, or compact fluorescent lamps (CFL), all of which emit zero NIR photons.[1060]

These artificial forms of light may thus be called "visible only" emitters, since they produce no infrared or UV light. This is an enormous loss of potential benefit for humans and, when combined with avoidance of sunlight, sunscreens, 'protective clothing,' and hats, results in devastating combined effects.

Once again, just as with vegetable oil avoidance, there is a simple solution. However, rather than avoidance, in this case, it is to embrace the sun and sunlight. In 1871, Ellen G. White wrote the following passage, published in *The Health Reformer*:

"The feeble one should press out into the sunshine as earnestly and naturally as do the shaded plants and vines. The pale and sickly grain

blade that has struggled up out of the cold of early spring, puts out the natural and healthy deep green after enjoying for a few days the health-and-life-giving rays of the sun. Go out into the light and warmth of the glorious sun, you pale and sickly ones, and share with vegetation its life-giving, health-dealing power."[1064]

We should also consider, if possible, the replacement of LED, OLED, and CFL bulbs with old-fashioned incandescent (tungsten) light sources, full-spectrum lamps that also produce NIR, candlelight, firelight, or other natural sources of light, along with frequent stints in the sun.

VITAMIN K2 – THE FINAL FAT-SOLUBLE VITAMIN TO COMPLETE THE "HEALTHY TRIO"

In the most simplified form, vitamins A and D function primarily as hormones, signaling cells to produce proteins, while vitamin K activates a subset of those proteins.[986][987] Thus, there is an exquisite synergy between these vitamins, the likes of which will probably never be fully appreciated.

In 1945, in the 2nd Edition of his book, *Nutrition and Physical Degeneration*, Weston A. Price described "a new vitamin like activator" which he maintained was important in the mineralization of teeth and bones, but which was also a critical factor in growth and development, reproduction, and much more.[1065] Price called this compound "*Activator X*" and he asserted that it was present in butterfat, the organs of animals consuming rapidly growing green grass, the milk of animals grazing on green grass, certain seafoods, and eggs.

Price found that cod liver oil, which was an excellent source of vitamins A and D, had little if any of this critical nutrient. Price was certain that "Activator X" played a fundamental role in the utilization of minerals to ossify teeth and bones, produce wide dental arches (with consequent straight teeth), and to prevent much degenerative disease.

He was able to relatively quantify the degree to which foods contained this nutrient via analysis of thousands of samples of dairy products from around the world. For example, he found the nutrient in "the milk of several species, varying with the nutrition of the animal," and he showed that it was only present when the animals were consuming rapidly growing green grass. Thus, "Activator X" was highest in cattle consuming green grass in the spring and fall, but during the winter, levels would fall precipitously.

Price provided a memorable example of the extraordinary effect of a proper whole foods diet, along with a carefully selected butter, when he chronicled the events of a young boy that a minister friend had referred to him. The minister had been called to the home of a desperate family during the Great Depression to baptize a dying child.[1066] The child was "in and out of convulsions," "badly emaciated," with "one leg in a cast" due to a fractured femur sustained two to three months previously, with "rampant tooth decay," and a "very bad bronchial cough." The complete fracture of the bone in the boy's thigh occurred while he was walking across the room, developed a convulsion, and fell to the floor. No healing of the fracture had occurred, requiring the continued cast. The diet of the boy "consisted of white bread and skimmed milk."

Price knew that the skimmed milk contained much of the necessary minerals, including calcium, phosphorous, and magnesium; however, with the fat almost entirely removed, it was greatly lacking in the fat-soluble vitamins (A, D, and "Activator X," or K2) which would work together to deposit the minerals into the bone. Price also reviewed that the convulsions were due to low calcium levels in the blood. He wrote the following regarding the dietary recommendation:

> "The program provided was a change from the white flour bread to wheat gruel made from freshly ground wheat and the substitution of whole milk for skimmed milk, with the addition of about a teaspoonful of a very high vitamin butter [obtained from cattle grazing on green grass] with each feeding."[1066]

After the dinner meal of whole, raw milk and "wheat gruel," which was essentially fresh whole ground wheat in hot water (a porridge), he "slept all night without a convulsion." He then "was fed the same food five times the next day and he did not have a convulsion. He proceeded rapidly to regain his health without recurrence of his convulsions. In a month the fracture was united." Six weeks after this dietary program was started, the boy was able to run and jump over the garden fence, affirming to Price that the femur had fully healed. Price wrote, "He was restored to health by the simple process of having Nature's natural foods restored to him."[1066]

The dietary essentials were, of course, provided in the whole raw milk and whole wheat, but not skimmed milk and white wheat flour, the latter two of which are nutrient deficient. The "high vitamin butter" provided the "Activator X" that Price knew was critical to the utilization of the minerals. Just these two whole foods (milk and wheat), carefully selected, along with butter from cattle grazing on green grass, provided all of the dietary essentials needed to not only save this boy's life, but to fully restore him to health.

For some 60 years following Price's death (in 1948), attempts to connect his "X factor" with a known nutrient had failed until colleague nutrition researcher, Chris Masterjohn, PhD, made the discovery in 2008 that the critical nutrient was vitamin K2.[987] Masterjohn reviewed in 2008 that there were long-standing misunderstandings about the functions of vitamins K1 and K2, even though they had both been chemically isolated in 1939.[1067] He wrote,

> "Although both K vitamins were discovered and characterized over the course of the 1930s, two fundamental misunderstandings about these vitamins persisted for over sixty years: the medical and nutritional communities considered blood clotting to be their only role in the body, and considered vitamins K1 and K2 to simply be different forms of the same vitamin."[987]

It wasn't until 1997 that the medical community determined that vitamin K had an additional role besides clotting[1068] – a concept that Weston A. Price was on the verge of discovering (with his "Activator X") shortly before his death in 1948.

Vitamin K1 is plentiful in leafy green plants (e.g., spinach, kale) and green vegetables (e.g., broccoli and Brussels sprouts),[1069] is variably converted to vitamin K2 in at least some animals,[1070][1071][1072] and is a critical component of blood clotting.[1073]

Vitamin K2 is abundant in cheese, curd, and natto (Japanese fermented soy),[1069] and relatively abundant in animal meats.[1074] Polygastric animals, such as beef and other ruminants, consume grasses containing vitamin K1, which is then fermented in their guts to vitamin K2, and which finally ends up in their milk and muscle.[1075][1076][1077][1078] Thus, milk, butter, cheese, and other dairy products are excellent potential K2 sources for human consumption.

Conversion of vitamin K1 to K2 has not been determined in humans, but it is abundantly clear that high vitamin K1 intakes have not solved the deleterious outcomes associated with deficiency of vitamin K2.[728] Furthermore, observational studies have found that higher intakes of vitamin K2 have been associated with greater reductions of vascular calcification and cardiovascular disease than comparable amounts of vitamin K1.[728] Japanese natto, the world's richest source of vitamin K2, has been a staple in their culture for nearly 1,000 years – about 30 generations – and this has been postulated as one of the reasons for not only their low cardiovascular risk but also their lower fracture risk and greater bone density than other nations.[1074]

Chris Masterjohn, PhD, in his review of Price's "Activator X", wrote the following:

> *"Vitamin K2 is the substance that makes the vitamin A- and vitamin D-dependent proteins come to life. While vitamins A and D act as signaling molecules, telling cells to make certain proteins, vitamin K2 activates these proteins by conferring upon them the physical ability to bind calcium… In all such cases, the proteins are only functional once they have been activated by vitamin K."*[987]

One of the best examples of this is osteocalcin, which is a protein that, once activated, results in deposition of calcium and phosphorous salts in bone and teeth. However, osteocalcin will not be produced unless cells receive signals from both vitamins A and D.[1079] Furthermore, osteocalcin will not accumulate in the extracellular matrix of bone and facilitate the deposition of calcium salts to create hardened bone unless it has been activated by vitamin K2.[1080]

Vitamins A and D are both responsible for regulating the expression of matrix gla protein (MGP), which, when activated by vitamin K2, results in the mineralization of bone (to create strong bones) as well as the protection of soft tissues, such as arteries, from calcification.[1081]

Simply put, with vitamins A, D, and K2 in optimal supply, teeth and bones are highly mineralized and strong, while arteries remain free of improper calcification. When vitamin K2 is deficient, arteries begin to calcify, which is yet another component of coronary heart disease. This has been called the "calcium paradox," which is the situation in which deficiency of vitamin K2 leads to both "lack of calcium in the bone and its storage in the vessel wall."[1082]

Thus, we have entire populations with both cardiovascular disease and osteoporosis – which indicates that they have calcification of vessel walls but lack of calcification in the bones, leaving them prone to heart disease and fractures. And the cardiovascular disease is closely tracked by the coronary artery calcium (CAC) score, which is a measure of calcification of the coronary arteries (see Chapter Four).[1083]

Deficiency of K2, therefore, drives both coronary artery calcification and osteoporosis, both of which are rampant in modern societies. Both conditions are due to deficiencies of fat-soluble vitamins – especially K2 – which is almost entirely secondary to the substitution of vegetable oils for animal fats.

Harumi Okuyama, PhD, Faculty of Pharmaceutical Sciences, Nagoya City University, Japan, along with colleagues, have shown profound correlations between seed oil consumption and chronic disease, that have common mechanisms of harm as certain anticoagulant medications. "These vegetable oils," they wrote, "and medicines such as statin and warfarin share, in part, a common mechanism to inhibit vitamin K2-dependent processes, which was interpreted to lead to increased onset of CVD [cardiovascular disease], DM [diabetes mellitus], chronic kidney disease, bone fracture and even mental disorder… High n-6/n-3 [omega-6/omega-3] fatty acid ratio of ingested foods, but not animal fats, was emphasized to be another risk factor for many of the diseases described above."[1084]

The latest available Dietary Reference Intake (DRI) from the Institute of Medicine (IOM) and U.S. National Academies Press (2001) recommends an Adequate Intake (AI) of vitamin K as 120 and 90 μg/day for men and women, respectively.[1085] However, the IOM fails to make any distinction between vitamins K1 and K2. The National Institutes of Health (NIH) Office of Dietary Supplements "Fact Sheet for Health Professionals," updated in 2021, also makes no distinction between vitamins K1 and K2, provides no specific recommendations for vitamin K2, and references the 2001 IOM recommendation.[1086] The NIH source of 2021 states, "Clinically significant vitamin K deficiency in adults is very rare and is usually limited to people with malabsorption disorders or those taking drugs that interfere with vitamin K metabolism."[1086]

Currently, one-third of the American population is dying of heart disease,[271] most of whom have moderate or severe coronary artery calcification (see Chapter One), and 54% of the U.S. population over age 50 has osteoporosis,[1087] both of which are conditions related in part to vitamin K2 deficiency. Yet we still have no official government recommendation for this extremely important vitamin.

Butter, eggs, whole milk, organ meats, fish, cod liver oil, the fatty content of meats, beef tallow, and, in general, the fat of many animals, all collectively and together provide pre-formed vitamins A, D, and K2, whereas 'vegetable oils' provide absolutely none.

The displacement of these vitamins is the final coup de grâce of seed oils – the disastrous end result of producing a pro-oxidative, pro-inflammatory, toxic, and finally, nutrient-deficient, biological milieu. The four of these components conspire together to exact disaster in a plethora of ways. Seed oils are indeed biological poisons – poisons that have primarily been in global diets mostly since the late 19th century. Removing them from every product to be consumed should be the primary goal of any diet.

SUGARS VS. SEED OILS: WHY ALES FROM SEED OILS ARE FAR WORSE THAN AGES FROM SUGARS

In recent decades, sugar has been implicated in obesity, hypertension, myocardial infarction (MI, or heart attack), cardiovascular disease, cancers, dyslipidemia (abnormal lipids), hypertension, diabetes, non-alcoholic fatty liver disease, pancreatitis, cognitive decline, and other chronic diseases.[1088][1089] It seems to have become fashionable to blame sugar for obesity and chronic disease, but the evidence for causality is far from proven.[1088][1090]

As mentioned previously, sugar is indeed a nutrient-deficient food, and we will argue that sugar in most forms should be minimized. It is our position that sugar-sweetened beverages (SSBs), sweets, candy, confectionery, and the like should generally be restricted or eliminated.[484][1090] Nevertheless, proper perspective is critical to constructing healthy diets that are simultaneously nutrient-dense, non-toxic, and satisfying.

One of the earliest critics of sucrose (table sugar) in the diet was John Yudkin, FRSC, Professor of the Department of Nutrition at Queen Elizabeth College, London, who published the book, *Pure, White and Deadly* in 1972.[1091] Then in 2002, Gary Taubes authored a cover story in *The New York Times Magazine* entitled, "What if It's All Been a Big Fat Lie?" which focused more on a low-carbohydrate approach to diet for health and weight loss.[1092] Taubes' article certainly garnered enormous attention, while it simultaneously enlightened millions regarding the epic failure of the "low fat is healthy" message.

In 2009, American physician and endocrinologist, Robert Lustig, MD, gave a lecture at the University of California San Francisco entitled, "Sugar: The Bitter Truth," which went viral. Lustig argued, in part, that the fructose component of sugar (sugar is a 50:50 mix of glucose and fructose) is a major cornerstone in the obesity epidemic and that fructose metabolism leads to de novo lipogenesis (liver fat production), hepatic insulin resistance, and all of the manifestations of the metabolic syndrome.[1093] Lustig, however, has also repeatedly blamed processed foods, as evidenced by the title of his book, *Fat Chance: Beating the Odds Against Sugar, Processed Food, Obesity, and Disease*.[1094]

In 2019, the World Health Organization persisted with its long-term position on sugar, recommending that consumption of "free sugars" (i.e., added sugars, but not fruit sugars) be less than 10% of calories for both adults and children, but additionally suggested, "a further reduction to <5% of total energy is encouraged for added health benefits."[1095]

Sugar is a marker of processed food, but so are seed oils, refined flours, and trans fats (the latter of which are components of seed oils, see Chapter One). Without question, in any population consuming processed foods, sugars and seed oils generally tend to track together. This often results in both food components correlating to overweight, obesity, and chronic disease. As such, drawing causal inference to disease is problematic in observational population studies, even in observational longitudinal studies where the two food groups are followed over time.

However, if we can track the two food groups (sugars and vegetable oils) far enough back in time to where disease prevalence is little or none and consumption of one of the two food groups is little or none, this should be most revealing. Fortunately, the U.S. is one of the very few countries where this is possible because we have known data on sugars, seed oils, diabetes, and obesity, all going back to the 19th century. See the bar graph on page 257 to contrast the prevalence of diabetes and obesity versus sugar and vegetable oil consumption in 1908, 1935, and 2016 ("U.S. Seed Oils and Sugar Vs. Diabetes and Obesity, 1908-2016").

As one can see from this most telling bar graph (and many previous graphs), in the U.S. in 1908, sugar consumption was already 325 cal/day (81 g/day), but seed oils were only 11 calories per day (1.2g/day).[4][3] In that year, obesity was only about 1.2%, diabetes was approximately 0.2% or perhaps far less (it was 0.0028% in 1890 and 0.37% in 1935), coronary heart disease (CHD) and heart attacks were virtually unknown, metabolic syndrome had never been described, the first case of Alzheimer's disease was diagnosed that same year (in Germany, but

U.S. Seed Oils and Sugar Vs. Diabetes and Obesity, 1908 - 2016

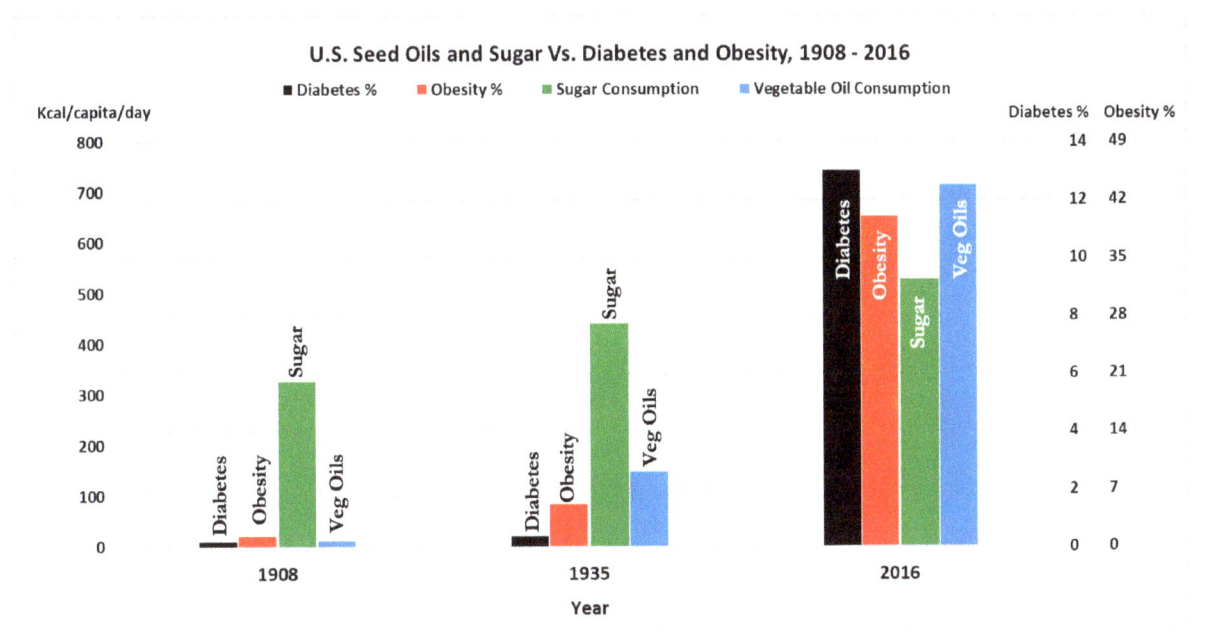

U.S. seed oil and sugar consumption vs diabetes and obesity prevalence, 1908-2016. References: 1) Vegetable Oil Data: Knobbe, Stojanoska. Medical Hypotheses: 2017;109:184-198 2) Sugar Data: Guyenet, Landen. *The Hungry Brain*. New York, Flatiron Books, 2017. 3) Obesity statistics, see references herein. 4) Diabetes statistics, see references herein. © C. Knobbe, 2022. Ancestral Health Foundation.

no known cases in the U.S.),[526] and age-related macular degeneration was an extraordinary medical rarity.[4]

If we assume that Americans of 1908 were consuming the same number of calories as Americans of 1971, which was 1,955 cal/day (NHANES 1971), sugar consumption in 1908 in the U.S. was already 16.6% of calories, which is far above the WHO recommendations today (10% maximum).

In 1935, sugar consumption had risen to 440 cal/day and seed oils were 146 cal/day, however, CHD had become the leading cause of death. Obesity is estimated at about 4.0 to 5.0% in 1935, based on the actual 1.2% obesity in 1900[449] [450] and the next actual data of 13.4% in 1960[451] (using Excel cumulative average yearly growth with a generated curvilinear increase).

Diabetes was only 0.37% in 1935[485] despite sugar consumption of 440 calories a day, which was approximately 22.5% of calories (same methodology as above). Metabolic syndrome had been described in the early 1920s by Kylin and Marañon, in Sweden and Spain, respectively, but no published cases existed in the U.S.[504] [505] Thus, in 1935 type 2 diabetes was still a medical rarity (or at least oddity), yet the sugar consumption was more than twice the current recommendations by the WHO. As one can see, in retrospect, it becomes almost impossible to blame obesity, metabolic syndrome, and diabetes on sugar.

In 2016, we observe that sugar consumption was 526 cal/day and vegetable oils were 713 cal/day, while diabetes and obesity had risen to an extraordinary 13.0% and 39.8%, respectively. If we observe the correlations in data between 1908 and 2016, we see a weakly positive but still trivial correlation between sugar consumption and obesity and diabetes, however, we see an extremely strong and positive correlation between vegetable oils, obesity, and diabetes.

For example, while sugar consumption (as a percentage of total calories) increased 62% between

1908 and 2016, vegetable oils increased 6,382%. During the same time-frame, obesity elevated 33-fold and diabetes rose about 4,000-fold!

Given this evidence and the evidence we've observed in virtually every analysis thus far, we would submit that perhaps 90% or more of the underlying cause of obesity is related to seed oil consumption. We currently estimate that seed oils and high omega-6 diets are responsible for more than 99% of the cause of diabetes and metabolic syndrome.

So while high blood sugar (hyperglycemia) is problematic, the main driver of excess sugar in the blood is not from overconsumption of carbohydrates or sugars, but rather, it is unquestionably from overconsumption of seed oils. Why? As reviewed previously, seed oils in excess drive an oxidatively destructive process involving the cardiolipin molecule in the electron transport chain (ETC), resulting in failed energy production, increased reactive oxygen species, and insulin resistance.[973][974][975]

This toxic reaction at the cellular level truly represents a microcosm of the devastation involving the entire body. And cellular insulin resistance drives whole-body insulin resistance, which ultimately leads to progressively increasing blood sugars as the condition progresses.

However, as stated previously, this does not exonerate added sugar consumption from exacting harm in other ways. First, there are no vitamins or minerals in added sugars and, therefore, substantial consumption can contribute to nutrient-deficiencies.[484] Second, sugar has been tied to the production of advanced glycation end products, or AGEs.[1096] AGEs occur when, sugar or more technically glucose, is in excess supply in the bloodstream, which then attaches to proteins in the body, a process referred to as glycation; however, the sugar can also attach to fats or even DNA.[1096]

When sugar binds to proteins this is referred to as the Maillard or browning reaction.[1097] The measurement of glycated hemoglobin in the blood is known as hemoglobin A1c (HgbA1c).[1098] This is a measure of the degree to which the elevated sugar in the blood has damaged oxygen-carrying protein hemoglobin. The higher the sugar level in blood, the higher HgbA1c will be, the latter of which represents damage to protein structures, with increasing HgbA1c representing increasingly damaged proteins. This all roughly correlates to the destructive effects that excess sugar has upon our bodies, i.e., it is driving and increasing some of the same processes we observe in aging.[1098]

However, increased sugar in our blood doesn't even begin to compare to the enormously destructive effects of seed oils, which markedly increase oxidation, inflammation, and toxicity, resulting in widespread destruction. As reviewed earlier, oxidation alone in the body is dramatically underestimated in terms of its disastrous effects, which are broad in scope and well-known to induce everything from cell death to obesity to every chronic disease known. Thus, the damaging insults of the advanced lipid oxidation end products (ALEs), which are driven primarily by seed oils, are dramatically worse than AGEs from excess sugars.

It is important to note that the body can handle far more sugar in the blood with dramatically reduced whole-body destructive effects, if one eliminates seed oils from the diet and keeps LA consumption exceedingly low. As examples of this, consider that diabetes independently tends to drive earlier heart disease, aging, etc., but for diabetics who smoke, which increases biological oxidation and insulin resistance, the combined effects of higher blood sugars and increased oxidation results in a far more rapid acceleration of diabetic complications.[1099][1100]

The worst-case scenario is the diabetic individual with poorly controlled (high) blood sugars (increased glycation), who smokes (increased oxidation and toxicity), and who also eats fast food regularly (vastly increased oxidation and toxicity), the latter, of course, containing huge amounts of seed oils. This is the "triple-whammy" of glycation, oxidation, and toxicity, at its worst. We've witnessed this scenario numerous times, and in these people, devastating disease may occur by age 20s or even sooner.

Sugars in the form of fruits, sweet potatoes, certain vegetables, whole raw milk, whole raw yogurt, natural maple syrup (in limited amounts), raw honey, molasses, and other natural foods we will submit are virtually never a problem and these foods, when well tolerated by the individual, are generally excellent sources of nutrition. Again, in many populations, consumption of natural sugars in whole, organic, natural foods has been shown to have an outstanding record of success as part of healthful, nutritious diets.

ANIMAL STUDIES – SEED OILS RAPIDLY INDUCE OBESITY, DIABETES, FATTY LIVER, INSULIN RESISTANCE, AND HEART FAILURE

Many animal studies have shown that diets high in omega-6 LA rapidly induce obesity and severe metabolic disease. One of the first well-controlled animal studies that investigated this was a study by David Pan and Leonard Storlien of the Garvan Institute of Medical Research in Sydney, Australia, in 1993.

In this study, the researchers put rats on three different isocaloric (equal calorie) high-fat diets, with identical amounts of fat (59%), protein (21%), and carbohydrate (20%).[1101] Rodents are omnivores with physiology that is extremely similar to humans.

In the study, adult but still growing rats weighing 250 grams at the beginning of the study were placed on each of three different diets, which varied only in the type of dietary fat and the LA% in the diet. The fat types and LA percentages were as follows: 1) Edible beef tallow, 4.4% LA, 2) Olive oil, 7.7% LA, and 3) Safflower oil, 36.6% LA (LA percent in terms of total calories, in keeping with typical methodology). Each major fat type accounted for 46.6% of calories while the remaining 12.4% of fat calories came from linseed oil, which made all diets also equal in omega-3 fatty acids.

Therefore, this was a very tightly controlled study in which omega-6 LA was the single variable, or as close as one might come to that. The animals were kept on each diet for just three weeks before the experiment was concluded and the animals analyzed (see table on page 260, "21 Day Animal Study: Isocaloric Diets (Equal Calories): Different Dietary LA%").

After just three weeks on the diet, as compared to the beef tallow group, the olive oil group gained 7.5% more weight, and the safflower oil group gained 12.3% more weight.[1101]

In human equivalents, as compared to the beef fat group, the olive oil group gained 12.8 pounds and the safflower oil group gained 21 pounds, in just three weeks! (See graph on page 261.)

And again, these were isocaloric (equal calorie) diets.[1101] See Figure 5.1 ("21 Day Animal Study: Isocaloric Diets (Equal Calories)"). The abdominal fat tissue showed that the LA percentage was

CHAPTER 5

FIG. 5.1

21 Day Animal Study: Isocaloric Diets (Equal Calories): Different Dietary LA%

Fat Source	Calories	Fat %	Om-6 %	Body Fat LA %
Beef Fat 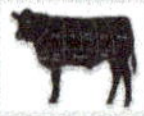	Same	59%	4.4%	10.3%
Olive Oil 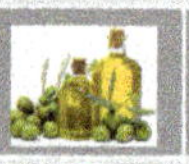	Same	59%	7.7%	15.2%
Safflower Oil 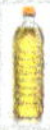	Same	59%	36.6%	54.5%

Pan DA. Dietary Lipid Profile is a Determinant of Tissue Phospholipid Fatty Acid Composition and Rate of Weight Gain in Rats. J Nutr. 1993;123(3):512-9.
© C. Knobbe. Ancestral Health Foundation, 2022.

10.3% in the beef fat group, 15.2% in the olive oil group, and 54.4% in the safflower oil group.

This single study turns the calories in versus calories out dogma of weight loss on its head, does it not? All of the animals received and verifiably consumed all of their food, and they each received a very slight calorie restriction to ensure that all food provisions were consumed.

Ergo, how can we account for the very large difference in weight gain between the three groups of animals, given that they all had the same weight initially, they all consumed the same number of calories, and they all consumed the same macronutrient ratios (proteins to carbohydrate to fat)? We will return to this question subsequently.

ANOTHER STUDY INDICATES THAT HIGH OMEGA-6 LA DIETS INDUCE OBESITY AND DISEASE IN RODENTS

In another study led by Poonamjot Deol, PhD, at the University of California, Riverside, along with six colleague researchers, soybean oil consumption in rodents was compared and contrasted with both the usual rodent chow diet, high fructose sugar, high soybean oil, and high soybean oil plus high fructose diets.[1102] In what might be the most well-designed, comprehensive, and sophisticated animal study of its kind, the researchers deeply addressed the issue of increased omega-6-rich oils in the diet, perhaps better than anyone in history. For the purposes of this book, only a brief synopsis will be given, as the depth and breadth of science from this study is far beyond the scope of this book.

In this study, after weaning at three weeks of age male mice were randomly assigned to one of five diets used in the study. The control diet was of standard rodent laboratory chow, which contained 13.5% fat, derived mostly from pork fat and fish meal, 58% carbohydrate, and 28.5% protein. The remainder of animals were randomized to one of four diets, which all contained 40% fat (typical of recent Americans), but varied the omega-6 LA percentage (by varying soybean oil and coconut oil content) and varied fructose sugar content, the latter of which has been the vilified component of sugar in the cause of insulin resistance and metabolic syndrome.[1103]

Four of these diets that we will compare and contrast may be summarized as 1) Rodent chow diet with 1.2% LA, 2) 4% soybean oil diet with 2.2% LA, 3) 19% soybean oil diet with 10% LA (typical of Americans currently, except without added sugar), and 4) 19% soybean oil plus 25.9% fructose diet (comparable to Americans for seed

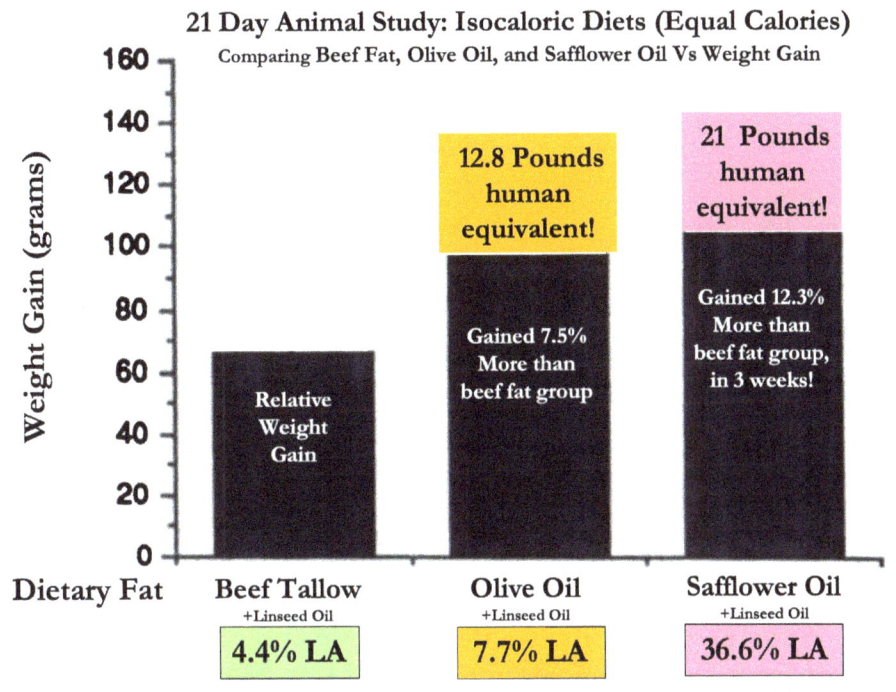

21 Day Animal Study: Isocaloric Diets (Equal Calories)
Comparing Beef Fat, Olive Oil, and Safflower Oil Vs Weight Gain

Dietary Fat	Beef Tallow +Linseed Oil	Olive Oil +Linseed Oil	Safflower Oil +Linseed Oil
% LA	4.4% LA	7.7% LA	36.6% LA
Result	Relative Weight Gain	Gained 7.5% More than beef fat group — 12.8 Pounds human equivalent!	Gained 12.3% More than beef fat group, in 3 weeks! — 21 Pounds human equivalent!

Pan DA. Dietary Lipid Profile is a Determinant of Tissue Phospholipid Fatty Acid Composition and Rate of Weight Gain in Rats. J Nutr. 1993;123(3):512-9. © C. Knobbe, 2022. Ancestral Health Foundation.

---

oils with a much higher concentration of fructose).

The most important consideration is that all of the experimental diets were isocaloric (equal calories), and the total amounts of fat, carbohydrate, and protein were constant in all diets except the control diet (as it was low fat).

As compared to the chow group (1.2% LA), the 4% soybean oil group (2.2% LA) gained about 30% more weight and the 19% soybean oil group (10% LA) gained about 63% more weight in just 32 weeks (about 7.5 months). If we compare these gains in the form of human equivalents using a 170 pound (77 kg) reference man for the chow group, the ending weights would be about 221 pounds (100 kg) for the 4% soybean oil group and 277 pounds (126 kg) for the 10% soybean oil group (see graph on page 262, "On Isocaloric (Equal Calorie) Diets, Soybean Oil Induces Severe Obesity!").

In a fourth diet used in this study, the soybean oil was kept at 19% in order to keep the dietary LA at 10%, however, as part of the carbohydrate component of the diet, a very high 25.9% fructose sugar was included.

In this dietary experiment, the addition of this massive amount of fructose was actually protective of weight gain. As we see in the graph on page 263, as compared to the 1.2% LA chow diet, the addition of 25.9% fructose to the 19% soybean oil diet led to an approximate 53% increase in weight, whereas the 19% soybean oil diet without added sugar led to an approximate 63% increase in weight.

In human equivalents, the high soybean oil and fructose diet resulted in an end weight of about 261 pounds, whereas the high soybean oil diet resulted in an end weight of about 277 pounds (as previously shown). See the graph on page 263 ("On Isocaloric Diets, Soybean Oil Worse than Soybean Oil with High Sugar!").

CHAPTER 5

On Isocaloric (Equal Calorie) Diets, Soybean Oil Induces Severe Obesity!
Diets of Standard Chow (1.2% LA), 4% Soybean Oil (2.2% LA) and 19% Soybean Oil (10% LA) for 32 Weeks

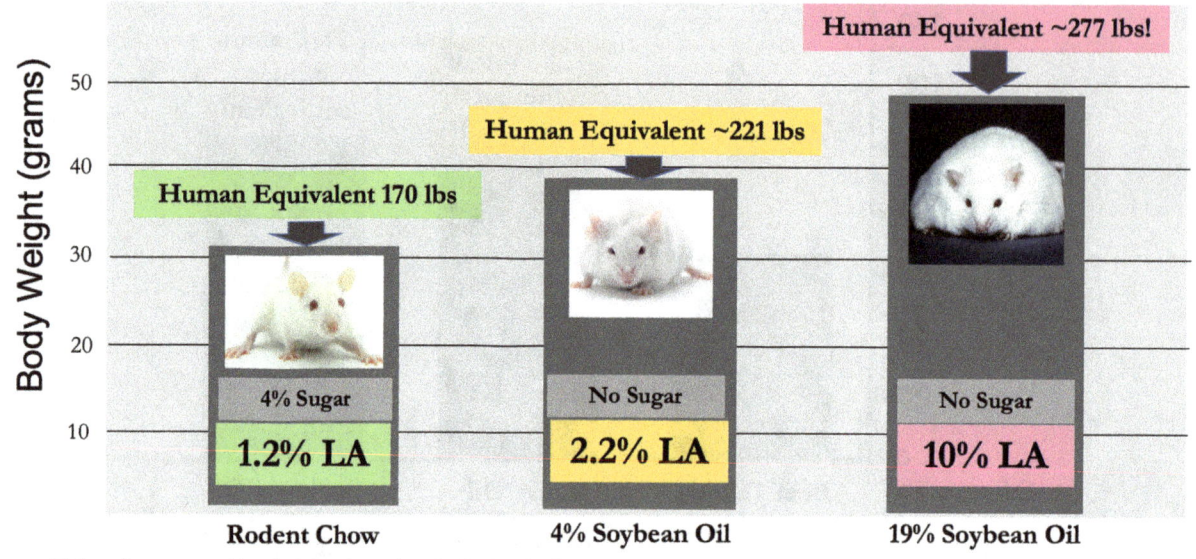

All three diets were equal in calories, study conducted in male mice after weening at three weeks of age, conducted for 32 weeks (7.5 months). Chow diet made with animal fat and was 13.5% fat, while the other diets were 40% fat, with equal amounts of carbohydrate and protein. The isolated variable was the linoleic acid (LA) percentage. Rodent images not from study. Reference: Deol P, et al. Soybean Oil is More Obesogenic and Diabetogenic than Coconut Oil and Fructose in Mouse: Potential Role for the Liver. PLoS ONE. 2015;10(7): e0132672. © C. Knobbe, 2022. Ancestral Health Foundation.

In this study, all diets that were higher in LA percent than the 1.2% chow diet resulted in far greater weight gain and metabolic disturbances. The worst outcome in this study in almost every metric was the 19% soybean oil diet, which was 10% LA. It should be reviewed that even this level of LA percentage is currently below the average dietary LA% in the U.S. (most recent data show 11.8% dietary LA in 2008, see Chapter One).

The 19% soybean oil diet resulted in the greatest weight gain, fat gain (adiposity), diabetes, glucose intolerance, and insulin resistance. As a matter of fact, the insulin resistance and glucose intolerance were even greater on the soybean oil diet without any added sugars than the 19% soybean oil and 25.9% fructose diet.

The high fructose diet (with 4% soybean oil, not presented above) in this study did seem to cause overweight/obesity; however, that was in a diet combined with 4% soybean oil. In that part of the dietary experiment, excessive fat deposition in the liver did occur, but no diabetes or insulin resistance was induced. The 19% soybean oil diet caused very large deposits of fat in the liver cells (hepatocytes) and "hepatocyte ballooning," suggesting potentially severe liver damage. This was noted at the 16-week time-point in the study but was severe at 35 weeks.

It may be worth the redundancy of restating that these were isocaloric (equal calorie) diets and, therefore, we absolutely cannot attribute any differences to calories. We also cannot attribute any deleterious outcomes on the soybean oil diet to carbohydrates or sugars, as the carbohydrate content was far lower in the 19% soybean oil diet than in the control (chow) diet and, of course, there were no added sugars to the 19% soybean oil diet. The

On Isocaloric Diets, Soybean Oil Worse than Soybean Oil with High Sugar!
Diets of Standard Chow (1.2% LA), 19% Soybean Oil + 25.9% Fructose (10% LA), and 19% Soybean Oil (10% LA) for 32 Weeks

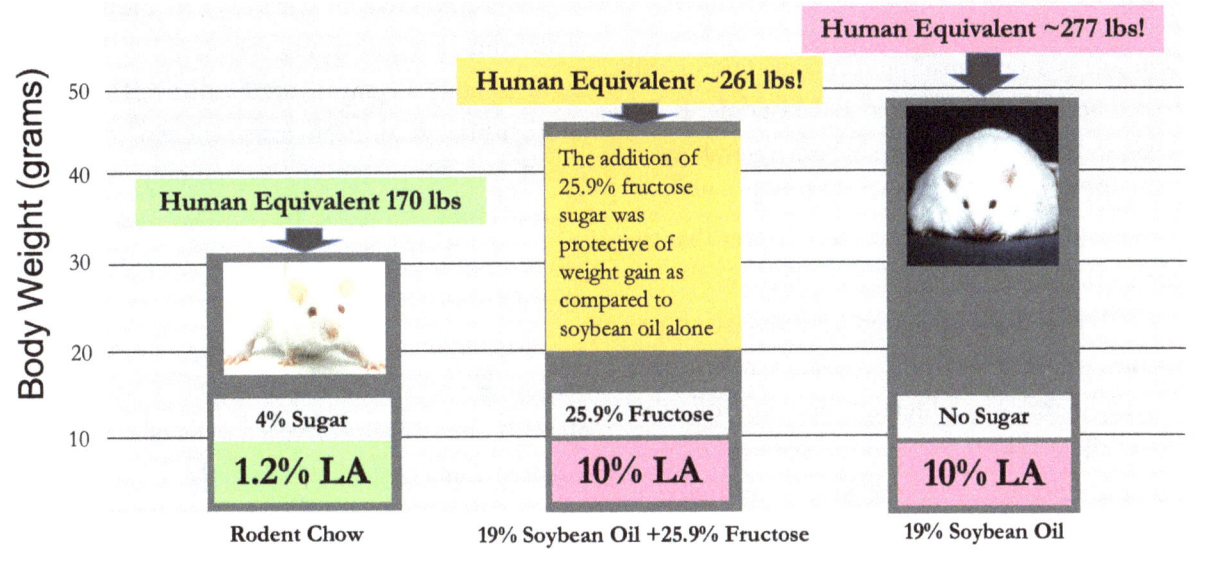

Human Equivalent ~277 lbs!

Human Equivalent ~261 lbs!

Human Equivalent 170 lbs

The addition of 25.9% fructose sugar was protective of weight gain as compared to soybean oil alone

4% Sugar
1.2% LA
Rodent Chow

25.9% Fructose
10% LA
19% Soybean Oil + 25.9% Fructose

No Sugar
10% LA
19% Soybean Oil

All three diets were equal in calories, study conducted in male mice after weening at three weeks of age, conducted for 32 weeks (7.5 months). Chow diet made with animal fat and was 13.5% fat, while the other diets were 40% fat, with equal amounts of carbohydrate and protein. The isolated variables were the linoleic acid (LA) percentage and the fructose sugar. Rodent images not from study. Reference: Deol P, et al. Soybean Oil is More Obesogenic and Diabetogenic than Coconut Oil and Fructose in Mouse: Potential Role for the Liver. PLoS ONE. 2015;10(7): e0132672. © C. Knobbe, 2022. Ancestral Health Foundation.

soybean oil diet, with 10% LA, was devastating to the health of these animals, period.

MORE ANIMAL STUDIES PROVE SEVERE WEIGHT GAIN, METABOLIC DISASTER, AND HEART FAILURE WITH SEED OILS

Quite a number of other studies have found similar results as those reviewed above, that is, diets high in seed oils and LA lead to obesity, fatty liver, and many metabolic disturbances.[1104][1105][1106][1107][1108]

One further study most deserving of mention was a study in which researchers divided experimental rats into two groups, one of which received normal lab chow, while the other group received normal lab chow that was supplemented with (soaked in) 20% sunflower oil (by weight), which is quite comparable to current U.S. consumption.[1109]

In just four weeks' time, in comparison to the group on lab chow, the group receiving the sunflower oil experienced a 32% reduction in cardiac output at "high afterloads," which indicates the cardiac output during the systolic (high pressure) phase of the heartbeat. In other words, in a period of just four weeks, the rats on the safflower ('vegetable') oil diet had already begun to experience heart failure.

The extraordinary dangers of high-PUFA seed oils were so well documented in these studies that one might think the government would move to ban these if our health were a concern. But instead, what we witness is continued endorsements of seed oils and advice to consume even more of these devastating oils.

CARNOSINE TO THE RESCUE – THE SACRIFICIAL SINK FOR AGES AND ALES

Carnosine is a very small protein consisting of only two amino acids, beta-alanine and histidine. It is a proven and powerful scavenger of both reactive oxygen species (ROS) and ALEs or OxLAMs.[1112][1113][1114]

Recall from the review in this chapter that the primary lipid oxidation products include 9- and 13-HODE and the advanced lipid oxidation end products (ALEs) 4-HNE, MDA, acrolein, carboxyethylpyrrole, and literally hundreds of other ALEs, all of which conspire in synergy to produce the devastating effects of cell dysfunction, cell death, and a myriad of disastrous biological impacts that contribute to chronic disease.

Carnosine, which is found almost entirely in the flesh of animal meats,[1117] has been shown both in laboratory and animal studies to prevent the formation of both ALEs and AGEs,[1110][1111][1117] thereby greatly deterring the onset of the many conditions that are induced by oxidation and glycation, such as diabetes, atherosclerosis, Alzheimer's disease, Parkinson's disease, cancers, etc.[1112][1113][1114][1117]

Carnosine has been shown to suppress the damage from HNE and MDA, which are two of the most prominent ALEs.[1117] Carnosine can also help prevent the glycation of LDL, a situation which may contribute to atherosclerosis and heart attacks.[1115] Therefore, the consumption of meat helps to reduce atherosclerosis, and this may even help to explain why, as meat consumption dropped in the U.S. from the late 19th century to reach a low point around the 1930s, coronary heart disease (CHD) became the leading cause of death (see Chapter One). Of course, vegetable oils are by far and away the primary drivers of CHD, but a reduction in meat consumption resulting in reduced carnosine consumption may have contributed.

Concentrations of carnosine in meats, especially ruminant meats, are very high;[1116] however, there is none in any plant foods.[1117] This is yet another biological mechanism wherein ancestrally raised animal meats are exceedingly protective against chronic disease. In contrast, lack of meat can be harmful, especially in the face of seed oil consumption.

Vegetarians have been shown to have reduced carnosine levels in their own muscle mass of up to 50%.[1118] Thus, vegans or vegetarians who consume no meat would both likely benefit from supplementation with the amino acid beta-alanine, which will raise carnosine levels in muscle.[1119] Beta-alanine is the rate-limiting raw nutrient and appears to be the most effective supplement to raise carnosine levels. Not only is carnosine (as a supplement) more expensive, but it has to be broken down to its constituent amino acids and be reformulated in the cell to produce carnosine.[1120]

Carnosine, which is prominent in muscle meats, has been shown to be protective against heart failure, diabetes, ischemia/reperfusion injury (e.g., the effects of heart attack or stroke), cancers, aging, neurodegenerative disorders such as Alzheimer's disease and Parkinson's disease, ophthalmic disorders, and delayed wound healing.[1117][1121] Animal muscle meat consumption may, therefore, be very protective against ALEs and AGEs, even providing some protection when seed oils and sugar consumption have been present and excessive.

WHAT THE DEEPER SCIENCE SAYS

CHAPTER 5: SUMMARY

The one single unifying factor that ties together all native, traditional, ancestral diets, whether derived exclusively from animal meats or derived almost entirely from plants, is that they're all very low in omega-6 LA. Analyses of such ancestral diets, which provide for excellent growth and extraordinary resistance to overweight and chronic disease, is that they generally all contain about 2 percent or less LA as a percentage of total calories in the diet and perhaps never more than about 3.5 percent of calories. On the other hand, westernized diets, which are inundated with seed oils, typically provide as much as 6 to 12% of the diet as LA.

Diets high in omega-6 linoleic acid (LA) almost exclusively exist in diets containing seed oils. Such diets result in marked accumulation of LA within cells, cell membranes, and mitochondrial membranes. Polyunsaturated fatty acids (PUFA) are highly prone to oxidation and, unlike monounsaturated and saturated fats, tend to undergo oxidation easily when exposed to free radicals in the body. Thus, high consumption of LA in the diet produces high levels of cellular accumulation of omega-6 LA, leading to highly pro-oxidative, pro-inflammatory, toxic, and nutrient-deficient states. Collectively, this is the "perfect storm" that sets the stage for the catastrophic lipid peroxidation cascade (CLIPS) and all chronic disease states.

High levels of LA consumption induce very high levels of LA in cells, cell membranes, and body fat (adipose). The accumulated excess of LA, being a polyunsaturated fat, then becomes a massive target for oxidation, which increases biological oxidative stress, mitochondrial dysfunction, and consequently results in a loss of energy production.

Markedly enhanced oxidation induced by seed oils results in degenerative changes in the mitochondria at the level of the electron transport chain (ETC), which immediately produces increased reactive oxygen species (ROS), which, in turn, generates even further ROS. The end result of this is increased insulin resistance at the cellular level, which may lead to progressively increasing blood sugar, metabolic syndrome, and eventually, type 2 diabetes.

Mitochondrial dysfunction may lead to various degrees of cellular energy failure. With crippled ability to properly burn fats for fuel, cells begin to abnormally store energy in the form of fats, leading to undesirable weight gain.

This may account for the massively increased body weight in experimental animals consuming higher omega-6 LA diets, even when such diets are isocaloric (equal in calories) to other experimental diets that are lower in LA, as has been shown in multiple studies. This evidence demonstrates that, when all other dietary components are equal, the animals on the higher omega-6-containing diets commonly gain tremendously more weight in the form of subcutaneous and visceral fat, while simultaneously developing metabolic disease, insulin resistance, diabetes, fatty liver disease, and heart failure. This is undeniable and indisputable evidence of causality.

Therefore, we absolutely, positively cannot conclude that weight gain is simply a calories in versus calories out equation. This evidence is the proof.

Seed oils will induce massive weight gain in animals and people, potentially without increasing caloric consumption.

But far worse, energy failure at the cellular level leads to a multitude of chronic diseases, including heart failure, cancers, Alzheimer's disease, Parkinson's disease, age-related macular degeneration (AMD), and a multitude of other chronic diseases.

High omega-6 diets, rich in LA, also lead to a pro-inflammatory biological milieu, and this inflammation further contributes to many disease states.

Toxicity from seed oils is a product not only of increased omega-6 LA consumption, but far higher consumption of the advanced lipid oxidation end products (ALEs) that are associated with seed oils, particularly seed oils that have been heated. The latter occurs anytime seed oils are used in cooking, especially fast food cooking, where seed oils may be heated and re-heated many times, for many days. The associated ALEs, including 4-hydroxynonenal (HNE), malondialdehyde (MDA), carboxyethylpyrolle (CEP), acrolein, and literally hundreds of other ALEs, collectively are cytotoxic, genotoxic, mutagenic, carcinogenic, thrombogenic, atherogenic, and obesogenic. Thus, the ALEs contribute greatly to all westernized, chronic diseases.

In the event seed oils are not heated, diets rich in omega-6 LA will still raise LA at the tissue level, producing a pro-oxidative environment that leads to endogenous production of ALEs. Thus, even if ALEs are not consumed exogenously from edible oils, high omega-6 LA diets will induce much higher ALEs production endogenously, that is, within the body.

Finally, seed oil consumption displaces natural animal fat consumption, which results in displacement of the fat-soluble vitamins, particularly vitamins A, D, and K2, and this alone leads to and further contributes to chronic, degenerative disease.

The most hazardous edible oils to avoid would include soybean, corn, canola, cottonseed, rapeseed, grapeseed, sunflower, safflower, and rice bran, though excluding nearly all edible oils would be the safest approach. If edible oils must be used, then the highly saturated oils, including coconut, palm kernel, and cacao butter would be best to use.

In summary, when seed oils are consumed to excess, which is almost any amount, a pro-oxidative, pro-inflammatory, toxic, and nutrient-deficient biological milieu is produced, potentially leading to abnormal weight gain and any number of chronic diseases. The simple avoidance of the highly polyunsaturated seed oils alone will produce marked resistance to undesirable weight gain and chronic disease and will begin to reverse these complications.

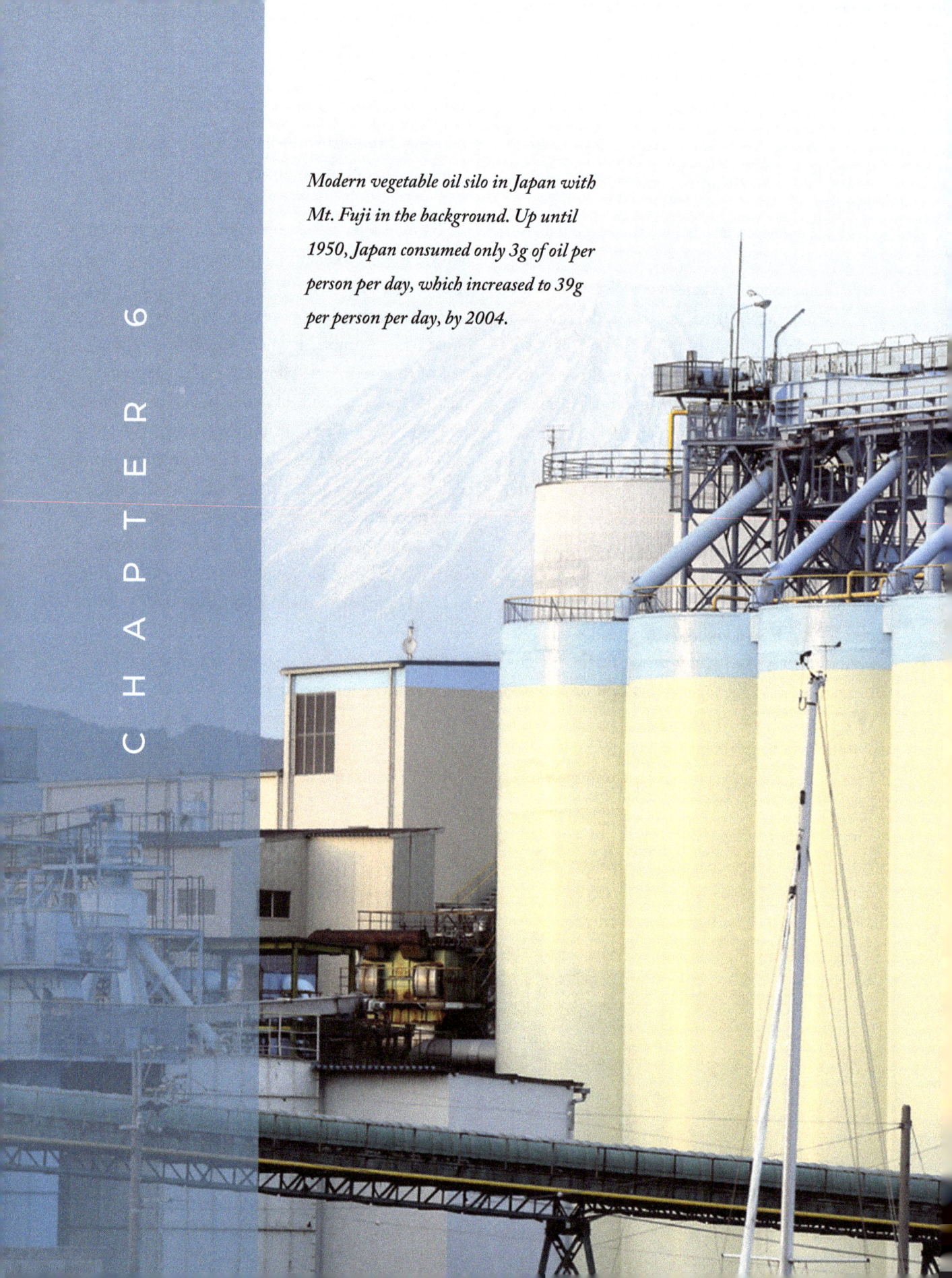

CHAPTER 6

Modern vegetable oil silo in Japan with Mt. Fuji in the background. Up until 1950, Japan consumed only 3g of oil per person per day, which increased to 39g per person per day, by 2004.

CHAPTER 6

THE MOST COMPELLING EVIDENCE OF ALL FOR THE SEED OIL HYPOTHESIS

"There is no expedient to which a man will not go to avoid the real labor of thinking."

— THOMAS A. EDISON (CIRCA 1895)

ANCESTRAL HEALTH FOUNDATION

CHAPTER 6

There's some real labor in deep thinking. There's certainly some deep thinking required to understand how and why diets are either beneficial or detrimental. But, with a little thought, contemplation, and investigation, one should rapidly be able to make logical, rational, and beneficial decisions regarding a healthy and individualized diet.

In this chapter, we will review what we believe to be some of the most compelling evidence of all in support of the seed oil hypothesis as the primary cause of chronic disease. This is the evidence implicating seed oils in the declining health of the Japanese, including the Okinawans, and similar evidence on a global scale. These final population reviews, combined with an understanding of the biological mechanisms of disease, should leave no doubt that the "seed oil hypothesis" is accurate, supported, and irrefutable.

SEED OILS ARE DEVASTATING THE HEALTH OF JAPANESE, INCLUDING OKINAWANS

The Japanese have a recent history that is consistent with perhaps the best health of virtually any country worldwide.[1122] Japanese women in 2013 still had the longest life expectancy in the world.[1122] The country is home to the Okinawans, who, at least at one time, were among the longest surviving people on the planet.[1123]

And while the Japanese continue to have relatively excellent longevity, in recent decades, there has been a tremendous loss of life, health, and vitality, associated with extraordinary increases in chronic disease (reviewed below). This, however, has paralleled increasing seed oil consumption with more compelling data, in fact, to indict seed oils than in any other country we are aware of.

The traditional diet in Japan was heavily influenced by the fact that the country is an archipelago with much access to seas, a rainy season, and subtropical temperatures. Traditionally, very minimal amounts of terrestrial animal meats were consumed, given that the region couldn't support many herbivorous ungulates (cattle).[1124] The single most important staple food for mainland Japanese, since at least 300 B.C., has been rice.[1125]

Naomichi Ishige, researcher of the history and culture of Japanese food and cuisine, wrote:

"Calculations based on national statistics for Japan in 1873 – when there had as yet been virtually none of the Western influence on dietary patterns that accompanied modernization – show that rice was the dominant source of both calories and protein. Specifically, on a per capita daily basis, rice provided 1,148 kilocalories [equivalent to "calories" in general nomenclature] or 65.5 per cent of calories received from staple crops (grains and potatoes), as well as 23.1 grams of protein [Koyama and Gotô 1985:491-2]. Such thorough reliance on rice was the chief feature of the Japanese diet from the introduction of rice cultivation some two millennia ago up to the 1960s, a time of great change in eating patterns, when large amounts of meat, dairy products and fats and oils began to be eaten, and both the amount of rice consumed and its importance as a protein source began to decline."[1126]

Rice, in the most traditional fashion, was boiled. However, rice was also ground into flour to make crackers, noodles, and dumplings, and pounded into rice cakes.[1127] Vegetable consumption in Japan was primarily based on soybean, from which they made flavoring paste (miso), tofu (bean curd), and soy sauce. Seafood – predominantly fish – and chicken eggs accounted for the primary animal foods.[1124] Other animal meat consumption was extremely minimal, for example, in 1900, "meat" consumption (mostly beef) accounted for only 800 g/person/year (1.76 lbs).[1128]

The traditional diet in Okinawa, which is the southernmost and westernmost prefecture, was based substantially on the sweet potato, which has been the primary carbohydrate of the diet from the 1600s until about 1960, accounting for greater than 50% of calories.[1129] The remainder of the traditional diet was based on marine foods, lean meats, fruit, green and yellow vegetables, soybean-based foods, tea, alcohol, and medicinal plants.[1136]

In the 20th century, caloric consumption became very low in war-torn Japan following World War II, and food shortages persisted for several years thereafter.[1130] The earliest data on food consumption in Japan that provides quantitative and qualitative evidence is from 1949-1950 and is derived, in part, from the Japan National Nutrition Survey, 1950.

This evidence shows that food shortages still existed as total caloric consumption was estimated at 2,068 cal/day in Japan in 1950 and 1,785 cal/day in Okinawa (the southernmost prefecture of Japan) in 1949.[1123] Total carbohydrates accounted for 79% of calories in Japan in 1950 and 85% of calories in Okinawa in 1949. Rice accounted for 54% of calories in Japan, but only 12% of calories in Okinawa, and sweet potatoes accounted for 3% of calories in Japan but a very high 69% of calories in Okinawa for the same years.[1123]

Total fat was extraordinarily low at only 6% of calories in mainland Japan, and 8% of calories in Okinawa in 1950 and 1949, respectively, and oils only accounted for 3 g/day for both populations for those same years, which was 1% of calories in Japan and 2% of calories in Okinawa.

By some accounts, Japan was fully recovered from WWII by 1952 following U.S. "rehabilitation of the state" with "widespread military, political, economic, and social reforms."[1131] By 1956, the once devastated economy had recovered to real per capita Gross Domestic Product (GDP) that was higher than the pre-war 1940 level.[1132]

American occupation of the state quickly began to induce westernized food consumption.[1133] In the late 1940s, Japanese children were served bread and milk in school lunches for the first time, and at the same time, the Japanese were introduced to hamburgers with cheese.[1134]

By 1958, total energy intake had increased to 2,837 calories per day, and most certainly suggests that the Japanese had all the food they desired.[1135] From that point, total caloric consumption steadily decreased to 2,202 cal/day by 1999[1135] and ~1,850 cal/day by 2010.[54] During the same approximate time frame (1958 to 1999), protein consumption elevated from 11% to 18%, fat consumption rose from 5% to 20%, and carbohydrate consumption steadily dropped from 84% to 62%.[1135]

Rice consumption alone dropped from a staggering 593 grams/day (2,372 calories) in 1958 to 236 grams/day (944 calories) in 1999.[1135] By 2010, carbohydrate consumption had dropped to 56%, and fat consumption had elevated to 27%.[54] Saturated fat was 2% of calories in 1950,[1123] (when food was restricted) but still extremely low in 2010

(Okinawa) at just 7% of calories,[1136] which is perhaps the lowest total fat and saturated fat of any country in the world.

The critical component during this entire period is the derivation of fat. During this same approximate time frame (~1950 to 2010), as mentioned, there was only 3 g/day of oils consumed in 1949-1950, either in mainland Japan or in Okinawa (type of oil not specified).[1123] High-PUFA seed oils then rose to 9 g/day by 1961, 37 g/day by 1999, and to 39 g/day by 2004.[4]

Thus, seed oils accounted for just 27 calories per day in 1950, but elevated to 351 calories by 2006, which is a 13-fold overall increase in edible oil consumption during this period. Edible oils in Japan recently are almost exclusively rapeseed (~21 %LA) and soybean oils (~53 %LA).[1137] The omega-6 as a percent of calories is estimated for each of these time periods (using Cronometer and all available data) and is confirmed to have risen from ~1.0% of calories in 1961 to ~7.8% of calories by 2010 (see table below, "Japan Nutrition Transition: 1949-2010").

In the graph on page 273 ("Japan Nutrition Transition: 1949 – 2010"), we visualize Japan's nutrition transition for the years 1949 to 2010. Notice that total calories and carbohydrate as a percent of the diet have both been falling since 1958, while sugar consumption has been falling since 1989. 'Vegetable oil' consumption has been rising since 1950 and was still climbing as of 2010.

Thus, the critical component of the nutrition transition of Japan is based on seed oils having supplanted other traditional foods. And what did this do to their health?

The prevalence of overweight and obesity (BMI ≥ 25) in Japan in men aged 60 to 69 years has soared from about 16% in 1978 to about 27% in 1998,[1138] while overweight and obesity in men aged 20 to 69 years of age elevated to 31.2% by 2010.[1139]

Women in Japan have had much more volatile fluctuations in weight since the 1970s; however, 25.2% of women aged 40 to 69 were overweight (BMI ≥ 25) in 1997, and that number dropped to 22.2% by 2010.[1139]

Japan Nutrition Transition: 1949 – 2010				
Year	1949-1950	1958-1961	1999	2004-2010
Total Calories (Kcal/cap/day)	1916	2837	2202	1850
Carbohydrate %	79	84	62	56
Fat %	8	5	20	27
Saturated Fat %	2	-	-	7
Vegetable Oils (Kcal/cap/day)	27	81	333	351
Sugars & Sweeteners (Kcal/cap/day)	-	198	329	283
Om-6 % (of total calories)	1.5	1.0	5.8	7.8

See references herein. © C. Knobbe, 2022. Ancestral Health Foundation.

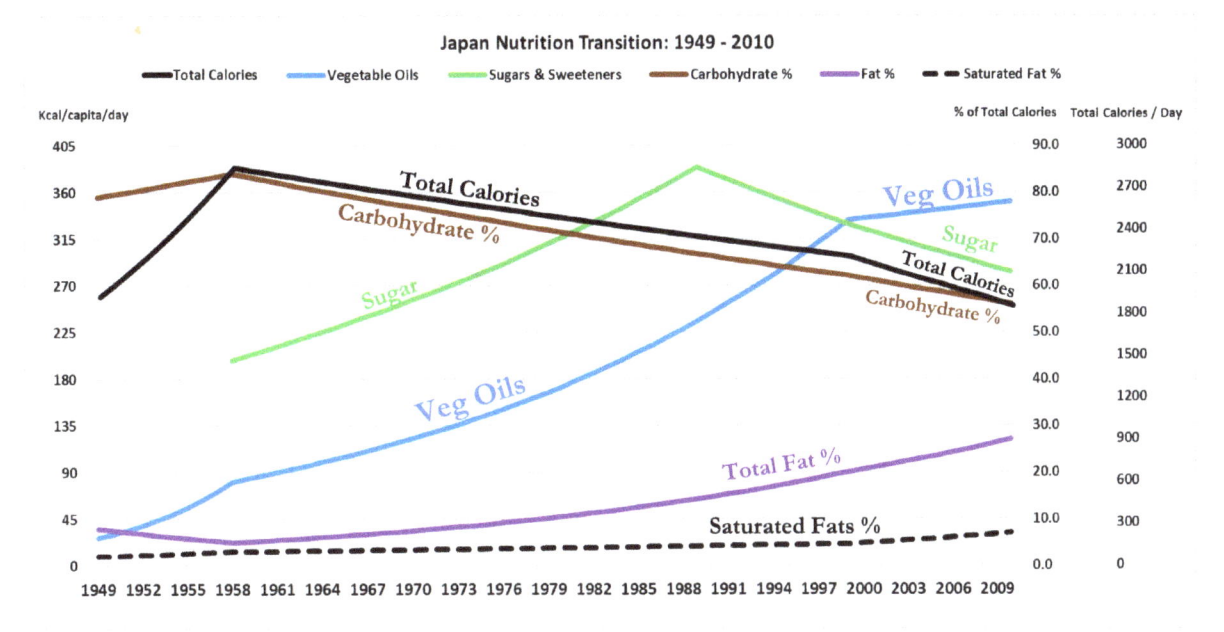

Japan Nutrition Transition: 1949 - 2010

Legend: Total Calories, Vegetable Oils, Sugars & Sweeteners, Carbohydrate %, Fat %, Saturated Fat %

Japan food consumption data, 1949 – 2010. See references cited herein. © C. Knobbe, 2022. Ancestral Health Foundation.

In Figure 6.1 ("High PUFA Vegetable Oils Driving Male Obesity in Japan: 1960-2010"), we observe overweight and obesity in men in Japan to have elevated from 16% in 1978 to 31.2% in 2010, during the same time interval that consumption of calories, carbohydrate, and even sugar, all declined (sugar steadily declined after 1989). Of course, the correlation with vegetable oils is positive, strong, and undeniable.

This is exactly what we have observed in a number of animal studies. As we have reviewed, even on isocaloric (equal calorie) diets, the higher the consumption of omega-6 LA, the greater the obesity and metabolic disease.

Diabetes in Japan has seen an explosive growth since the 1950s. Researcher, Takeshi Kuzuya, at the Jichi Medical School in Japan, reviewed all available diabetes prevalence data in Japan back to 1954, and found that diabetes was extremely rare at that time.

Although Kuzuya did not give the prevalence of diabetes for 1954, we have used the methodology within the paper to estimate diabetes for that year. Using the same conversion factor Kuzuya used to estimate the total number of diabetics (as well as the prevalence) in 1972, we estimated that the prevalence of diabetes in Japan was 0.02% in 1954.[1140] It then elevated to 0.027% in 1972, 0.88% by 1987,[1140] 5.5% in 1997, and 6.9% in 2007.[1141] This indicates that diabetes in Japan escalated about 345-fold between 1954 and 2007.

In Figure 6.2 ("High PUFA Vegetable Oils Driving Diabetes in Japan: 1960-2010"), we observe an extraordinary relationship between diabetes and vegetable oil consumption, very similar to obesity. Notably, high-PUFA edible oils and diabetes having risen in striking correlation, while calories, carbohydrates, and most recently, sugar, have all declined (sugar declined steadily after 1989).

The breast cancer incidence rate in Japan was 21.7 per 100,000 people in 1975 and elevated nearly 5-fold to 101.4 per 100,000 in 1999.[1142] There are similarly very large increases in the incidence rates of cancers

CHAPTER 6

FIG. 6.1

High PUFA Vegetable Oils Driving Male Obesity in Japan: 1960 – 2010 *

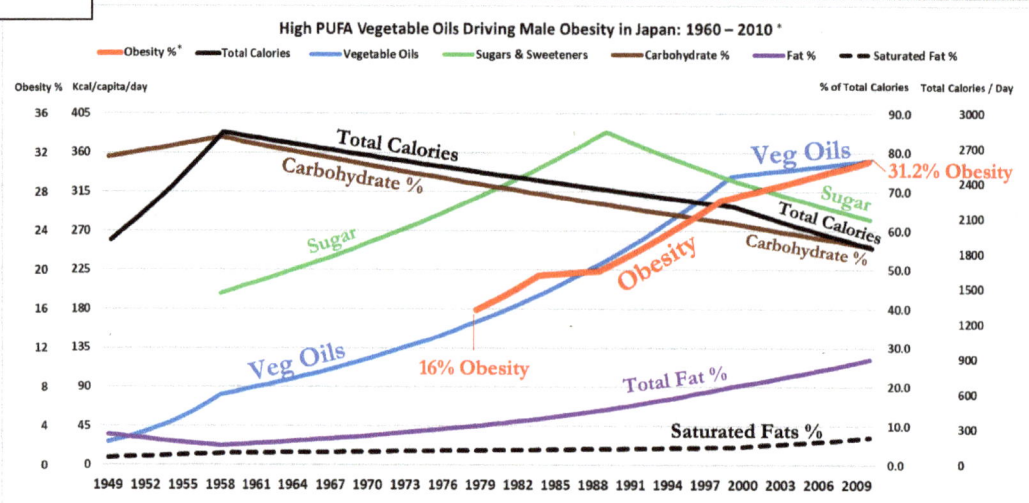

*"Obesity" as used in this graph represents the prevalence of both overweight and obesity (BMI ≥ 25) in males in Japan only. References: 1) Yoshiike N, Kaneda F, Takimoto H. Epidemiology of obesity and public health strategies for its control in Japan. Asia Pacific J Clin Nutr. 2002;11(Suppl):S727-S731. 2) Nishi N. Monitoring Obesity Trends in Health Japan 21. J Nutr Si Vitaminol. 2015;61:S17-S19. 3) Food consumption data: see references herein. © C. Knobbe, 2022. Ancestral Health Foundation.

FIG. 6.2

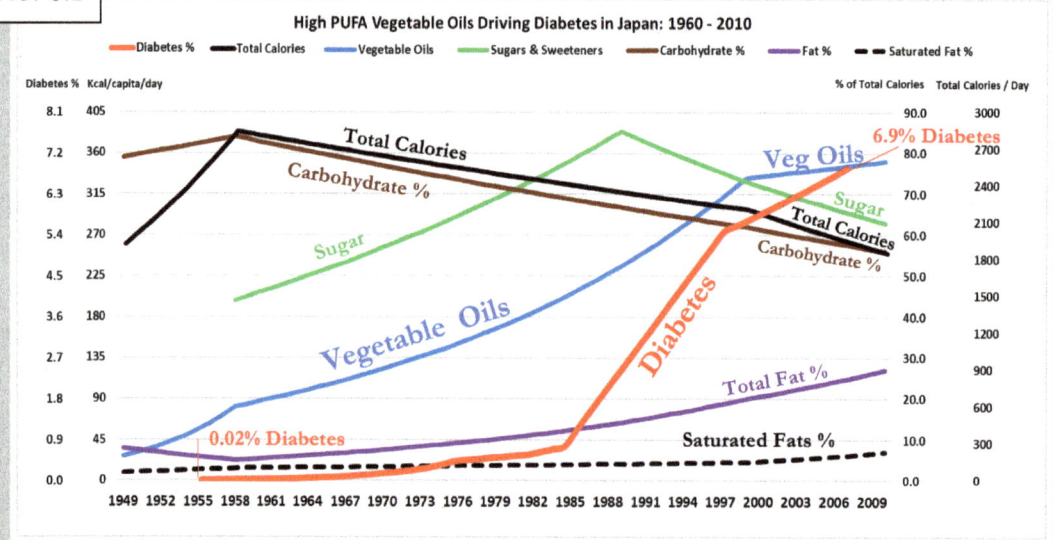

High PUFA Vegetable Oils Driving Diabetes in Japan: 1960 - 2010

References: 1) Diabetes statistics 1954-1987: Diabetes Research and Clinical Practice. 1994;24 Suppl:S15-S21. 2) Diabetes statistics 1997-2007: Nani A, Shimazu T, Takachi R. Dietary patterns and type 2 diabetes in Japanese men and women: the Japan Public Health Center-based Prospective Study. Eur J Clin Nutr. 2013;67:18-24 3) Food consumption data: see references herein. © C. Knobbe, 2022. Ancestral Health Foundation.

THE MOST COMPELLING EVIDENCE OF ALL

FIG. 6.3

High PUFA Vegetable Oils Driving Breast Cancer in Japan: 1975 - 1999

Legend: Breast Cancer/100k — Total Calories — Vegetable Oils — Sugars & Sweeteners — Carbohydrate % — Fat % — Saturated Fat %

- 101.4/100K Breast CA
- 21.7/100K Breast CA

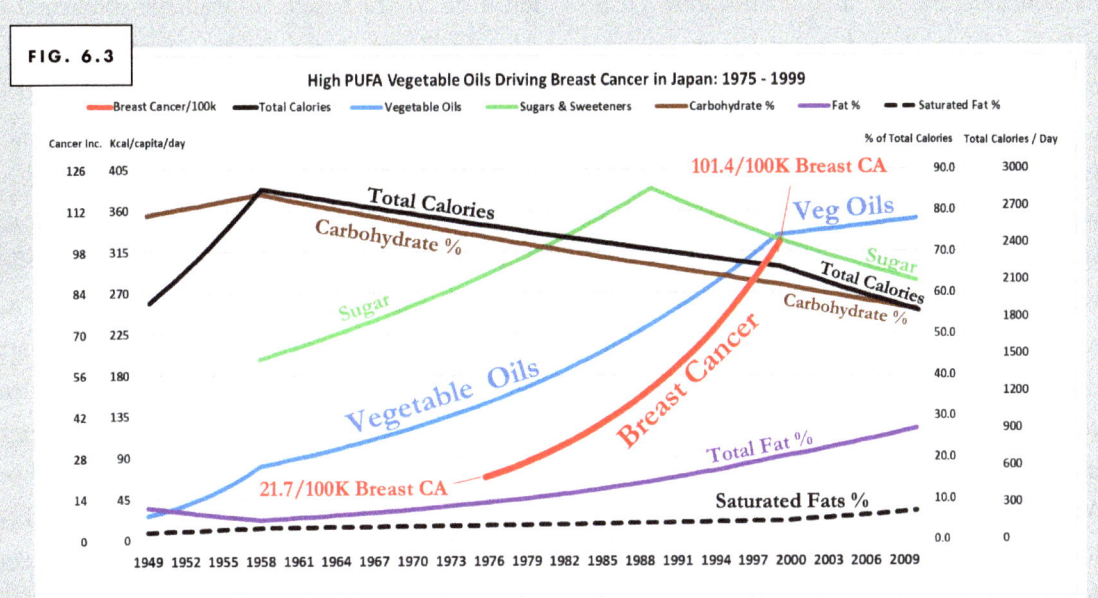

References: 1) Cancer statistics: Saika K, Sobue T. Epidemiology of Breast Cancer in Japan and the US. JMAJ. 2009;52(1):39-44 2) Food consumption data: see references herein. © C. Knobbe, 2022. Ancestral Health Foundation.

FIG. 6.4

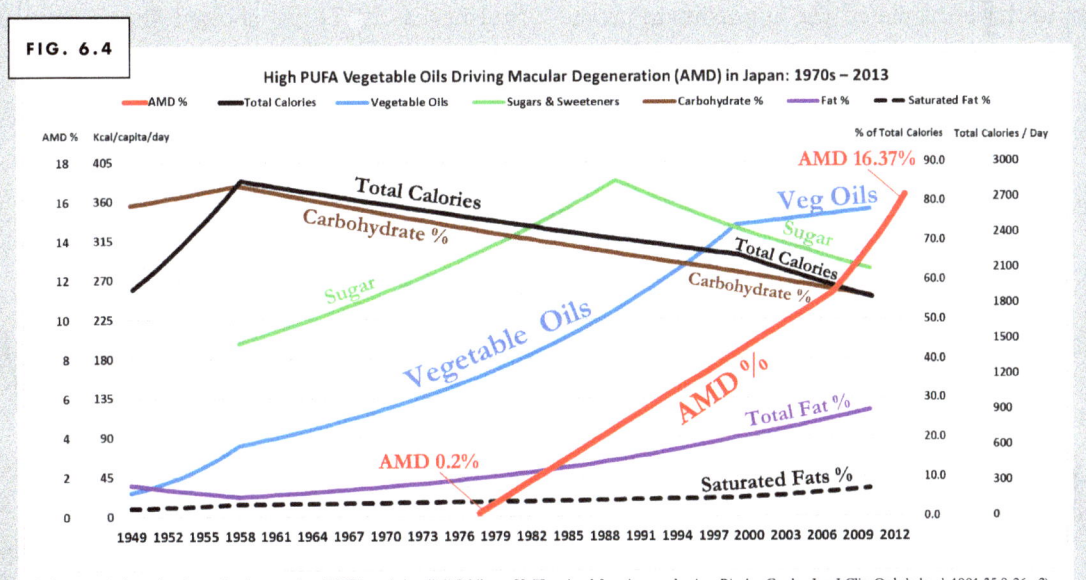

High PUFA Vegetable Oils Driving Macular Degeneration (AMD) in Japan: 1970s – 2013

Legend: AMD % — Total Calories — Vegetable Oils — Sugars & Sweeteners — Carbohydrate % — Fat % — Saturated Fat %

- AMD 16.37%
- AMD 0.2%

References: 1) Age-related macular degeneration (AMD) statistics: 1) 1) Ichikawa H. The visual functions and aging, Rinsho Ganka. Jpn J Clin Ophthalmol. 1981;35:9-26. 2) Hoshino M, Mizuno K, Ichikawa H. Aging alterations of retina and choroid of Japanese: light microscopic study of macular region of 176 eyes. Jpn J Ophthalmol. 1984;28(1):89-102. 3) Knobbe CA, Stojanoska M. The 'Displacing Foods of Modern Commerce' Are the Primary and Proximate Cause of Age-Related Macular Degeneration: A Unifying Singular Hypothesis. Medical Hypotheses. 2017;109:184-198. 4) Yasuda M, Kiyohara Y, Hata Y, at al. Nine-year incidence and risk factors for age-related macular degeneration in a defined Japanese population: the Hisayama study. Ophthalmology. 2009;116(11):2135-40. 5) Nakata I, Yamashiro K, Nakanishi H, et al. Prevalence and characteristics of age-related macular degeneration in the Japanese population: the Nagahama study. Am J Ophthalmol. 2013;156(5):1002-1009. 2) Food consumption data: see references herein. © C. Knobbe, 2022. Ancestral Health Foundation.

of the colon, lung, and rectum (data not shown here). Thus, the incidence of four major cancers has risen markedly between the years of 1960 and 1995.

Once again, we observe that yet another chronic condition – cancer – in this case, breast cancer and three other major cancers – all elevated markedly, while calories, carbohydrates, and even sugar, all declined. Note again the strong positive relationship to seed oils, with both breast cancer and vegetable oils having risen in lockstep (see Figure 6.3, "High PUFA Vegetable Oils Driving Breast Cancer in Japan: 1975-1999").

Age-related macular degeneration (AMD), the leading cause of irreversible vision loss and blindness in people over the age of 60 worldwide, has elevated exponentially in Japan just since the 1970s. For the period between 1974 and 1979 in Japan, we have calculated the approximate prevalence of AMD based on available published evidence, arriving at a figure of approximately 0.2% during the years from 1974 to 1979.[1143][1144] AMD elevated to affect 11.4% of those aged 40 and above in 2007 (the Hisayama Study).[1145]

This indicates a 57-fold increase in the prevalence of AMD in a period of just 30 years. In 2013, however, the Nagahama Study found that total AMD prevalence among those 50 to 59 years of age was 16.37%,[1146] which indicates an approximate 82-fold increase in AMD in the 34-year period between 1979 and 2013. Once again, we observe AMD to have risen in lockstep with seed oil consumption. See Figure 6.4, "High PUFA Vegetable Oils Driving Macular Degeneration (AMD) in Japan: 1970s -2013."

In our previously published research (Knobbe, Stojanoska, 2017), we showed strong correlations

Japan Nutrition Transition & Health Between Approximately 1960 and 2004	
Calories Down 31%	Male Obesity Elevates: 16% to 31.2%
Carbohydrate Down 28%	4 Major Cancers Markedly Up
Seed Oils Up 333%	Type 2 Diabetes Up 345-Fold (1954 – 2007)
Fat Up 440%	Age-Related Macular Degeneration Up 82-Fold
Saturated Fat Only 7% (2004)	Metabolic Syndrome 30.2% of Men/10.3% of Women and Half of Okinawan men are obese (2004)
Om-6 Up 680% (1% to 7.8%)	Blood Pressure Meds Increase 3% to 20%
Sugar falling after 1989	Smoking rate decreases from 68.5% to 45.2%

While total calories and carbohydrates decrease and sugar falls after 1989, but seed oils escalate from 1961 to 2004, many chronic diseases escalate exponentially. See references herein. © C. Knobbe, 2022. Ancestral Health Foundation.

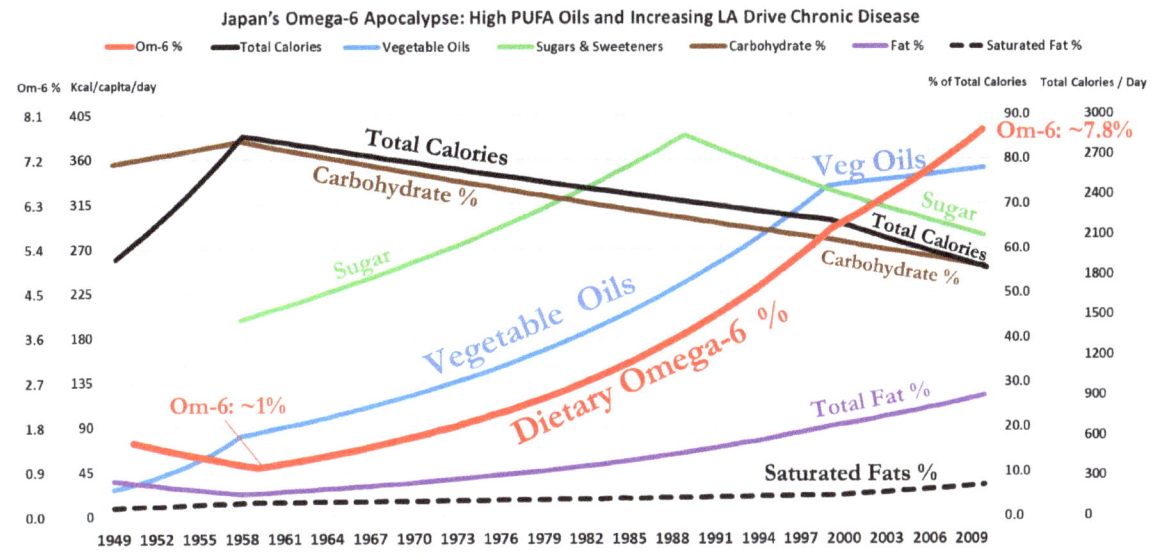

Japan's Omega-6 Apocalypse: High PUFA Oils and Increasing LA Drive Chronic Disease

Japan food consumption data, 1949 – 2010. Omega-6 percentage of diet calculated from food consumption data (Cronometer). See references cited herein.
© C. Knobbe, 2022. Ancestral Health Foundation.

between high-PUFA seed oils, processed foods, and AMD, with data from 25 nations all in support.[4]

There are many other chronic disease considerations in Japan related to their markedly increasing seed oil consumption. For example, diastolic blood pressure (the lower number) elevated on average from 73.5 to 82 mm Hg, between 1958 and 1999.[1135]

For this same time frame, the use of blood pressure medicines elevated from 3% to 20%, body mass index increased from 21.7 to 23.7 (kg/m²), while smoking rate decreased from 68.5% to 45.2%.[1135] As of 2004, metabolic syndrome affected 30.2% of men and 10.3% of women in Okinawa, and half of the men over 40 years were obese (BMI ≥ 25).[1147] Additionally, life expectancy in Okinawa has fallen sharply for men in recent decades, especially as compared to other prefectures in Japan.[1148]

In the table on page 276 ("Japan Nutrition Transition & Health Between Approximately 1960 and 2004"), we've summarized the most pertinent changes in nutrition and the effects on health.

Finally, we should observe the marked increase in omega-6 consumption in Japan since 1960, with rising omega-6 percentage from about 1% in 1960 to 7.8% in 2010. See the graph above, "Japan's Omega-6 Apocalypse: High PUFA Oils and Increasing LA Drive Chronic Disease." This absolute increase of 6.8% in omega-6 consumption is, in our opinion, practically the sole driver of their extraordinary increase in overweight, obesity, and numerous chronic diseases. And in this country, there appears to be no other competing theories of explanation.

Japan is the quintessential nation to test almost every hypothesis on the nutritional basis of chronic disease. In Japan, we have observed calories and carbohydrates declining steadily since 1961, and sugar declining since 1989, while obesity, diabetes, cancers, and age-related macular degeneration (AMD), all escalated exponentially.

The one component of the diet, however, that is positively correlated to overweight and these chronic diseases is the 4.3-fold increase in seed oils between 1961 and 2004. This is further represented by an approximate 7-fold increase in the omega-6 percentage of the diet.

Japan represents yet another population in which we observe an increasingly westernized, processed food-laden diet, with devastating effects in what Weston A. Price referred to as "Nature's laboratory."[28] Six decades of evidence in this country alone should convince us of the disastrous effects of seed oils.

INCREASING GLOBAL CHRONIC DISEASE PARALLELS THE RISE IN VEGETABLE OIL CONSUMPTION HISTORICALLY

Next, we will examine the relationship between carbohydrate consumption, sugar consumption, and total 'vegetable oil' consumption in correlation to global obesity. First, we should note that the United States has the highest rate of obesity of any high-income country in the world,[1149][1150] and we also have the highest per capita 'vegetable oil' consumption of any country in the world. The most recent data show U.S. vegetable oil consumption at approximately 79g/day (2018) (see Figure 6.5).[1151]

Out of the 38 OECD (high-income) countries alone, the U.S. has the highest obesity while consuming the most seed oil per capita of any nation in the world.[1152] Shouldn't our 'heart healthy' seed oil consumption – the one single dietary component that has changed the most in the past 155 years – be the prime target of interest?

An article from *Harvard Public Health* prominently displays a graph of U.S. vs worldwide obesity with the title, "The world is getting heavier, and America leads the way."[1150] Curiously, the Harvard School of Public Health has been one of the most outspoken advocates of consuming 'heart healthy' 'vegetable oils.'

For example, since August 20, 2019, the Harvard School of Public Health has prominently displayed an article on their website with the headline, "No need to avoid healthy omega-6 fats," which displays an image beneath showing a bottle pouring vegetable oil into a frying pan.[1153] The article's first line reads, "Omega-6 fats from vegetable oils—like their cousins, the omega-3 fats from fish – are good for the heart."[1153]

In the graph on page 279 ("Total disease burden by cause, World, 1990 to 2019"), courtesy of Our World In Data, we observe that the global burden of chronic disease has been escalating every year since 1990, which is every year since data became available.

A very recent paper published by the Institute for Health Metrics and Evaluation (IHME) reviewed a scientific paper published in *The Lancet*, characterizing the "perfect storm of rising chronic disease" as well as the "global crisis of chronic disease and failure of public health."[1154] And as we have reviewed throughout this book, historical references back to the 19th century confirm that the chronic disease burden has escalated exponentially since the late 19th century.

Thus, we've established that global obesity and chronic diseases have been rising incessantly for a century or more on a global scale. Now let's take a look at the worldwide production of vegetable oil in relation to this. In the graph on page 280 ("Total Vegetable Oil Consumption – World"), our team of colleagues has collectively evaluated all available evidence to prepare global 'vegetable oil' consumption going back to 1865.

THE MOST COMPELLING EVIDENCE OF ALL

FIG. 6.5

Share of adults that are obese, 1975 to 2016

Obesity is defined as having a body-mass index (BMI) equal to, or greater than, 30. BMI is a person's weight (in kilograms) divided by their height (in meters) squared.

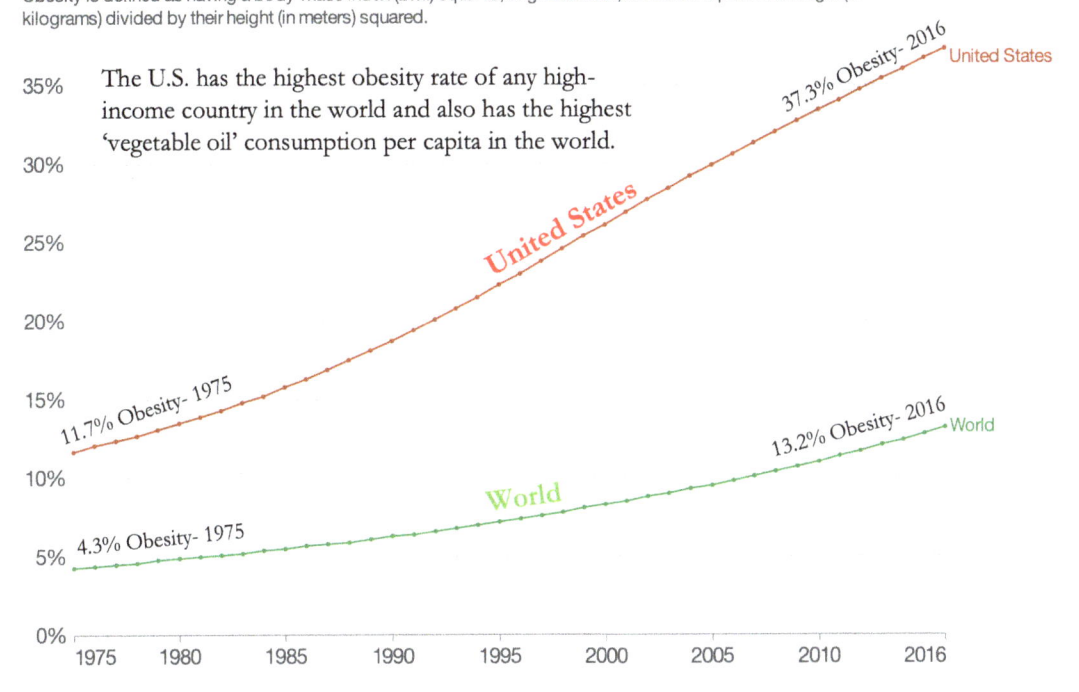

The U.S. has the highest obesity rate of any high-income country in the world and also has the highest 'vegetable oil' consumption per capita in the world.

- United States: 11.7% Obesity - 1975 → 37.3% Obesity - 2016
- World: 4.3% Obesity - 1975 → 13.2% Obesity - 2016

Source: WHO, Global Health Observatory
OurWorldInData.org/obesity • CC BY

References: 1) Obesity data: OurWorldInData.org. 2) Vegetable oil consumption: https://www.fao.org/faostat/en/#home.
© C. Knobbe, 2022. Ancestral Health Foundation.

Total disease burden by cause, World, 1990 to 2019

Total disease burden measured as Disability-Adjusted Life Years (DALYs) per year. DALYs measure the total burden of disease – both from years of life lost due to premature death and years lived with a disability. One DALY equals one lost year of healthy life.

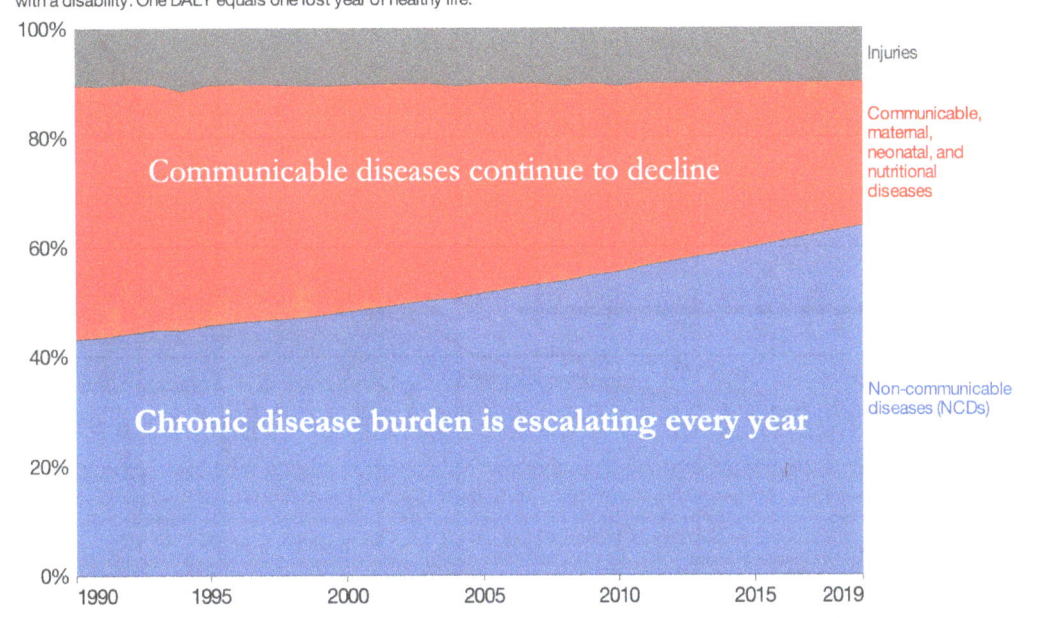

- Injuries
- Communicable diseases continue to decline — Communicable, maternal, neonatal, and nutritional diseases
- Chronic disease burden is escalating every year — Non-communicable diseases (NCDs)

Source: IHME, Global Burden of Disease
CC BY

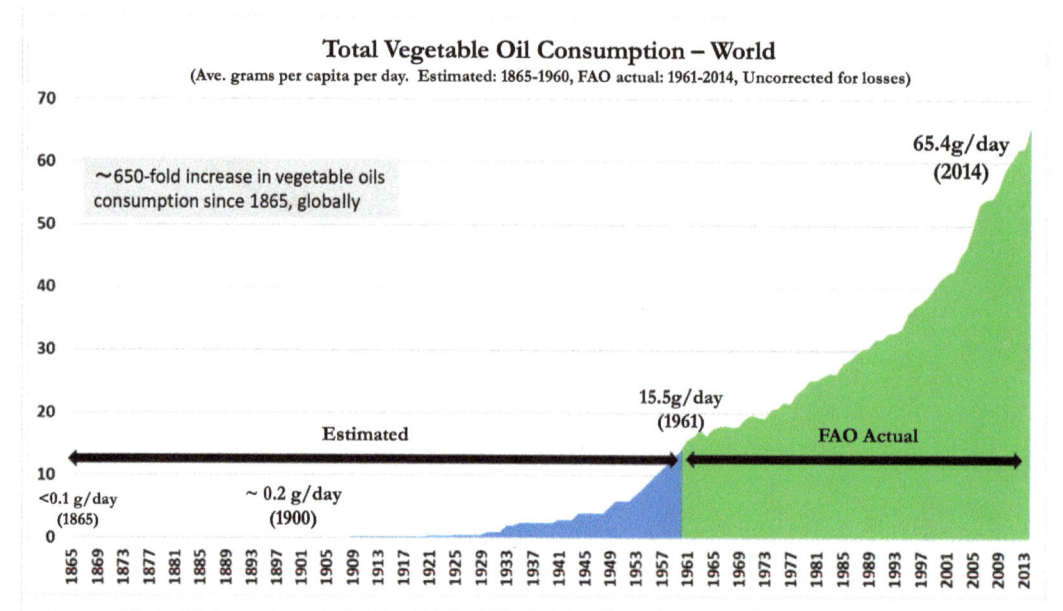

CHAPTER 6

Total Vegetable Oil Consumption – World
(Ave. grams per capita per day. Estimated: 1865-1960, FAO actual: 1961-2014, Uncorrected for losses)

~650-fold increase in vegetable oils consumption since 1865, globally

65.4 g/day (2014)

15.5 g/day (1961)

Estimated — FAO Actual

<0.1 g/day (1865)   ~ 0.2 g/day (1900)

References: 1) Food and Agriculture Organization (FAO) FBS, Retrieved 2 Sep 2021. Available: http://knoema.com/FAOFBS2017/food-balance-sheets. 2) Graph element from 1961 – 2014 retrieved from Our World In Data. 3). Knobbe CA, Richer SP, Freilich BD, et al. Westernized Diet, Vegetable Oil, Nutrient Deficiency and Omega-6 Apocalypse: Can We Explain Age-Related Macular Degeneration and Associated Chronic Diseases - Obesity, Coronary Heart Disease, Cancers, Metabolic Disease, Diabetes, Alzheimer's, and More – With a Unifying Hypothesis? Manuscript submitted for publication, Ancestral Health Foundation, Boulder, CO, USA, 2022. Data and graph not corrected for losses. © C. Knobbe, 2022. Ancestral Health Foundation.

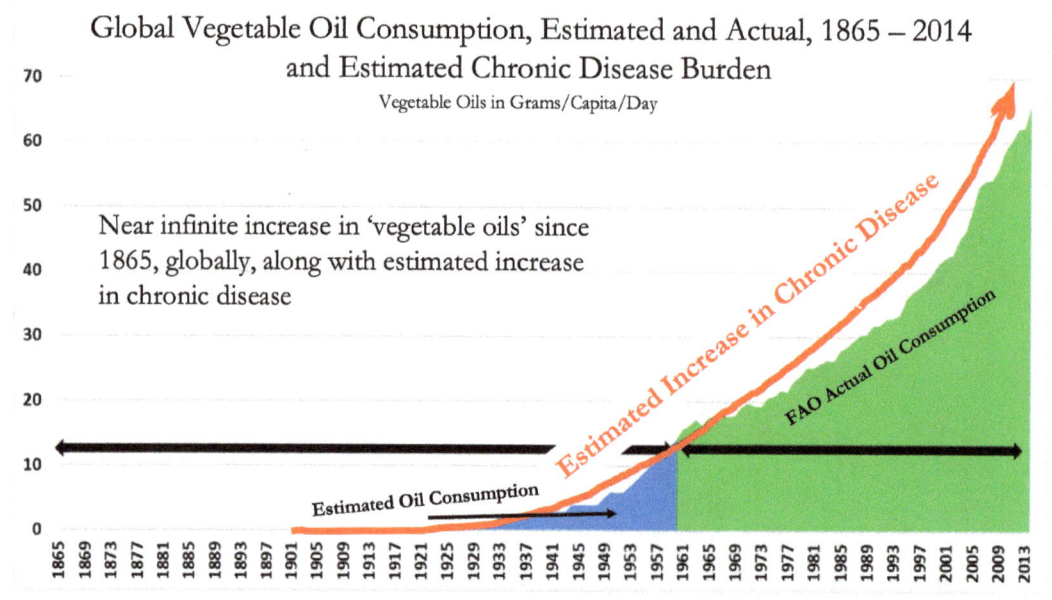

Global Vegetable Oil Consumption, Estimated and Actual, 1865 – 2014 and Estimated Chronic Disease Burden

Vegetable Oils in Grams/Capita/Day

Near infinite increase in 'vegetable oils' since 1865, globally, along with estimated increase in chronic disease

Estimated Oil Consumption — Estimated Increase in Chronic Disease — FAO Actual Oil Consumption

References: 1) Food and Agriculture Organization (FAO) FBS, Retrieved 2 Sep 2021. Available: http://knoema.com/FAOFBS2017/food-balance-sheets. 2) Graph element from 1961 – 2014 retrieved from Our World In Data. 3). Knobbe CA, Richer SP, Freilich BD, et al. Westernized Diet, Vegetable Oil, Nutrient Deficiency and Omega-6 Apocalypse: Can We Explain Age-Related Macular Degeneration and Associated Chronic Diseases - Obesity, Coronary Heart Disease, Cancers, Metabolic Disease, Diabetes, Alzheimer's, and More – With a Unifying Hypothesis? Manuscript submitted for publication, Ancestral Health Foundation, Boulder, CO, USA, 2022. Data and graph not corrected for losses. © C. Knobbe, 2022. Ancestral Health Foundation.

We have estimated 'vegetable oil' consumption data for years 1865 to 1960 (shown in blue) based on available historical data and available records.[3] This was stitched together with the known data from the FAO, which runs from years 1961 to 2014. In 1865, 'vegetable oil' consumption worldwide approached zero, but it is indeed not quite zero and wouldn't have been exactly zero even thousands of years ago.[3] The known data for vegetable oil consumption was published by the FAO, beginning in 1961 and ending in 2014 (shown in green) and was obtained in the most useable format courtesy of Our World In Data (OurWorldInData.org).

On page 280 is a graph of global vegetable oil consumption and the estimated increase in chronic disease in correlation (see "Global Vegetable Oil Consumption, Estimated and Actual, 1865-2014 and Estimated Chronic Disease Burden"). Recollect that we have seen increases, for example, in coronary heart disease, diabetes, Alzheimer's disease, dementia, and age-related macular degeneration that are, at a minimum, at least thousands of fold.

OBESITY AND CHRONIC DISEASE ESCALATE EXPONENTIALLY WORLDWIDE, WHILE CARBS ARE STABLE, SUGARS RISE 5%, AND 'VEGETABLE OILS' APPROXIMATELY DOUBLE: 1975-2014

In Fig. 6.6, we observe that global obesity (BMI ≥ 30) has increased in adult men from an average of 3.2% in 1975 to 10.8% in 2014 (see "Vegetable Oil and Sugar Consumption Vs Global Adult Obesity, Men – 1975-2014").[1155] Obesity increased in women from 6.4% in 1975 to 14.9% in 2014 (see Fig. 6.7, "Vegetable Oil and Sugar Consumption Vs Global Adult Obesity, Women – 1975-2014").[1155]

During the same period of time, on a global scale, sugar consumption elevated just 5%, while vegetable oils increased by 85%, which is a near doubling.

We also observe that the global body mass index (BMI), calculated as mass (weight) divided by height squared (BMI = mass (kg)/height (m)^2), in relation to vegetable oils and sugar. In populations other than Asians, overweight is considered a BMI at or above 25 and obesity is a BMI at or above 30.

Of note, people may have relatively high BMIs without being overweight or obese since BMI does not take into account actual body fat. However, as a broad measure of overweight or obesity in entire populations, BMI is a quite accurate predictor[1156] and has been shown to track predictably with body fat (adiposity).[1157]

On a global scale, the BMI of men increased on average from 21.7 in 1975 to 24.2 in 2014 and in women from 22.1 in 1975 to 24.4 in 2014[1155] (see graphs on page 283). In these plots, we observe a near-perfect correlation between increasing BMI and increasing vegetable oil consumption, but during the same interval of time, carbohydrate consumption declined slightly.

Globally, we've observed an enormous increase in diabetes which, of course, parallels the worldwide consumption of vegetable oils (see "Global Vegetable Oil and Sugar Consumption Vs Diabetes Prevalence, Men: 1980-2014," on page 284). The NCD Risk Factor Collaboration Group determined in their analyses of data from 200 countries that diabetes prevalence has increased from 4.3% in 1980 to 9.0% in 2014 in men, and from 4.0% to 7.9% for the same years in women[1158] (see page 284). During this same time frame (1980 to 2014), sugar consumption decreased from 236 kcal/day to 232 kcal/day (down 1.7%), while vegetable oil consumption increased from 180 cal/day to 279 cal/day (up 55%, or 1.55-fold).

CHAPTER 6

FIG. 6.6

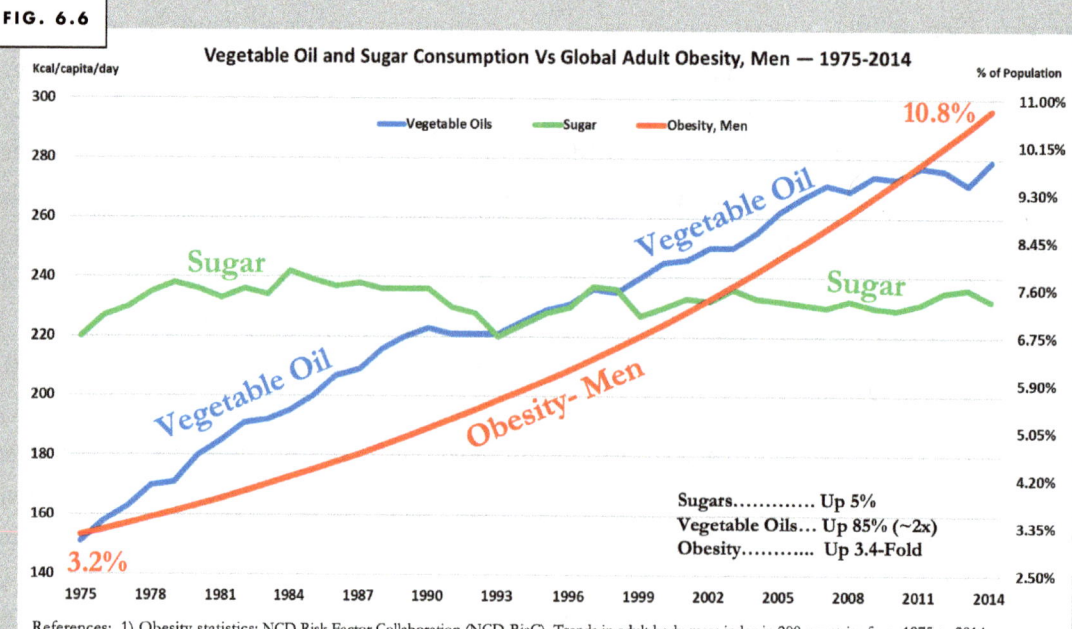

Vegetable Oil and Sugar Consumption Vs Global Adult Obesity, Men — 1975-2014

- Vegetable Oils: Up 85% (~2x)
- Sugars: Up 5%
- Obesity: Up 3.4-Fold
- Obesity Men: 3.2% → 10.8%

References: 1) Obesity statistics: NCD Risk Factor Collaboration (NCD-RisC). Trends in adult body-mass index in 200 countries from 1975 to 2014: a pooled analysis of 1698 population-based measurement studies with 19.2 million participants. The Lancet. 2016;387(10026):P1377-1396. 2) Food and Agriculture Organization (FAO) FBS, Retrieved 2 Sep 2021. Available: http://knoema.com/FAOFBS2017/food-balance-sheets. © C. Knobbe, 2022. Ancestral Health Foundation.

FIG. 6.7

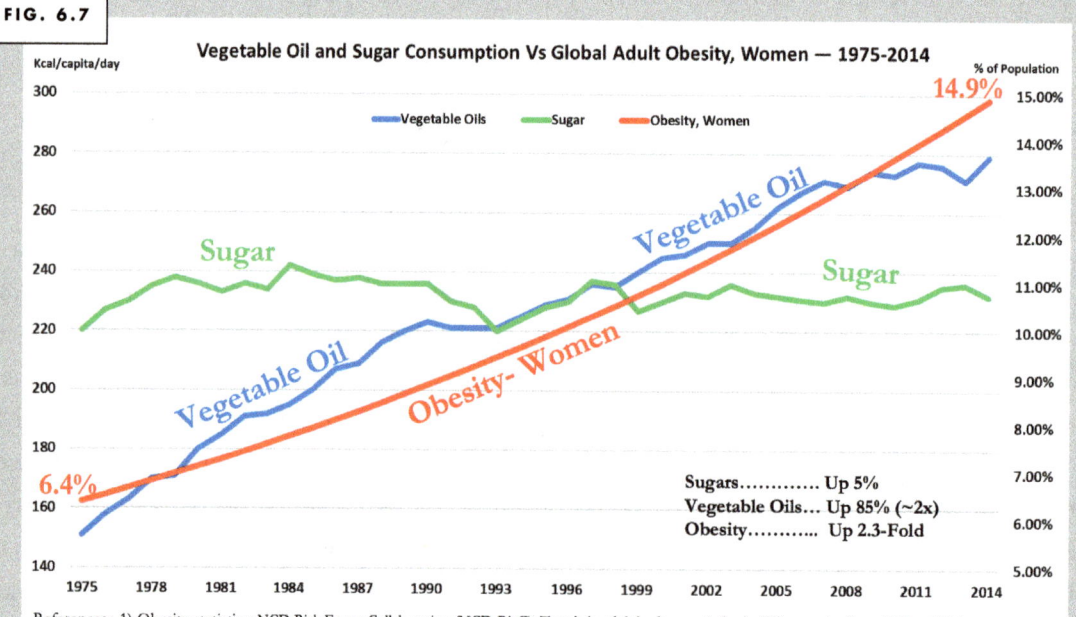

Vegetable Oil and Sugar Consumption Vs Global Adult Obesity, Women — 1975-2014

- Vegetable Oils: Up 85% (~2x)
- Sugars: Up 5%
- Obesity: Up 2.3-Fold
- Obesity Women: 6.4% → 14.9%

References: 1) Obesity statistics: NCD Risk Factor Collaboration (NCD-RisC). Trends in adult body-mass index in 200 countries from 1975 to 2014: a pooled analysis of 1698 population-based measurement studies with 19.2 million participants. The Lancet. 2016;387(10026):P1377-1396. 2) Food and Agriculture Organization (FAO) FBS, Retrieved 2 Sep 2021. Available: http://knoema.com/FAOFBS2017/food-balance-sheets. © C. Knobbe, 2022. Ancestral Health Foundation.

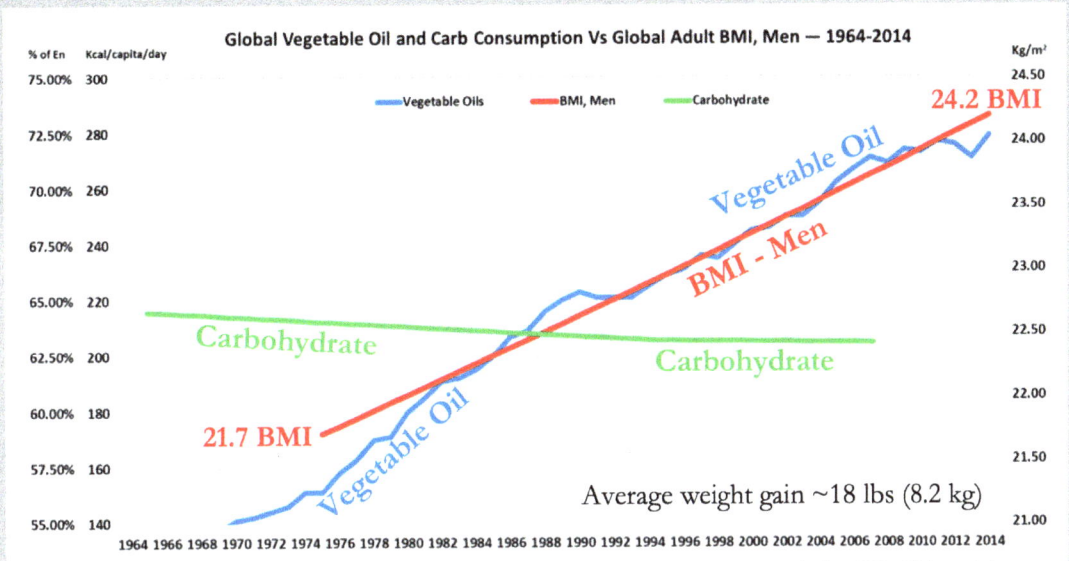

THE MOST COMPELLING EVIDENCE OF ALL

Global Vegetable Oil and Carb Consumption Vs Global Adult BMI, Men — 1964-2014

- Vegetable Oils
- BMI, Men
- Carbohydrate

21.7 BMI → 24.2 BMI

Average weight gain ~18 lbs (8.2 kg)

References: 1) BMI statistics: NCD Risk Factor Collaboration (NCD-RisC). Trends in adult body-mass index in 200 countries from 1975 to 2014: a pooled analysis of 1698 population-based measurement studies with 19.2 million participants. The Lancet. 2016;387(10026):P1377-1396. 2) Food and Agriculture Organization (FAO) FBS, Retrieved 2 Sep 2021. Available: http://knoema.com/FAOFBS2017/food-balance-sheets. © C. Knobbe, 2022. Ancestral Health Foundation.

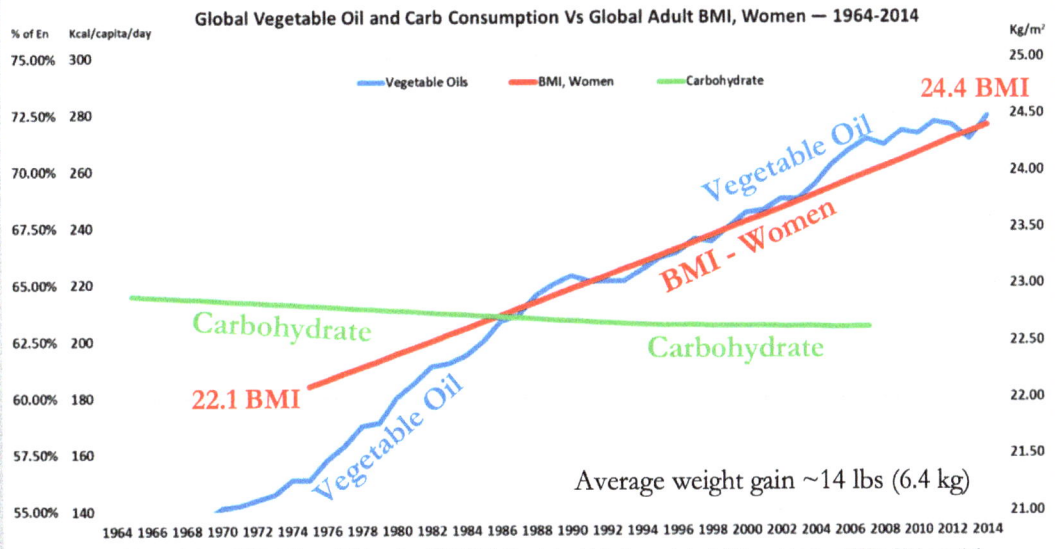

Global Vegetable Oil and Carb Consumption Vs Global Adult BMI, Women — 1964-2014

- Vegetable Oils
- BMI, Women
- Carbohydrate

22.1 BMI → 24.4 BMI

Average weight gain ~14 lbs (6.4 kg)

References: 1) BMI statistics: NCD Risk Factor Collaboration (NCD-RisC). Trends in adult body-mass index in 200 countries from 1975 to 2014: a pooled analysis of 1698 population-based measurement studies with 19.2 million participants. The Lancet. 2016;387(10026):P1377-1396. 2) Food and Agriculture Organization (FAO) FBS, Retrieved 2 Sep 2021. Available: http://knoema.com/FAOFBS2017/food-balance-sheets. © C. Knobbe, 2022. Ancestral Health Foundation.

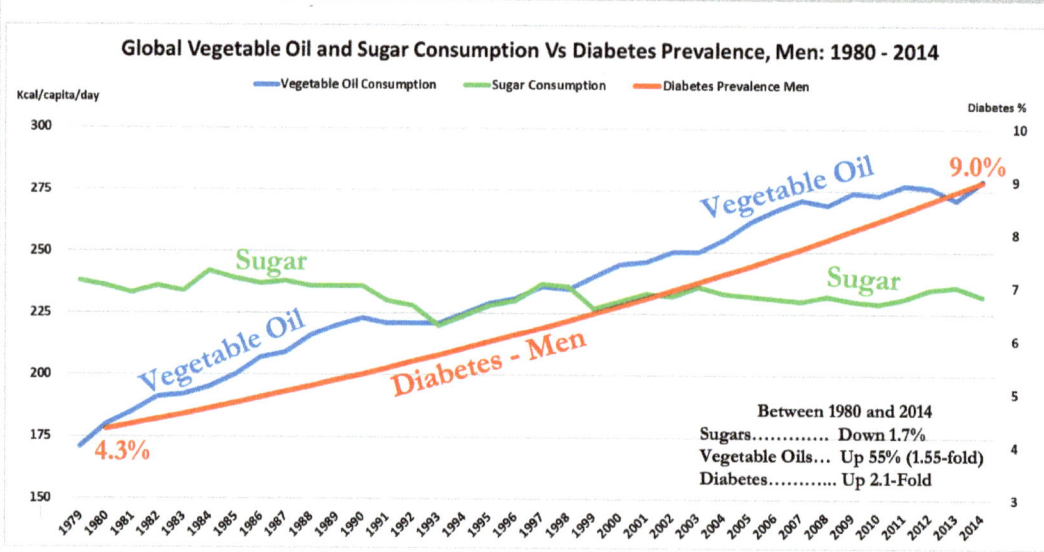

CHAPTER 6

Global Vegetable Oil and Sugar Consumption Vs Diabetes Prevalence, Men: 1980 - 2014

Between 1980 and 2014
Sugars............ Down 1.7%
Vegetable Oils... Up 55% (1.55-fold)
Diabetes........... Up 2.1-Fold

References: 1) Diabetes data: NCD Risk Factor Collaboration (NCD-RisC). Worldwide trends in diabetes since 1980: a pooled analysis of 751 population-based studies with 4.4 million participants. The Lancet. 2016;387:1513-30. 2) Vegetable oil and sugar consumption data: Food and Agriculture Organization (FAO) FBS, Retrieved 2 Sep 2021. Available: http://knoema.com/FAOFBS2017/food-balance-sheets. © C. Knobbe, 2022. Ancestral Health Foundation.

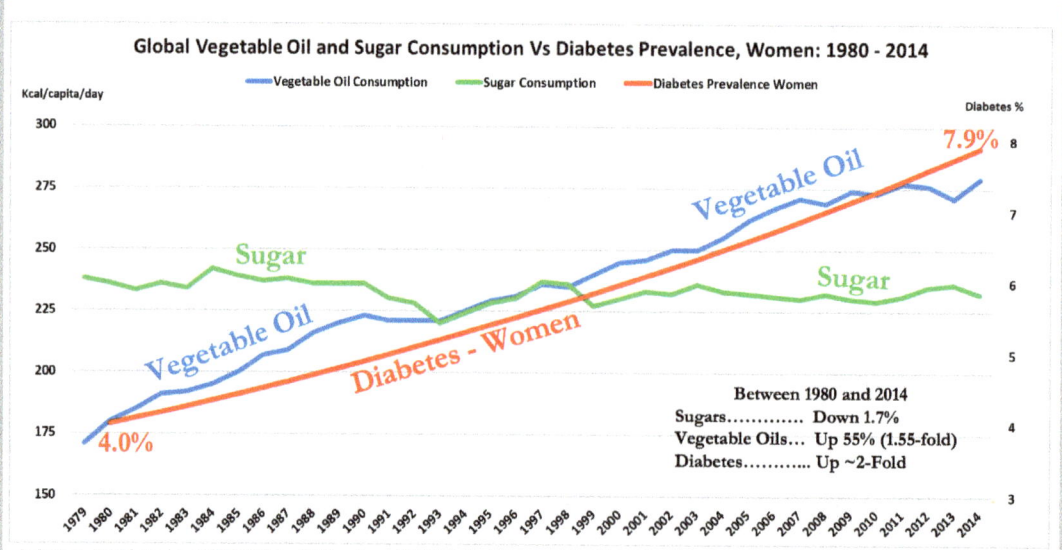

Global Vegetable Oil and Sugar Consumption Vs Diabetes Prevalence, Women: 1980 - 2014

Between 1980 and 2014
Sugars............ Down 1.7%
Vegetable Oils... Up 55% (1.55-fold)
Diabetes........... Up ~2-Fold

References: 1) Diabetes data: NCD Risk Factor Collaboration (NCD-RisC). Worldwide trends in diabetes since 1980: a pooled analysis of 751 population-based studies with 4.4 million participants. The Lancet. 2016;387:1513-30. 2) Vegetable oil and sugar consumption data: Food and Agriculture Organization (FAO) FBS, Retrieved 2 Sep 2021. Available: http://knoema.com/FAOFBS2017/food-balance-sheets. © C. Knobbe, 2022. Ancestral Health Foundation.

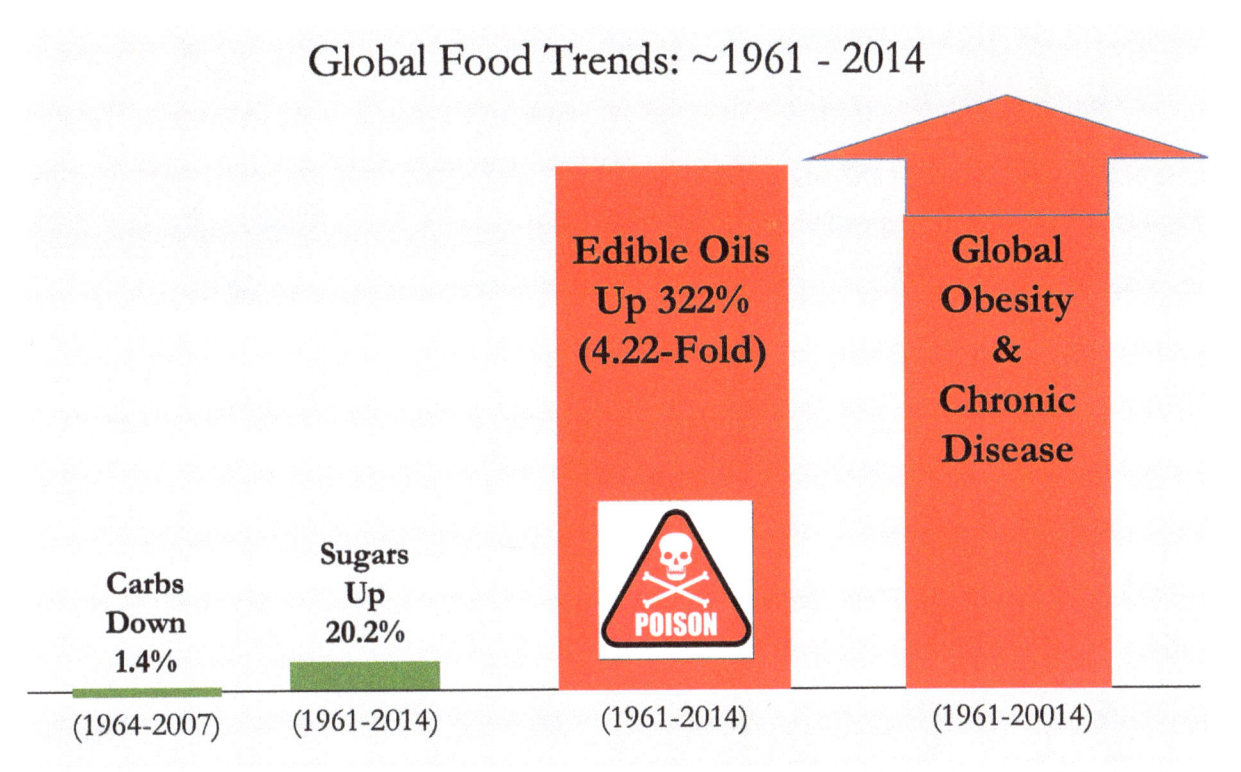

Global Food Trends: ~1961 - 2014

Carbs Down 1.4% (1964-2007)

Sugars Up 20.2% (1961-2014)

Edible Oils Up 322% (4.22-Fold) (1961-2014) — POISON

Global Obesity & Chronic Disease (1961-20014)

FAO Statistics Division 2010, *Food Balance Sheets*, Food and Agriculture Organization of the United Nations, Rome, Italy, viewed 17th March, 2011. Retrieved: http://faostat.fao.org/. © C. Knobbe, 2022. Ancestral Health Foundation.

On a global scale, sugar consumption increased 20.2% between 1961 and 2014.[1159] Worldwide, as a percentage of total calories, carbohydrate consumption was 64.5% in 1964, 63.2% in 1994,[1160] and 63.1% in 2007.[1161]

Thus, carbohydrate consumption declined by 1.4% globally between 1964 and 2007. However, total vegetable oil consumption increased, on a per capita basis, from 15.5 g/capita/day in 1961 to 65.4 g/day in 2014, which is an increase of 322%, or 4.22-fold (see "Global Food Trends: ~1961 – 2014" above).

HEALTHY POPULATIONS: WHAT DO THEY NOT CONSUME?

This will be the shortest segment of the entire book, as it's that simple. Healthy populations and individuals do not consume substantial amounts of refined sugars, refined flours, seed oils, or trans fats. In a nutshell, they do not consume man-made, processed, nutrient-deficient, and toxic foods.

This has been reviewed with respect to the traditional living people of many populations, including 19th century Americans, Maasai, early 20th century Ugandans, Tokelauans, Papua New Guineans of Tukisenta, South Pacific Islanders, New Zealand Maori, Australian Aboriginals, Greenland Inuit ('Eskimos'), and the Japanese. The same can be confirmed in all hunter-gatherer populations, where none of them would have ever had any such processed foods, and certainly would not have had any seed oils except in exceedingly rare circumstances.

HEALTHY BABIES AND CHILDREN: RAISING THEM ANCESTRALLY

Infants, toddlers, and nearly all children have little choice but to consume the foods we provide, whether those foods are provided by parents, caretakers, educational systems, restaurants, or other commercial sources of food. We have a moral and ethical obligation to provide the foods for our children that will nurture and promote the most precious gifts of all, which are the gifts of healthy bodies, minds, and spirits. This can only be accomplished in this day and age with careful attention to our food choices.

Giving birth to healthy children begins long before conception, and both the mother and father are important, although the mother's nutrition is far more critical.[1162] Although we won't be able to review this section in detail, it should be clear that entirely ancestral diets in future mothers-to-be or expectant mothers are absolutely and fundamentally critical to preventing birth defects and giving birth to healthy infants.

For example, a deficiency of folate (vitamin B9) in the mother, particularly around the time of conception, may result in neural tube defects such as spina bifida, which is a condition typically resulting in permanent paralysis of the lower limbs.[1163] Rich sources of folate include dark green leafy vegetables, beans, fresh fruits, whole grains, liver, and seafood.

Deficiency of vitamin B12 (rich sources include liver, beef, fish, and clams, but there is virtually none in plants) and elevated homocysteine (often due to folate deficiency) may induce birth defects and pregnancy complications including spontaneous abortions, placental abruption, pre-eclampsia, and low birth weight infants.[1163] Deficiency of vitamin A is known to induce congenital spinal deformities.[1164]

Vitamin D deficiency during pregnancy may impact the development of chronic conditions in adulthood including asthma, multiple sclerosis (MS), and other neurological disorders.[1165] These are just a few examples, but the effects of nutrient deficiencies in the mother could have devastating and life-long impacts on the child.

Infants should be breast-fed if at all possible and until they can be weaned to whole foods. It should be appreciated that feeding from the mother's breast, historically, has been an "obligatory requirement for all mammals for their survival."[1166] In fact, this was also true of humans until very recently.

The WHO considers breast-feeding so vital to infant and childhood health that the subject has received considerable attention for decades. In 1979, a WHO article declared, "Breast-feeding is an integral part of the reproductive process, the natural and ideal way of feeding the infant and a unique biological and emotional basis for child development. This, together with its other important effects on the prevention of infections, on the health and well-being of the mother, on child spacing, on family health… It is therefore the responsibility of a society to promote breast-feeding and to protect pregnant and lactating mothers from any influences that could disrupt it."[1166]

Historically, "wet nursing," which is the practice of utilizing "a woman who breastfeeds another's child," was practiced for thousands of years when the mother, for any number of reasons, including disease and death, could not nurse the infant or toddler.[1167] However, in the 19th century, "artificial feeding became a feasible substitute for wet nursing" due to advancements in the development of the feeding bottle as well as the availability of animal's milk.[1167]

Breast milk is perhaps the most complex, nutritious, and wholesome of all foods and should always be considered the "gold standard" for feeding of the infant or toddler.[1168 1169 1170] If the lactating mother is well nourished, and in many cases, even if she is not, breast milk is infinitely superior to manufactured (man-made) formula and should always be the preferred nutrition for infants and young children, whenever possible.[1171]

It should be obvious that the mother's nutrition deeply affects her breast milk, and ancestrally-minded researchers recommend exclusive breastfeeding for the first 6 months of life with continued breastfeeding combined with whole complementary foods up to 2 years of age or beyond.[1172] Certainly, concentrations of both fat-soluble vitamins (A, D, E, K) and water-soluble vitamins (B vitamins and C), and especially vitamins A, C, B6, and B12 have been found to reflect the dietary nutrient intakes of the maternal diet.[1172]

Several studies have evaluated the effects of higher LA consumption on the developing infant brain. LA accumulates in maternal milk just as it does in body fat, with higher levels in mothers who are consuming higher levels of seed oils.[1173] The typical breast milk fatty acid composition has increased from 7% LA in 1970 to 12% LA in 2000.[1173 1174 1175] The value of 12% LA of total fatty acids corresponds to 8% of total energy consumed. Even a growing infant may only need 1% to 2% of energy from LA, thus driving contemporary westernized diets to far exceed the necessary LA, potentially up to 4- to 8-fold.[1173]

One study found that high maternal breast milk LA percentage (greater than 9.7% of energy) was associated with both reduced motor function and cognitive scores in 2- to 3-year-old children.[1176] In another study, children who were breastfed had higher IQ scores by an average of 4.5 points; higher LA levels in breast milk were associated with lower verbal IQ scores, and children given breast milk higher in LA and lower in DHA (the long-chain omega-3s) had lower IQs.[1177]

Infant formula may prove disastrous to the health of infants and children, even precipitating a much higher likelihood of sudden infant death (SIDS)[1178] and necrotizing enterocolitis (NEC), the latter of which is an inflammatory condition of the bowel that may lead to sepsis and death in up to 50% of affected infants.[1179] Knowledgeable experts in infant nutrition have stated,

"Currently, infant formula-feeding is widely practiced in the United States and appears to contribute to the development of several common childhood illnesses, including atopy [allergic disorders], diabetes mellitus, and childhood obesity."[1167]

Formula feeding of infants even in the first week of life has been shown to be correlated with increased risk of obesity decades later.[1180] Formula feeding has also been associated with rapid weight gain in early infancy[1181 1182] as well as greater risk of obesity in childhood and adolescence.[1183 1184] In one study, formula-fed infants had undetectable levels of vitamin K2, which would predict poor outcomes for both teeth and bones, at a minimum.[1185]

But why and how could baby formula be so unhealthy and dangerous? The most parsimonious answer is that the natural animal fats of processed baby formula have been removed (or never provided) while seed oils have been substituted. In short, baby formula is one of the single most processed foods there is.

Researchers of infant formula have confirmed the following, which references the most egregious mistake for the health of infants:

"Like human milk, fat provides approximately 40-50% of energy in cow's milk-based infant formula. In infant formula, butterfat from whole cow's milk is removed and replaced with a combination of vegetable oils..."[1168]

This, of course, drives a very high omega-6 LA consumption in infants and children consuming formula. As early as the 1970s, infant formula provided up to a staggering 58% of fatty acids as LA.[1186] Infants fed this formula had only 1 to 3% body fat LA at birth, and this was shown to rise to about 25% at one month and 32 to 37% by four months. It has also been common practice to prepare formulae in which all the cow's milk has been removed and replaced with corn oil.

Similac Advance Infant Formula, a product of Abbott Nutrition, was the top-ranked baby formula sold in the U.S. in 2016.[1187] While the container labeling promotes the product with the phrases, "Brain Nourishing," "Eye Health," "Growth and Development," and "OptiGRO," the formula ingredients are listed as "Nonfat Milk [powdered milk], Lactose, High Oleic Safflower Oil, Whey Protein Concentrate, Soy Oil, Coconut Oil..."[1188] The fat content is approximately 50% of total calories, which is similar to maternal milk. However, maternal milk contains 100% of the fat from a mammal – the mother – whereas this prototypical infant formula contains 100% vegetable oil. Is it any wonder our children's health is so severely compromised?

Does this high level of LA in mother's milk as well as infant and toddler diets contribute to obesity? Gérard Ailhaud, of the French Institute of Health and Medical Research, would surely answer yes to this question. He and colleague researchers, for example, have shown in mice that pups from wild-type mothers who were fed high LA diets (LA:ALA ratio 59:1) were 40% heavier just one week after weaning, as compared to pups raised on low LA diets (LA:ALA ratio 2:1), even when the diets were isocaloric (equal in calories).[1189] Furthermore, this weight difference in the pups was maintained into adulthood. Ailhaud asserted that the marked increases in LA in westernized diets in recent decades "may be responsible at least in part for the dramatic rise in the prevalence of childhood overweight and obesity."[1189]

In 2008, Ailhaud and colleagues wrote, "At least in rodent models, the relative intake of *n-6* to *n-3* [omega-6:omega-3] PUFA is clearly emerging as a new factor in this development [of adipose fat cell size and number]. In these models, higher linoleate [LA] intake raises tissue arachidonic acid (AA), which increases prostacyclin production and, in turn, stimulates signaling pathways implicated in adipogenesis [increased number and size of fat cells]. Thus, by 2008, these French researchers had already established solid evidence implicating seed oils and high omega-6 consumption in the rising prevalence of overweight and obesity.

In the medical textbook, *Primary Prevention by Nutrition Intervention in Infancy and Childhood*, Ailhaud and colleagues wrote,

"Childhood obesity can be considered a non-infectious epidemic...the importance of qualitative changes (i.e., the fatty acid composition of fats) has been largely disregarded despite a

dramatic alteration in the balance of essential polyunsaturated fatty acids (PUFAs). Since the 1960s, indiscriminate recommendations have been made to substitute vegetable oils, high in n-6 [omega-6] PUFAs and low in n-3 [omega-3] PUFAs, for saturated fats. Moreover significant changes in animal feed and in the food chain have been introduced. For example, the n-6/n-3 ratios in food commonly consumed in the American diet range from 17 to 41, largely above official recommendations. Among the consequences, these changes have led to a 4-fold increase in the supply of dietary arachidonic acid [AA] in the last 50 years."[1190]

In 2013, British researchers at the University Hospital Southampton, Southampton, U.K., published the results of an examination of 293 mother-child pairs who had undergone complete measurements of maternal plasma PUFA concentrations in late pregnancy, followed by an examination of their children's body composition at ages 4 and 6 years.[1191] The results showed that maternal plasma omega-6 PUFA concentration positively predicted their children's fat mass at both 4 ($p = 0.01$) and 6 years ($p = 0.04$) of age. The maternal plasma omega-3 concentration showed no association with the children's fat mass, however.

Thus, it is clear that increasing omega-6 consumption in mothers drives greater fat mass development in children, likely through multiple mechanisms.

It also appears that excess LA and its breakdown products, the ALEs, along with loss of pituitary melatonin production, are major factors in early menarche (first menstruation, or female "period").[1192] According to researchers,

"The age of puberty has dropped from mid- to late teens in the late 1800s, to pre-teens today."[1193]

This is deemed secondary to increasing LA consumption, which increases the longer-chain omega-6 arachidonic acid (AA) and prostaglandin #E2, which increases sex hormone production, weight gain, and early menarche. Once again, we see the correlation to seed oil consumption and perhaps many other factors of westernization of the diet.

My co-author, Suzanne Alexander, breastfed both of her daughters until they were nearly three years old and then continued to feed them whole, natural foods throughout their teenage years while they lived at home. Neither of them ever missed a single day of school from kindergarten through their senior year of high school, never required a single antibiotic, never had a cavity, and were 14 and 16 years old at menarche (first period).

Summing up, our advice is for expectant parents to consume ancestral diets well before conceiving and continue such throughout pregnancy. It is also best, if possible, to exclusively breastfeed for six months, minimum, followed by some degree of breastfeeding as desired for up to 2 years or more, in conjunction with whole, natural foods. We believe that breastfeeding should be the norm, should be culturally desirable, and should be encouraged for all mothers who are able.

Animal meats, eggs, fish, fruit, vegetables, whole grains, etc., all preferably ancestrally raised and organic, can rapidly become the infant's diet which will continue into childhood. Babies, just four to six months old, should generally eat animal meats, poultry, and fish that have been pureed, along with pureed or very small pieces of fruits and vegetables, all with butter, eggs, or other healthy animal fats.

Infants, toddlers, and children should consume ancestral diets, which means that man-made, processed foods, including seed oils, should not be a part of the diet. When children are raised on ancestral diets, they'll generally be far more likely to continue the same as teenagers, young adults, and even into their elder years.

VEGANISM AND VEGETARIANISM: WHAT CAN WE LEARN? ADVICE AND CAUTIONS

There is much to be learned regarding both the benefits as well as the risks involved from those who have followed either vegan or vegetarian diets. For those not familiar with the terms, "vegan" diets are considered to be entirely plant-based, that is, without any animal foods or animal products. Vegetarian diets generally differ from vegan diets in that some animal products are consumed, e.g., dairy, milk, eggs, cheese, and honey.

Veganism is purported to be about twice as popular today as it was five years ago.[1194] In the U.S., 9.7 million people are estimated to be vegan, which is approximately 2.9% of the population. In Germany, vegans account for about 0.1% to 1% of the population.[1203] The estimated percentage of the population that is vegan in other countries includes 1.2% in Austria, 1% in Australia, and more than 5% in Israel.[1193]

Vitamin B12 deficiency (absence) is the most obvious detrimental result of a vegan diet and was first described in 1849; in fact, the disorder was generally considered to be fatal until 1926, when the deficient diet was supplemented with liver, which either cured or slowed the degenerative disorder.[1195] Liver, of course, is high in vitamin B12.

In 1918, nutrition researcher E.V. McCollum, wrote the following excerpt:

"...the Chinese, Japanese and the peoples of the Tropics generally, have employed the leaves of plants as almost their sole protective food. They likewise eat eggs and these serve to correct their diet... Those people who have employed the leaf of the plant as their sole protective food are characterized by small stature, relatively short span of life, high infant mortality, and...

"The peoples who have made liberal use of milk as a food, have, in contrast, attained greater size, greater longevity, and have been much more successful in the rearing of young. They have been more aggressive than the non-milk using peoples, and have achieved much greater advancement in literature, science and art.

"They have developed in a higher degree educational and political systems which offer the greatest opportunity for the individual to develop his powers. Such development has a physiological basis, and there seems every reason to believe that it is fundamentally related to nutrition."[1196]

In his global travels during the 1930s, Weston A. Price searched long and hard to find even a single population surviving and thriving on a diet that was entirely plant-based, but on five continents, he found none.[28] It appears that this was a disappointment to Price, though we cannot be certain. In 1935, he described in great detail how he searched for vegans in the deep inland hills of the South Sea Islands, where the sea would be most difficult to reach. Price described his journey and findings as follows:

"One of the purposes of this trip was to find, if possible, native dietaries consisting entirely of plant foods which were competent for providing all the factors needed for complete and normal physical development without the use of any animal tissues or product.

"A special effort was accordingly made to penetrate deeply into the interior of the two largest Islands where the inhabitants were living quite remote from the sea, with the hope that groups of individuals would be found living solely on a vegetarian diet. Not only were no individuals or groups found, even in the interior, who were not frequently receiving shell fish from the sea, but I was informed that they recognized that they could not live over three months in good health without getting something from the sea."[1197]

In his 1939 textbook, *Nutrition and Physical Degeneration*, Price wrote,

"It will be noted that vitamin D, which the human does not readily synthesize in adequate amounts [in the absence of sunlight exposure], must be provided by foods of animal tissues or animal products. As yet I have not found a single group of primitive racial stock which was building and maintaining excellent bodies by living entirely on plant foods. I have found in many parts of the world most devout representatives of modern ethical systems advocating the restriction of foods to the vegetable products. In every instance where the groups involved had been long under this teaching, I found evidence of degeneration in the form of dental caries [cavities], and in the new generations in the form of abnormal dental arches [producing misaligned teeth, etc.] to an extent very much higher than in the primitive groups who were not under this influence."[1198]

Populations couldn't survive on entirely plant-based diets prior to the advent of vitamin and possibly mineral supplements, as the B12 deficiency alone would have proven lethal. The usual sources of vitamin B12 are all animal foods, including meats, milk, eggs, fish, and shellfish.[1199] There are only a very few plant sources of B12, such as dried green and purple lavers (nori), although most other edible algae contain either none or just trace amounts.[1198] Most blue-green algae contain "pseudo-vitamin B12," which is clearly inactive in humans. Thus, deficiency of vitamin B12 in vegan diets is the rule, unless supplemented.

According to nutrition researchers, Fiona O'Leary and Samir Samman, University of Sydney, Australia, "Vitamin B12 deficiency is common, mainly due to limited dietary intake of animal foods or malabsorption of the vitamin. Vegetarians are at risk of vitamin B12 deficiency as are other groups with low intakes of animal foods or those with restrictive dietary patterns. Malabsorption of vitamin B12 is most commonly seen in the elderly secondary to gastric achlorhydria [low stomach acid]. The symptoms of sub-clinical deficiency are subtle and often not recognized. The long-term consequences of sub-clinical deficiency are not fully known but may include adverse effects on pregnancy outcomes, vascular, cognitive, bone and eye health."[1194]

In a study by Wolfgang Hermann and colleagues, published in the American Journal of Clinical Nutrition in 2003, some 174 apparently healthy people living in Germany and the Netherlands were evaluated for vitamin B12 deficiency. They found that, in those who took no vitamin supplements, 92% of the vegans, 77% of the lacto-ovo-vegetarians, and 11% of the omnivores had vitamin B12 deficiency (holo-transcobalamin II < 35 pmol/L).[1200]

Obviously, like many individual nutrients, large segments of the population are deficient, including the meat eaters. But again, we must recall that today, the average omnivore is consuming a diet composed of 75% processed, nutrient-deficient foods. And consumption of red meat in the U.S. has been on the decline since about 1975 (see Chapter Two).

Symptoms of vitamin B12 deficiency include anemia (low red blood cell counts), fatigue, weakness, nausea, constipation, numbness, tingling in the hands and feet, balance issues, ataxia (unsteady gait), memory problems, and depression.[1201] Curiously, these same symptoms and many more occur in iron deficiency, which is very common in vegan, vegetarian, and even omnivorous diets.[1202, 1203]

The German Nutrition Society (DGE), on the basis of current scientific literature, developed the following position on the vegan diet:

> *"With a pure plant-based diet, it is difficult or impossible to attain an adequate supply of some nutrients. The most critical is vitamin B12. Other potentially critical nutrients in a vegan diet include protein respecting indispensable amino acids, long-chain omega-3 fatty acids, other vitamins (riboflavin, vitamin D) and minerals (calcium, iron, iodine, zinc and selenium). The DGE does not recommend a vegan diet for pregnant women, lactating women, infants, children or adolescents."*[1204]

It is our collective experience that, while vegan diets may prove beneficial initially, many who persist with long-term vegan diets may eventually succumb to various maladies due to many nutrient deficiencies, particularly vitamin B12, but perhaps also to deficiencies of the fat-soluble vitamins, A, D, and K2, and deficiencies of riboflavin (B2), zinc, iron, iodine, and calcium, almost exactly as reviewed by the German Nutrition Society.

It is also our experience that those who pursue strict vegan diets, if removing processed foods and seed oils, may experience substantial benefits initially. However, over a period of a few months to a few years, many will ultimately develop deficiencies that may prove dangerous or even life-threatening.[1205, 1206, 1207] With respect to minerals in the diet, it should be acknowledged that, despite the fact that many minerals are abundant in plant sources, the bioavailability (intestinal absorption) of those nutrients may be poor due to the presence of oxalates, lectins, and phytates in the foods, which may bind the minerals and markedly reduce absorption.[1208]

Infants and children raised on strict vegan diets will suffer from malnutrition which may end in childhood death and parents charged with neglect.[1209, 1210] Reviews on such cases include "Vegan Child Abuse,"[1211] "Vegan parents on trial for baby's death, allegedly from malnutrition,"[1212] "US vegan parents who eat only raw fruit and vegetable are charged with MURDER for the starvation death of their 18-month old son...,"[1213] "Vegan Parents on Trial, Charged with Neglect, After Baby's Death,"[1214] and "Parents sentenced over neglect of child on vegan-only diet."[1215]

Many will argue that the above cases represent misdirected, poorly planned, and inadequately supplemented vegan diets, which is likely true, however, one should consider that even small amounts (e.g., less than 10%) of animal foods (e.g., whole, raw milk, and eggs) may correct nutrient deficiencies, which is especially and critically important for infants and growing children. Veganism and vegetarianism will generally be better tolerated in adults, when properly supplemented, however, bio-individuality is key to success or failure.

The Papua New Guineans of the highlands of Tukisenta, reviewed in Chapter Four, are perhaps the closest ancestrally living population to being vegan, who had no supplements. As reviewed, more than 90% of their diet was provided by sweet potatoes, yet they were very healthy. They did, however, occasionally feast on pork and, very rarely, consumed chicken. Once again, all ancestrally surviving populations consumed some amount of animal foods, perhaps as little as just a few percent of the diet, just as Weston A. Price found.

In the 1930s, when Price found and treated individuals suffering from nutrient deficiencies, he treated them with a variety of whole foods, always including animal sources, especially whole raw milk, eggs, butter, cod liver oil, and "bread and cereal grains freshly ground to retain the full content of the embryo or germ…"[1216] In 1939, he wrote,

> *"The foods selected for reinforcing the deficient nutrition [of individuals] have always included additional fat-soluble vitamins [e.g. whole raw milk, butter, cod liver oils] and a liberal source of minerals in the form of natural food. Human beings cannot absorb minerals satisfactorily from inorganic chemicals [supplements]. Great harm is done, in my judgment, by the sale and use of substitutes for natural foods [emphasis added]."*[1217]

While some may thrive on vegan or vegetarian diets when properly supplemented, others may severely falter. Thus, we should exercise great caution in the expectation of proper absorption and utilization of vitamins and minerals from supplements alone, instead of whole foods. Nevertheless, it is our goal to collectively educate, assist, support, and encourage all individuals who, for moral, ethical, religious, or health reasons, choose any dietary plan.

HEALTHY POPULATIONS: MACRONUTRIENT RATIOS DO NOT MATTER!

Thomas A.B. Sanders, PhD, Emeritus Professor of Nutrition and Dietetics, King's College London, United Kingdom, in a chapter he authored in the medical textbook *Functional Dietary Lipids (2016),* wrote,

> *"There is little evidence from longitudinal cohort studies to show that the relative proportions of fat and carbohydrate have changed as obesity has become more prevalent…*
>
> *Yet there is good evidence, using double-labeled water to measure energy expenditure, to show that obese individuals do not have low energy requirements… Meta-analyses [analyses of many studies] of trials of dietary advice to reduce fat intake show a statistically significant effect on weight. However, the reduction in weight is generally modest, on average a reduction in BMI of 0.51 kg/m² [1.1 lbs/m²] in the longer-term studies [emphasis added]."*[640]

If we're to investigate the root causes of a disease or condition, we should heed the words of Dr. Sanders. By now, you probably have already realized that

Population	Carbohydrate %	Health
Inuit ('Eskimos') (1908)	8	Excellent
Maasai	17	Excellent
Tokelauans	24	Excellent
Japan (~1960)	~84	Excellent
Okinawa (~1960)	~84	Excellent
Tukisenta, Papua New Guinea	94.6	Excellent

References cited within. © C. Knobbe, 2022. Ancestral Health Foundation.

Population	Total Fat %	Health
Maasai	66	Excellent
Tokelauans	53	Excellent
Inuit ('Eskimos) (1908)	47	Excellent
Japan (~1960)	~5	Excellent
Okinawa (~1960)	~5	Excellent
Tukisenta, Papua New Guinea	3.0	Excellent

References cited within. © C. Knobbe, 2022. Ancestral Health Foundation.

there are populations that consume very low levels of fat and very high levels of fat, or alternatively stated, very high levels of carbohydrate and very low levels of carbohydrate, or anywhere in between, and yet they're all healthy. So if we desire to get at the root cause of the obesity and chronic disease epidemic, we should logically question whether macronutrient ratios – the ratios of carbohydrates to proteins to fats – are even important.

In fact, if the relative proportions of fat and carbohydrate have not changed as obesity has escalated, why should we believe that either too much carbohydrate or too much fat is the root cause of the problem? Even if a low fat diet or a low carbohydrate diet works in an individual or in a study, could it be that there is a confounding variable, which is the true underlying lynchpin of the effect?

We will assert, of course, that the confounding variable, in this case, is the presence of seed oils, primarily, which are controlling omega-6 LA consumption. In the two tables on page 294, we have listed just some of the populations presented in this book along with their respective macronutrient ratios, and their health while consuming their native, traditional, ancestral diets.

As we have observed repeatedly, there is virtually no relationship between either the percentage of carbohydrate or fat consumption and overweight, obesity, or chronic disease. In fact, it is only logical to conclude that macronutrient ratios make little, if any, difference to overweight or health.

OMEGA-6 LA IN HEALTHY VERSUS CHRONIC DISEASE-RIDDLED POPULATIONS

Within this book, we have reviewed the dietary omega-6 LA content of the following ancestrally living populations (in the table below, "Dietary Omega-6 Linoleic Acid (LA) in Ancestral Vs Westernized Populations"). Notice that, in general, populations consuming ancestral diets have less than about 2% of dietary calories as LA, whereas westernized populations, as reviewed repeatedly, have dietary LA currently ranging from about 7% up to 12% LA (all references previously provided).

WHY DO LOW CARB DIETS WORK (WHEN THEY DO)?

The question one might ask then is, why do low carbohydrate diets work? There is some evidence that low carbohydrate diets induce greater weight loss than low fat diets.[1218] In a meta-analysis of 38 studies comparing low fat versus low carbohydrate diets, those that went on the low carbohydrate diets lost an average of 1.3 kg (2.86 lbs) more weight.[1219] The average difference is not much, but obviously, some have far greater results than others. And some certainly have no benefit or continue to gain weight.[1220] Over the longer term (e.g., three months to two years), there is substantial evidence

Dietary Omega-6 Linoleic Acid (LA) in Ancestral Vs Westernized Populations

Ancestral Populations Dietary LA% (All less than 2.0% Dietary LA)		Westernized Populations Dietary LA% (Since ~ 1990)
1908 Inuit	0.6%	
1970 Tukisenta, Papua New Guineans	0.6%	7 – 12%
1960 Japan	0.6%	
1865 Americans	1.0%	
1968 Tokelau	1.6%	
1972 Maasai	1.7%	

References cited within. Dietary Om-6 linoleic acid (LA) is generally under 2% in populations consuming ancestral diets that contain little or no seed oils. Westernized diets contain about 7-12% LA. © C. Knobbe, 2022. Ancestral Health Foundation.

U.S. Diet 2005-06: Food Sources of Linoleic Acid (LA) in Descending Order

Rank	Food Item	Contribution to Intake (%)	Cumulative Contribution	High Carbohydrate?
1	Chicken/Chicken mixed dishes	9.3	9.3	Yes
2	Grain-based desserts	7.5	16.8	Yes
3	Salad dressing	7.4	24.2	
4	Potato/corn/other chips	6.9	31.1	Yes
5	Nuts/seeds & nut/seed mixes	6.5	37.6	
6	Pizza	5.3	42.9	Yes
7	Yeast breads	4.5	47.4	Yes
8	Fried white potatoes	3.5	50.9	Yes
9	Pasta and pasta dishes	3.5	54.4	Yes
10	Mexican mixed dishes	3.3	57.7	Yes
11	Mayonnaise	3.1	60.8	
12	Quickbreads	3.0	63.8	Yes
13	Eggs and egg mixed dishes	2.8	66.6	
14	Popcorn	2.6	69.2	Yes
15	Sausage, franks, bacon, ribs	2.1	71.3	

Ref: Table 3. Food sources of linoleic acid (PFA 18:2), listed in descending order by percentages of their contribution to intake, based on NHANES 2005-2006.

that low carbohydrate diets show no greater weight loss or health advantages over other diets.[1221]

But even if low carbohydrate diets do, indeed, work better for weight loss, the question is why? We will submit that the primary reason that 'low carb' diets work, when they do, is because those that follow them unknowingly and unwittingly, simultaneously reduce their LA consumption.

There is quite strong evidence of this, for example, above is a list of the top 15 sources (listed in descending order) of LA in the American diet, based on the 2005-2006 NHANES study.[1222] The second column provides the LA contribution to the average American's intake, the third column the cumulative contribution from all sources listed, and the fourth column addresses whether the respective food source tends to be high or low in carbohydrates. Notice that 10 of the 15 sources of LA in the U.S. diet also tend to be high in carbohydrates!

Thus, when reducing high carbohydrate foods, such as french fries, hamburger buns, potato chips, and grain-based desserts, just as examples, one will simultaneously tend to substantially reduce LA, and again, unknowingly and unwittingly. This, we will submit, is the primary reason that low carbohydrate diets do indeed have more success. And again, not intrinsically because they're low in carbohydrates, but because they're lower in LA.

WHY ARE SEED OILS STILL IN THE FOOD SUPPLY?

We asked this very question of our friend and colleague, investigative science journalist, Nina Teicholz, who spent a decade researching and writing her book, *The Big Fat Surprise - Why Butter, Meat, and Cheese Belong in a Healthy Diet.*[1223] Here is Teicholz' answer:

"In the last century, consumption of vegetable oils (canola, sunflower, safflower, corn, etc.) has grown more than any other food stuff. From a consumption level of nearly zero in 1900, vegetable oils have risen to become, now, some 30% of all calories we consume. It's important to understand that these oils are not natural; they're the result of an industrialized process that, after squeezing oil from a bean or seed, creating a grey, nutrient-free liquid that must be treated with a solvent, then bleached, distilled, degummed, deodorized, winterized, stabilized, and treated with a chelate to remove toxic metals, among other things.

"This artificial product, which had previously been used to lubricate machinery, was inserted into the American food supply in the form of Crisco, in 1911. From there, its consumption skyrocketed. For one, it quickly became cheaper than the traditional alternatives, butter and lard, used in Western cooking for thousands of years. "The biggest boost, however, came from the American Heart Association (AHA), which, in 1961, told Americans to consume vegetable oils, which lower cholesterol, as a measure of protection against heart disease. The AHA was highly influential, especially at a time when Amer- icans were in a panic over the rising tide of heart disease, and no one knew the cause.

"The reality is that the AHA had long been receiving major financial support from Procter & Gamble, the maker of Crisco and Crisco oil, and the company supports the AHA to this day. With the AHA endorsement, vegetable oil companies could market their products as a kind of heart-healthy drug.

"To preserve that image, Mazola, Wesson, Conagra, Unilever and other vegetable oil businesses got into the business of supporting nutrition researchers, conferences, and scientific events. The US government also got on board in 1980, telling Americans to replace natural fats with vegetable oils; this is why only these oils can be used in school lunches, hospital meals, and in most other institutional food. Vegetable oils also became the backbone of the food industry; they are the fat used in cookies, crackers, chips and most ultra-processed foods. The food behemoths manufacturing these products, such as Nestle and Mondelez (formerly Kraft) depend on these oils for all their goods, and these companies have collectively spent billions of dollars to 'own' the food-and-health space that convinces us these oils are crucial for heart-disease prevention."[1224]

HAVE WE ESTABLISHED CAUSALITY? CAN WE CONVICT SEED OILS FOR OBESITY & CHRONIC DISEASE?

In Chapter One we asked the question: When does correlation rise to the level of causation?

In 1965, Sir Austin Bradford Hill, English epidemiologist and statistician, set forth nine criteria that have become the gold standard for establishing causal inference between a presumed cause and an observed effect in epidemiologic studies. By utilizing these criteria and evaluating the evidence, including epidemiologic studies, experimental evidence, the dose-response relationship, counterarguments, biological plausibility, and the other characteristics of Bradford Hill's criteria, we can further examine the basis for determining whether we may make the leap from correlation, to *causation*.

Let's just very briefly examine Sir Austin Bradford Hill's criteria for attempting to prove causality with regard to seed oils and chronic disease.[21]

1) Strength of the association.

Have we observed that seed oils lead to coronary heart disease, hypertension, overweight, obesity, diabetes, metabolic syndrome, Alzheimer's disease, AMD, and so much more, in population after population? Indeed we have. Have we established any confounders? We've observed in population after population that, for example, sugar and even carbohydrates have been on the decline while numerous chronic diseases elevated, always in parallel with seed oils.

Japan is the quintessential example: As seed oils elevated, obesity and chronic disease elevated, even while total calories, carbohydrates, and sugar all declined.

We have observed macronutrient ratios that vary all across the board while populations remain brilliantly healthy.

We have also observed saturated fat consumption that varies from negligible (around 1% of calories), for example, in the Papua New Guineans of Tukisenta, to approximately 50% of calories, in the Maasai and the Tokelauans, but all three populations were very healthy, without any appreciable degree of obesity, CHD, or diabetes.

However, the one single factor that is consistently observed is that, as seed oil and LA consumption increase, obesity and chronic diseases elevate dramatically. The fact that seed oil consumption has elevated infinitely while chronic diseases have often elevated thousands of fold is indicative of great strength of the association.

For comparison, smoking cigarettes increases the risk of lung cancer or dying from lung cancer by 15- to 30-fold.[1225] Put another way, non-smokers get lung cancer too, however, their risk is about 1/15th to 1/30th the risk of smokers.

In contrast, we have observed increases of coronary heart disease, type 2 diabetes, metabolic syndrome, age-related macular degeneration, Alzheimer's disease, and dementia, which are all thousands of fold greater today than they were in the 19th century. All of these chronic diseases have risen in direct correlation to an extraordinary increase in seed oil consumption.

2) Consistency of the evidence.

In every single case, as we observe seed oils elevate in any given population, we observe parallel increases in overweight and chronic disease. This seems to be an inviolable certainty. There is not, to our knowledge, a single population that violates this principle. On the other hand, for populations that do not consume seed oils, such as hunter-gatherers, we observe virtually none of these chronic diseases. The evidence is remarkably consistent.

3) Specificity.

Hill's criterion as it relates to specificity originally suggested that one exposure caused only one disease. For example, the bacterium *Mycobacterium tuberculosis* is required to develop tuberculosis.

One "exposure" – one disease. Cigarette smoking, on the other hand, increases the risk of many cancers, CHD, stroke, chronic obstructive pulmonary diseases, other lung diseases, diabetes, and many other diseases, because it poisons the entire body.[1226]

Like cigarette smoking, seed oil consumption is implicated in virtually every chronic disease there is.

Systemic toxins or poisons don't affect just one biological system. They affect many.[1227] Why? Because they poison entire organ systems throughout the body. For example, cyanide poisons every cell of the body by interfering with the cell's ability to utilize oxygen. Seed oils, similarly, are systemic toxins that produce widespread adverse biological effects.

Thus, seed oils do not specifically induce a single disease. They induce a much higher risk of innumerable chronic diseases. Hill's "specificity" criterion, in the case of systemic toxins such as cigarette smoking, whole-body radiation, or seed oil consumption, might be broadened in scope to "induce myriad chronic diseases."

4) Temporal sequence.

This criterion must always be met in order to establish causal inference. The cause must precede the effect temporally. Do we observe dramatic increases in chronic diseases in populations before they consume seed oils? No, we generally do not see obesity and most all chronic diseases in hunter-gatherers, for example, who do not consume processed foods and edible oils. The seed oils have proximate cause – they always come first. It is rarely the other way around. In essence, no seed oils – little or no chronic disease. Massive seed oils – massive disease. But again, seed oil consumption *precedes the onset* of most all chronic diseases. We've established the temporal relationship.

It is possible to develop such chronic diseases without the presence of seed oils, and this does not violate causal inference as it relates to temporal sequence or any other of Hill's criteria. In other words, there may be other causalities, especially in complex biological systems, with marked genetic susceptibilities and numerous other environmental factors, albeit their roles may be diminutive in contrast to seed oil exposure (consumption). However, we repeatedly observe a very strong temporal relationship between seed oil "exposure" – consumption – and increases in chronic disease.

It is also clear that very long latency periods exist between the "exposure" (consumption) of seed oils and the development of many chronic diseases. For example, heart attacks, Alzheimer's disease, dementia, and age-related macular degeneration (AMD), are all examples of disease conditions with very long latency periods between exposure and development of disease. This is also known as the "incubation period" for a disease.

The incubation period may be three days after exposure to an adenovirus that might produce a cold, for example, whereas continued consumption of seed oils for four or five decades or more will generally be required to produce a heart attack, Alzheimer's disease, or AMD, for example. Long incubation periods are known and expected in biological science.[1228] [1229] [1230] In general, it has been suggested that the earliest or typical age of onset might be the incubation period, as the exposure may begin in the prenatal period.[1231]

Very long incubation periods for chronic diseases make it impossible to study the effects of diets on such diseases using randomized controlled trials. This is true because controlling the entire diet in people requires the holding of subjects within a metabolic ward where all foods are carefully prepared, analyzed, and tracked in a metabolic kitchen; the longest of such studies, to our knowledge, has lasted no more than a few months.[1232][1233] Thus, it should be clear that we should never expect randomized controlled clinical trials (RCCTs) to properly and formally address dietary intervention in humans with respect to chronic diseases that have decades-long incubation periods.

5) Biological gradient (dose-response effect).

In his classic paper, Hill wrote, "if a dose-response is seen, it is more likely that the association is causal."[21] Over and over, we've observed this: More oils, more disease. In many countries, we observe that heart disease, overweight, obesity, diabetes, macular degeneration, etc., are all either very low in prevalence or virtually non-existent, and as seed oil consumption gradually elevates, so does obesity and chronic disease. More oils equals more poison, and more disease. The biological gradient is established.

The recent history in Japan represents the quintessential example to illustrate the biological gradient. Seed oils consumption gradually elevated from 3 g/day in 1950 to 39 g/day by 2004, with marked increases in every chronic disease measured, including an increase in diabetes prevalence of 345-fold and an increase in AMD prevalence of 82-fold.

In the United States, CHD, diabetes, metabolic syndrome, obesity, and Alzheimer's disease, among many other conditions, were all either unknown or medical rarities in 1890, when seed oil consumption averaged about one gram per day. However, when seed oil consumption averaged 80 g/day in 2010, all of these conditions increased dramatically, and, in the case of diabetes, up to a 4,643-fold increase between 1890 and 2016.

In some cases, the dose-response effect achieves a threshold effect, above which further increases in "dose" produce little or no further increases in disease. For example, as shown by Clement Ip, diets achieving omega-6 LA content above 4.4% in laboratory animals failed to produce substantially increased risk in terms of cancer development. The same threshold effects may prove to be true with regard to CHD or other chronic diseases. Perhaps many populations have already surpassed the threshold effect for many diseases.

Furthermore, there are many other factors besides seed oil consumption upon which entire diets may or may not induce disease. For example, diets higher in antioxidants would be expected to be protective for those consuming more seed oils. And some people will have greater genetic susceptibility to one disease versus another.

Thus, the dose-response relationship is neither linear nor stochastic (random). But, the dose-response effect as it relates to seed oils is exceedingly strong, directional, and quite predictable in its devastating effects. This is strong evidence moving us further towards causal inference.

The observation of populations in epidemiologic studies over extended periods of time is what Weston A. Price referred to as "Nature's laboratory."[28] This is indeed the best possible evidence of all upon which we may make causal inference for disease conditions that take decades to develop, since entire diets cannot be controlled in people except over very short periods of time. In Nature's laboratory, we may observe dietary patterns and transitions in populations over many decades of time and, in the case of some populations, such as the U.S., over a period of more than one-and-a-half centuries.

6) Plausibility/Biological rationale.

We have reviewed what is called the "pathophysiology," that is, the biological mechanisms via which seed oils exact their destruction. Seed oils, via both high omega-6 LA content and the presence of ALEs, induce a markedly pro-oxidative, pro-inflammatory, toxic, and nutrient-deficient biological milieu. Each of these works independently and in synergy to exact widespread destruction.

There is tremendous evidence to indicate reasons for both a highly pro-oxidative and pro-inflammatory state, for example, with diets rich in seed oils. There is also tremendous evidence that seed oils produce high levels of toxic ALEs. Seed oils also displace animal fats resulting in nutrient deficiencies since edible oils contain neither vitamins A, D, or K2. In short, the plausible biological mechanisms have been reviewed in great detail.

7) Coherence.

With this criterion of Hill, we must ask, is the postulated causal relationship consistent with what is known about the disease/disorder? Does the story make coherent sense in light of all evidence? Indeed, overweight, obesity, CHD, cancers, type 2 diabetes, and virtually all chronic diseases are unified by physiological state that is pro-oxidative, pro-inflammatory, toxic, and nutrient-deficient. Furthermore, nearly all such chronic diseases are unified by mitochondrial dysfunction, which is yet another disastrous end result of seed oil consumption.

8) Experimental evidence.

Have we observed experimental evidence in animals to further support causality? Indeed, much evidence has been reviewed in support, including obesity, metabolic disease, diabetes, heart failure, etc., all in animals given seed oil diets in amounts comparable to westernized populations. We have observed in these studies very rapid development of metabolic disease and obesity, for example, in rodents given high omega-6 LA-containing diets, as compared to similar rodents on isocaloric (equal calorie) low LA diets.

Thus, experimental evidence in omnivorous animal models closely parallels what we have observed in humans at the population level.

9) Analogous evidence.

Have we observed in other biological systems that, for example, highly pro-oxidative states lead to chronic disease? Most certainly. Arsenic poisoning, for example, exacts its destruction by inducing a severely pro-oxidative state with an end result akin to the effects of seed oils.[1234][1235][1236] Arsenic poisoning induces atherosclerosis,[1237] cancers, liver disease, diabetes,[1238] obesity, glucose intolerance, insulin resistance, increased blood lipids (e.g., triglycerides),[1239] metabolic syndrome,[1240] and other chronic disease conditions.

However, both seed oils and arsenic exact their toll primarily via inducing a more pro-oxidative state and, we can therefore conclude that both toxicants would be expected to produce similar metabolic and disease outcomes, which they do. This is further evidence that the "seed oil hypothesis of chronic disease" is correct.

Have we established causality? We will conclude with our final thoughts on this question in the chapter summary.

CHAPTER 6: SUMMARY

We will submit that the heuristic value of observing the dietaries of populations over many decades of time while comparatively correlating chronic disease prevalence in Nature's laboratory is the most valuable evidence available in the discipline of Nutrition. Accordingly, this is why a great emphasis on population studies has been made throughout this book.

We have observed in Japan that, while calories, carbohydrates, and sugar have all declined, overweight, obesity, diabetes, cancers, and age-related macular degeneration have all increased exponentially. Seed oils and the omega-6 percentage of the diet, however, steadily increased during this entire period of time.

In Japan and Okinawa, fat consumption elevated from 5% in about 1960 to 20% by 1999, while both carbohydrate and sugar consumption dropped, and saturated fat consumption increased only to a maximum of 7% in 2004, which is still amongst the lowest levels in the world. High-PUFA vegetable oils, however, increased from 9 grams a day in 1961 to 39 g/day by 2004, which was associated with omega-6 LA consumption rising from 1% in 1960 to 7.8% in 2004.

With this westernized dietary transition, characterized by marked increases in seed oil consumption, obesity doubled in men, diabetes elevated 345-fold, age-related macular degeneration increased 82-fold, and metabolic syndrome rose to 30.2% in men and 10.3% in women, all over a period of about a half-century.

Thus, in Japan, which includes Okinawa, many chronic disease conditions increased exponentially in correlation to a marked increase in seed oil and omega-6 LA consumption.

Based on the best historical evidence, on a global scale, vegetable oil consumption was close to zero in 1865, having risen to an average of 65.4 g/day (589 cal/day) by 2014, which is a near infinite increase. In parallel with that, we've observed a near infinite increase in chronic disease, as evidenced by the history of coronary heart disease, cancers, diabetes, metabolic syndrome, Alzheimer's disease, dementia, age-related macular degeneration (AMD), autoimmune diseases, and a plethora of rare, chronic diseases that seem to have no prior record in medical history.

On a global scale, we have observed that, from the period of 1964 to 2007, carbohydrate consumption fell 1.4 percent. During the period of 1961 to 2014, sugars increased 20.2 percent. However, during that same time period of 1961 to 2014, vegetable oil consumption increased 322 percent, which is 4.22-fold. During that interval, we have observed marked increases in overweight, obesity, diabetes, and the before mentioned litany of chronic disease on a worldwide basis.

Seed oils are devastating the health of populations worldwide. Is there any other logical conclusion that we can draw?

You must be the judge as to whether we have established causality. You cannot afford to allow anyone else to decide, except yourself.

With regard to the Bradford-Hill criteria, we have demonstrated 1) strength of the evidence, 2) consistency of the evidence, 3) specificity, 4) temporal sequence, 5) biological gradient (dose-response relationship), 6) biological rationale, 7) coherence, 8) experimental evidence, and 9) analogous evidence.

Without the slightest reservation, it is our assertion that *we have met the Bradford Hill criteria for establishing causality. This is not just correlation, but causation. We have met every criterion to 'prove' causality.*

Seed oils are indeed poison. By far and away, seed oils hold the enormous bulk of responsibility for inducing obesity and virtually every major chronic disease there is, and perhaps nearly all of the unusual chronic diseases as well.

Being poisoned results in widespread and disastrous destruction, with myriad devastating consequences. Poisons are not selective to a given disease or organ system. They do not discriminate. They poison most any cell of any organ system resulting in widespread chronic disease.

We've been poisoned, slowly and surely, with poisons euphemistically named 'vegetable oils,' which we've been told are 'heart healthy' and desirable. They are, instead, the single most noxious components of our food supply, without exception.

Removal of processed foods and seed oils is the only answer to prevent and treat overweight, obesity, and the whole host of chronic diseases that are ravaging us individually and globally. These include coronary heart disease, heart attacks, hypertension, strokes, cancers, metabolic syndrome, type 2 diabetes, Alzheimer's disease, dementia, age-related macular degeneration, autoimmune diseases, overweight, obesity, and a myriad of rare chronic diseases. The solution is elegantly straightforward, simple, and effective. But, prevention is key.

This entire ancestral nutrition model should be considered canonical theory in the fields of both Nutrition and Medicine. In other words, the omega-6 LA theory, perhaps better termed the "seed oil theory of chronic disease," should be considered a fundamental law of Nutrition that should forever serve as a foundational guide to physicians, clinicians, scientists, and the lay public.

In light of this, we recommend that each of you begin immediately with the introduction of an ancestral diet. Simply consume the foods of our ancestors, which includes primarily meats, fowl, fish, seafood, eggs, and dairy, all ancestrally raised, if possible, as well as fruits, vegetables, tubers, lentils, and whole grains, all organically raised and prepared, if available and affordable.

The benefits will begin immediately and will accumulate over time, with the ultimate rewards being beyond comprehension. This is one of the greatest gifts that you can give to yourself and your family. Never underestimate the potential of an ancestral diet. Never.

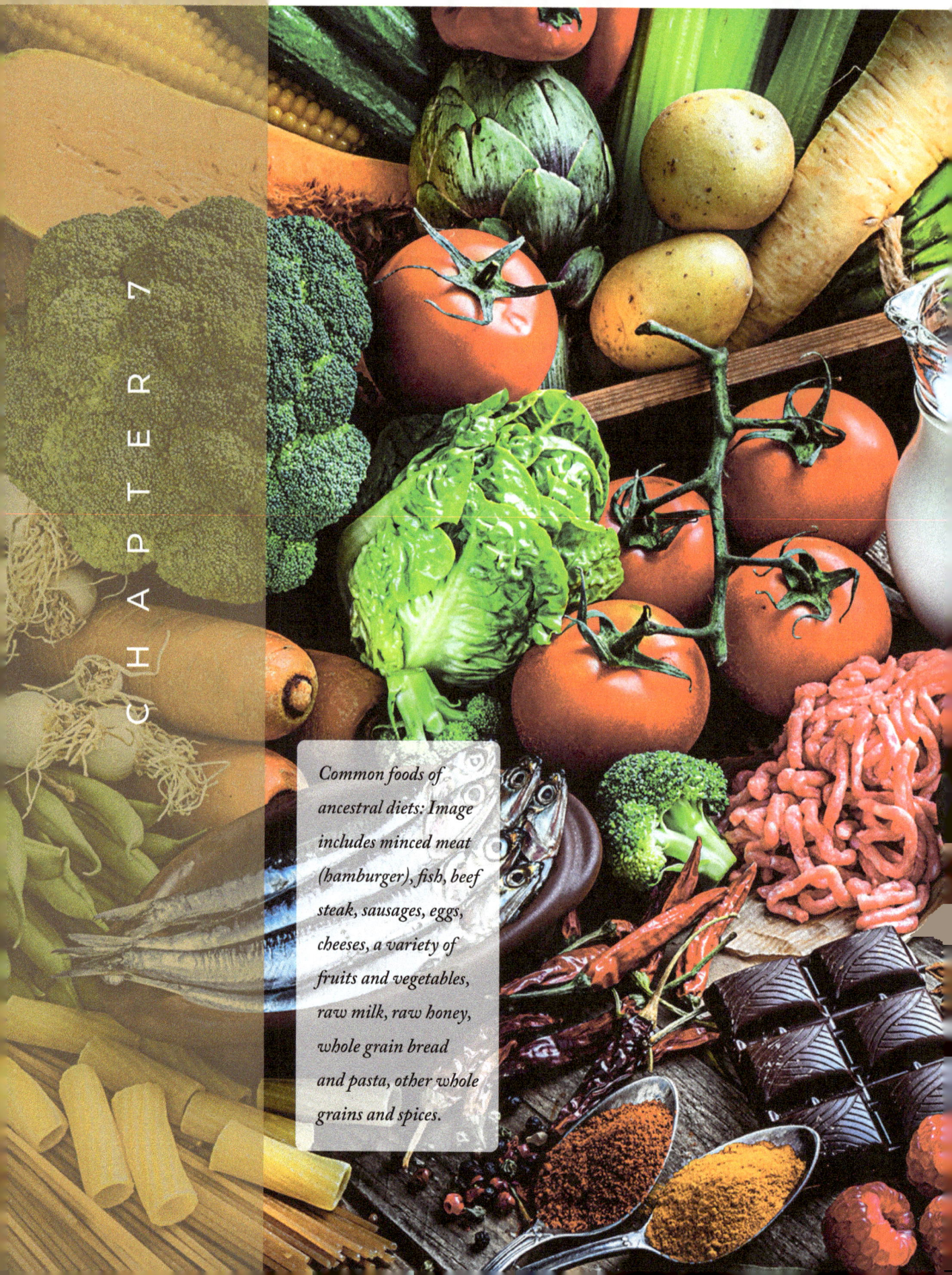

CHAPTER 7

Common foods of ancestral diets: Image includes minced meat (hamburger), fish, beef steak, sausages, eggs, cheeses, a variety of fruits and vegetables, raw milk, raw honey, whole grain bread and pasta, other whole grains and spices.

CHAPTER 7

THE ANCESTRAL DIET PROTOCOL

"Unthinking respect for authority is the greatest enemy of truth."

— ALBERT EINSTEIN

It behooves us to respect our own logic and intuition, and not to blindly respect the opinions of 'authorities,' (even us) just because they appear to be authoritative and perhaps represent authoritative institutions – including Harvard School of Public Health, Tufts University's Department of Nutrition, Mayo Clinic's Department of Nutrition, and the like. Authorities may have biases and hidden agendas.

Think they don't? Consult Nina Teicholz's book, *The Big Fat Surprise*, for a true eye-opener on this subject. We advise that, rather than to simply respect an individual or an institution, instead respect the evidence, the history, and the science. And what is science? It is essentially a search for the truth. Science seeks to explain evidence found in the natural world. In this chapter, we will review some of the hands-on practicality of consuming a nutrient-dense, low LA diet.

PROCESSED FOODS – MUST AVOID!

Processed foods may almost entirely be defined by the presence of four characteristics: added sugars, refined flours, seed oils, and trans fats. Add to this short list the so-called "mystery ingredients" such as artificial flavors and sweeteners that are the concoctions of food scientists who work for Big Food manufacturers, and now you have nearly the complete picture of processed foods.

Look at any packaged food, and if it has any of these four ingredients, it's likely a processed food. In the U.S. today, there are more than 600,000 food items available, but think about this – only a relatively small number of those foods would be whole foods, that is, God-given foods or what we might call the foods of Nature. Such foods would essentially consist of meats, fowl, fish, eggs, dairy, fruits, vegetables, whole grains, nuts and seeds (in extremely limited quantities), herbs, and spices. These are the whole foods and the list is pretty simple.

Processed foods in the U.S. currently consist of about 21% sugar, 17% refined wheat flour, 24 to 32% seed oils, and perhaps around 0.5 to 1% trans fats, all as a percentage of calories.[3][4] Many people currently believe that trans fats have been removed from the U.S. food supply due to the U.S. FDA removal of trans fats from GRAS (Generally Regarded As Safe) status in 2015. However, trans fats exist within seed oils of many types and are not being considered as being in violation of food policy by the U.S. FDA (reviewed in Chapter One).

In fact, complete removal of industrially produced trans fats from the food supply would require comprehensive and absolute elimination of seed oils, or at least those requiring deodorization (the stage of processing in which trans fats are primarily produced). However, as anyone can see, seed oils hold the bulk of our fat consumption in numerous westernized nations. In many westernized societies, seed oils account for more calories consumed than either animal meats or fruits and vegetables combined. Yet, they're a highly manufactured, processed, dangerous, and entirely unnatural component of the food supply, which had a minuscule part of food systems prior to 1865. Just look at almost any processed food and you'll find that the fat within the food is not butter, lard, or beef tallow, but rather, it is almost always from one or more of the highly polyunsaturated oil varieties.

THE ANCESTRAL DIET PROTOCOL

Cooking Oil	% Linoleic Acid (LA) Approximate Average Value (Range in parentheses)
Safflower	75%
Grape seed	70%
Sunflower	68%
Corn	58%
Cottonseed	55%
Soybean	53%
Rice bran	35%
Peanut	32%
Canola	21%
Lard (CAFO – corn/soy fed)	20%
Linseed (flaxseed)	16%
Avocado	14%
Olive oil	10% (3% - 27%)
Palm oil	10%
Beef tallow (CAFO, corn/soy fed)	3%
Butter (CAFO, corn/soy fed)	2%
Palm kernel oil	2%
Coconut oil	2%
Lard (Ancestrally raised)	2%
Beef tallow (100% Grass fed)	2%
Butter (100% Grass fed)	1.4%

HIGH PUFA SEED ('VEGETABLE') OILS TO AVOID

The high PUFA seed oils include soybean, corn, canola, rapeseed, grapeseed, sunflower, safflower, rice bran, and a few others of far lesser consumption. These are, of course, the most dangerous edible oils. They're the most highly processed and, therefore, have the most ALEs, but also have extraordinarily high LA.

The table on page 307 provides a fairly comprehensive list of the most commonly consumed oils and their approximate LA content.[1241,1242,1243] In general, the lowest LA-containing fats would be the fats of choice. However, we would ask, why not avoid all oils? Why not revert to the cooking fats of our ancestors – traditionally raised lard, butter, and beef tallow? These would be approximately the lowest in LA but will also provide the fat-soluble vitamins A, D, and K2.

One should consider close examination of this table and note that virtually none of the edible oils ('vegetable oils') ever existed in the enormous majority of populations consuming ancestral diets.

In fact, olive oil and coconut oil would be two of the oils that indeed have a multi-millennial history of consumption (albeit on a very small scale globally), both of which also have been associated with far better health.[1244,1245] Note their approximate LA content is 10% and 2%, respectively. Thus, once again, what we see is that authentic olive oil, at approximately 10% LA on average, should indeed be associated with better health than the typical seed oils, most of which are in the 21% to 78% range of LA. These levels of LA are impossible to obtain in virtually any native, traditional diets.

But nevertheless, seed oils are already highly oxidized by the time they hit the bottle and will oxidize further within the human body, producing even greater quantities of ALEs.

The production of ALEs occurs frequently in food preparation, particularly in most fast-food restaurants where cooking oils are heated for many hours and days, with repeat cooking of french fries, chicken "nuggets," fried fish, etc., which is standard procedure for fast-food. In fact, many such restaurants are notorious for heating and cooking with such oils for many days and even up to a week or more before discarding! Lipid scientists have discovered enormous quantities of ALEs in the typical seed oil fryer vats used in fast food restaurants as we have reviewed.

With respect to the omega-6 content of such oils, just one tablespoon of safflower oil with about 78% LA, contains about 10 grams of LA. Sunflower oil contains about 9 g LA per tablespoon, corn and soybean oils about 7 g, and sesame oil about 6 g. Now consider this: A typical ancestral diet would contain about 5 grams or less of LA per day, in total!

FRUIT OILS – COCONUT, PALM, PALM KERNEL, OLIVE, AND AVOCADO OILS – FAR SAFER

The fruit oils are consistently associated with far better health outcomes in population studies – and for good reason.[1246] As reviewed, first of all, they're dramatically lower in LA content. As one can see from the table on page 307, coconut oil is about 2% LA, palm kernel oil about 2.3%, palm oil is about 10%, olive oil about 10% (but with a range of 3.34% to 27.12%)[1247] and avocado oil about 14% (with a range of 10.5% to 15.15%).[1248]

Once again, the lower the LA content, in general, the lower the risk of chronic disease. Furthermore, all of the fruit oils can be extracted from their respective fruits primarily with simple mechanical pressing and without the use of high heat, hexane solvents, or any form of chemical refining. This means that even the small amounts of omega-6 LA and omega-3 ALA in such oils are much more greatly protected from oxidation, i.e., ALEs are drastically lower.

However, when using olive oil one needs to be hyper-vigilant because tests reveal anywhere from 69% to 73% percent of the olive oils sold in American grocery stores and restaurants have failed to meet the International Olive Oil Council (IOC) sensory standards for Extra Virgin Olive Oil (EVOO).[1249] This indicates that the oils were either adulterated with cheap, oxidized, omega-6 vegetable oils, such as sunflower oil or peanut oil, or non-human grade olive oils, which are harmful to health in a number of ways.[1250]

Adulteration of olive oil began in the 19th century and continues to this day. As such, if choosing olive oil, be wary of the possibility of adulteration and seek out olive oil companies with impeccable reputation and high standards for quality and authenticity.

Even so-called "extra virgin olive oil" is often diluted with other less expensive oils, including hazelnut, soybean, corn, sunflower, palm, sesame, grape seed and/or walnut.[1248] These added oils will not be listed on the label, nor will most people be able to discern that such 'olive oil' is not 100 percent pure. Chances are, you've been eating poor-quality olive oil for so long — or you've never tasted a pure, genuine, high-quality olive oil to begin with — so you may not be aware that there is anything wrong with it.

In January 2016, 60 Minutes revealed how the olive oil business has been corrupted by what the Italians refer to as the "Agromafia."[1251] According to journalist Tom Mueller, featured in the 60 Minutes' report, the Mafia has infiltrated virtually all areas of the olive oil business, including harvesting, pricing, transportation and the supermarkets.

In the brief documentary, Mueller stated, "Last month police in Italy nabbed 7,000 tons of phony olive oil. Much of it was bound for American stores… Branded as 'Italian extra virgin.' The scam was cooked up by organized crime." That's enough fraudulent olive oil to fill approximately 14 million 0.5 liter bottles of oil.

And this was just one fraudulent scam. The reality is that olive oil, which would generally be one of the safest oils, has been the subject of one of the greatest frauds. And this is because EVOO is an expensive oil to produce, it is easily adulterated, and the market is enormous, all of which makes this an alluring opportunity for organized crime.

In essence, food scammers have infiltrated the entire food chain "from farm to fork," to use Mueller's phrase.[1250] The fraud is massive; at least half of all the extra virgin olive oil sold in Italy is adulterated as well. That's pretty astonishing, considering the reverence Italians have for olive oil. In the U.S., chances of getting the real McCoy are even slimmer, with as much as 80 percent of olive oil being adulterated.[1252]

Forbes interviewed olive oil expert, David Neumann on the subject, who said, "America is the dumping ground of all of those fraudulent operations. There are not enough resources to control the over 350,000 tons of olive oil entering the country. That's why, even after the scandals, adulterated olive oil bottles are still on supermarket shelves."[1251]

Quality can also be seriously compromised by the fact that olive oil is shipped by boat, which takes a long time. It is then stored and distributed to grocery stores, where the oil may sit on the shelf for another several months. Unlike fine wine, olive oil does not get better with age.

Olive oil is similar to fresh-squeezed orange juice, meaning it has a rather short shelf life. Pure olive oil that's minimally processed contains health-promoting antioxidants and phenolics, provided the oil hasn't oxidized — and oxidation is an enormous risk for olive oil. By the time you buy and use it, the olive oil may already be on the verge of going bad.

If you purchase and consume an excellent quality, fresh, artisanal extra virgin olive oil (EVOO), you're probably pretty safe with that. We would recommend visiting the olive oil company that you intend to buy from to ask questions and make every possible attempt to confirm that you're buying fresh, authentic EVOO. Additionally, we recommend only purchasing EVOO that is sold in dark green or dark brown colored bottles, never in clear glass bottles, given that light increases oxidation of the PUFAs in the oils. We recommend looking for a quality certification seal from the International Olive Oil Council (IOC) or California Olive Oil Council (**https://cooc.com/certified-oils**).

Keep in mind that there are very substantial variations in LA content between EVOOs and very few of them will have ever had multiple fatty acid analyses to determine a typical LA concentration. This could be accomplished by submitting your own sample(s), but the expense may be significant. Studies have shown that EVOO has an LA range from a low of 3.34% to a high of 27.12%, with an average of around 10 to 11%.[1246] It's quite interesting that a number of samples of Greek olive oils tested had LA concentrations ranging from 6.35 to 11.52%.[1253]

EVOO samples from the island of Crete, Greece (Cretan cultivars) were found to have LA concentrations ranging from 5.05 to 7.02, with an average LA of 5.79%.[1254] Are such olive oils one of the reasons that people from Ikaria, Greece are among the longest living people in the world? These are exceedingly low LA levels for olive oil and such cultivars might be a consideration for those who desire the lowest LA EVOO.

If you've been consuming westernized foods and seed oils at all, you will need a lengthy period of time on an ancestral diet – up to two to three years or more – to get your body fat (adipose) LA composition back to an ancestral level. During this transition period, even typical olive oils may be too high in LA to achieve goals. During this time, consumption of foods lower in LA, such as butter, ghee, ancestrally raised (non-soy-fed) eggs, grass-fed beef, tallow, wild-caught Alaskan salmon or Sockeye salmon, etc., would all be very beneficial in terms of reaching such goals.

In the table on page 311, we've provided a guide to help prove the authenticity and quality of olive oil, should you choose to use it.

Extra Virgin Olive Oil (EVOO)
Selection and Consumption Guide

Certification	The North American Olive Oil Association (NAOOA) is the nation's largest and most comprehensive olive oil testing and certification program. Consider using the NAOOA's certified list available at AboutOliveOil.org to find EVOO that meets strict criteria. The California Olive Oil Council and the Australian Olive Oil Association also require olive oil to meet quality standards.
Labeling Terms	We recommend to consume only "extra virgin" olive oils, since all other categories will have been processed, which will reduce antioxidants and increase oxidation.
Evaluation	If using EVOO regularly, if possible, we recommend visiting the olive grove from which you buy. Confirm that the olives are pressed quickly after harvest and stored in stainless steel containers, preferably topped with nitrogen gas to prevent oxygen from coming in contact with the oil.
Color and Flavor	Many fresh EVOOs will be of a nearly luminescent green color, however, others will naturally be a pale straw to gold color, neither of which is necessarily concerning. The oil should smell and taste fruity, possibly herbaceous, and may even be bitter or spicy, the latter of which is indicative of high (and healthy) levels of antioxidants.
Storage and Use	Olive oil should be kept in a cool and dark place. The cap or cork should be replaced immediately after pouring, in order to reduce exposure to oxygen. Olive oil should best be used within six weeks of purchase.
Containers	Olive oil is best kept in bottles or steel containers that protect against exposure to light. If bottled, be sure the glass is darkened, however, if the glass is clear the bottle should be otherwise protected from light, e.g., inside a cardboard box.

NUTS AND SEEDS ARE IMMENSE SOURCES OF OMEGA-6 LA: PROCEED WITH CAUTION!

If you review allopathic medicine's health resources it is likely you are regularly informed that nuts and seeds are beneficial for your health and there is often the suggestion to consume them because they're "heart healthy."[1255] The American Heart Association, for example, recommends eating approximately four servings (1.5 ounces per serving) of unsalted nuts per week, because nuts are low in saturated fat, high in polyunsaturated fats and, therefore, in their view, "lower the bad cholesterol."[1256] Once again, high omega-6 diets do indeed lower the measured cholesterol just exactly the same as high seed oil diets, but is this beneficial? In our opinion, absolutely not.

Nuts/Seeds	% Linoleic Acid (LA)
Poppy seed	62%
Pine nut	62%
Walnut	60%
Sunflower seed	59%
Hemp seed	57%
Wheat germ	55%
Pecan nut	50%
Sesame seed	48%
Brazil nut	43%
Pumpkin seed	37%
Peanut	33%
Pistachio	33%
Almond nut	27%
Cashew nut	21%
Filbert nut	17%
Macadamia nut	2.5%

Nuts and seeds are as much as 85% fat, in fact, the enormous majority of calories in nuts and seeds come from fat, but of course, it's not the fat that's the problem. It's the kind of fat. As may be observed in the table above, the LA content of nuts and seeds is exceedingly high. In fact, pecans are 50% LA, Brazil nuts 43% LA, and walnuts come in at a whopping 53% LA.[1257] From the perspective of LA content, nuts and seeds rival the LA in many seed oils.

Thus, a 1.5 oz. serving (about a handful) of almonds provides 6 g of LA, while the same serving size of pecans provides 12 g, sunflower seeds 15 g, and walnuts provide 17 g LA! Once again, native, traditional diets, almost none of which contain nuts and seeds as staple foods, generally provide less than or equal to about 5 g LA per day.

So while nuts and seeds do not contain ALEs to any significant degree, unlike the high PUFA seed oils, they certainly can contribute tremendously to the LA content of the diet. This will then drive up the LA content of our body fat, cells, and cell membranes, resulting in untoward effects. As such, nuts and seeds should be greatly minimized or even eliminated, especially if one has consumed seed oils in recent years.

LINOLEIC ACID (LA) IN ANCESTRALLY RAISED VS CAFO-RAISED, CORN & SOY-FED ANIMALS

Just as the LA concentration in olive oil can range from about 3 to 27%, the LA in animal meats may vary tremendously depending on the fodder. In every case, not only will the LA content be lower, but the overall nutrient density will be higher in animals raised ancestrally than in animals fed grains, corn, soy, and genetically modified organism (GMO) corn and soy. The latter two are almost exclusively what animals are being fed in concentrated animal feeding operations (CAFOs).

Green America, an organization that works toward a more sustainable society, states that "98% of GM soy and 49% of GM corn goes to feeding livestock and poultry."[1258] It has also been established that 70-90% of the harvested genetically engineered (GE) crops are fed to food-producing animals.[1259]

ANCESTRALLY-FED VS CORN- AND SOY-FED BEEF – THE MAIN PROBLEM WITH CAFO BEEF

It should be intuitively obvious that none of the animals being fed GMO corn, soy, or the like, or even animals fed non-GMO corn and soy, are consuming their native, traditional, ancestral diet. In monogastric animals, like chicken and pork, feed that is high in LA (corn and soy) will drive very high body fat LA, just as we see in humans.[1260]

In polygastric (multiple stomach) ruminants, such as cattle, buffalo, sheep, goats, deer, elk, etc., the high consumption of unsaturated fats that occurs with consumption of high LA feed, such as corn and soy, does not end up producing high LA in their milk and body fat.[1261]

In fact, ruminants have very low concentrations of LA in both their meat and milk, no matter what they eat.[1260]

This is true because the polygastric stomach of ruminants contains a "biohydrogenation chamber," that is, a compartmentalized stomach, part of which contains bacteria that can convert high omega-6 LA containing feed into saturated and monounsaturated fats. Thus, in terms of LA in the body fat of ruminants, there is only about 0.5% dif-

Omega-6 Linoleic Acid (LA) in Grass-Fed Vs Corn/Soy-Fed Beef
(Expressed as % of Total Fat)

Cattle Type	100% Grass-Fed Beef	Grain-Fed Beef
Mixed Cattle	2.01%	2.38%
Angus Steers	3.41%	3.93%

Daley et al, A review of fatty acid profiles and antioxidant content in grass-fed and grain-fed beef. Nutrition Journal, 2010;9:10.
© C. Knobbe, 2022. Ancestral Health Foundation.

ference in LA between 100% grass-fed cattle and GMO corn and soy-fed animals.[1261]

As is shown on page 313, typical 100% grass-fed cattle often have about 2.01 to 3.41% linoleic acid in their fat, whereas corn- and soy-fed (grain-fed) beef still only have about 2.38 to 3.93% LA in their body fat (both as a percentage of total fat).[1262]

The issue of consuming GMO corn- and soy-fed beef (or other ruminant meat) then, is not so much the LA difference, but primarily a matter of the accumulation of glyphosate herbicide – the noxious poison of Roundup – in the meat of the CAFO-raised animals. Glyphosate accumulates in the "Roundup ready" GMO plants sprayed with Roundup, which are then consumed by the animals (or humans) consuming them.[1263] In turn, animals accumulate glyphosate in their flesh and milk, which is then consumed by humans feeding upon them. The potential for devastating health outcomes is marked and severe.[1264]

ANCESTRALLY FED VERSUS CORN- AND SOY-FED CHICKEN

Chicken and fowl are monogastric omnivorous animals and, therefore, are highly susceptible to developing high levels of body fat LA when fed a high LA diet, just like humans.[1259] Contrary to what grocery store labels would have us believe, chickens are not vegans or vegetarians. They are omnivores, and just like any omnivore, they eat the flesh of other animals. Chickens on pasture will eat insects, worms, grubs, etc., and will eat from carcasses of many animals when available.

On the island of Tokelau, Ian Prior and colleagues assessed the body fat LA in chickens that were consuming ancestral diets (non-corn or soy-fed), and determined that the LA was 2.5% of total fatty acids (total fat).[17] However, in USDA studies of GMO corn and soy-fed, i.e., typical "grocery store" chicken, LA content was 18.0% of fatty acids.[1265] Thus, CAFO-raised chicken in westernized countries has become yet another substantial source of LA.

Ashley Armstrong, PhD, and her sister, Sarah Armstrong, of Angel Acres Farm in Marcellus, Michigan, (no affiliation) raise a relatively small flock of chickens on ancestrally fed diets (without corn or soy) for the purpose of producing healthy, nutritious, low LA eggs (see further detail under eggs in this chapter). An independent fatty acid analysis of the skinless, boneless chicken breasts and thighs from Angel Acres Farm chickens versus CAFO (Tyson and Gold Leaf) raised corn- and soy-fed chickens was completed in early 2022 at the University of Michigan.

As shown in the table on top of page 315, a typical 6-ounce (170 gram) skinless chicken breast from chicken raised on corn and soy (Tyson store bought) had an average of 0.42 grams of

Omega-6 Linoleic Acid (LA) in Ancestrally Fed Vs Corn/Soy-Fed Chicken
(Expressed as % of Total Fat)

Ancestrally-Fed	GMO Corn / Soy Fed
2.5%	18.0%

Ancestrally-Fed: Prior IA, et al. Cholesterol, coconuts, and diet on Polynesian atolls: a natural experiment: the Pukapuka and Tokalau Island studies. Amer. J Clin Nutr. 1981;34(8):1552-1561. 2) GMO Corn/Soy Fed: USDA Food Data Central. Chicken, broiler or fryers, breast, skinless, boneless, meat only, cooked, braised. https://fdc.nal.usda.gov/fdc-app.html#/food-details/331960/nutrients. © C. Knobbe, 2022. Ancestral Health Foundation.

Omega-6 Linoleic Acid (LA) in Corn- and Soy-Fed (CAFO) Chicken Vs Ancestrally Fed Chicken

	Skinless Chicken Breast (6 Oz or 170 grams muscle meat)		~2 Skinless Chicken Thighs (6 Oz or 170 grams muscle meat)	
	Tyson Store-Bought Corn & Soy Fed	Angel Acres Farm Ancestrally Raised	Gold Leaf Corn & Soy Fed	Angel Acres Farm Ancestrally Raised
Total Linoleic Acid (LA) in Grams	0.42	0.06	2.79	0.53

Independent fatty acid analysis per The Fenton Lab, Michigan State University, with samples provided by Angel Acres Farm, Marcellus, Michigan. © C. Knobbe, 2022. Ancestral Health Foundation.

LA, whereas an ancestrally raised chicken breast (from Angel Acres Farm) had only 0.06 grams of LA. For the lean, skinless meat of approximately two chicken thighs (6 ounces, or 170 grams), the CAFO-raised corn- and soy-fed chicken thighs had 2.79 grams of LA whereas the ancestrally raised chicken thighs had only 0.53 grams of LA.

Thus, the CAFO-raised corn- and soy-fed chicken breast had 7 times as much LA as did the ancestrally raised chicken breasts, and the latter had only a trivial amount of total LA (0.07 grams). The LA content was also 5.3 times greater in the CAFO-raised (Gold Leaf) skinless chicken thighs and, importantly, the higher total fat content in the CAFO-raised chicken produced a very substantial amount of LA in just two thighs without the skin (2.79 grams).

One can see that store-bought, CAFO-raised, corn- and soy-fed chicken can be a very substantial source of LA, however, we also observe that the LA content of the skinless chicken breast, which is a lean cut of muscle meat, has a relatively low level of LA. As such, if ancestrally raised chicken is not affordable or available, consuming the leanest cuts of muscle meat from chicken, such as the chicken breast, would be the safest approach.

ANCESTRALLY FED VERSUS CORN- AND SOY-FED PORK

Pigs are monogastric omnivorous animals, just like humans, and also develop very high levels of LA in their body fat when fed GMO corn and soy.[1259] When consuming their traditional diet on the island of Tokelau, for example, pigs were found by Ian Prior and colleagues to have a body fat LA of just 2.0%.[17]

In contrast, pigs fed GMO corn and soy have been shown to develop body fat LA up to 20.0%[1266] and even 26.0%.[1259] Karl Holovach, of Frog Eye Meats, Knoxville, Maryland (no affiliation), raises

Omega-6 Linoleic Acid (LA) Ancestrally-Fed Vs Corn/Soy-Fed Pork
(Expressed as % of Total Fat)

Ancestrally Fed	Grain (Corn / Soy) Fed
2.0 – 4.25%	20.0%

1) Ancestrally fed: Prior IA, et al. Cholesterol, coconuts, and diet on Polynesian atolls: a natural experiment: the Pukapuka and Tokalau Island studies. Amer. J Clin Nutr. 1981;34(8):1552-1561. 2) Data courtesy of Karl Holovach, Frog Eye Meats, Medallion Labs Independent Analysis, 3 Mar 2021. © C. Knobbe, 2022. Ancestral Health Foundation.

a small herd of pork and cattle in ancestral fashion, without feeding corn and soy. The pigs are fed whole milk, fruits, and whatever they can forage on pasture, which might include grubs, insects, and even small animals. Holovach's pork samples were independently analyzed (Medallion Labs, Minneapolis, MN) and found to have just 4.25% LA, which is the lowest level that we're currently aware of in the U.S.[1267]

LA CONCENTRATION IN BEEF BURGERS VERSUS PLANT-BASED 'BURGERS'

Meat replacement 'burgers' have become more popular, perhaps out of unwarranted fear that meat drives overweight or chronic disease. However, once again, replacement of meat is proven potentially harmful. Researchers at the University of Padova, Legnaro, Italy, analyzed 24 samples of "meat-based burgers" and 27 different samples of "plant-based burgers" for fatty acid content.[1268]

The median (~average) meat-based burger contained 2.65% linoleic acid (LA) while the median plant-based burger contained 15.66% LA.[1267] Thus, for any given weight of total fat for each of the two, the plant-based burger will contain about six times more LA than the beef burger and also will contain no naturally present fat-soluble vitamins (A, D, or K2) or other important micronutrients like carnosine, carnitine, creatine, or vitamin B12.

ANCESTRAL VERSUS OTHER VARIETIES OF EGGS

Eggs are one of the most nutrient-dense foods available, containing all of the fat-soluble vitamins, A, D, K1, K2, and E, as well as thiamine (B1), riboflavin (B2), niacin (B3), pantothenic acid (B5), pyridoxine (B6), biotin (B7), folate (B9), cyanocobalamin (B12), choline, and a number of minerals.[1269] [1270] The shells can be eaten for calcium, either by eating the shell in its whole form or grinding it into a powder.

Eggs, however, are subject to accumulation of substantial amounts of LA when chickens (or other fowl, presumably) are fed a non-ancestral diet of corn and soy, which is the case in almost all CAFOs.

Ashley Armstrong, PhD, proprietor of Angel Acres Farms in Marcellus, Michigan, reviewed previously, runs a small flock of entirely ancestrally fed chickens for the purposes of producing nutrient-dense "low LA eggs." These eggs are also beyond organic, without a shred of chemicals in the feed or pasture.

Unlike CAFO-raised chickens that are nearly always fed GMO corn and soy, the Angel Acres chickens are raised traditionally, free to roam on pasture, while being fed an entirely organic diet of peas, barley, alfalfa, fresh grass, raw organic liver, beef tallow, and minerals, as well as insects, worms, small animals, etc. – whatever they can find on pasture. They're also exposed to an abundance of fresh air and natural sunlight.

Omega-6 Linoleic Acid (LA) % in 100% Beef Vs Plant-Based 'Burger'	
Meat-Based (Beef) Burger	**Plant-Based 'Burger'**
2.65%	15.66%

De Marchi M, Costa A, Pozza M, et al. Detailed characterization of plant-based burgers. Scientific Reports. 2021;11:2049.
© C. Knobbe, 2022. Ancestral Health Foundation.

Omega-6 Linoleic Acid (LA) % In Chicken Eggs (by Feed & Environment)
(Expressed as % of Total Fat)

	Ancestral Eggs (Diet of peas, barley, alfalfa, fresh grass, raw liver, beef tallow, worms, insects, minerals)	**"Pasture Raised"** (Diet of Non-GMO corn and soy)	**"Cage Free"** (Diet of GMO corn and soy)	**"CAFO Eggs"** (Typical grocery store eggs fed GMO corn and soy, kept in concentrated quarters)
LA (mg/egg)	176	465	585	734
Ratio of LA Expressed as Multiple of Ancestral Eggs	1.0	2.6	3.3	4.2

Data courtesy of Angel Acres Farm, Marcellus, Michigan. References: 1) Egg analyses for all groups except the "CAFO Eggs" independently performed at The Fenton Lab, Michigan State University. Data for "CAFO Eggs": USDA, FoodData Central. Eggs, Grade A, Large, egg whole.
© C. Knobbe, 2022. Ancestral Health Foundation.

The Angel Acres eggs ("Ancestral Eggs") and other groups were tested independently at The Fenton Lab, Michigan State University. Simultaneously, two more groups were tested, including, "pasture-raised" eggs from chickens fed a diet of non-GMO corn and soy (("Pasture-Raised"), and "Cage-Free" grocery store eggs fed a diet of GMO corn and soy. Finally, these groups were contrasted against grocery store "CAFO Eggs" fed a diet of GMO corn and soy where animals were kept in confined feeding operations (USDA studies).

In the table above, note that the Angel Acres eggs produced only 176 mg LA per egg, versus 465 mg/egg in the "Pasture-Raised" group, 585 mg/egg in the "Cage-Free" group, and 734 mg/egg in the "CAFO Eggs." Thus, as compared to the ancestrally raised eggs, the "Pasture-Raised" eggs contained 2.6 times more LA, the "Cage-Free" eggs 3.3 times more LA, and the "CAFO Eggs" produced 4.2 times more LA per egg (see table above).

The ancestrally raised eggs (Angel Acres Farms eggs) also are more nutrient-dense in a number of nutrients. For example, the ancestral eggs, as compared to "Cage-Free" eggs, contained 20% more B1, 55% more B3, 82% more B5, and 129% more vitamin E. Vitamin K1 (phylloquinone) was undetectable in the "Cage-Free" eggs but 0.09 µg/egg yolk in the ancestral eggs.

As previously reviewed, we recommend a goal of keeping LA at 2% of calories or less in our daily diets. On a 2,250 calorie/day diet, this amounts to 5 grams (45 calories) worth of LA. The ancestrally raised eggs (Angel Acres) produced only 0.70g LA in a total of four eggs, which is just 14% of the daily goal of LA. Contrast that to 1.86 g LA (37% of goal) for the "Pasture-Raised" eggs, 2.34 g LA (47% of goal) for the "Cage-Free" eggs, and 2.94 g LA (59% of goal) for the CAFO eggs. With this data, one can see how traditionally raised ancestral eggs provide tremendous nutrition with very little LA, while corn- and soy-fed chicken eggs rapidly devour one's daily LA goal. (See the table on page 318.)

WILD-CAUGHT VERSUS FARM-RAISED CORN- AND SOY-FED FISH

The complexities of consuming fish, whether farmed or wild-caught, is beyond the scope of this review. In general, we will assert that there are benefits to

CHAPTER 7

Daily Goal: Consume Less than or Equal to 5.0 g/LA/Day

Assume 4 Egg Breakfast: Total LA by Egg Type and Percent of Daily Goal

Egg Type	Grams LA in 4 Eggs	% of Daily LA Goal
Ancestral Eggs	0.70	14%
"Pasture Raised"	1.86	37%
"Cage-Free"	2.34	47%
CAFO Eggs	2.94	59%

Data courtesy of Angel Acres Farm, Marcellus, Michigan. References: 1) Egg analyses for all groups except the "CAFO Eggs" independently performed at The Fenton Lab, Michigan State University. Data for "CAFO Eggs": USDA, FoodData Central. Eggs, Grade A, Large, egg whole. © C. Knobbe, 2022. Ancestral Health Foundation.

consuming seafood and fish, however, wild-caught will almost always be safer. Fish that are farmed are typically fed a variety of plants, grains, soy, and vegetable oils, which is obviously not an ancestral diet for any type of fish.[1271] The deleterious changes in the fatty acid profiles of farm-raised versus wild-caught fish are so obvious in a given species that researchers can determine the fodder of a given fish based on the fatty acid profile. Farmed commercial fish have lower omega-3, higher omega-6, higher LA, and higher omega-6 to omega-3 ratios, as compared to their wild-caught counterparts.[1272]

Brazilian researchers analyzed the fatty acids in 21 species of wild-caught fish and 11 species of farmed fish, finding that the omega-6 to omega-3 ratio was generally between 1.0 and 2.0 in the wild-caught species whereas the farmed fish ratios were between 3.4 to 9.8.[1271]

Researchers from UiT The Arctic University of Norway, completed extensive fatty acid analyses of Atlantic salmon, which is one of the most commonly consumed salmon types.[1273] The researchers tested a large sample of wild-caught Atlantic salmon, farmed Atlantic salmon, and "escaped salmon," the latter group of which was comprised of 17 of the fish that were expected to be of the wild-caught variety but which had actually escaped from the farm. The "escaped salmon" were evaluated as a separate group.

The Norwegian researchers found that the wild-caught salmon had only 1.35% LA, versus 14.38% in the farmed group, and 12.8% in the escaped group. The LA content, in grams per 100g of fatty acids, was only 0.1g in wild-caught salmon, 2.5g in farmed, and 1.6g in the escaped. It is worth pointing out that the total LA content was 25 times higher in the farmed salmon than in the wild-caught! The total fat was also far lower in the wild-caught salmon at just 6g per 100 grams muscle, versus 17.9 g in the farmed, and 12.0 grams in the escaped. See the table on page 319 ("LA Content: Wild-Caught vs Farmed vs Escaped Salmon").

This is a striking difference in body fat in the

LA Content: Wild-Caught vs Farmed vs Escaped Salmon

	Wild-Caught	Farmed	Escaped
LA % (as % of total fatty acids)	1.35	14.38	12.8
LA Amount (g/100g muscle)	0.1	2.5	1.6
Total Fat (g/100 g muscle)	6.0	17.9	12.0

Jensen I-J. Eilertsen K-E, Otnaes CHA, et al. An Update on the Content of Fatty Acids, Dioxins, PCBs and Heavy Metals in Farmed, Escaped and Wild Atlantic Salmon (*Salmo salr* L.) in Norway. Foods. 2020;9:1901; doi:10.339/foods9121901.
© C. Knobbe, 2022. Ancestral Health Foundation.

fish on the high omega-6 diet, and strongly suggests that fish may develop many of the same complications from high omega-6 non-traditional diets, as do humans and other animals. With respect to the omega-6 LA in the fish as well as higher levels of omega-3 ALA, the authors wrote, "The high content of LA (18:2*n*-6) and alpha-linolenic acid (ALA (18:3*n*-3) in the farmed salmon illustrates the substantial inclusion of vegetable oils in the feed."[1272]

This is a very beneficial study because it concludes that the farming of fish, which includes soy and high omega-6 diets, not only produces high LA levels in the flesh of the fish, but makes the animals gain substantial fat, just as we've observed in humans and other animal studies. The "escaped" fish are also very intriguing because we can observe that, in just a short time in the ocean (less than one year) consuming a natural diet, body fat declined markedly, and LA content of the body fat also dropped precipitously.

It is extraordinary that the farmed salmon consuming the high omega-6 diet had three times as much body fat in their muscle as did the wild-caught salmon. However, as has been observed repeatedly, this is precisely what we see in humans, chickens, pork, and rodents. At least for monogastric animals, this appears to be a unifying negative effect on physiology.

An area of significant concern regarding fish consumption is the presence of heavy metal contaminants, particularly mercury.[1272] In nearly all cases, larger species have far higher mercury concentrations, as they have longer lives, consume more mercury, and accumulate more in their flesh.[1274] For example, the U.S. EPA tables show that salmon, a relatively small fish, has only 0.02 parts per million (ppm), whereas other fish had the following levels: Chilean sea bass at 0.35, Albacore tuna at 0.35, shark at 0.98, swordfish at 0.99, and Tilefish (Mexico) at 1.45.[1275]

Thus, even a typical Albacore tuna might have 17.5 times as much mercury as compared to salmon. A good rule of thumb is to primarily consume smaller fish, such as anchovies, sardines, salmon, cod, herring, mackerel, and flounder. Large fish such as tuna, shark, and swordfish consumption on a regular basis would be extraordinarily more likely to produce toxicity.

One final consideration is that animals in concentrated animal feeding operations (CAFOs) are treated inhumanely and without regard for their welfare. They are subjected to extraordinary confinement, inappropriate diets, and forced to live in unsanitary and polluted conditions. Such animals are treated with blatant disregard for their natural socialization, maternal instincts, or natural habitat. Omnivorous humans should, if possible, vote for sustainable, regenerative farmers and ranchers with your purchasing dollars. It's better for the animals and us.

THE BENEFITS OF A LOW LA ANCESTRAL DIET

Many people rapidly begin to lose undesirable weight and become healthier within just a few days or weeks of beginning a low LA diet. Furthermore, by completely eliminating seed oils from our diets, oxidation products (ALEs) in our blood will rapidly diminish, oxidized LDL (ox-LDL) will be reduced, and inflammatory mediators in the blood, such as eicosanoids, prostaglandins, leukotrienes, and thromboxanes, will all be reduced.[1276][1277][1278][1279] Collectively, this will result in reduced inflammation and a generalized reduction of heart attack and stroke risk, all within just hours or a few days of beginning such a diet.

Despite the fact that the half-life of LA in the body is 600 to 680 days,[664] which means that there could be a large reservoir of LA in our bodies (for those who have been consuming high LA diets), the longer we consume a low LA diet, the more active we are, and the more nutrient-dense our diet is, the better off we'll be.

Much like giving up smoking, the benefits of reducing LA in the diet may continue to accrue for perhaps eight to ten years! During this time, you will likely continue to become leaner (if needed), your risks of heart disease, stroke, cancers, and many other chronic diseases will progressively dissipate, and your energy and health should have tremendous overall improvements. Thousands of personal testimonials cannot be wrong.

For those who desire to quantify the amount of LA in their diet, we suggest considering the use of Cronometer (no affiliation), which is a downloadable free "app" (a small fee is required for mobile phone use) that allows one to enter food types and quantities in order to get a close approximation of nutrient consumption, including the amount of omega-6 LA in the diet. There are issues with any attempts to quantify LA consumption, however.

For example, as we've reviewed in this chapter, there are marked differences in LA content between ancestrally raised animals and CAFO raised animals (that are fed GMO corn and soy), which not only affects their meat, but also affects their milk, butter, and eggs. Pork lard, for example, derived from pigs raised in CAFOs, will likely be in the 20% LA range, but pork lard from ancestrally raised pigs, will be in the 2 to 4% range. There are also significant ranges in the LA content of oils, especially olive oil (3-27% LA). All such considerations are very important to health outcomes in our complicated food environment today

Cronometer will provide a fairly accurate assessment of omega-6 LA consumption if data is carefully entered. Furthermore, one can rank order foods with the highest omega-6 content by right clicking on the number, which will allow one to identify problem foods quickly. It is important to realize that Cronometer will only report total omega-6, so the omega-6 LA content is about 80 to 90% of the total omega-6.

CHAPTER 7: SUMMARY

Following "The LA Protocol" is remarkably simple but requires vigilance and a bit of time to plan and prepare foods. Processed foods almost by definition include the presence of either sugars, refined flours, seed oils, or combinations of these. This is why the first major step in moving to a low LA diet is to remove processed foods, which means eliminating all fast foods, many restaurant foods, and foods that are already packaged, prepared, boxed, or canned.

Preparing your own food is the best way to be certain of what you're consuming, and, with a little knowledge, you can make tremendous improvements in your diet very easily and rapidly, with extraordinary rewards.

Avoiding the high PUFA oils of soybean, corn, canola, rapeseed, grapeseed, sunflower, safflower, rice bran, and a few others is easy to accomplish if you prepare your own food. If you do not prepare your food, avoidance of these oils is not only strongly recommended, but it is without a doubt the key consideration to achieving high levels of vitality, health, and freedom from disease.

Cooking with butter (or clarified butter/ghee) works well in almost every case. Butter is low in LA (~2%), high in saturated and monounsaturated fats, and contains vitamins A, D, and K2, making this perhaps the healthiest cooking fat. Coconut and palm kernel oils are exceedingly low in LA and should be considered healthy alternatives to butter. However, keep in mind that coconut oil, palm kernel oil, and macadamia nut oil, all of which are very low in LA, do not contain any vitamins A, D, or K2. Cacao butter (2% LA)[1280] is nearly equivalent to coconut and palm kernel oils, but because it may have a slight chocolate and/or nutty flavor, it might best be used in desserts.

Nuts and seeds and their oils should be considered as large potential sources of LA and we recommend greatly restricting, or better yet, eliminating these. Nuts and seeds, as well as their oils, are certainly less harmful than seed oils, but overall, cannot "hold a candle" to traditionally raised butter or beef tallow. Cooking with traditionally raised grass-fed butter or beef tallow is strongly recommended as both will be exceedingly low in LA. Pork lard from traditionally raised swine on pasture, which consume all-natural diets (e.g., animals left to forage), will result in exceedingly low LA levels as well.

Unfortunately, it is quite challenging to find these types of foods, as they are not typically commercially available. Use of the website EatWild.com (no affiliation) and the Weston A. Price Foundation's associated website, RealMilk.com (no affiliation), will both be beneficial in this regard. To the best of our knowledge, there are no relatively large-scale commercial chicken farm operations that do not provide corn and soy fodder, which, of course, results in the high LA levels. Fortunately, however, there are now a number of smaller farming operations raising chickens on pasture that are both corn and soy free, and we would strongly recommend considering these if chicken is consumed regularly.

The evidence is overwhelming that consuming ancestrally raised animals and their products results in far less LA consumption. This is most critical when we consume monogastric animals, including pork, fowl, and fish. The difference in the case of ruminant animals, with regard to LA content, between 100% grass-fed and corn- and soy-fed, is not that substantial. Therefore, we would submit that consuming CAFO-raised beef, at approximately 3% LA in the fat, would be far superior to consuming most vegetable oil fat, which generally ranges from about 10% to 78% LA. Olive oil, of course, averages around 10% LA.

A low LA diet will rapidly begin to produce positive results for everyone, reducing the risk of heart attacks and strokes, perhaps within hours to days of beginning such a diet. Within a few weeks, most people will begin to have improvements in their body composition. The long-term results are beyond comprehension or description.

Though prevention is never as glamorous or exciting as intervention, in our view, preventing heart disease, heart attacks, strokes, cancers, metabolic disease, type 2 diabetes, overweight, and so much more, reigns king. But remember, almost all cases of overweight and most types of chronic disease are reversible. The earlier we begin and the more consistent we are, the better the results.

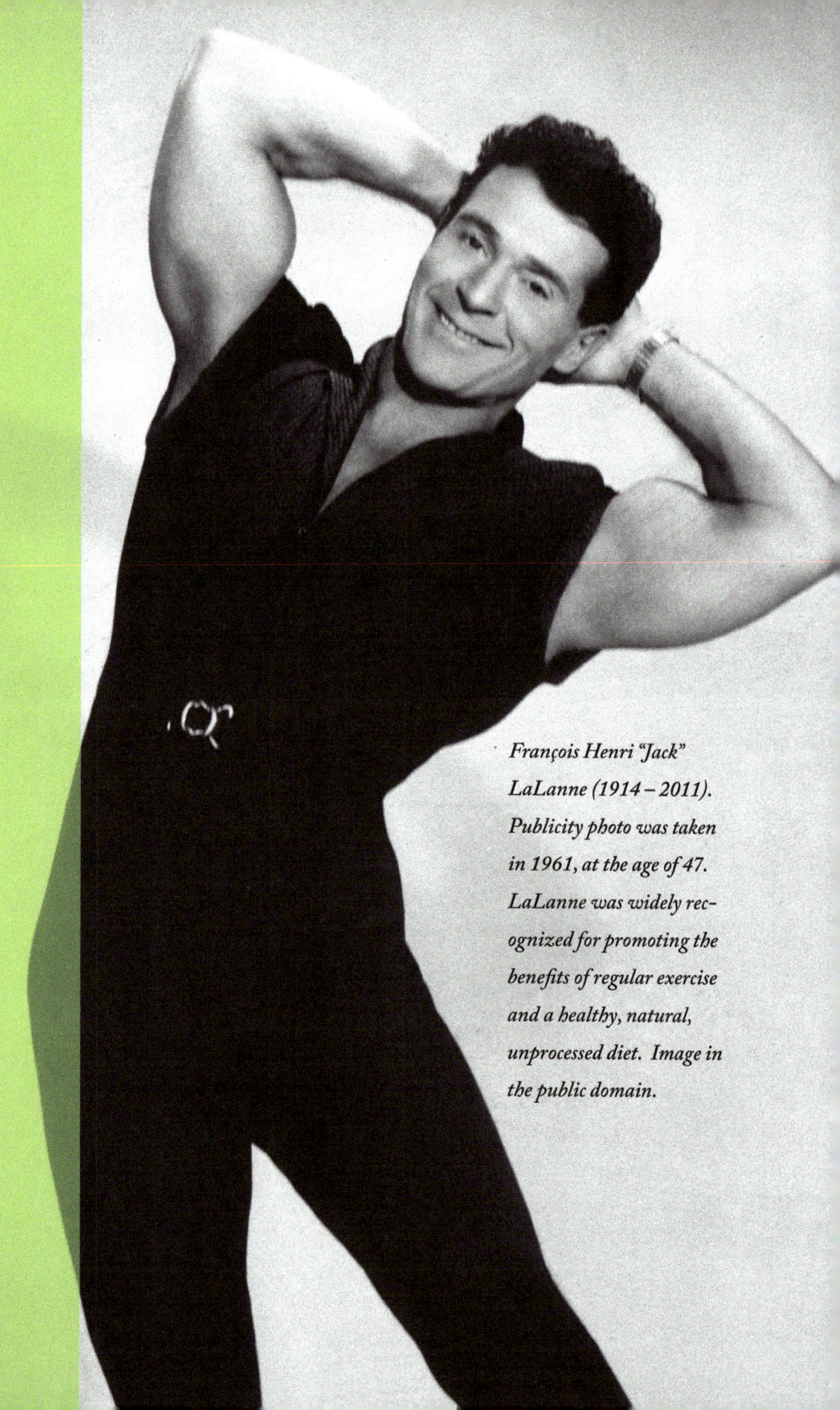

CHAPTER 8

François Henri "Jack" LaLanne (1914 – 2011). Publicity photo was taken in 1961, at the age of 47. LaLanne was widely recognized for promoting the benefits of regular exercise and a healthy, natural, unprocessed diet. Image in the public domain.

CHAPTER 8

EAT ANCESTRALLY AND MOVE

"If man made it, don't eat it."

— JACK LALANNE

As simple as ancestral diets are, our world has presented so many obstacles to consuming such diets that deep thought, investigation, and consideration are critical to maintaining not only our own health but also the health of our loved ones. If we could travel back in time to the year 1865, consuming a densely nutritious, safe, ancestral diet would have been extremely simple. Practically all one would have to do is eat a variety of foods!

Today, the food environment is chock full of culinary land mines. Navigating around these dangers, we will admit, is not easy. However, the rewards from understanding and implementing an ancestral diet are beyond description. It will undoubtedly be gratifying and potentially lifesaving, while producing vitality, energy, and increasing longevity. Spreading the message to your family and friends might do the same for them.

ELIMINATE PROCESSED FOODS – IT'S WORTH REPEATING

Though we've probably beaten this one to death, drastically reducing or eliminating processed foods is the most fundamental objective to lose undesirable weight, enhance health, and prevent or reverse chronic disease rapidly and permanently. Processed foods exact their destructive toll on your mind and body through two synergizing effects: 1) Nutrient deficiency and 2) Toxicity.

Processed foods, which are essentially refined sugars and flours, seed oils, and artificially produced trans fats, collectively are almost entirely devoid of vitamins and minerals which are contained in whole, natural foods, such as meats, fowl, fish, fruits, vegetables, eggs, dairy, and whole grains. Secondly, seed oils and trans fats are enormous sources of toxicity that exact their destructive effects through pro-oxidative, pro-inflammatory, toxic, and nutrient-depleting effects.

If we eliminate processed foods in one fell swoop, our health begins to improve within hours to days. This sounds simple and indeed it is, but if one has become accustomed to consuming the foods of modern commerce, then reverting to an all-natural diet that is made up exclusively of ancestrally raised animal meats (which include beef, pork, poultry, and fish) and eggs, plus fruits, vegetables, whole grains, and dairy, may prove to be a challenging task. However, the rewards may be so rapid and gratifying that the task will soon become second nature.

In order to simplify this process, however, we might suggest beginning with a stepwise approach. First, invoke the 80/20 rule. In this case, we believe that 80% of the benefits can be achieved with just 20% of the effort, and that 20% of the effort is simply to eliminate all seed oils from your diet. The easiest approach to keep this exceedingly simple is to avoid all foods with oils in them. If this is a bit overwhelming, then we suggest eliminating all oils with the exception of coconut, palm kernel, macadamia nut, or cacao butter, all of which are about 2% LA. Remember that butter and beef tallow are even safer and far superior in the vital fat-soluble vitamins A, D, and K2, which, of course, are not present in coconut oil, palm kernel oil, macadamia nut oil, or cacao butter (or any vegetable oils).

FRACTALS OF HEALTH: TAKE THE NEXT BIG STEPS

Once elimination of seed oils has been successfully accomplished, you might soon begin to appreciate obvious and marked improvements in your health, including desirable weight loss and notable improvements in the signs or symptoms of any chronic disease. At this point, the next steps are to remove most processed foods, refined sugars, refined flours, and then, finally, attempt to entirely remove genetically modified (GMO) foods.

Removing sugars in our diets does not include removing the naturally occurring sugars in fruits, raw honey, and pure maple syrup (made from 100% maple sap), but this does involve eliminating foods with added sugars. Eliminating sugar-sweetened beverages, including fruit juices with added sugars, will almost always be beneficial. Increasing natural, whole fruit consumption, however, has often been shown to be beneficial to weight loss.[1281][1282][1283]

Added processed sugars are indeed "empty calories," and may contribute to nutrient deficiencies if the remainder of the diet is not nutrient-dense. Removing (or reducing) sugars is, therefore, an excellent second step after removing seed oils. In fact, if one eliminates both seed oils and sugars, these two steps alone may achieve 90% or more of the benefits of moving towards a more ancestral diet.

Following the removal of seed oils and sugars, the next step is to remove refined flours. This step eliminates foods that contain "white flour," "enriched white wheat flour," or other similar refined flours, opting instead for whole grain flours, if well tolerated. Whole grain flour, which includes the bran and germ of the wheat kernel, provides natural B vitamins, minerals, small amounts of omega-3 and omega-6 fatty acids, and proteins.

Whole grains are whole foods and, once again, such a diet modification increases nutrient-density, which may benefit health in many ways. Some people, of course, may have gut disturbances associated with wheat or gluten, such as those with celiac disease, and elimination of wheat (all forms), rye, and barley may be a requirement for both general health and gut health.[1284]

Next, we suggest removing genetically modified organism (GMO) type foods, which include almost all currently produced non-organic soybeans, corn, sugar beets, canola, and cottonseed oil.[1285] Some fresh fruits and vegetables are also available in GMO varieties, including certain potatoes, summer squash, apples, and papayas. GMO-based foods are exceedingly likely to produce deleterious effects on health, as they not only have been sprayed with and contain the herbicide glyphosate (Roundup weed spray), but perhaps the modified food itself is also problematic.[1285]

Choosing to eat only organic foods will help reduce exposure to the pervasive dietary toxin glyphosate (as well as other herbicides and pesticides). The best resource for this is the book *Toxic Legacy* written by our friend and colleague, Stephanie Seneff, PhD, who is a senior scientist at Massachusetts Institute of Technology (MIT).[1286]

The American Academy of Environmental Medicine (AAEM) concludes that GMO foods induce serious health risks, including infertility, immune dysfunction, accelerated aging, insulin dysregulation, and altered functions of major organs, particularly the gastrointestinal system.[1287] The AAEM concludes that this is not a casual association, but rather, rises to the level of undeniable causation. Avoiding GMOs is the next big step to a healthier lifestyle and the beneficial effects may even preserve life.

Another consideration to ancestral health may be time-restricted feeding (TRF), which has been touted for its many benefits.[1288] The cycling of feasting (feeding) and famine (fasting) is believed by many to mimic the eating habits of our ancestors and, thereby, to restore our physiology to a more natural state that allows a whole host of biochemical benefits to occur. There is some evidence that TRF may facilitate weight loss[1289] but also helps to reduce the risk of chronic diseases like Type 2 diabetes,[1290] heart disease,[1291] cancer,[1292] and Alzheimer's disease.[1293]

While there are many variations, TRF typically involves not eating for about 12 to 14 consecutive hours a day. In general, this means that one would eat all meals for the day within an 8 to 12-hour window, or even less. For example, if the last meal of the day is consumed by 7:00 PM and the next meal is consumed at 9:00 AM, this has provided a 14-hour fast. Among the many benefits of TRE is the upregulation of autophagy and mitophagy — natural cleansing processes necessary for optimal cellular renewal and function.[1294]

TRF should not be universally practiced since many people, especially women, may have maladaptive responses to a short eating window. For example, Ramadan fasting, where participants refrain from eating or drinking from dawn to sunset, has been shown to increase nocturnal cortisol (stress hormone) levels,[1295][1296] reduce melatonin production,[1297][1298] decrease rapid eye movement (REM) sleep (indicating reduced sleep benefits),[1299] depress thyroid hormone T4 in those with hypothyroidism,[1300] and may even induce excessive menstrual bleeding (menorrhagia) or cause a reduction or elimination of menses (oligomenorrhea).[1301]

However, even though this eating technique is not universally beneficial, some may experience significant benefits. Therefore, TRF may be a consideration for some, and it appears that, in general, men may tolerate TRF better than women. In all cases, we suggest "listening" to your body and making individual judgments as to the benefits of a restricted eating window.

MORE OPTIMAL HEALTH: CONSUME PASTURE-RAISED ANIMALS AND WILD-CAUGHT FISH

The next step in achieving more optimum health will be to consume pasture-raised animals, which have consumed their own native, traditional diets. For beef, buffalo, and bison, this is 100% organically grown grass. Ancestrally raised pigs and chickens, which are both omnivores, normally consume diverse diets of plants, insects, earthworms, small animals, roots, fruits, and grains while living on pasture, exposed to sunshine, and allowed to forage, root in the soil, and freely roam.[1302][1303] All such animals in nature consume far lower LA in their diets and thus have lower LA in their own fat. This makes them far healthier for us to consume.

Wild-caught fish, likewise, have far healthier fatty acid profiles as compared to farm-raised fish, which are typically fed GMO soy and vegetable oils, very similar to land animals held in concentrated animal feeding operations (CAFOs).[1304] Wild-caught fish have markedly lower omega-6 LA, much more long-chain omega-3 EPA and DHA, more of a number of minerals, and, of course, markedly lower levels of the Roundup herbicidal poison, glyphosate, because they've not consumed GMO soy like most farm-raised fish today.[1303][1305]

MOST OPTIMAL HEALTH: ADD OFFAL, COD LIVER OIL, FISH EGGS, AND OTHER NUTRIENT-RICH SOURCES OF VITAMINS AND MINERALS

One of the last major steps in achieving our highest level of health, which also benefits overweight and chronic disease (if the latter exists), is to consume the foods that are the most nutrient-dense sources of vitamins and minerals. As reviewed, it is the fat-soluble vitamins A, D, and K2 that are the most difficult to get but which also have the most significant impact on health and disease.

These three fat-soluble vitamins are not widely distributed in the food supply and, therefore, understanding their food sources is of critical importance. **As shown by E.V. McCollum and Weston A. Price, the foods richest in these three fat-soluble vitamins are primarily grass-fed butter, eggs, fish roe (eggs), whole raw milk, cod liver oil, and offal, the latter of which are the organs of animals, especially the liver.**

Beef fat (tallow or suet) is a close second to these other animal fats in terms of supplying the critical fat-soluble vitamins, however, pork lard alone does not contain enough of these vitamins to properly support growth or maintain health in adulthood. Ancestrally raised pigs obviously will produce low LA meat, but since pork lard alone is not sufficient for obtaining all of the fat-soluble vitamins, other sources of these vitamins (as listed above) should be consumed as well.

Weston A. Price found that many traditionally living cultures considered such foods to be sacred. In fact, their "accumulated wisdom," as Price called it, had been passed down through many generations with teachings that such foods were indeed the key to healthy babies, proper growth and development in children, and the prevention of disease in adulthood.[28] Price found that all healthy, traditionally living people regularly consumed one or more of the above list of foods that are so rich in these critically important fat-soluble vitamins.

Fat-soluble vitamins are critical to the utilization of minerals in the body. As reviewed previously, Price found that no amount of minerals could provide benefit without proper amounts of fat-soluble vitamins (see quote below). Once these are provided in sufficient quantity, adequate consumption of all the minerals and trace minerals becomes of great importance, and this would include calcium, phosphorous, iron, sodium, chloride, potassium, zinc, magnesium, copper, and many others. In 1939, Price wrote the following:

"It is possible to starve for minerals that are abundant in the foods eaten because they cannot be utilized without an adequate quantity of the fat-soluble activators [vitamins A, D, and K2 (Price's Activator X")].[1306]

The evidence for this is ubiquitous and perhaps the best current example is the extraordinary use and consumption of calcium supplements, but with ever-increasing osteoporosis due to both vitamin D and K2 deficiency.[1307] One of the major functions of vitamin D is to drive calcium absorption in the gut (intestine).[1308] Vitamin K2 drives calcium into teeth and bones, while deficiency causes calcium to be deposited into soft tissues, such as arterial walls.[1082] Hence, in part, the current epidemic of osteoporosis and calcified arteries (the latter of which is an aspect of atherosclerosis).

With respect to mineral *utilization* (not the minerals themselves), the best foods to eat would be organic, ancestrally raised organs. Typically, beef liver or chicken liver would be the most common sources. While a few ounces a week may be extremely beneficial for a period of time, the amount consumed over the long-term will depend entirely on an individual's condition and initial degree of deficiency (if such exists). Over the long-term, consumption may need to be substantially reduced if nutrient sufficiency is achieved. In fact, organ meats may not be required at all once optimal nutrient status has been attained.

We believe, however, that long-term consumption of just small amounts of liver is very beneficial, for example, consumption of just 0.5 ounces (~ 15 grams) of 100% grass-fed liver per day, several times per week. When consumed chronically, we believe one should likely not consume more than three to four ounces of beef liver per week.

It is most difficult and perhaps impossible to make broad recommendations for consumption of dense sources of the fat-soluble vitamins, as bio-individuality, past consumption, acute and chronic stressors, and many other factors must be taken into consideration. However, we might suggest that for most people, consuming 2 to 4 ounces of organ meats per week may be very beneficial. A suggestion may be to alternate between consuming sources of beef liver, chicken liver, and fish liver (e.g., smoked cod liver).

Many people object to the taste of organ meats such as liver and may desire to choose foods such as liverwurst, which has added spices to enhance palatability. Consumption of organ meats (such as liver) mixed into meatloaf may be another easy way to increase consumption while improving flavor.

For those not consuming organ meats, cod liver (e.g., smoked cod liver), cod liver oil (CLO), or extra virgin cod liver oil (EVCLO) might well be considered. However, fish oils of any type are fragile molecules that may oxidize easily. The fact that the oils may oxidize might well be deemed harmful, however, there are further considerations here. First, the oils are best extracted cold and should be bottled in dark glass, kept out of light, stored in cool conditions, and consumed soon after bottling. Second, the purpose of CLO, or the more favorable EVCLO, is to provide vitamins A and D.

Vitamins A and D are best obtained through other sources, especially eggs, butter, whole raw milk, and organ meats, plus sunlight exposure of bare, 'unprotected' skin (for vitamin D). However, for those who are not consuming these foods and getting some sunlight exposure regularly, EVCLO may be the next best option.

If used, dosing of EVCLO will depend on age, body weight, previous nutrition, degree of stress, current condition (recent illness or infection will increase the need for vitamin A), and other factors. However, according to the Weston A. Price Foundation, as a general rule-of-thumb, children 3 months to 12 years of age may benefit from ½ to 1 teaspoon per day.[1309] Children over age 12 years up to adults may require long-term dosing of 1 to 2 teaspoons per day. Pregnant and nursing women may greatly benefit from 2 to 4 teaspoons daily.

Another valuable option for obtaining the fat-soluble vitamins A, D, and K2, for those who are unable for any reason to consume fresh organs, is to consume desiccated (dried) organs. Excellent sources of desiccated organs to consider include Heart & Soil Supplements, which is an organization founded by Paul Saladino, MD, and Paleovalley Supplements (no affiliation with either organization). Each of these organizations produces desiccated organ supplements from cattle that are 100% grass-fed and pasture raised.

FINAL DIETARY TWEAKS: BASED ON NUTRIENT TESTING

In some cases, even when the diet appears to be sufficient and optimal in every regard and is consumed for a prolonged duration, health status may remain sub-par. Perhaps one still has fatigue, dry skin, dry eyes, joint pains, arthritis, gut disturbances, wobbly gait, "brain fog," poor libido, poor exercise tolerance, or any number of other signs and symptoms that haven't resolved while consuming an ancestral diet. In this scenario, we strongly advise completing a wide variety of nutritional tests in order to assess such status.

Then, in many such cases, one can target deficiencies or sub-optimal status to improve or resolve such issues. An argument can be made to do the aforementioned testing initially, however, this is an individual decision that we believe is best made based on one's individual circumstances.

Testing of the nutritional status can be broadly-based or fine-tuned. A broadly-based nutrient status may include a complete blood count (CBC), complete metabolic profile (CMP), serum levels of vitamins A, D, K, B1, B2, B3, B5, B9, B12, iron panel, serum levels of copper, selenium, and zinc, RBC-magnesium, blood lipid panel including oxidized LDL (Ox-LDL), TSH, free T4, fasting serum insulin, glucose, hemoglobin A1c (HgbA1c), and heavy metal panel. This is a very basic evaluation but may uncover many potential deficiencies, sub-optimal nutrient levels, or toxicities (only heavy metals in this case). Unfortunately, evaluation of adipose (body fat) fatty acids to assess LA is only completed in scientific studies.

The great majority of conventionally trained physicians (medical doctors or osteopathic physicians) will not be familiar with vitamin and mineral testing and, in some cases, consultation with a functional medicine practitioner, integrative medical practitioner, naturopath, holistic physician, nutrition practitioner, nutritional therapy practitioner, certified nutritionist, nutritional therapist or comparable, may be very beneficial, provided they have experience and expertise in this area.

EXERCISE AND FITNESS: FINAL CRITICAL COMPONENTS OF HEALTH

As discussed in previous chapters, many ancestrally living populations were extremely fit, often described as being lean and muscular even into their elder years. Thus, the need to discuss the importance of maintaining or increasing muscle mass as we age is very important.

The benefits of exercise are perhaps beyond description, but according to researchers, it is clear that exercise helps to "reduce the risk of all-cause mortality, chronic disease, and premature death."[1310] Regular exercise, including aerobic, resistance, and stretching exercises are all important to maintaining strength, balance, coordination, and avoidance of falls.

In fact, there is an abundance of solid evidence that exercise is an effective preventative strategy against more than 25 chronic medical conditions, including cardiovascular disease, stroke, hypertension, colon cancer, breast cancer, and type 2 diabetes.[1311]

Loss of muscle mass, or sarcopenia, which is often associated with aging, may contribute to weakness, frailty, much greater risk of falls, and even increase the risk for chronic diseases.[1312] Sarcopenia and degenerative conditions of muscle may lead to loss of insulin sensitivity, which may contribute to metabolic disorders including diabetes.[1313] Conversely, the development of diabetes may contribute to a decline in muscle mass, strength, and function leading to increased risk of physical disability, fractures, and mortality.[1314] [1315] [1316]

Any kind of exercise is better than none. For those who have been sedentary for years, who are aging, or plagued with disabilities, our advice is to focus on what you can realistically accomplish. This might include taking walks and perhaps mild resistance exercises, such as body weight squats, climbing a few stairs, sit-ups, and lifting very light dumbbells.

For those who are capable, it is our belief that resistance exercise may be more beneficial than "cardio" type exercise, the latter of which might include walking, jogging, treadmills, elliptical machines, and the like. Resistance exercise is, without question, the best way to increase or maintain muscle mass. Such exercise types might include body-weight exercises, such as squats, push-ups, pull-ups, and sit-ups.

For more elite athletes, a much more aggressive workout plan may include weightlifting, including heavy squats, deadlifts, bench presses, curls, pull-ups, and a variety of abdominal exercises. Athletes in this category may well want to include high-intensity interval training (HIIT), which includes brief episodes of intense physical activity (usually 15 to 30 seconds) followed by very short intervals of rest (e.g., 10 seconds), over a period of approximately three to four minutes. Multiple sets may be accomplished for maximum effect. Such exercise regimens may help to produce favorable body composition changes, that is, loss of body fat combined with muscle gain, which are more effective than moderate-intensity continuous training regimens.[1308] [1317]

OPTIONS FOR FARM FRESH PRODUCE AND ANCESTRALLY FED MEATS

If you live in the U.S., the following (non-affiliated) organizations may help to locate farm-fresh, organic, and ancestrally raised foods (listed in alphabetical order):

American Grassfed Association (AGA)

The goal of the American Grassfed Association is to promote the grass-fed industry through government relations, research, concept marketing, and public education. Their website also allows one to search for AGA-approved producers certified according to strict standards that include being raised on a diet of 100 percent forage; raised on pasture and never confined to a feedlot; never treated with antibiotics or hormones; and born and raised on American family farms.

Community Involved in Sustaining Agriculture (CISA)

CISA is dedicated to sustaining agriculture and promoting the products of small farms.

Demeter USA

Demeter-USA.org provides a directory of certified Biodynamic farms and brands, which create healthy soils using compost and crop and grazing rotations. This directory can also be found on BiodynamicFood.org.

Eat Well Guide

Wholesome Food from Healthy Animals — The Eat Well Guide is a free online directory of sustainably raised meat, poultry, dairy, and eggs from farms, stores, restaurants, inns, hotels, and online outlets in the United States and Canada.

EatWild.com

EatWild.com provides lists of farmers known to produce raw dairy products as well as grass-fed beef and other farm-fresh produce (although not all are certified organic). Here you can also find information about local farmers markets, as well as local stores and restaurants that sell grass-fed products.

Farmers Markets

A national listing of farmers markets: **https://www.ams.usda.gov/services/local-regional**.

Grassfed Exchange

The Grassfed Exchange has a listing of producers selling organic and grass-fed meats across the U.S.

Local Harvest

This website will help you find farmers markets, family farms, and other sources of sustainably grown food in your area where you can buy produce, grass-fed meats, and many other naturally raised foods.

RealMilk.com

If you're still unsure of where to find raw milk, check out Raw-Milk-Facts.com and RealMilk.com. These sites provide up-to-date status on the legal requirements for raw milk by state and a listing of raw dairy farms in your area. The Farm to Consumer Legal Defense Fund also provides a state-by-state review of raw milk laws. California residents can also find raw milk retailers using the store locator available at **www.OrganicPastures.com**.

The Cornucopia Institute

The Cornucopia Institute maintains web-based tools rating all certified organic brands of eggs, dairy products, and other commodities based on their ethical sourcing and authentic farming practices separating CAFO "organic" production from authentic organic practices.

Weston A. Price Foundation

The Weston A. Price Foundation has local chapters in most states. Many of them are connected with buying clubs in which you can easily purchase organic foods, including grass-fed raw dairy products like milk and butter.

OUR 10 MAJOR RULES TO TAKE CHARGE OF YOUR HEALTH DESTINY

Listed in order of most to least important, here are our top ten recommendations to lose undesirable weight and prevent or even reverse most chronic disease.

1. Avoid all High-PUFA 'Vegetable Oils'

The oils of soybean, corn, canola, cottonseed, rapeseed, grapeseed, sunflower, safflower, and rice bran should be strictly eliminated when possible. Sesame and peanut oils are definitely safer but not recommended. Palm oil and avocado oils are far safer still. Given issues with adulteration, olive oil should only be consumed if one can verify that it is authentic and extra virgin (EVOO); however, cooking with olive oil is best avoided, that is, it is better consumed fresh and without cooking. Coconut and palm kernel oils are the safest oils but are not as nutrient-dense as animal fats.

In order to strictly avoid seed oils, carefully read every label on foods you purchase and be especially cautious when you are eating out. If you want to take it to the advanced level, use Cronometer.com, carefully enter all your consumed foods, and aim for a goal omega-6 LA intake of less than or about 2% of your calories. This will require calculating your own omega-6 LA consumption and recall that LA is approximately 90% of total omega-6 consumed.

2. Animal Fats Are Best for Cooking

When high heat cooking is used, animal fats, such as grass-fed butter, ghee, beef tallow, suet, or pasture-raised ancestrally fed lard (rendered pork fat) are all best. If such animal fats are not available or a vegan or vegetarian diet is preferred, coconut oil, palm kernel oil, or macadamia nut oils are the next best options.

3. Markedly Reduce or Eliminate Processed Foods

This will include the reduction or elimination of manufacturer prepared foods, such as packaged, boxed, canned, and otherwise ready-to-eat foods. Fast foods and many restaurant foods that contain seed oils should also be eliminated if at all possible.

4. Reduce or Eliminate Refined Sugars and Flours

Such reduction may include the removal of added sugars from sugar-sweetened beverages such as sodas, fruit juices, tea, and coffee, but also most commercially prepared desserts, cookies, cakes, candies, and other confectioneries.

5. Must-Have Sources of Fat-soluble Vitamins (A, D, and K2)

These vitamins are not widely distributed in the food-supply, and one must be vigilant to be sure that the diet is plentiful. The best dietary sources include grass-fed butter, whole raw (unpasteurized) milk, ancestrally raised chicken eggs, a variety of organ meats (e.g., beef liver, chicken liver, and fish liver), raw cheeses and hard cheeses, fish eggs (roe), and extra virgin cod liver oil. The need for such vitamins will vary tremendously depending on past consumption and various stressors. Muscle meats from ancestrally raised cattle, pigs, chicken, fish, and shellfish can be consumed as desired; for omnivores, these foods should generally anchor the diet.

6. Whole Food Sources of Fruits, Vegetables, Tubers (e.g., potatoes, yams, taro), Legumes, and Whole Grains

These foods may range in consumption from smaller amounts of the diet or nearly the entire diet and either approach is consistent with a healthy, ancestral, traditional diet. Use of these foods will depend entirely on which foods are most compatible with one's desired cuisine. In all cases, attention to ancestral detail of preparation is important. For example, grains are best consumed whole and after sprouting.

7. Regular Sun Exposure and Sleep

In addition to increasing one's vitamin D level, regular sun exposure will help to optimize circadian rhythm as well as to provide one with near infrared light, which will improve mitochondrial health and blood pressure by increasing your nitric oxide levels. Sun exposure is proven to help with sleep, which is essential for optimum health and should also be a top priority.

8. Exercise

Regular movement throughout the day is ideal rather than a simple 30-60-minute visit to the gym. Resistance exercise is preferred over traditional "cardio" type exercises, as resistance exercise better preserves muscle mass. However, all forms of exercise are beneficial, and variety and enjoyment should be the focus.

9. If Affordable, Eat Organic Foods

Eating organic is one of the easiest ways to optimize our nutrition without supplementation. Studies have repeatedly shown that organic foods have much lower pesticide residues and contain higher amounts of health-promoting nutrients.

10. If 100% Grass-fed, Pastured, and Organic Foods Are Not Affordable – Not to Worry!

It is our belief that 80% of the problem in our modern-day food supply is the ubiquitous presence of seed oils alone. Simply by eliminating the toxic and dangerous oils and most processed foods will produce extraordinary benefits.

As such, if ancestrally raised animal meats (e.g., beef, pork, chicken, fish, and shellfish) are not available for any reason, it is our advice to strongly consider cuts of beef (even CAFO raised) as the primary animal meat consumed, since the LA content will always be low, even when corn- and soy-fed (e.g. in CAFOs). Second, in this same scenario (if choosing CAFO raised), choose leaner cuts of pork and fowl (e.g., chicken breasts and lean pork), which will further reduce omega-6 LA consumption. Finally, consuming conventionally raised produce is far better than consuming processed, nutrient-deficient foods.

CHAPTER 8: SUMMARY

Ancestral diets are made up primarily of whole, unprocessed foods, including meats, fowl, fish, eggs, raw dairy, fruits, vegetables, and whole grains. With these fundamental ingredients and any desired herbs and spices, virtually any type of food can be prepared in traditional fashion. Vegetable oils will have no place in any such diet and refined sugars and flours will be substantially minimized or eliminated.

With such a simple philosophy, literally any recipe can be made in traditional, ancestral fashion. Whether one desires American, French, Chinese, Japanese, German, Korean, Mexican, or any other cuisine, simply prepare the dish using ancestrally appropriate ingredients. If the recipe calls for any type of vegetable oil, simply substitute a good quality, ancestrally raised butter, lard, or beef tallow, or perhaps use coconut oil, macadamia nut oil, or palm kernel oil for the safest low LA cooking.

For cooking under high heat, animal fats will generally be safest, however, if large amounts of cooking fats are needed and animal fats are unavailable, coconut oil or palm kernel oil might be the best options. For nearly all cooking, we almost exclusively use high-quality 100% grass-fed butter, beef tallow, or suet, all of which are derived from cattle that graze only on organic grasslands. If no cooking fat is desired, use of filtered or spring water may also be beneficial.

GMO foods should be carefully avoided, if possible, by choosing non-GMO and preferably organic options. This is key in avoiding the risks of the pervasively present poisonous herbicide, glyphosate, as well as many other toxic herbicides and pesticides.

Consuming pasture-raised, 100% grass-fed ungulates (cattle, bison, elk, deer, etc.) and ancestrally fed animals such as chicken, fowl, pig, fish, and shellfish are all ways to further reduce omega-6 consumption. In all cases, the animals we eat should, preferably, have consumed their own native, traditional diet. The avoidance of CAFO-raised animals, whether cattle, pigs, chicken, fish, or other fauna, is another major step towards a healthier, lower LA diet.

However, if the cost of 100% grass-fed, grass-finished, organically raised cattle, or ancestrally raised animals such as chicken, pigs, or wild-caught fish is unaffordable, we would advise to simply choose conventionally raised forms of these animals. And in this case, conventionally raised beef (or other ruminants) will have the lowest LA given that they are polygastric animals. When choosing the meats of conventionally raised chicken, pigs, or farm-raised fish, it would generally be wisest to choose the leanest cuts in order to further reduce LA consumption.

Regular exercise and, particularly, resistance exercise, is very beneficial to overall health and achievement of health goals. Furthermore, regular sun exposure of 'unprotected' skin is a critical component of health.

Implementing an ancestral diet is actually very simple but will require vigilance and persistence. By far and away, the best way to accomplish this is by preparing all or nearly all of your own food, which has been procured by yourself, utilizing the knowledge gained herein.

Take charge of your health destiny. Be a positive influence and example to your children, family, friends, and colleagues. Most of all, stay focused on one simple law of Nutrition and Medicine: Eating only the foods provided by God in Nature will deliver nourishment to your mind and body that will provide for a long, healthy life, full of vitality. It's the greatest investment you will ever make in yourself and your family.

EPILOGUE

It has been our pleasure and honor to write and present this book to you. We hope and pray that we have been able to convey a substantial slice of our knowledge regarding ancestral health to you and that this will impact not only your life but the lives of your beloved families, friends, and colleagues. We thank you for not only buying this book but for spreading this message. We've seen the devastation of westernized diets and seed oils not only in our medical, health, and nutrition practices, but also in our friends and in our own families. The suffering and premature death are not only unnecessary, but also, tragic. It is, furthermore, a travesty because the pain, suffering, misery, and death are entirely preventable with ancestral diets.

The take-home messages of *The Ancestral Diet Revolution* are elegantly simple: Drastically reduce or eliminate all seed oils from the diet and greatly limit added sugars and refined flours. In a nutshell, avoid man-made, processed foods. The easiest way to accomplish this, and perhaps the only way for most people, is to prepare your own food so that you are in control of the ingredients.

We hope that you will appreciate that our goals are altruistic and humanitarian. Among our goals include research efforts that we hope will forever transform modern medicine. These goals are, in part, centered around plans for a broad-based 21st century version of Weston A. Price's studies. Such studies will compare the health and diets of 5 or 6 populations around the world who are still consuming ancestral diets to their genetic cohorts in urbanized areas who have westernized their diets.

These studies will evaluate heart disease, hypertension, stroke, cancers, type 2 diabetes, metabolic syndrome, Alzheimer's disease, dementia, age-related macular degeneration (AMD), overweight/obesity, and more. Such studies will cost many millions of dollars, will be directed by myself (Knobbe) and may take five years or more to complete. Such studies will be funded via philanthropic charitable contributions through Ancestral Health Foundation and Cure AMD Foundation, both of which are entirely nonprofit organizations based in Colorado. Please consider supporting these foundations and our efforts for the greater good of all. Donations can be made at either foundational website: Information located on page 341.

WHERE TO FIND US

FOUNDATIONAL WEBSITES

ANCESTRALHEALTHFOUNDATION.ORG

&

CUREAMD.ORG

SOCIAL MEDIA

ANCESTRAL HEALTH FOUNDATION
& CURE AMD FOUNDATION

YOUTUBE CHANNEL: CHRIS KNOBBE MD

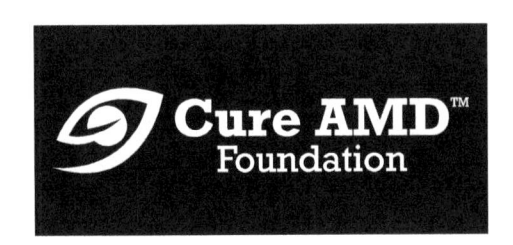

A FEW OF OUR FAVORITE QUOTES

WESTON A. PRICE WROTE,

"Life in all its fullness is Mother Nature obeyed."

THEOPHRAST PARACELSUS, PARAPHRASED,

"The dose makes the poison."

EDWARD STANLEY WROTE,

"Those who think they have no time for healthy eating will sooner or later have to find time for illness."

THOMAS EDISON SAID,

"The doctor of the future will give no medication but will interest his patients in the care of the human frame, in diet and in the cause and prevention of disease."

BENJAMIN FRANKLIN SAID,

"He's the best physician that knows the worthlessness of most medicines."

THOMAS JEFFERSON WROTE,

"Without health there is no happiness. An attention to health, then, should take the place of every other object."

MARGARET MEAD, ANTHROPOLOGIST, WROTE,

"Never doubt that a small group of thoughtful, committed citizens can change the world; indeed, it's the only thing that ever has."

A QUOTE FROM EACH OF US

"The Big Food and Edible Oil industries operate almost solely based on profit margins, rather than the health and well-being of consumers, producing chronic illnesses that are nothing but diseases of greed. Consumers are merely innocent victims of misinformation and a toxic, nutrient-deficient food supply."

— SUZANNE ALEXANDER, M.Ed.

"Seed oils are not blatantly, obviously, and directly killing us, tantamount to the Jewish Holocaust, but rather, one by one, maiming, debilitating, and eventually bringing our demise, en masse, in the most oblique, clandestine, and imperceptible manner, disguised as 'healthy food.'"

— CHRIS KNOBBE, MD

ENDNOTES

1. Dyer JM, Stymne S, Green AG, Carlsson AS. High-value oils from plants. The Plant Journal. 2008;54:640-655.

2. USDA Economic Research Service (ERS). Food Availability (Per Capita) Data System. 2018. Retrieved from: **https://www.ers.usda.gov/data-products/food-availability-per-capita-data-system/**

3. Knobbe CA, Richer SP, Freilich BD, Kent D, Cripps JR, Reynolds TM, Dito JJ, Walgama JP, Hunter JD, Henderson T, Stojanoska M, Barry JT, Kiwara AL, Sommer R, Ross RD, Kaushal S, Luff AK. Westernized Diet, Vegetable Oil, Nutrient Deficiency and Omega-6 Apocalypse: Can We Explain Age-Related Macular Degeneration and Associated Chronic Diseases - Obesity, Coronary Heart Disease, Cancers, Metabolic Disease, Diabetes, Alzheimer's, and More – With a Unifying Hypothesis? Manuscript submitted for publication. University of Texas Southwestern Medical Center, Dallas, U.S., 2022.

4. Knobbe CA, Stojanoska M. The 'Displacing Foods of Modern Commerce' Are the Primary and Proximate Cause of Age-Related Macular Degeneration: A Unifying Singular Hypothesis. Medical Hypotheses. 2017;109:184-198.

5. Blasbalg TL, Hibbeln JR, Ramsden CE, et al. Changes in consumption of omega-3 and omega-6 fatty acids in the United States during the 20th century. Amer J Clin Nutr. 2011;93(5):950-962.

6. Guyenet SJ, Carlson SE. Increase in Adipose Tissue Linoleic Acid of US Adults in the Last Half Century. Advances in Nutrition. 2015;6(6):660-664.

7. Mead, James F, Fulco, Armand J. The Unsaturated and Polyunsaturated Fatty Acids in Health and Disease. Springfield, IL, Charles C. Thomas, 1976, pp. 104-114.

8. Ramsden CE, Ringel A, Feldstein AE, et al. Lowering dietary linoleic acid reduces bioactive oxidized linoleic acid metabolites in humans. Prostaglandins, Leukotrienes and Essential Fatty Acids. 2012;87(4-5):135-141.

9. Greene JF, Hammock BD. Toxicity of linoleic acid metabolites. Adv Exp Med Biol. 1999;469:471-7.

10. Cury-Boaventura MF, Gorjão, Martins de Lima T, et al. Comparative toxicity of oleic and linoleic acid on human lymphocytes. Life Sci. 2006;78(13):1448-56.

11. Moran JH, Nowak G, Grant DF. Analysis of the Toxic Effects of Linoleic Acid, 12,13-cis-Epoxyoctadecenoic Acid, and 12,13-Dihydroxyoctadecenoic Acid in Rabbit Renal Cortical Mitochondria. Toxicol Applied Pharmacol. 2001;172(2):150-61.

12. U.S. Department of Agriculture. Agriculture Research Service. Nutrient intakes from food: mean amounts consumed per individual, by gender and age. Available: **http://www.ars.usda.gov/ba/bhnrc/fsrg**. Accessed 7 Jul 2019.

13. Mead, James F, Fulco, Armand J. The Unsaturated and Polyunsaturated Fatty Acids in Health and Disease. Springfield, IL, Charles C. Thomas, 1976, pp. 3-16.

14. Whelan J. The health implications of changing linoleic acid intakes. Prostaglandins Leukot Essent Fatty Acids. 2008;79(3-5):165-7.

15. Harris, Randall E. Epidemiology of Chronic Disease: Global Perspectives, Second Edition. Burlington, MA, Jones & Bartlett Learning, 2020.

16. Araujo de Vizcarrondo C, Carrillo de Padilla F, Martin E. Fatty acid composition of beef, pork, and poultry fresh cuts, and some of their processed products. Arch Latinoam Nutr. 1998;48(4):354-8.

17. Prior IA, Davidson F, Salmond CE, Czochanska Z. Cholesterol, coconuts, and diet on Polynesian atolls: a natural experiment: the Pukapuka and Tokelau Island studies. Amer J Clin Nutr. 1981;34(8):1552-1561.

18. Holovach K. Unpublished data. Medallion Labs. Grocery store pork samples, Report #39408.1, Medallion Labs, Minneapolis, MN, 4 Mar 2021.

19. De Marchi M, Costa A, Pozza M, et al. Detailed characterization of plant-based burgers. Scientific Reports. 2021;11:2049.

20. Howell RW, Collins FI. Factors Affecting Linolenic and Linoleic Acid Content of Soybean Oil. Agronomy Journal. 1957;49(11):593-597.

21. Hill AB. The environment and disease: association or causation? Proc R Soc Med. 1965;58:293-300.

22. van Reekum R, Streiner DL, Conn DK. Applying Bradford Hill's Criteria for Causation to Neuropsychiatry. Journ Psychiatry and Clin Neurosciences. 2001;13:3:318-25.

23. Price WA. New Light From Primitive Races On Modern Degeneration – Physical, Mental, and Moral. Rhein Memorial Lecture, read before the First District Dental Society, Jan 15, 1940, New York City, New York.

24. Price, WA. Light From Primitive Races On the Relation of Nutrition to Individual and National Development. The Journal of the American Dental Association. 1939;26:938-948.

25. Price, WA. Eskimo and Indian Field Studies in Alaska and Canada. The Journal of the American Dental Association. 1936;23:417-437.

26. Price, WA. Why Dental Caries With Modern Civilizations? V. An Interpretation of Previously Reported Field Studies. Dental Digest, July, 1933.

27. Price, WA. New Light on the Cause and Control of Tooth Decay in Man, from Field Studies of Primitive Districts Providing Immunity. Communication for the Eighth Australian Dental Congress, Adelaide, South Australia, Aug, 1933. Proceedings of Congress.

28. Price, Weston A. Nutrition and Physical Degeneration. Lemon Grove, CA: The Price-Pottenger Nutrition Foundation Inc; 1939.

29. Ibid. p. 246.

30. Price, Weston A. Nutrition and Physical Degeneration. Lemon Grove, CA: The Price-Pottenger Nutrition Foundation Inc; 1939, p. xvi.

31. Price, Weston A. Nutrition and Physical Degeneration. Lemon Grove, CA: The Price-Pottenger Nutrition Foundation Inc; 1939, p. 452, pp. 246-8.

32. Monteiro CA, Cannon G, Levy RB, et al. Ultra-processed foods: what they are and how to identify them. Public Health Nutrition, 2019;22(5):936-941.

33. Koehn, NF. Henry Heinz and Brand Creation in the Late Nineteenth Century: Making Markets for Processed Food. Business History Review. 1999;(3). https:rsm.idm.oclc.org/login?url=http://search.ebscohost.com/login.aspx?direct=true&db=-congale&AN=edsgcl.59013836&site=eds-live&scope=site. Accessed March 30, 2019.

34. Petrick GM. Feeding the masses: H.J. Heinz and the creation of industrial food. Endeavour. 2009;33(1):29-34. Doi:10.1016/j.endeavour.2008.11.002.

35. Muhammad KG. The sugar that saturates the American diet has a barbaric history as the 'white gold' that fueled slavery. The New York Times Magazine. 14 Aug 2019. Retrieved: https://www.nytimes.com/interactive/2019/08/14/magazine/sugar-slave-trade-slavery.html. Accessed 3 Mar 2022.

36. "Profiling Food Consumption in America." USDA Economic Research Service, Factbook, Chapter 2. ND. Available at http://www.usda.gov/factbook.chapter2.pdf.

37. Nixon HC. The Rise of the American Cottonseed Oil industry. J Political Econ. 1930;38(1):73-85.

38. Dean LD, Davis JP, Sanders TH. Groundnut (Peanut) Oil. In: Gunstone F, ed. Vegetable Oils in Food Technology: Composition, Properties and Uses. West Sussex, UK, 2011, p. 225.

39. Bedigian D, Harlan JR. Evidence for cultivation of sesame in the ancient world. Economic Botany. 1986;40(2):137-154.

40. Vossen P. Olive Oil: History, Production, and Characteristics of the World's Classic Oils. American Society for Horticultural Science. 2007;42(5):1093-1100.

41. Shankar P. Coconut oil: A review. Agro Food Industry Hi Tech. 2013;24(5):62-64.

42. Henson IE. A Brief History of the Oil Palm. In Lai OM, Tan CP, Akoh CC, editors. Palm Oil – Production, Processing, Characterization, and Uses. Urbana, IL, USA: AOCS Press; 2012: pp. 1-29.

43. Hamm H, Hamilton RJ, Calliauw G. Edible Oil Processing, Second Edition. West Sussex, UK: Wiley-Blackwell, 2013.

44. "How It's Made – Canola Oil." Discovery and Science Channel. 11 March 2012. Retrieved Aug 15, 2021, Available at https://www.youtube.com/watch?v=Cfk2IXlZdbI.

45. Hoffman G. The Chemistry and Technology of Edible Oils and Fats and Their High Fat Products. San Diego, CA, Academic Press Inc., 1989.

46. Tompkins, D.A. Cotton Seed Oil, History and Commercial Features. Charlotte, N.C., Presses Observer Printing House. 1902, p.4.

47. Trademark Registration by N.K. Fairbank & Company for Cottolene brand Fatty, Oleaginous, or Unctuous Food Substances. U.S. Library of Congress. Created 11 Oct 1887. Images in the Public Domain.

48. Ganz, Robert (Robert Ganz & Co., Proprietors). The

Manufacture of Cottonseed Oil and Allied Products. New York, The National Provisioner Publishing Co., 1897, p.1

49 Ganz, Robert (Robert Ganz & Co., Proprietors). The Manufacture of Cottonseed Oil and Allied Products. New York, The National Provisioner Publishing Co., 1897, pp.78-88.

50 Ramsey D, Graham T. How Vegetable Oils Replaced Animal Fats in the American Diet. The Atlantic. 26 April 2012.

51 Rider AF. The Search for Vegetable Oils. Business Digest and Investment Weekly. 13 Mar, 1918;5(11):345.

52 USDA Economic Research Service (ERS). Food Availability (Per Capita) Data System. 2018. Retrieved from: **https://www.ers.usda.gov/data-products/food-availability-per-capita-data-system/**

53 FAO/WHO. Fats and Oils in Human Nutrition Report of a Joint Expert Consultation. Food and Agriculture Organization of the United Nations and the World Health Organization. FAO Food Nutr Pap. 1994;57:1-147.

54 Okuyama H, Langsjoen PH, Ohara N, et al. Medicines and Vegetable Oils as Hidden Causes of Cardiovascular Disease and Diabetes. Pharmacology. 2016;98(3-4):134-70.

55 U.S. Department of Agriculture. Agriculture Research Service. Nutrient intakes from food: mean amounts consumed per individual, by gender and age. Available: **http://www.ars.usda.gov/ba/bhnrc/fsrg**. Accessed 7 Jul 2019.

56 Speth JD, Spielmann KA. Energy Source, Protein Metabolism, and Hunter-Gatherer Subsistence Strategies. Journal of Anthropological Archaeology. 1983;2:1-31.

57 Leheska JM, Thompson LD, Howe JC, Hentges E, et al. Effects of conventional and grass-feeding systems on the nutrient composition of beef. Journ Animal Science. 2008;86:3575-85.

58 Ford ES, Dietz WH. Trends in energy intake among adults in the United States: findings from NHANES. Am J Clin Nutr. 2013;97(4):848-53.

59 Blasbalg TL, Hibbeln JR, Ramsden CE, et al. Changes in consumption of omega-3 and omega-6 fatty acids in the United States during the 20th century. Amer J Clin Nutr. 2011;93(5):950-962.

60 Guyenet SJ, Carlson SE. Increase in Adipose Tissue Linoleic Acid of US Adults in the Last Half Century. Advances in Nutrition. 2015;6(6):660-664.

61 Molfino A, Gioia G, Fanelli FR, Muscaritoli M. The Role for Dietary Omega-3 Fatty Acids Supplementation in Older Adults. Nutrients. 2014;6(10):4058-4072.

62 Deol, P, Fahrmann J, Yang J, et al. Omega-6 and omega-3 oxylipins are implicated in soybean oil-induced obesity in mice. Scientific Reports. 2017;7:12488. DOI:10.1038/s41598-017-12624-9.

63 Deol P, Evans JR, Dhahbi J, et al. Soybean Oil Is More Obesogenic and Diabetogenic than Coconut Oil and Fructose in Mouse: Potential Role for the Liver. PLOS ONE. 2015;10(7): e0132672. Doi:10.1371/journal.pone.0132672.

64 Pan DA, Storlien LH. Dietary Lipid Profile Is a Determinant of Tissue Phospholipid Fatty Acid Composition and Rate of Weight Gain in Rats. J Nutr. 1993;123(3):512-9. Doi: 10.1093/jn/123.3.512.

65 Simopoulos AP. An Increase in the Omega-6/Omega-3 Fatty Acid Ratio Increases the Risk for Obesity. Nutrients. 2016;8:128. Doi:10.3390/nu8030128.

66 Kearney J. Food consumption trends and drivers. Phil Trans R Soc. 2010;365:2793-2807.

67 Ham H, Hamilton RJ, Calliauw G. Edible Oil Processing. Second ed. West Sussex, UK: Wiley-Blackwell; 2013.

68 James EM. The refining and bleaching of vegetable oils. J Amer Oil Chemist's Society. 1958;35(2):76-83.

69 Afshar PG, Honarvar M, Gharachorloo M, et al. Bleaching of vegetable oils using press mud obtained from sugar industry. Eur J Experiment Biol. 2014;4(1):677-684.

70 Gupta MK. Practical Guide to Vegetable Oil Processing, Second Edition. London, UK, Academic Press and AOCS Press; 2017.

71 Zehnder CT. Chapter 14 – Deodorization. Practical Handbook of Soybean Processing and Utilization. 1995, pp. 239-257.

72 Trautman NM, Carlsen WS, Krasny ME, Cunningham CM. Assessing Toxic Risk. Arlington, VA. NSTA Press, 2001.

73 Campbell GM. Roller Milling of Wheat. Chapter 7. Handbook of Powder Technology, Volume 12. Oxford, UK, Elsevier BV, 2007, 383-419.

74. Slavin JL, Jacobs D, Marquart L. Grain processing and nutrition. Crit Rev Biotechnol. 2001;21(1):49-66.

75. Shewry PR. Wheat. J Exp Bot. 2009;60(6):1537-1553.

76. Wheat: Wheat's Role in the U.S. Diet. USDA Economic Research Service. 19 Jun 2013. Available: https://www.ers.usda.gov/topics/crops/wheat/wheats-role-in-the-us-diet.aspx. Retrieved 24 Aug 2021.

77. Benchley R, Spannagl M, Pfeifer M, et al. Analysis of the bread wheat genome using whole genome shotgun sequencing. Nature. 2012;491:705-710.

78. Cordain L, Eaton SB, Sebastian A, et al. Origins and evolution of the Western diet: health implications for the 21st century. Am J Clin Nutr. 2005;81:341-354.

79. Kantor L, Blazejczyk A. Food Availability (Per Capita) Data System. USDA, Economic Research Service. July 2021. Retrieved: https://www.ers.usda.gov/amber-waves/2016/december/a-look-at-calorie-sources-in-the-american-diet. Accessed 24 Aug 2021.

80. Wheat Sector at a Glance. USDA Economic Research Service. ND. Retrieved: https://www.ers.usda.gov/topics/crops/wheat/wheat-sector-at-a-glance/. Accessed 25 Aug 2021.

81. Whole Grain Statistics. Oldways Whole Grains Council. July 2021. Retrieved: https://wholegrainscouncil.org/newsroom/whole-grain-statistics. Accessed 24 Aug 2021.

82. Schisgall O. Eyes on Tomorrow – the Evolution of Proctor & Gamble. New York, NY: Doubleday and Company; 1981, p. 63-72

83. List GR, Jackson MA. Giants of the past: The battle over hydrogenation (1903-1920). Inform. 2007;18:403-405.

84. Semma M. Trans fatty acids: properties, benefits and risks. J Health Sci. 2002;48(1):7-13.

85. Schleifer D. The Perfect Solution: How Trans Fats Became the Healthy Replacement or Saturated Fats. Technology and Culture, Johns Hopkins University Press. 2012;53(1):94-119.

86. Neil, Marion Harris. A Calendar of Dinners with 615 Recipes Including the Story of Crisco. Proctor & Gamble Co., 1914.

87. Veit, Helen Zoe. How Crisco Made Americans Believers in Industrial Food. Smithsonian Magazine. 23 Dec 2019. Retrieved: https://www.smithsonianmag.com/innovation/how-crisco-made-americans-believers-industrial-food-180973845/. Accessed 16 Dec 2021.

88. Norris S. Trans Fats: The Health Burden. Library of Parliament, Science and Technology Division. PRB 05-21E. 21 Jun 2007. https://epe.lac-bac.gc.ca/100/200/301/library_parliament/backgrounder/2007/trans_fats-e_revised/PRB0521-2e.pdf. Accessed 8 Nov 2021.

89. Gebauer SK, Baer DJ. Trans-Fatty Acids: Health Effects, Recommendations, and Regulations. Encyclopedia of Human Nutrition (Third Ed.). 2013;288-292.

90. Brouwer IA, Wanders AJ, Katan MB. Trans fatty acids and cardiovascular health: research completed? Eur J Clin Nutr. 2013;67:541-547.

91. Field CJ, Hosea Blewett H, Proctor S, Vine D. Human health benefits of vaccenic acid. Applied Physiology, Nutrition, and Metabolism. 2009;34(5):979-91.

92. Koba K, Yanagita T. Health benefits of conjugated linoleic acid (CLA). Obesity Research & Clinical Practice. 2014;8(6):e525-e532.

93. Lee KW, Lee HJ, Cho HY, Kim YJ. Role of the Conjugated Linoleic Acid in Prevention of Cancer. Critical Rev Food Sci Nutr. 2005;45(2):135-144.

94. Johnston PV, Johnson OC, Kummerow FA. Occurrence of Trans Fatty Acids in Human Tissue. Science, New Series. 1957;126(3276):698-699.

95. Kummerow FA. Role of Butterfat in Nutrition and In Atherosclerosis: A Review. Journal of Dairy Science. 1957;40(10):1350-1359.

96. Dennis, B. Fred Kummerow, U. of I. professor who fought against trans fats, dies at 102. Chicago Tribune. 2 June 2017. Retrieved: https://www.chicagotribune.com/news/obituaries/ct-fred-kummerow-obituary-wapomet-20170602-story.html. Accessed 14 Nov 2021.

97. Watson, Elaine. Researcher files lawsuit vs FDA after it ignored his petition calling for ban on artificial trans fats. Food Navigator USA. 12 Aug 2013.

98. Final Determination Regarding Partially Hydrogenated Oils. Federal Register; FDA. 17 Jun 2015.

99. Final Determination Regarding Partially Hydrogenated Oils. Federal Register; FDA. 21 May 2018.

100. Remig V, Franklin B, Margolis S, et al. Trans Fats in America: A Review of Their Use, Consumption, Health Implications, and Regulation. J Amer Diet Assoc. 2010;110(4):585-592.

101. Song J, Park J, Jung J, et al. Analysis of Trans Fat in Edible Oils with Cooking Process. Toxicol Res. 2015;31(3):307-312.

102. Ackman RG, Mag TK. Trans fatty acids and the potential for less in technical products. In J. I. Sebedio, & W.W. Christie (Eds), Trans fatty acids in human nutrition. Dundee: The Oily Press, 1998;35-58.

103. Ceriani R, Meirelles AJA. Formation of trans PUFA during deodorization of canola oil: a study through computational simulation. Chemical Engineering and Processing. 2007;46(5):375-385.

104. Devinat G, Scamaroni I, Naudet M. Isomerisation de l'acide linolenique Durant la desodorisation des huiles de colza et de soja. Revue Francaise des Corps Gras. 1980:27:283-287.

105. Grandigirard A, Sebedio JL, Fleury J. Geometrical isomerization of linolenic acid during heat treatment of vegetable oils. JAOCS. 1984;61(10):1563-1568.

106. Hénon G, Kemény Zs, Recseg K, et al. Deodorization of vegetable oils. Part I: Modelling the geometrical isomerization of polyunsaturated fatty acids. JAOCS. 1999;76(1):73-81.

107. Ackman RG, Hooper SN. Linolenic Acid Artifacts from the Deodorization of Oils. J Amer Oil Chem Soc. 1974;51:42-49.

108. Wolff RL. Trans-Polyunsaturated Fatty Acids in French Edible Rapeseed and Soybean Oils. JAOCS. 1992;69(2):106-110.

109. Wolff RL. Further studies on artificial geometrical isomers of alpha-linolenic acid in edible linolenic acid-containing oils. JAOCS. 1993;70(3):219-224.

110. O'Keefe S, Gaskins-Wright S, Wiley V, Chen I. Levels of Trans Geometrical Isomers of Essential Fatty Acids in Some Unhydrogenated U.S. Vegetable Oils. J Food Lipids.

111. De Greyt W, Radanyi O, Kellens M, Huyghebaert A. Contribution of trans-Fatty Acids from Vegetable Oils and Margarines to the Belgian Diet. Eur J Med Res. 1995;1(2):105-8.

112. Hou JC, Wang F, Wang Y-T, et al. Assessment of trans fatty acids in edible oils in China. Food Control. 2012;25:211-215.

113. Mossoba MM, Azizian H, Tyburczy C. Rapid FT-NIR Analysis of Edible Oils for Total SFA, MUFA, PUFA, and Trans FA with Comparison to GC. J Am Oil Chem Soc. 2013;90:757-770.

114. Rauber F, Campagnolo PD, Hoffman DJ, Vitolo MR. Consumption of ultra-processed food products and its effects on children's lipid profiles: a longitudinal study. Nutrition, Metabolism and Cardiovascular Diseases. 2015;25(1):116-122.

115. Yudkin, John. Pure, White and Deadly: How Sugar Is Killing Us and What We Can Do to Stop It. London, Davis-Poynter, 1972.

116. Guyenet, Stephan. The Hungry Brain: Outsmarting the Instincts That Make Us Overeat. New York, Flatiron Books, 2017, pp. 77-78.

117. Cordain L, Eaton SB, Sebastian A, et al. Origins and evolution of the Western diet: health implications for the 21st century. Am J Clin Nutr. 2005;81:341-354.

118. Toussant-Samat M. A History of Food. Cambridge, MA, Blackwell Publishers, 1987, pp.217-221.

119. Carter, NC. San Diego Olives: origins of a California industry. J San Diego Hist. 2008;54(3):138-40.

120. Grigg D. The European diet: regional variations in food consumption in the 1980s. Geoforum. 1993;24:277-289.

121. Toussant-Samat M. A History of Food. Cambridge, MA, Blackwell Publishers, 1987, p. 211.

122. Carter, NC. San Diego Olives: origins of a California industry. J San Diego Hist. 2008;54(3):138-40.

123. Ramsey D, Graham T. How Vegetable Oils Replaced Animal Fats in the American Diet. The Atlantic. 26 Apr 2012.

124. "Energy from vegetable oils." Knoema World Data Atlas. Food Balance Sheets. Retrieved: **https://knoema.com/atlas/topics/Agriculture/Food-Supply-Total-Energy-kcalcapitaday/Energy-from-vegetable-oils**. Accessed: 15 Nov 2021.

125. Orsavova J, Misurcova L, Ambrozova JV, et al. Fatty Acids Composition of Vegetable Oils and Its Contribution to Dietary Energy Intake and Dependence of Cardiovascular Mortality on Dietary Intake of Fatty Acids. Int J Mol Sci. 2015;16:12871-12890.

126. Guyenet S J, Carlson SE. Increase in Adipose Tissue Linoleic Acid of US Adults in the Last Half Century. Adv Nutr. 2015;6(6):660-4.

127. Raederstorff D, Wyss A, Calder PC, et al. Vitamin E function and requirements in relation to PUFA. Br J Nutr. 2015;114:1113-1122.

128. Harris PL, Quaife ML, Swanson WJ. Vitamin E Content of Foods. Journ Nutr. 1950;40(3):367-381.

129. Murphy SP, Subar AF, Block G. Vitamin E intakes and sources in the United States. AJCN. 1990;52(2):361-367.

130 Food and Nutrition Board IoM. Dietary Reference Intake for Vitamin C, Vitamin E, Selenium, and Carotenoids. Washington, DC: National Academies Press, 2000.

131 Traber MG, Stevens JF. Vitamins C and E: beneficial effects from a mechanistic perspective. Free Radic Biol Med. 2011;51:1000-1013.

132 Traber MG. Vitamin E inadequacy in humans: causes and consequences. Adv Nutr. 2014;5:503-514.

133 Sokol RJ. Vitamin E deficiency and neurologic disease. Annu Rev Nutr. 1988;8:351-373.

134 Gohil K, Vasu VT, Cross CE. Dietary alpha-tocopherol and neuromuscular health: search for optimal dose and molecular mechanisms continues! Mol Nutr Food Res. 2010;54:693-709.

135 Troesch B, Hoeft B, McBurney M, et al. Dietary surveys indicate vitamin intakes below recommendations are common in representative Western countries. Br J Nutr. 2012;108:692-698.

136 Krauss RM, Eckel RH, Howard B, et al. AHA Dietary Guidelines – Revision 2000: A Statement for Healthcare Professionals From the Nutrition Committee of the American Heart Association. Circulation. 2000;102:2284-2299.

137 Tindall AM, Peterson KS, Skulas-Ray AC, et al. Replacing Saturated Fat With Walnuts or Vegetable Oils Improves Central Blood Pressure and Serum Lipids in Adults at Risk for Cardiovascular Disease: A Randomized Controlled -Feeding Trial. JAHA. 2019;8:e011512.

138 Whole Wheat Flour. Nutrition Coordinating Center Food & Nutrient Database (NCCDB). University of Minnesota. Accessed 18 Nov 2021.

139 Wheat Flour, White, All-Purpose, Unenriched. USDA. Accessed 18 Nov 2021.

140 Jonnalagadda S, Harnack L, Liu R, et al. Putting the whole grain puzzle together: health benefits associated with whole grains—summary of American Society for Nutrition 2010 satellite symposium. J Nutr. 2011;141(5):1011S-22S.

141 Slavin JL, Jacobs D, Marquart L, Wiemer K. The role of whole grains in disease prevention. J Am Diet Assoc. 2001;101:780-5.

142 Slavin J. Why whole grains are protective: biological mechanisms. Proc Nutr Soc. 2003;62:129-34.

143 Bruce B, Spiller GA, Klevay LM, Gallagher SK. A diet high in whole and unrefined foods favorably alters lipids, antioxidant defenses, and colon function. J Am Coll Nutr. 2000;19:61-7.

144 Thompson LU. Antioxidants and hormone-mediated health benefits of whole grains. Crit Rev Food Sci Nutr. 1994;34:473-97.

145 Slavin JL, Martini MC, Jacobs DR, Marquart L. Plausible mechanisms for the protectiveness of whole grains. Am J Clin Nutr. 1999;70:S459-63.

146 Fardet A, Canlet C, Gottardi G, et al. Whole-Grain and Refined Wheat Flours Show Distinct Metabolic Profiles in Rats as Assessed by a ^{1}H NMR-Based Metabonomic Approach. Journal of Nutrition. 2007;137(4):923-929.

147 Forman HJ, Zhang H, Rinna A. Glutathione: Overview of its protective roles, measurement, and biosynthesis. Mol Aspects Med. 2009;30(1-2):1-12.

148 McCollum, E.V. The Newer Knowledge of Nutrition – The Use of Food For the Preservation of Vitality and Health. New York, The MacMillan Company, 1919.

149 McCollum, E.V. 1919, p. 16.

150 Osborne, Thomas B., Mendel, Lafayette B. Further Observations of the Influence of Natural Fats Upon Growth. Journal of Biological Chemistry. 1915:20(3):379-390.

151 McCollum, E.V. 1919, p. 29.

152 McCollum, E.V. 1919, p. 31.

153 Funk, C. J State Med. 1912;xx,341; Biochem Bull, 1915, iv, 304.

154 Piro A, Tagarelli G, Lagonia P, et al. Casimir Funk: His Discovery of the Vitamins and Their Deficiency Disorders. Ann Nutr Metab. 2010;57:85-88.

155 McCollum, E.V., Kennedy C. Jour Biol Chem. 1916;xxiv, 491.

156 McCollum, E.V. 1919, p.32.

157 Alothman M, Hogan SA, Hennessy D, et al. The "Grass-Fed" Milk Story: Understanding the Impact of Pasture Feeding on the Composition and Quality of Bovine Milk. Foods. 2019;8(8):350.

158 Ward NE. Chapter 20 – Vitamins in Eggs. Egg Innovations and Strategies for Improvements. 2017;207-220.

159 Beef Liver Nutrition Coordinating Center Food & Nutrient Database (NCCDB). University of Minnesota. Accessed 18 Nov 2021.

160 Olafsdottir AS, Wagner KH, Thorsdottir I, Elmadfa I.

Fat-Soluble Vitamins in the Maternal Diet, Influence of Cod Liver Oil Supplementation and Impact of the Maternal Diet on Human Milk Composition. Ann Nutr Metab. 2001;45:265-272.

161. Nordic Naturals Cod Liver Oil. Chris Masterjohn, PhD. Retrieved: **https://chrismasterjohnphd.com/advanced-results-mk-4/entry/229605**. Accessed: 28 Nov 2021.

162. VitaK Test Results. The Weston A. Price Foundation. Nov 24, 2015. Retrieved: **https://www.westonaprice.org/health-topics/cod-liver-oil/vitak-test-results/**. Link: minKMeasurements120315-WestonPriceFoundation-foodsamples1. Accessed: 28 Nov 2021.

163. Vegetable Oil. Nutrition Coordinating Center Food & Nutrient Database (NCCDB). University of Minnesota. Accessed 18 Nov 2021.

164. Sakai K, Kino S, Takeuchi M, et al. Analysis of antioxidant activities in vegetable oils and fat soluble vitamins and biofactors by the PAO-SO method. Methods Mol Biol. 2010;594:241-50.

165. Household USDA Food Facts Sheet. "Oil, Vegetable." USDA. Oct, 2012. Retrieved from: **http://www.fns.usda.gov/sites/default/files/HHFS_OIL_VEGETABLE_100440Oct2012.pdf**

166. FoodData Central, Oil, soybean. USDA. Published 12/16/2019. Retrieved from: **https://fdc.nal.usda.gov/fdc-app.html#/food-details/748366/nutrients**

167. Olive Oil. Nutrition Coordinating Center Food & Nutrient Database (NCCDB). University of Minnesota. Accessed 18 Nov 2021.

168. Almond Oil. Nutrition Coordinating Center Food & Nutrient Database (NCCDB). University of Minnesota. Accessed 18 Nov 2021.

169. Lard. Nutrition Coordinating Center Food & Nutrient Database (NCCDB). University of Minnesota. Accessed 18 Nov 2021.

170. The National Diet-Heart Study. American Heart Association Monograph No. 18, American Heart Association, New York, 1968.

171. Grundy SM, Denke MA. Dietary influences on serum lipids and lipoproteins. J Lipid Res. 1990;31:1149-1172.

172. Mattson FH, Grundy SM. Comparison of effects of dietary saturated, monounsaturated, and polyunsaturated fatty acids on plasma lipids and lipoproteins in man. J Lipid Res. 1985;26:194-202.

173. Wilson TA. Ausman LM, Lawton CW, et al. Comparitive Cholesterol Lowering Properties of Vegetable Oils: Beyond Fatty Acids. J Amer Coll Nutr. 2000;19(5):601-607.

174. Dubois V, Breton S, Linder M, et al. Fatty acid profiles of 80 vegetable oils with regard to their nutritional potential. Eur J Lipid Sci Techn. 2007;109(7):710-732.

175. Reaven P, Parthasarathy S, Grasse BJ, et al. Effects of Oleate-rich and Linoleate-rich Diets on the Susceptibility of Low Density Lipoprotein to Oxidative Modification in Mildly Hypercholesterolemic Subjects. 1993;91:668-676.

176. Parthasarathy S, Raghavamenon A, Garelnabi MO, Santanam N. Oxidized Low-Density Lipoprotein. Methods Mol Biol. 2010;610:403-417.

177. Parthasarathy S, Litvinov D, Selvarajan K, et al. Lipid peroxidation and decomposition—conflicting roles in plaque vulnerability and stability. Biochim Biophys Acta. 2008;1781:221-231.

178. Haberland ME, Olch CL, Folgelman AM. Role of lysines in mediating interaction of modified low density lipoproteins with the scavenger receptor of human monocyte macrophages. J Biol Chem. 1984;259:11305-11.

179. Haberland ME, Fogelman AM, Edwards PA. Specificity of receptor-mediated recognition of malondialdehyde-modified low density lipoproteins. Proc Natl Acad Sci USA. 1982;79:1712-6.

180. DiNicolantonio JJ, O'Keefe JH. Omega-6 vegetable oils as a driver of coronary heart disease: the oxidized linoleic acid hypothesis. Open Heart. 2018;5:e000898. Doi:10.1136/openhrt02018-000898.

181. West R, Beeri MS, Schmeidler J, et al. Better Memory Functioning Associated With Higher Total and Low-Density Lipoprotein Cholesterol Levels in Very Elderly Subjects Without the Apolipoprotein e4 Allele. Amer J Ger Psych. 2008;16(9):781-785.

182. Jacobs EJ, Gapstur SM. Cholesterol and Cancer: Answers and New Questions. Cancer Epidem Biomarkers Prevent. 2009;18(11):2805-2806.

183. Weverling-Rijnsburger AWE, Blauw GJ, Lagaay AM, et al. Total cholesterol and risk of mortality in the oldest old. The Lancet. 1997;350(9085):1119-1123.

184. Huang X, Chen H, Miller WC, et al. Lower low-density lipoprotein cholesterol levels are associated with Parkinson's disease. Movement Disorders. 2007;22(3):377-381.

185 Horwich TB, Hamilton MA, MacLellan WR, Fonarow GC. Low serum total cholesterol is associated with marked increase in mortality in advanced heart failure. Journ Cardiac Failure. 2002;8(4):216-224.

186 Tedders SH, Fokong KD, McKenzie LE, et al. Low cholesterol is associated with depression among US household population. Journ Affective Disorders. 2011;135(1-3):115-121.

187 Fiedorowicz JG, Haynes WG. Cholesterol, mood, and vascular health: Untangling the relationship. Curr Psychiatr. 2010;9(7):17-A.

188 Golomb BA, Stattin H, Mednick S. Low cholesterol and violent crime. Journ Psychiatric Res. 2000;34(4-5):301-309.

189 Zampelas A, Magriplis E. New Insights into Cholesterol Functions: A Friend or an Enemy? Nutrients. 2019;11(7):1645.

190 Kelley RI, Hennekam RCM. The Smith-Lemli-Opitz syndrome. Journ Med Genetics. 2000;37:321-335.

191 Vegetable Oil Market: Global Industry Analysis and Trends. Maximize Market Research Pvt. Ltd. Retrieved: **https://www.maximizemarketresearch.com/market-report/global-vegetable-oil-market/108821/**. Accessed 30 Nov 2021.

192 Energy From Vegetable Oils. Knoema. Retrieved: **https://knoema.com/atlas/topics/Agriculture/Food-Supply-Total-Energy-kcalcapitaday/Energy-from-vegetable-oils**. Accessed: 15 Aug 2021.

193 Waldman M, Lamb M. Dying For A Hamburger. New York, Thomas Dunne Books, 2005.

194 Dementia. World Health Organization (WHO). 2 Sep 2021. Retrieved: **https://www.who.int/news-room/fact-sheets/detail/dementia**. Accessed 9 Sep 2021.

195 Ahmed AM. History of Diabetes Mellitus. Saudi Med J. 2002;23(4):373-378.

196 Hitzenberger K, Richter-Quittner M. Ein Beitrag zum Stoffwechsel bei der vaskulären Hypertonie. Weiner Arch Innere Med. 1921;2:189-216.

197 Kylin E. Hypertonie and zuckerkrankheit. Zentralblatt für Innere Medizin. 1921;42:873-877.

198 Kucharz EJ, Shampo MA, Kyle RA. Casimir Funk—Polish-Born American Biochemist. Mayo Clinic Proceedings. 1994;69(7):656.

199 List, Gary R. The History of Lipid Science & Technology. AOCS Lipid Library. Retrieved: **https://lipidlibrary.aocs.org/resource-material/the-history-of-lipid-science-and-technology**. Accessed 4 Aug 2021.

200 "Fitness Guru Jack LaLanne Dies at 96." USA Today (online). ND. Retrieved: **https://usatoday30.usatoday.com/yourlife/fitness/exercise/2011-01-25-lalanneobit24_ST_N.htm**. Accessed: 5 Dec 2021.

201 Olver, Lynne. The Food Timeline. FoodTimeline.org. Dec 2021. Retrieved: **https://foodtimeline.org/**. Accessed 18 Dec 2021.

202 Refrigerating apparatus. Patent application, US1126605A, filed April 7, 1913. United States Patent Office. Retrieved at Google Patents: **https://patents.google.com/patent/US1126605**.

203 Casto R. The Typical American Family Diet in 1908. Livestrong (Livestrong.com). ND. Retrieved: **https://www.livestrong.com/article/461209-the-typical-american-family-diet-in-1908/**. Accessed 4 Dec 2021.

204 Olver, Lynne. The Food Timeline – FAQs: Popular 20th Century American Foods. Home menus, 1901. FoodTimeline.org. ND. Retrieved: **https://www.foodtimeline.org/fooddecades.html#1900s**. Accessed: 1 Nov 2021.

205 Healthy diet. World Health Organization. ND. Retrieved: **https://www.who.int/health-topics/healthy-diet#tab=tab_1**. Accessed: 15 Nov 2021.

206 Noncommunicable diseases. World Health Organization. 13 Apr 2021. Retrieved: **https://www.who.int/news-room/fact-sheets/detail/noncommunicable-diseases**. Accessed 15 Nov 2021.

207 Ultra-processed food and drink products in Latin America: Trends, impact on obesity, policy implications. 2015. Retrieved: **https://www3.paho.org/hq/index.php?option=com_content&view=article&id=11153:ultra-processed-food-and-drink-products&Itemid=1969&lang=en**. Accessed: 30 Nov 2021.

208 Simopoulos AP. Importance of the Ratio of Omega-6/Omega-3 Essential Fatty Acids: Evolutionary Aspects. World Review of Nutrition and Dietetics. 2003;92:1-22.

209 Eaton SB, Konnor M, Shostak M. Stone agers in the fast lane: chronic degenerative diseases in evolutionary perspective. Am J Med. 1988;84:739-749.

210 Ilich, JZ, Kelly OJ, Kim Y, Spicer MT. Low-grade chronic inflammation perpetuated by modern diet as a promoter of obesity and osteoporosis. Arh Hig Rada Toksikol. 2014;65(2):139-48.

211 Stuckler D, Nestle M. Big Food, Food Systems, and Global Health. PLoS Med. 2012;9(6): e1001242. Doi: 10.1371/journal.pmed.1001242.

212 Poti JM, Braga B, Qin B. Ultra-processed Food Intake and Obesity: What Really Matters for Health – Processing or Nutrient Content? Current Obesity Reports. 2017;6:420-431.

213 Popkin BM. Global nutrition dynamics: the world is shifting rapidly toward a diet linked with noncommunicable diseases. Am J Clin Nutr. 2006;84:289-98.

214 Carrera-Bastos P, Fontes-Villalba M, O'Keefe JH, Lindeberg S, Cordain L. The western diet and lifestyle and diseases of civilization. Research Reports in Clinical Cardiology. 2011;;2:15-35.

215 Tilman D, Clark M. Global diets link environmental sustainability and human health. Nature. 2014;515:518-522.

216 O'Keefe JH, Cordain L. Cardiovascular Disease Resulting From a Diet and Lifestyle at Odds With Our Paleolithic Genome: How to Become a 21st-Century Hunter-Gatherer. Mayo Clin Proc. 2004;79:101-108.

217 Lustig RH, Schmidt LA, Brindis CD. The toxic truth about sugar. Nature. 2012;482:27-29.

218 Simopoulos AP. Importance of the Ratio of Omega-6/Omega-3 Essential Fatty Acids: Evolutionary Aspects. World Review of Nutrition and Dietetics. 2003;92:1-22

219 Fuso A, Domenichelli C. Diet, Epigenetics, and Alzheimer's Disease. Handbook of Nutrition, Diet, and Epigenetics. 2018:987. Doi:10.1007/978-3-319-55530-0pass:[_}99.

220 Kanoski SE, Davidson TL. Western diet consumption and cognitive impairment: Links to hippocampal dysfunction and obesity. Physiology & Behavior. 2011;103(1):59-68.

221 Swaminathan A, Jicha GA. Nutrition and prevention of Alzheimer's dementia. Front Aging Neurosci. 2014;Vol.6, Article 282:1-13.

222 Gardener AL, Rainey-Smith SR, Barnes MB, et al. Dietary patterns and cognitive decline in an Australian study of ageing. Mol. Psychiatry. 2015;20:860-866.

223 Chiba M, Nakane K, Komatsu M. Westernized Diet is the Most Ubiquitous Environmental Factor in Inflammatory Bowel Disease. The Permanente Journal. 2019;23. Doi:10.7812/TPP/18-107.

224 Jacka FN, Pasco JA, Mykletun A, et al. Association of Western and Traditional Diets With Depression and Anxiety in Women. Amer J Psychiatry. 2010;167(3):305-11.

225 Cordain L, Eaton SB, Brand-Miller J, Lindeberg S, Jensen C. An evolutionary analysis of the aetiology and pathogenesis of juvenile-onset myopia. Acta Ophthalmologica Scandinavica. 2002;80:125-135.

226 Moodie R, Stuckler D, Monteiro C, et al. Profits and pandemics: prevention of harmful effects of tobacco, alcohol, and ultra-processed food and drink industries. The Lancet. 2013;381(9867):670-679.

227 Moodie R, Stuckler D, Monteiro C, The Lancet NCD Action Group. Profits and pandemics: prevention of harmful effects of tobacco, alcohol, and ultra-processed food and drink industries. Lancet 2013;381:670-79.

228 Saksena MJ, Okrent AM, Anekwe TD, et al. America's Eating Habits: Food Away From Home, EIB-196. U.S. Department of Agriculture, Economic Research Service, September 2018.

229 Guyenet, Stephan. The Hungry Brain – Outsmarting the Instincts That Make Us Overeat. New York, Flatiron Books, 2017, pp. 75-76.

230 Baraldi LG, Steele EM, Canella DS, et al. Consumption of ultra-processed foods and associated sociodemographic factors in the USA between 2007 and 2012: evidence from a nationally representative cross-sectional study. BMJ Open. 2018;8,e020574.

231 Moubarac JC, Batal M, Louzada ML, et al. Consumption of ultra-processed foods predicts diet quality in Canada. Appetite. 2017;108:512-520.

232 Rauber F, Louzada MLDC, Steele EM, et al. Ultra-Processed Food Consumption and Chronic Non-Communicable Diseases-Related Dietary Nutrient Profile in the UK (2008-2014). Nutrients. 2018;10(5):587; **https://doi.org/10.3390/nu10050587**.

233 USDA Economic Research Service, 2009; **www.ers.usda.gov/publications/ElB33; www.ers.usda.gov/Data/FoodConsumption/FoodGuideIndex.htm#-calories** and https://www.ers.usda.gov/data-products/food-availability-per-capita-data-system/

234 Chronic Disease In America. Centers for Disease

Control and Prevention (CDC). ND. Retrieved: **https://www.cdc.gov/chronicdisease/resources/infographic/chronic-diseases.htm**. Accessed 2 Dec 2021.

235   Gerteis J, Izrael D, Deitz D, et al. Multiple Chronic Conditions Chartbook: 2010 Medical Expenditure Panel Survey Data. Washington, DC: Dept of Health and Human Services, Agency for Healthcare Research and Quality; 2014.

236   Alfranca O, Rama R, Tunzelmann N. Technological fields and concentration of innovation among food and beverage multinationals. International Food and Agribusiness Management Review, International Food and Agribusiness Management Association, 2003;5(2):1-14.

237   Harrison, T.R. Harrison's Principles of Internal Medicine. Philadelphia, The Blakeston Company, 1950.

238   Loscalzo J, Fauci A, Kasper D, Hauser S, Longo D, Jameson J. eds. Harrison's Principles of Internal Medicine 21e. McGraw Hill: 2021.

239   University of Michigan Center for Managing Chronic Disease. "About Chronic Disease." University of Michigan. ND. Retrieved: **https://cmcd.sph.umich.edu/about/about-chronic-disease/**. Accessed: 30 Nov 2021.

240   Sav A, King MA, Whitty JA, et al. Burden of treatment for chronic illness: a concept analysis and review of the literature. Health Expect. 2015;18(3):312-324.

241   Stafford RS, Davidson SM, Davidson H, et al. Chronic Disease Medication Use in Managed Care and Indemnity Insurance Plans. Health Serv Res. 2003;38(2):595-612.

242   Hyman MA, Ornish D, Roizen M. Lifestyle Medicine: Treating The Causes of Disease. Altern Ther Health Med. 2009;15(6):12-14.

243   Carrera-Bastos P, Fontes-Villalba M, O'Keefe JH, Lindeberg S, Cordain L. The western diet and lifestyle and diseases of civilization. Research Reports in Clinical Cardiology. 2011;;2:15-35

244   O'Keefe JH, Cordain L. Cardiovascular Disease Resulting From a Diet and Lifestyle at Odds With Our Paleolithic Genome: How to Become a 21st-Century Hunter-Gatherer. Mayo Clin Proc. 2004;79:101-108.

245   Trowell, H.C. and Burkitt, D.P. Western Diseases: their emergence and prevention. Harvard University Press, Cambridge, Massachusetts, 1981, p.xiv-xv.

246   Trowell H.C. Hypertension, obesity, diabetes mellitus and coronary heart disease. In: Trowell, H.C. and Burkitt, D.P. Western Diseases: their emergence and prevention. Harvard University Press, Cambridge, Massachusetts, 1981:3-32.

247   Konnor M, Eaton SB. Paleolithic Nutrition – Twenty-Five Years Later. Nutrition in Clinical Practice. 2010;25(6):594-602.

248   Cordain L, Brand Miller J, Eaton SB, et al. Plant-animal subsistence ratios and macronutrient energy estimations in worldwide hunter-gatherer diets. Am J Clin Nutr. 2000;71:682-92.

249   Sharma S. Assessing diet and lifestyle in the Canadian Arctic Inuit and Inuvialuit to inform a nutrition and physical activity intervention programme. J Hum Nutr Diet. 2010;23 (Suppl. 1):5-17.

250   Krogh, August and Krogh, Marie. A study of the diet and metabolism of Eskimos undertaken in 1908 on an expedition to Greenland. 1913. Retrieved: **https://babel.hathitrust.org/cgi/pt?id=uiuo.ark:/13960/t7qp3mp15&view=1up&seq=9**. Accessed 13 Jan 2021.

251   Sinnett PF, Whyte HM. Epidemiological Studies In A Total Highland Population, Tukisenta, New Guinea. J Chron Dis. 1973;26:265-290.

252   Lee RB. What hunters do for a living, or, how to make out on scarce resources. In: Lee RB, DeVore I, eds. Man the hunter. Chicago, Aldine, 1968:30-48.

253   Lee, Richard Borshay. The !Kung San: Men, Women, and Work in a Foraging Society. New York, Cambridge University Press, 1979.

254   Gaulin SJC, Konner M. On the natural diet of primates, including humans. In: Wurtman RJ, Wurtman JJ, eds. Nutrition and the Brain. Vol 1. New York, Raven Press, 1977:1-86.

255   Woodburn J. An Introduction to Hadza Ecology. In: Lee RB, Devore I, eds. Man the Hunter. Chicago, Aldine, 1968:49-55.

256   Tanaka J. The San, hunter-gatherers of the Kalahari: a study in ecological anthropology. New York, Columbia University Press, 1980.

257   Mann GV, Spoerry A, Gray M, Jarashow D. Atherosclerosis In the Masai. Am J Epidemiol. 1972;95:26-37.

258   Robson JRK, Yen DE. Some Nutritional ?Aspects of the Philippine Tasaday Diet. Ecol Food Nutr. 1976;5:83-89.

259 Fernandez CA, Lynch F. The Tasaday: Cave-Dwelling Food Gatherers of South Cotabato, Mindanao. Philippine Sociological Review. 1972;20(3):279-313.

260 Hawkes K, Hill K, O'Connell JF. Why Hunter Gather: Optimal Foraging and the Aché of Eastern Paraguay. American Ethnologist. 1982;9(2):379-398.

261 Lindeberg S, Lundh B. Apparent absence of stroke and ischaemic heart disease in a traditional Melanesian island: a clinical study in Kitava. J Int Med. 1993;233(3):269-275.

262 Egeland GM, Charbonneau-Roberts G, Kuluguqtuq J, et al. Back to the future – using traditional food and knowledge to promote a healthy future among Inuit. In: Kuhnlein HV, Erasmus B, Spigelski D, editors. Indigenous Peoples' Food Systems: The Many Dimensions of Culture, Diversity, Environment and Health. New York, NY: Food and Agriculture Organization of the United Nations (FAO; 2009. Retrieved: **https://arctichealth.org/media/pubs/295969/i0370e02.pdf**. Accessed 2 Oct 2021.

263 Shaffer PA. Antiketogenesis. II. The ketogenic antiketogenic balance in man. J Biol Chem. 1921;47:463-73.

264 Bang HO, Dyerberg J. Chp 1: Lipid Metabolism and Ischemic Heart Disease in Greenland Eskimos. In: Draper, H.H. (ed): Advances in Nutritional Research. New York, Springer Science +Business, 1980:1-22.

265 Ho KJ, Biss K, Mikkelson B, et al. The Masai of East Africa: Some Unique Biological Characteristics. Arch Path. 1971;91:387-410.

266 Simopoulos AP. Evolutionary aspects of diet, the omega-6/omega-3 ratio and genetic variation: nutritional implications for chronic diseases. Biomed Pharmacotherapy. 2006;60(9):502-507.

267 Simopoulos AP. Importance of the Omega-6/Omega-3 Balance in Health and Disease: Evolutionary Aspects of Diet. Simopoulos AP (ed): Healthy Agriculture, Healthy Nutrition, Healthy People. World Rev Nutr Diet. Basel, Karger, 2011, Vol 102:pp.10-21.

268 Feil, Harold. History of the Treatment of Heart Disease in the 19th Century. Bulletin of the History of Medicine. 1960;34(1):19-28. JSTORE, **www.jstor.org/stable/44446656**.

269 Grimes DS. An epidemic of coronary heart disease. QJ Med. 2012;105:509-518.

270 Johanss BW, Nicol PA. Swedish report on acute myocardial infarction in 1859. BMJ. 1982;284:888-9.

271 Jones DS, Podolsky SH, Greene JA. The Burden of Disease and the Changing Task of Medicine. N Engl J Med. 2012;366:2333-2338. DLI: 10.1056NEJMp1113569.

272 Osler, William. The Principles and Practice of Medicine. Edinburgh & London, Young J. Pentland, 1892.

273 Osler, William. The Principles and Practice of Medicine. Edinburgh & London, Young J. Pentland, 1892, pp. 655-656.

274 Nieto FJ. Cardiovascular Disease and Risk Factor Epidemiology: A Look Back at the Epidemic of the 20th Century. Amer J Pub Health. 1999;89(3):292-4.

275 Boudoulas H. Etiology of valvular heart disease. Expert Review of Cardiovascular Therapy. 2003;1:4:523-532.

276 Herrick JB. Clinical Features of Sudden Obstruction of the Coronary Arteries. JAMA. 1912;LIX(23):2015-2022. Doi:10.10001/jama.1912.04270120001001.

277 Roberts CS. Herrick and Heart Disease. In: Walker HK, Hall WD, Hurst JW, editors. Clinical Methods: The History, Physical, and Laboratory Examinations. 3rd Edition. Boston, Butterworths; 1990. Retrieved: **https://www.ncbi.nlm.nih.gov/books/NBK714/**. Accessed 15 Nov 2021.

278 Olszewski TM. James Herrick (1861-1954): Consultant physician and cardiologist. J Med Biography. 2018;26(2):132-136.

279 Herrick JB, Nuzum FR. Angina pectoris: Clinical experience with two hundred cases. JAMA. 1918;10:67-70.

280 Herrick JB. Thrombosis of the coronary arteries. JAMA. 1919;72:387-90.

281 Osler, William and McCrae, Thomas. The Principles and Practice of Medicine, Eighth Edition. D. Appleton and Company, 1915, p. 836.

282 Causes of Death Over 100 Years. Office for National Statistics (UK). 18 Sep 2017. Retrieved from: **https://www.ons.gov.uk/peoplepopulationandcommunity/birthsdeathsandmarriages/deaths/articles/causesofdeathover100years/2017-09-18** Accessed 3 Jun 2020.

283 American Heart Association. Heart disease and stroke statistics 2013 update. Circulation. 2013;127:e6-e245.

284 Silverman ME. Maurice Campbell: first editor of Heart. Heart. 2003;89(12):1379-1381.

285 Campbell M. Death rates from diseases of the heart: 1876 to 1959. BMJ. 1963;ii:528-35.

286 Unal B, Critchley JA, Capewell S. Explaining the decline in coronary heart disease mortality in England

and Wales between 1981 and 2000. Circulation. 2004;109:1101-7.

287 UK Department of Health. The National Service Framework for Coronary Heart Disease: Winning the War on Heart Disease. London, The Stationary Office, 2004.

288 Appleby J. Does poor health justify NHS reform? Brit Med J. 2011;342:10(d566).

289 Smoking Statistics. Action on Smoking and Health. ASH.org.uk. Retrieved: **https://ash.org.uk/wp-content/uploads/2019/10/SmokingStatistics.pdf**. Accessed 1 Nov 2021.

290 Pitts M, Dorling D, Pattie C. Oil for food – the global story of edible lipids. Journal of World-Systems Research. 2007;13:12-32.

291 Dalen JE, Alpert JS, Goldberg RJ, Weinstein RS. The Epidemic of the 20th Century: Coronary Heart Disease. The American Journal of Medicine. 2014;127:807-812.

292 Mann GV. Wheeler ED, Stare FJ. Cholesterol and Arteriosclerosis. Proc Third Research Conf., Council on Research, American Meat Institute. 1951.

293 Recent trends in mortality from heart disease. Stat Bull Metropol Life Insur Co. 1975;56:2-6.

294 Rogers DE, Blendon RJ. The changing American health scene – Sometimes things get better. JAMA. 1977;237(16):1710-1714.

295 Herkner H, Arrich J, Havel C, Müllner M. Bed rest for acute uncomplicated myocardial infarction. Cochrane Database Syst Rev. 2007;2007(2): CD003836.

296 Adnet F, Renault R, Jabre P, et al. Incidence of acute myocardial infarction resulting in sudden death outside the hospital. Emerg Med J. 2011;28(10):884-6.

297 Ford ES, Ajani UA, Croft JB, et al. Explaining the Decrease in U.S. Deaths from Coronary Disease, 1980-2000. NEJM. 2007;356:2388-2398.

298 Mensah GA, Wei GS, Sorlie PD, et al. Decline in Cardiovascular Mortality: Possible Causes and Implications. Circ Res. 2017;120(2):366-380.

299 Yazdanyar A, Newman AB. The Burden of Cardiovascular Disease in the Elderly: Morbidity, Mortality, and Costs. Clin Geriatr Med. 2009;25(4):563-577.

300 Curtin SC. Trends in Cancer and Heart Disease Death Rates Among Adults Aged 45-64: United States, 1999-2017. National Vital Statistics Reports, CDC. 2019;68(5):1-9. 22 May, 2019. Retrieved: **https://www.cdc.gov/nchs/data/nvsr/nvsr68/nvsr68_05-508.pdf**.

301 Lloyd-Jones DM, Larson MG, Beiser A, Levy D. Lifetime risk of developing coronary heart disease. The Lancet. 1999;353(9147):89-92.

302 Coronary Heart Disease, Myocardial Infarction, and Stroke – A Public Health Issue. Centers for Disease Control and Prevention (CDC). ND. Retrieved: **https://www.cdc.gov/aging/publications/coronary-heart-disease-brief.html**. Accessed: 20 Dec 2021.

303 Report by the Central Committee for Medical and Community Program of the American Heart Association. Dietary Fat and Its Relation to Heart Attacks and Strokes. JAMA. 1961;175(5):389-391.

304 Teicholz, Nina. The Big FAT Surprise – Why Butter, Meat, and Cheese Belong in a Healthy Diet. New York, Simon & Schuster. 2014, p336.

305 Hamley S. The effect of replacing saturated fat with mostly n-6 polyunsaturated fat on coronary heart disease: a meta-analysis of randomized controlled trials. Nutrition Journal. 2017;16(1):30.

306 Siri-Tarino P, Sun Q, Hu F, Krauss R. Meta-analysis of prospective cohort studies evaluating the association of saturated fat with cardiovascular disease. Am J Clin Nutr. 2010;91:535-46.

307 Schwingshackl L, Hoffman G. Dietary fatty acids in the secondary prevention of coronary heart disease: a systematic review, meta-analysis and meta-regression. BMJ Open. 2014;4:e004487.

308 Saturated Fat. American Heart Association. ND. Retrieved: **https://www.heart.org/en/healthy-living/healthy-eating/eat-smart/fats/saturated-fats**. Accessed 14 Nov 2021.

309 American Heart Association. "Healthy Cooking Oils." ND. Retrieved: **https://www.heart.org/en/healthy-living/healthy-eating/eat-smart/fats/healthy-cooking-oils**. Accessed 15 Nov 2021.

310 Per capita availability of chicken higher than that of beef. USDA Economic Research Service (ERS). 14 Jan 2021. Retrieved: **https://www.ers.usda.gov/data-products/chart-gallery/gallery/chart-detail/?chartId=58312**. Accessed 15 Nov 2021.

311 Horowitz, Roger. Putting Meat On the American Table. Baltimore, The Johns Hopkins University Press, 2006, pp. 11-12.

312 Daniel CR, Cross AJ, Koebnick C, Sinha R. Trends in meat consumption in the USA. Public Health Nutr. 2011;14(4):575-83.

313 Hilliard, Sam Bowers. Hot Meat and Hoecake. Athens and London, The University of Georgia Press, 2014, p.41.

314 Ogle, Maureen. In Meat We Trust – An Unexpected History of Carnivore America. Boston, Houghton Mifflin Harcourt, 2013, pp. 3-4.

315 Rigotti NA, Pasternak RC. Cigarette Smoking and Coronary Heart Disease. Cardiology Clinics. 1996;14(1):P51-68.

316 Achievements in Public Health, 1900-1999: Tobacco Use – United States, 1900-1999. CDC MMWR. Retrieved: https://www.cdc.gov/mmwr/preview/mmwrhtml/mm4843a2.htm. Accessed 10 Dec 2021.

317 Jha P. The hazards of smoking and the benefits of cessation: A critical summation of the epidemiological evidence in high income countries. eLife Sciences 9. DOI::10.7554/eLifes.49979.

318 U.S. Department of Health and Human Services (USDHHS). Let's Make the Next Generation Tobacco-Free: Your Guide to the 50th Anniversary Surgeon General's Report on Smoking and Health (Consumer Booklet). Atlanta, GA: U.S. Department of Health and Human Services, Centers for Disease Control and Prevention, National Center for Chronic Disease Prevention and Health Promotion, Office on Smoking and Health; 2014.

319 Stallones RA. The association between tobacco smoking and coronary heart disease. Int J Epidemiol. 2015:735-743.

320 Lands WEM, Libelt B, Morris A, et al. Maintenance of lower proportions of (n-6) eicosanoid precursors in phospholipids of human plasma in response to added dietary (n-3) fatty acids. Biochimica et Biophysica Acta (BBA) – Molecular Basis of Disease. 1992;1180(2):147-162.

321 Lands WEM. Diets could prevent many diseases. Lipids 2003;38(4):317-21.

322 Caramia G. [The essential fatty acids omega-6 and omega-3: from their discovery to their use in therapy]. Minerva Pediatr. 2008;60(2):219-33.

323 Mariamenatu AH, Abdu EM. Overconsumption of Omega-6 Polyunsaturated Fatty Acids (PUFAs) versus Deficiency of Omega-3 PUFAs in Modern-Day Diets: The Disturbing Factor for Their "Balanced Antagonistic Metabolic Functions" in the Human Body. Journ of Lipids. 2021;2021:8848161. Doi: 10.1155/2021/8848161.

324 Eaton SB, Konner M, Shostak M. Stone Agers in the Fast Lane: Chronic Degenerative Diseases in Evolutionary Perspective. Amer J Med. 1988;84:739-749.

325 Cordain L, Martin C, Florant G, Watkins BA. The fatty acid composition of muscle, brain, marrow and adipose tissue in elk: Evolutionary implications for human dietary lipid requirements. World Rev Nutr Diet. 1998;83:225-226.

326 Kuipers RS, Luxwolda MF, Dijck-Brouwer DA, et al. Estimated macronutrient and fatty acid intakes from an East African Paleolithic diet. Br J Nur. 2010;104:1666-1687.

327 "Artemis Simopoulos, MD." American Nutrition Association. ND. Retrieved: https://theana.org/scientific-advisors/Simopoulos. Accessed 1 Feb 2022.

328 Simopoulos AP, Leaf A, Salem N. Essentiality of and Recommended Dietary Intakes for Omega-6 and Omega-3 Fatty Acids. Ann Nutr Metab. 1999;43:127-130.

329 Institute of Medicine (IOM). Dietary fats: Total fat and fatty acids. In: Dietary Reference Intakes for Energy, Carbohydrate, Fiber, Fat, Fatty Acids, Cholesterol, Protein, and Amino Acids; National Academies Press: Washington DC, USA, 2005;pp. 470-472, 030908525X (pbk) 0309085373 (hardcover).

330 Simopoulos AP. The importance of the omega-6/omega-3 fatty acid ratio in cardiovascular disease and other chronic diseases. Experimental Biology and Medicine. 2008;233(6):674-688.

331 Simopoulos AP. An increase in the omega-6/omega-3 fatty acid ratio increases the risk for obesity. Nutrients. 2016;8(3):128.

332 Simopoulos AP. Evolutionary aspects of the diet, the omega-6/omega-3 ratio and genetic variation: nutritional implications for chronic diseases. Biomedicine & Pharmacotherapy. 2006;60(9):502-507.

333 Couet C, Delarue J, Ritz P, et al. Effect of dietary fish oil on body fat mass and basal fat oxidation in healthy adults. Int J Obes Relat Metab Disord. 1997;21:637-643.

334 Fontani G, Corradeschi F, Felici A, et al. Blood profiles, body fat and mood state in healthy subjects on different diets supplemented with omega-3 polyunsaturated fatty acids. Eur J Clin Investig. 2005;35:499-507.

335 Hill AM, Buckley JD, Murphy KJ, Howe PR. Combining fish-oil supplements with regular aerobic exercise improves body composition and cardiovascular disease risk factors. Am J Clin Nutr. 2007;85:1267-1274.

336 Belury MA, Mahon A, Banni S. The conjugated linoleic acid (CLA) isomer, t10c12-CLA, is inversely associated with changes in body weight and serum leptin in subjects with type 2 diabetes mellitus. J Nutr. 2003;133:257S-260S.

337 Chan DC, Watts GF, Nguyen MN, Barrett PH. Factorial study of the effect of n-3 fatty acid supplementation and atorvastatin on the kinetics of HDL apolipoproteins A-I and A-II in men with abdominal obesity. Am J Clin Nutr. 2006;84:37-43.

338 Simopoulos AP. The Impact of the Bellagio Report on Healthy Agriculture, Healthy Nutrition, Healthy People: Scientific and Policy Aspects and the International Network of Centers for Genetics, Nutrition and Fitness for Health. J Nutrigenet Nutrigenom. 2015;7:189-209.

339 Yang H, Hu FB, Manson JE. Marine Omega-3 Supplementation and Cardiovascular Disease: An Updated Meta-Analysis of 13 Randomized Controlled Trials Involving 127 477 Participants. J Amer Heart Assoc. 2019;8:e013543.

340 Silaste M, Rantala M, Alfthan G, et al. Changes in dietary fat intake alter plasma levels of oxidized low-density lipoprotein and lipoprotein(a). Arterioscler Thromb Vasc Biol. 2004;24(3):498-503.

341 Trowell, H.C. and Burkitt, D.P. Western Diseases: their emergence and prevention. Harvard University Press, Cambridge, Massachusetts, 1981, p.26.

342 Shaper AG, Jones KW. Serum-Cholesterol, Diet, and Coronary Heart Disease In Africans and Asians in Uganda. The Lancet. 1959;274(7102):534-537.

343 Clark LT, Ferdinand KC, Flack JM, et al. Coronary heart disease in African Americans. Heart Dis. 2001;3(2):97-108.

344 Noncommunicable Diseases Country Profiles 2018. World Health Organization (WHO). 2018. Retrieved: **file:///Users/chrisknobbe/Downloads/9789241514620-eng.pdf**. Accessed 15 Dec 2021.

345 Health Nutrition and Population Statistics. Original data: **https://datacatalog.worldbank.org/dataset/health-nutrition-and-population-statistics**. Data retrieved: Knoema.com, CC by 4.0 Creative Commons Attribution.

346 Mpoke S, Johnson KE. Baseline survey of pregnancy practices among Kenyan Maasai. West J Nurs Res. 1993;15(3):298-310.

347 "The Maasai People." Maasai Association. ND. Retrieved: **http://www.maasai-association.org/maasai.html**. Accessed: 27 Dec 2021.

348 Ho KJ, Biss K, Mikkelson B, Lewis LA, Taylor CB. The Masai of East Africa: some unique biological characteristics. Arch Pathol. 1971;91(5):387-410.

349 Markiewicz-Keszycka M, Czyzak-Runowska G, Lipinska P, Wójtowski J. Fatty Acid Profile of Milk – A Review. Bull Vet Inst Pulawy. 2013;57:135-139.

350 Mann GV, Spoerry A, Gray M, Jarashow D. Atherosclerosis in the Masai. Am J Epidemiol. 1972;95(1):26-37.

351 Biss K, Ho KJ, Mikkelson B, et al. Some Unique Biological Characteristics of the Masai of East Africa. NEJM. 1971;284(13):694-699.

352 Galvin KA, Beeton TA, Boone RB, Burnsilver SB. Nutritional Status of Maasai Pastoralists under Change. Hum Ecol Interdiscip J. 2015;43(3):411-424.

353 Trowell, Hugh. Hypertension, obesity, diabetes mellitus and coronary heart disease. In: H.C. Trowell, D.P. Burkitt, eds. Western Diseases: their emergence and prevention. Cambridge, Massachusetts, Harvard University Press, 1981;p.6.

354 Trowell, Hugh. Hypertension, obesity, diabetes mellitus and coronary heart disease. In: H.C. Trowell, D.P. Burkitt, eds. Western Diseases: their emergence and prevention. Cambridge, Massachusetts, Harvard University Press, 1981;p.22.

355 McLarty DG, Swai AB, Kitange HM, et al. Prevalence of diabetes and impaired glucose tolerance in rural Tanzania. Lancet. 1989;1:871-875.

356 Masaki S, Ngoye A, Petrucka P, Buza J. Type 2 Diabetes Prevalence and Risk Factors of Urban Maasai in Arusha Municipality and Rural Maasai in Ngorongoro Crater. Journal of Applied Life Sciences International. 2015;3(4):157-168.

357 Food Balance Sheets. Knoema. Vegetable Oils, Sugars, United Republic of Tanzania. Retrieved: **http://www.fao.org/faostat/en/#data/FBS**. Accessed 27 Dec 2021.

358. U.S. Food & Drug Administration. Added Sugars on the New Nutrition Facts Label. 25 Feb 2022. Retrieved: https://www.fda.gov/food/new-nutrition-facts-label/added-sugars-new-nutrition-facts-label#:~:text=Added%20sugars%20include%20sugars%20that,concentrated%20fruit%20or%20vegetable%20juices. Accessed: 25 May, 2022.

359. Food and Agriculture Organization of the United Nations. Added sugars: Definition and estimation in the USDA Food Patterns Equivalents Databases [2017]. ND. Retrieved: https://agris.fao.org/agris-search/search.do?recordID=US201700215889. Accessed 25 May 2022.

360. Voet D, Voet JG. Biochemistry. New York, J. Wiley & Sons. 2010, p. 957.

361. O'Leary FO, Samman S. Vitamin B12 in Health and Disease. Nutrients. 2010;2(3):299-316.

362. Wessen, Albert F (ed.), Hooper A, Huntsman J, Prior IAM, Salmond CE. Migration and Health in a Small Society: The Case of Tokelau. New York, Oxford University Press, 1992, p.361.

363. Brittanica, The Editors of Encyclopedia. "Breadfruit." Encyclopedia Brittanica, 26 Jan 2021. Retrieved: https://www.britannica.com/plant/breadfruit. Accessed: 26 Dec 2021.

364. Prior IAM, Stanhope JM, Grimley Evans J, Salmond CE. The Tokelau Island Migrant Study. Int J Epidemiol. 1974;3(3):225-232.

365. Seneviratne KN, Jayathilaka N. Coconut Oil Chemistry and Nutrition. Battaramulla, Sri Lanka, Lakva Publishers, 2016, pp. 55, 89.

366. Prior IA, Davidson F, Salmond CE, Czochanska Z. Cholesterol, coconuts, and diet on Polynesian atolls: a natural experiment: the Pukapuka and Tokelau Island studies. Amer J Clin Nutr. 1981;34(8):1552-1561.

367. Orsavova J, Misurcova L, Ambrozova JV, et al. Fatty Acids Composition of Vegetable Oils and Its Contribution to Dietary Energy Intake and Dependence of Cardiovascular Mortality on Dietary Intake of Fatty Acids. Int J Mol Sci. 2015;16:12871-12890.

368. Nettleton JA. "Fatty Acids in Cultivated and Wild Fish." ResearchGate. January, 2000. Retrieved from: https://www.researchgate.net/publication/239572046_Fatty_Acids_in_Cultivated_and_Wild_Fish. Accessed 23 Jun 2020.

369. The Facts on Fats – 50 Years of American Heart Association Dietary Fats Recommendations. American Heart Association (AHA) and American Stroke Association. June 2015.

370. Dietary Guidelines for Americans 2020 – 2025. USDA. Retrieved: https://www.dietaryguidelines.gov/sites/default/files/2020-12/Dietary_Guidelines_for_Americans_2020-2025.pdf. Accessed 26 Dec 2021.

371. Healthy Diet. World Health Organization (WHO). 2018;Fact Sheet No 394. Retrieved: https://www.who.int/nutrition/publications/nutrientrequirements/healthy_diet_fact_sheet_394.pdf?ua=1. Accessed 26 Dec 2021.

372. Hughes, Robert G. Diet, Food Supply and Obesity in the Pacific. World Health Organization (WHO), Regional Office for the Western Pacific. 2003.

373. Pollock, Nancy J. These Roots Remain: Food Habits in Islands of the Central and Eastern Pacific Since Western Contact. The Institute for Polynesian Studies, University of Hawaii, 1992.

374. Burrows, William. Some Notes and Legends of a South Sea Island. Fakaofo of the Tokelau or Union Group. Journal of the Polynesian Society. 1923;32: No 127:143-173.

375. Malolo M, Matenga-Smith T, Hughes R. Pacific Foods – The Staples We Eat. Secretariat of the Pacific Community, Noumea, New Caledonia, 1999.

376. "Tokelau learns from Samoa." Food and Agriculture Organization of the United Nations (FAO). FAO Regional Office for Asia and the Pacific. ND. Retrieved: https://www.fao.org/asiapacific/news/detail-events/en/c/1133599/. Accessed 10 Jan 2022.

377. McGregor A, Sheehy M. Food security in the atoll countries of the South Pacific – with particular reference to Tuvalu: A report prepared for IFAD to assist in the preparation of funding proposal to the Global Agriculture and Food Security Program. 8 Sep 2019.

378. "Coconut Oil." The Nutrition Source. Harvard T.H. Chan School of Public Health. ND. Retrieved: https://www.hsph.harvard.edu/nutritionsource/food-features/coconut-oil/. Accessed 5 Jan 2022.

379. "How much do Tokelauans consume – and throw away – in one year? A study of 2014 imports by the Tokelau National Statistics Office, 2015/16, summary version 2. Retrieved: https://www.tokelau.org.nz/site/tokelau/files/TokelauNSO/WhatTokelauansConsumedIn2014-15jul16.pdf. Accessed 20 Jan 2022.

380 Trowell, H.C. and Burkitt, D.P. Western Diseases: their emergence and prevention. Harvard University Press, Cambridge, Massachusetts, 1981, p.255.

381 Estimates of Age-Standardized Prevalence of Diabetes in the Word, Regions, and 200 Countries. Available online: https://www.ncdrisc.org/data-downloads-diabetes.html. Accessed: 10 Jan 2022.

382 IDF Diabetes Atlas – Sixth Edition. International Diabetes Federation. 2013. Online version IDF Diabetes Atlas: http://www.idf.org/diabetesatlas.

383 Zimmet P, Whitehouse S. Chapter 15: Pacific Islands of Nauru, Tuvalu and Western Samoa. In: Trowell, H.C. and Burkitt, D.P. Western Diseases: their emergence and prevention. Harvard University Press, Cambridge, Massachusetts, 1981, p.208-9.

384 Winter-Smith J, Selak V, Harwood M, et al. Cardiovascular disease and its management among Pacific people: a systematic review by ethnicity and place of birth. BMC Cardiovascular Disorders. 2021;21, Article number: 515. https://doi.org/10.1186/s12872-021-02313-x.

385 FAO Expert Consultation Workshop. Enhancing evidence-based decision making for sustainable agriculture sector development in Pacific Islands Countries. FAO Sub-regional Office for the Pacific Islands. 20-22 October 2010. Retrieved: https://www.fao.org/publications/card/en/c/2a39b2bc-e27b-5246-8c15-41e9469a330b/. Accessed 10 Jan 2022.

386 Naiken, Loganaden. "FAO Methodology for Estimating the Prevalence of Undernourishment. Keynote Paper Abstract." FAO.org. ND. Retrieved: https://www.fao.org/3/y4250E/y4250e03.htm. Accessed 10 Jan 2022.

387 Strong, Wendell M. Is Cancer Mortality Increasing? The Journal of Cancer Research. 1921;6(3):251-256

388 "Fact Book Fiscal Year 2012." National Institutes of Health, National Heart, Lung, and Blood Institute. Feb 2013.

389 Lag R, Eisner MP, Kosary CL, et al. eds. SEER Cancer Statistics Review, 1973-1997. Bethesda: National Cancer Institute, 2000.

390 Deapen D, Lihua L, Perkins C, et al. Rapidly rising breast cancer incidence rates among Asian-American women. Int J Cancer. 2002;99:747-750.

391 Press Release No. 263 – Latest global cancer data: Cancer burden rises to 18.1 million new cases and 9.6 million cancer deaths in 2018. International Agency for Research on Cancer / World Health Organization. 12 Sep 2018. Retrieved from: https://www.who.int/cancer/PRGlobocanFinal.pdf

392 Global Burden of Disease Collaborative Network. Global Burden of Disease Study 2016 (GBD 2016) Results. Seattle, United States: Institute for Health Metrics and Evaluation (IHME), 2017. Data retrieved: OurWorldInData.org: https://ourworldindata.org/how-many-people-in-the-world-die-from-cancer. Accessed 28 Dec 2021.

393 Food Balance Sheets, Sugar & Sweeteners, Knoema, 1961-2017. Retrieved: http://www.fao.org/faostat/en#data/FBS. Accessed 27 Dec 2021.

394 Tung HT, Tsukuma H, Tanaka H, et al. Risk factors for breast cancer in Japan, with special attention to anthropometric measurements and reproductive history. Jpn J Clin Oncol. 1999;29:137-46.

395 Wakai K, Suzuki S, Ohno Y, et al. Epidemiology of breast cancer in Japan. Int J Epidemiol. 1995;24:285-91.

396 Matsuda T, Saika K. Cancer burden in Japan based on the latest cancer statistics: need for evidence-based cancer control programs. Ann Cancer Epidemiol. 2018;2(2):1-15, doi: 10.21037/ace.2018.08.01.

397 Trowell, H.C. and Burkitt, D.P. Western Diseases: their emergence and prevention. Harvard University Press, Cambridge, Massachusetts, 1981, pp. 337-351.

398 Matsumoto, N. "Is the Japanese Diet a Melting Pot? Japan as Seen in Food Culture." Japan's Food Culture. Japan Spotlight: Economy, Culture & History. 2008;27(4):30-31. Retrieved:

399 Chen W, Zheng R, Baade PD, et al. Cancer Statistics in China, 2015. CA Cancer J Clin. 2016;00:00-00. Doi: 10.3322/caac.21338. Available online at cacancerjournal.com.

400 Ministry of Health, the People's Republic of China. Report on the Third National Sampling Survey of Causes of Death. Beijing: The People's Health Press, 2008.

401 Zhao P, Dai M, Chen W, Li N. Cancer Trends in China. Jpn J Clin Oncol. 2010;40(4):281-285.

402 Global Burden of Disease Cancer Collaboration. Global, regional, and national cancer incidence, mortality, years of life lost, years lived with disability, and disability-adjusted life-years for 29 cancer groups, 1990

to 2017: a systematic analysis for the global burden of disease study. JAMA Oncol. 2019;5(12):1749-1768.

403 Global Burden of Disease Collaborative Network. Global Burden of Disease Study 2016 (GBD 2016) Health-related Sustainable Development Goals (SDG) Indicators 1990-2030. Seattle, United States: Institute for Health Metrics and Evaluation (IHME), 2017. Retrieved: **http://ghdx.healthdata.org/record/global-burden-disease-study-2016-gbd-2016-health-related-sustainable-development-goals-sdg**. Data and graph: OurWorldInData.org.

404 Parkin DM, Bray F, Ferlay J, Pisani P. Global Cancer Statistics, 2002. CA A Cancer Journal for Clinicians. 2005;55:74-108.

405 Parkin DM, Bray F, Ferlay J, Pisani P. Global Cancer Statistics, 2002. CA A Cancer Journal for Clinicians. 2005;55:74-108.

406 Chen JG, Zhang SW. Liver cancer epidemic in China: Past, present and future. Semin Cancer Biol. 2011;21(1):59-69.

407 Wang Z, Chen Z, Zhang L, et al. Status of hypertension in China: results from the China hypertension survey, 2012-2-15. Circulation. 2018;137(22):2344-2356.

408 Tao S, Zhou B. Epidemiology of hypertension in China. Chin Med J. 1999;112(10):878-882.

409 Liu M, Liu SW, Wang LJ, et al. Burden of diabetes, hyperglycaemia in China from 1990 to 2016: findings from the 1990 to 2016, global burden of disease study. Diabetes Metab. 2019;45(3):286-293. Doi:10.1016/j.diabet.2018.08.008.

410 Liu S, Li Y, Zeng X, et al. Burden of cardiovascular diseases in China, 1990-2016: findings from the 2016 global burden of disease study. JAMA Cardiology. 2019;4(4):342-352. Doi:10.1001/jamacardio.2019.0295.

411 Saklayen MG. The Global Epidemic of the Metabolic Syndrome. Current Hypertension Reports. 2018;20(12). **https://doi.org/10.1007/s11906-018-0812-z**.

412 Gu XY, Chen ML Vital Statistics, health services in Shanghai Country. Am J Public Health. 1982;72:19-23.

413 The World Bank. China: Long-Term Issues and Options in the Health Transition. Washington, DC: The World Bank; 1990.

414 Bai R, Wu W, Dong W, et al. Forecasting the Populations of Overweight and Obese Chinese Adults. Diabetes Metab Syndr Obes. 2020;13:4849-4857.

415 Food Supply, Vegetable Oils, Sugars: China. Knoema World Data Atlas. Food Balance Sheets. Retrieved: **http://www.fao.org/faostat/en/#data/FBS** (original data).

416 Food Balance Sheets. Sugar and Sweeteners, Food Supply. Knoema, 2018. Retrieved: **https://knoema.com/FAOFBS2017/food-balance-sheets**. Accessed 2 Jan 2022.

417 UN Food and Agriculture Organization (FAO), Data measures the food available for consumption at the household level but does not account for any food wasted or not eaten at the consumption level. OurWorldInData.org/food-supply. Accessed: 27 Dec 2021.

418 WHO calls on countries to reduce sugars intake among adults and children. WHO. 4 March 2015. Retrieved: **https://www.who.int/news/item/04-03-2015-who-calls-on-countries-to-reduce-sugars-intake-among-adults-and-children**. Accessed 28 Dec 2021.

419 Dunning WF, Curtis MR, Maun ME. The Effect of Dietary Fat and Carbohydrate on Diethystilbestrol-induced Mammary Cancer in Rats. Cancer Research. 1949;9(6):354-361.

420 Engel RW, Copeland DH. Mammary, Ear-Duct, and Liver Tumors in Rats Fed 2-Acetylaminofluorense. Cancer Research. 1951;11(3):180-183.

421 Duan Y, Zeng L, Zheng C, et al. Inflammatory Links Between High Fat Diets and Diseases. Front Immunol. 2018 Nov 13;9:2649. Doi: 10.3389/fimmu.2018.02649.

422 Carroll KK, Khor HT. Effects of Dietary Fat and Dose Level of 7,12-Dimethylbenz(α)-anthracene on Mammary Tumor Incidence in Rats. Cancer Research. 1970;30:2260-2264.

423 Carroll KK, Khor HT. Effects of level and type of dietary fat on incidence of mammary tumors induced in female Sprague-Dawley rats by 7,12-dimethylbenz(α) anthracene. Lipids. 1971;6(6):415-420.

424 Carroll KK, Hopkins GJ. Dietary Polyunsaturated Fat Versus Saturated Fat in Relation to Mammary Carcinogenesis. Lipids. 1979;14(2):155-158.

425 Engel RW, Copeland DH. Protective Action of Stock Diets against the Cancer-Inducing Action of 2-Acetyl-

aminofluorene in Rats. Cancer Research. 1952;12:211-215.

426 Tannenbaum A, Silverstone H. Nutrition and the Genesis of Tumours. In: R.W. Raven (ed.), Cancer. London, Butterwoth & Co., Ltd., 1957;Vol 1:pp.306-334.

427 Carroll KK. Experimental Evidence of Dietary Factors and Hormone-dependent Cancers. Cancer Research. 1975;35:3374-3383.

428 Carroll KK. Dietary fat and breast cancer. Lipids. 1992;27:793-797.

429 Bartsch H, Nair J, Owen RW. Dietary polyunsaturated fatty acids and cancers of the breast and colorectum: emerging evidence for their role as risk modifiers. Carcinogenesis. 1999;20(12):2209-2218.

430 Carroll KK. Summation: Which fat/how much fat—Animals. Preventive Medicine. 1987;16(4):510-515.

431 Kromhout D. The importance of N-6 and N-3 fatty acids in carcinogenesis. Med Oncol & Tumor Pharmacother. 1990;7:173.

432 Moral R, Escrich R, Solanas M, et al. Diets high in corn oil or extra-virgin olive oil differentially modify the gene expression profile of the mammary gland and influence experimental breast cancer susceptibility. Eur J Nutr. 2016;55:1397-1409.

433 Solanas M, Grau L, Moral R, et al. Dietary olive oil and corn oil differentially affect experimental breast cancer through distinct modulation of the p21Ras signaling and the proliferation-apoptosis balance. Carcinogenesis. 2010;31(5):871-879.

434 Escrich E, Solanas M, Moral R. Chp 15: Olive Oil, and Other Dietary Lipids, in Cancer: Experimental Approaches. In: Quiles JL, Ramirez-Tortosa MC, Yaqoob P (editors), Olive Oil & Health. CABI Publishing, Oxfordshire, UK, 317-360.

435 Chan PC, Ferguson KA, Dao TL. Effects of different dietary fats on mammary carcinogenesis. Cancer Res. 1983;43:1079-1083.

436 Tinsley IJ, Schmitz JA, Pierce DA. Influence of dietary fatty acids on the incidence of mammary tumors in the C3H mouse. Cancer Res. 1981;41:1460-1465.

437 Eynard AR, Quiroga P, Silva R, Munoz SE. Effect of dietary polyunsaturated fatty acids (PUFA) on metastatic and growth capability of a murine mammary gland adenocarcinoma. J Exp Clin Cancer Res. 1991;10:65-69.

438 Eynard AR, Manzur T, Moyano A, et al. Dietary deficiency or enrichment of essential fatty acids modulates tumorigenesis in the whole body of cobalt-60-irradiated mice. Prostaglandins, Leukotrienes and Essential Fatty Acids. 1997;56(3):239-244.

439 Ngo TH, Barnard J, Cohen P, et al. Effect of Isocaloric Low-Fat Diet on Human LAPC-4 Prostate Cancer Xenografts in Severe Immunodeficient Mice and the Insulin-like Growth Factor Axis. Clin Cancer Res. 2003;9(7):2734-2743.

440 Ip, C. Fat and Essential Fatty Acids in Mammary Carcinogenesis. Amer J Clin Nutr. 1987;45(1):218-224.

441 Zock PL, Katan MB. Linoleic acid intake and cancer risk: a review and meta-analysis. Am J Clin Nutr. 1998;68:142-153.

442 Pellizzon MA, Ricci MR. The common use of improper control diets in diet-induced metabolic disease research confounds data interpretation: the fiber factor. Nutr Metab (Lond). 2018;15:3. Doi: 10.1186/s12986-018-0243-5.

443 "Rats and Mice." Indiana Department of Health. In.gov. ND. Retrieved: **https://www.in.gov/health/erc/infectious-disease-epidemiology/rats-and-mice**. Accessed 30 Dec 2021.

444 Fiolet T, Srour B, Sellem L, et al. Consumption of ultra-processed foods and cancer risk: results from NutriNet-Santé prospective cohort. BMJ. 2018;360:k322.

445 Pickens MK, Yan JS, Ng RK, et al. Dietary sucrose is essential to the development of liver injury in the methionine-choline-deficient model of steatohepatitis. J Lipid Res. 2009;50:2072-2082.

446 Lustig RH. Fructose: Metabolic, Hedonic, and Societal Parallels with Ethanol. American Dietetic Association. 2010; doi: 10.1016/j.jada.2010.06.008.

447 Temple, Norman J, Burkitt, Denis P. Western Diseases – Their Dietary Prevention and Reversibility. Totowa, New Jersey, Humana Press, 1994, p. viii (Preface).

448 Trowell, H.C. and Burkitt, D.P. Western Diseases: their emergence and prevention. Harvard University Press, Cambridge, Massachusetts, 1981, p.15.

449 Carson SA. Racial differences in body mass indices of men imprisoned in 19th Century Texas. Economics & Human Biology. 2009;7(1):121-27.

450 Carson SA. Black and White Body Mass Index Values In Developing Nineteenth Century Nebraska. Journ

451 Fryar CD, Carroll MD, Ogden CL. Prevalence of Overweight, Obesity, and Extreme Obesity Among Adults: United States, Trends 1960-1962 Through 2009-2010. CDC, Division of Health and Nutrition Examination Surveys. Sep 2012.

452 Hales CM, Carroll MD, Fryar CD, Ogden CL. Prevalence of Obesity Among Adults and Youth: United States, 2015-2016. CDC National Health and Nutrition Examination Survey. NCHS Data Brief, No. 288, Oct 2017.

453 Fryar CD, Carroll MD, Afful J, Division of Health and Nutrition Examination Surveys. Prevalence of Overweight, Obesity, and Severe Obesity Among Adults Aged 20 and Over: United States, 1960-1962 Through 2017-2018. NCHS Health E-Stats. 2020.

454 Ward ZJ, Bleich SN, Cradock AL, et al. Projected U.S. State-Level Prevalence of Adult Obesity and Severe Obesity. N Engl J Med. 2019;381:2440-2450.

455 WHO Expert Consultation. Appropriate body-mass index for Asian populations and its implications for policy and intervention strategies. Lancet. 2004;363(9403):157-163.

456 Jih J, Mukherjea A, Vittinghoff E, et al. Using appropriate body mass index cut points for overweight and obesity among Asian Americans. Preventive Medicine. 2014;65:1-6. Doi: 10.1016/j.ypmed.2014.04.010.

457 Centers for Disease Control. "Obesity epidemic increases dramatically in the United States: CDC director calls for national prevention effort." CDC. Retrieved: https://www.cdc.gov/media/pressrel/r991026.htm. Accessed 3 Nov 2021.

458 Dietary Guidelines for Americans. "1980 Dietary Guidelines for Americans." DGA (Official website of the United States government). Retrieved: https://www.dietaryguidelines.gov/about-dietary-guidelines/previous-editions/1980-dietary-guidelines-americans. Accessed 15 Nov 2021.

459 Komlos J, Brabec M. "The evolution of BMI values of US adults: 1882-1986." VoxEU.org. 31 Aug 2010. Retrieved: https://voxeu.org/article/100-years-us-obesity. Accessed 5 Jan 2022.

460 Food Availability (Per Capita) Data System. USDA Economic Research Service (ERS). Loss Adjusted Food Availability: Calories. 26 Aug 2019. Retrieved: https://www.ers.usda.gov/data-products/food-availability-per-capita-data-system/. Accessed 4 Dec 2021.

461 "Healthy Cooking Oils." American Heart Association. ND. Retrieved: https://www.heart.org/en/healthy-living/healthy-eating/eat-smart/fats/healthy-cooking-oils. Accessed 2 Dec 2021.

462 "No need to avoid healthy omega-6 fats." Harvard Health Publishing, Harvard Medical School. 20 Aug 2019. Retrieved: https://www.health.harvard.edu/newsletter_article/no-need-to-avoid-healthy-omega-6-fats. Accessed 2 Dec 2021.

463 "Replacing Saturated Fat with Vegetable Oil Linked to Lower Heart Risk." Tufts University Health & Nutrition Letter. 2 Jan 2015. Retrieved: https://www.nutritionletter.tufts.edu/healthy-eating/fats/replacing-saturated-fat-with-vegetable-oil-linked-to-lower-heart-risk/. Accessed 2 Dec 2021.

464 "Mayo Clinic Minute: 5 tips for cooking with healthier oils." Mayo Clinic News Network. 20 Nov 2018. Retrieved: https://newsnetwork.mayoclinic.org/discussion/mayo-clinic-minute-5-tips-for-cooking-with-healthier-oils-2/. Accessed 2 Dec 2021.

465 Atkins, Robert C. Dr. Atkins' Diet Revolution. New York, NY, Bantam Books (Random House, Inc), 1972.

466 Source List: 1) UN Food and Agriculture Organization FAOSTAT food balance sheets: http://www.fao.org/faostat/en/#home. 2) Calculation of Energy Content of Foods, http://www.fao.org/docrep/006/Y5022E/y5022e04.htm. 3) Daily Caloric Supply Derived from Carbohydrates, Protein, and Fat, United States, 1961 to 2013. Our World In Data.org. Retrieved: https://ourworldindata.org/grapher/daily-caloric-supply-derived-from-carbohydrates-protein-and-fat?country=~USA.

467 Damms-Machado A, Weser G, Bischoff SC. Micronutrient deficiency in obese subjects undergoing low calorie diet. Nutrition Journal. 2012;11, Article number: 34.

468 Schneider A. Malnutrition with Obesity. Ernährungsmedizin A. 2008;33:280-283.

469 Grzybek A, Klosiewicz-Latoszek L, Targosz U. Changes in the intake of vitamins and minerals by men and women with hyperlipidemia and overweight during dietetic treatment. Eur J Clin Nutr. 2002;56:1162-1168.

470 Aasheim ET, Hofso D, Hjelmesaeth J, et al. Vitamin

471 Ernst B, Thurnheer M, Schmid SM, Schultes B. Evidence for the necessity to systematically assess micronutrient status prior to bariatric surgery. Obes Surg. 2009;19:66-73.

472 Xanthakos SA. Nutrient deficiencies in obesity and after bariatric surgery. Pediatr Clin North Am. 2009;56:1105-1121.

473 CDC National Health and Nutrition Examination Survey. 1999-2000. Retrieved: https://www.cdc.gov/nchs/data/nhanes/databriefs/calories.pdf. Accessed 15 Nov 2021.

474 Obesity Update / OECD Obesity Update 2017. Organization for Economic Cooperation and Development (OECD). 29 May 2017. Retrieved: https://www.oecd.org/health/health-systems/Obesity-Update-2017.pdf. Accessed 1 Dec 2021.

475 Popkin BM, Doak CM. The Obesity Epidemic Is a Worldwide Phenomenon. Nutr Rev. 1998;56(4):106-114.

476 Obesity Rates by Country 2021. World Population Review. 2021. Retrieved: https://worldpopulationreview.com/country-rankings/obesity-rates-by-country. Accessed: 2 Dec 2021.

477 Ha DTP, Feskens EJM, Deurenberg P, et al. Nationwide shifts in the double burden of overweight and underweight in Vietnamese adults in 2000 and 2005: two national nutrition surveys. BMC Public Health. 2011;11:62. https://doi.org/10.1186/1471-2458-11-62.

478 Elflein J. Prevalence of overweight and obesity worldwide in 2000 and 2016, by age. Statista. 21 Jul 2020. Retrieved: https://www.statista.com/statistics/1065611/share-of-overweight-and-obese-people-worldwide/. Accessed 2 Dec 2021.

479 Shetty P, Schmidhuber J. Introductory Lecture: The Epidemiology and Determinants of Obesity in Developed and Developing Countries. Inj J Vitam Nutr Res. 2006;76(4):157-162.

480 MacCracken J, Hoel D. From ants to analogues: Puzzles and promises in diabetes management. Postgrad Med. 1997;101:138-140, 143-5, 149-50.

481 Ahmed AM. History of Diabetes Mellitus. Saudi Med J. 2002;23(4):373-378.

482 Reed JA. Aretaeus, the Cappadocian. Diabetes. 1954;3:419-421.

483 Osler, William. The Principles and Practice of Medicine. New York, D. Appleton and Co., 1893. Special Edition privately printed for the members of The Classics of Medicine Library. Delanco, New Jersey. Publisher: Leslie B. Adams, Jr. 1978, p.296.

484 Johnson RJ, Sánchez-Lozada LG, Andrews P, Lanaspa MA. Perspective: A Historical and Scientific Perspective of Sugar and Its Relation with Obesity and Diabetes. Adv Nutr. 2017;8:412-422.

485 Kenny SJ, Aubert RE, Geiss LS. Prevalence and Incidence of Non-Insulin Dependent Diabetes. In: Diabetes In America, 2nd Edition. National Institutes of Health, National Institute of Diabetes and Digestive and Kidney Diseases. NIH Publication No. 95-1468, 1995, p. 49.

486 "Long-term Trends in Diabetes." CDC's Division of Diabetes Translation. United States Diabetes Surveillance System. April, 2017. Available at: http://www.cdc.gov/diabetes/data. Retrieved from: https://www.cdc.gov/diabetes/statistics/slides/long_term_trends.pdf

487 "National Diabetes Statistics Report, 2017." CDC Division of Diabetes Translation. Available from: https://www.cdc.gov/diabetes/pdfs/data/statistics/national-diabetes-statistics-report.pdf

488 Centers for Disease Control and Prevention. National Diabetes Statistics Report, 2020. Atlanta, GA: Centers for Disease Control and Prevention, U.S. Dept of Health and Human Services; 2020.

489 National Diabetes Statistics Report – 2020: Estimates of Diabetes and Its Burden in the United States. U.S. Department of Health and Human Services, CDC. Atlanta, GA. 2020. Retrieved: https://www.cdc.gov/diabetes/pdfs/data/statistics/national-diabetes-statistics-report.pdf. Accessed 1 Dec 2021.

490 Fang M. Trends in the Prevalence of Diabetes Among U.S. Adults: 1999-2016. Am J Prev Med. 2018;55(4):497-505.

491 Pinhas-Hamiel O, Zeitler P. The Global Spread of Type 2 Diabetes Mellitus In Children and Adolescents. J Pediatr. 2005;146:693-700.

492 Type 2 Diabetes. Centers for Disease Control (CDC). ND. Retrieved: https://www.cdc.gov/diabetes/basics/type2.html. Accessed 2 Jan 2022.

493 "Symptoms & Causes of Diabetes." NIH, National

Institute of Diabetes and Digestive and Kidney Diseases. ND. Retrieved: **https://www.niddk.nih.gov/health-information/diabetes/overview/symptoms-causes**. Accessed 2 Jan 2022.

494 Ford ES, Dietz WH. Trends in energy intake among adults in the United States: findings from NHANES. Am J Clin Nutr. 2013;97(4):848-853.

495 Panzam G. Mortality and survival in type II (non-insulin dependent) diabetes mellitus. Diabetologia. 1987;30:30:123-131.

496 Garcia MJ, McNamara PM, Gordon T, Kannell WB. Morbidity and mortality in diabetics in the Framingham population. Sixteen year follow-up study. Diabetes. 1974;23:105-111.

497 Hanefield M, Leonhardt W. Das metabolische syndrome. Dt. Gesundh-Wesen. 1981;36:545-551.

498 "Gerald Reaven, scientist who coined 'Syndrome X,' dies at 89." Stanford Medicine. 20 Feb 2018. Retrieved: **https://med.stanford.edu/news/all-news/2018/02/gerald-reaven-stanford-scientist-who-coined-syndrome-x-dies-at-89.html**. Accessed 14 Dec 2021.

499 Reaven GM. Banting Lecture 1988. Role of insulin resistance in human disease. Diabetes. 1988;37:1595-1607.

500 Mendizábal Y, Llorens S, Nava E. Hypertension in Metabolic Syndrome: Vascular Pathophysiology. Int J Hypertens. 2013;2013:230868. Doi: 10.1155/2013/230868.

501 Eckel RH, Grundy SM, Zimmet PZ. The metabolic syndrome. Lancet. 2005;365(9468):1415-28.

502 Cornier MA, Dabelea D, Hernandez TL, et al. The metabolic syndrome. Endocr Rev. 2008;29(7):777-822.

503 O'Neill S, O'Driscoll L. Metabolic syndrome: a closer look at the growing epidemic and its associated pathologies. Obes Rev. 2015;16(1):1-12.

504 Hitzenberger K, Richter-Quittner M. Ein Beitrag zum Stoffwechsel bei der vaskulären Hypertonie. Wiener Arch Innere Med. 1921;2:189-216.

505 Hitzenberger K. Über den Blutdruck bei Diabetes Mellitus. Wiener Arch Innere Med. 1921;2:461-466.

506 Kylin E. Hypertonie and zuckerkrankheit. Zentralblatt für Innere Medizin. 1921;42:873-877.

507 Marañón G. Über hypertonie and zuckerkrankheit. Zentralblatt für Innere Medizin. 1922;43:169-176.

508 Himsworth HP. Diabetes mellitus. A differentiation into insulin-sensitive and insulin-insensitive types. Lancet. 1936;1:127-130.

509 Himsworth HP, Kerr RB. Insulin-sensitive and insulin-insensitive types of diabetes mellitus. Clin Sci. 1939;4:119-151.

510 Gale EAM. The discovery of type 1 diabetes. Diabetes. 2001;50:217-26.

511 Gale EAM. Commentary: The hedgehog and the fox: Sir Harold Himsworth (1905-93). Int J Epidemiol. 2013;42(6):1602-1607.

512 Vague J. La differentiation sexuelle. Facteur determinant des formes de l'obesite. Presse Med. 1947;55:339-341.

513 Vague J. The degree of masculine differentiation of obesities. A factor determining predisposition to diabetes, atherosclerosis, gout and uric calculus disease. Am J Clin Nutr. 1956;4:20-34.

514 Samsell L, Regier M, Walton C, Cottrell L. Importance of Android/Gynoid Fat Ratio in Predicting Metabolic and Cardiovascular Disease Risk in Normal Weight as well as Overweight and Obese Children. J Obes. 2014;2014:846578. Doi: 10.1155/2014/846578.

515 Ford ES, Giles WH, Dietz WH. Prevalence of the metabolic syndrome among US adults: findings from the Third National Health and Nutrition Survey. JAMA. 2002;287:356-359.

516 Alexander CM, Landsman PB, Teutsch SM, Haffner SM. NCEP-defined metabolic syndrome, diabetes, and prevalence of coronary heart disease among NHANES III participants age 50 years and older. Diabetes. 2003;52:1210-1214.

517 Mozumdar A, Liguori G. Persistent Increase of Prevalence of Metabolic Syndrome Among U.S. Adults: NHANES III to NHANES 1999-2006. Diabetes Care. 2011;34(1):216-219.

518 Cook S, Weitzman M, Auinger P, Nguyen M, Dietz WH. Prevalence of a metabolic syndrome phenotype in adolescents: findings from the third National Health and Nutrition Examination Survey, 1988-1994. Arch Pediatr Adolesc Med. 2003;157:821-827.

519 Grundy SM. A constellation of complications: the metabolic syndrome. Clin Cornerstone. 2005;7:36-45.

520 Araújo J, Cai J, Stevens J. Prevalence of Optimal Metabolic Health in American Adults: National Health and Nutrition Examination Survey 2009-2016. Metab Syndr Relat Disord. 2019;17(1):45-52.

521 O'Hearn M, Lauren BN, Wong JB, et al. Trends and

Disparities in Cardiometabolic Health Among U.S. Adults, 1999-2018. J Am Coll Cardiol. 2022;80(2):138-151.
522 Eckel RH, Grundy SM, Zimmet PZ. The metabolic syndrome. Lancet. 2005;365:1415-28.
523 Ogurtsova K, Fernandes JD, Huang Y, et al. IDF Diabetes Atlas: global estimates for the prevalence of diabetes for 2015 and 2040. Diabetes Research and Clinical Practice. 2017;128:40-50.
524 Maurer K, Volk S, Gerbaldo H. Auguste D and Alzheimer's disease. Lancet. 1997;349(9064):1546-9.
525 Hippius H, Neundörfer. The discovery of Alzheimer's disease. Dialogues Clin Neurosc. 2003;5(1):101-8.
526 Waldman M, Lamb M. Dying For A Hamburger – Modern Meat Processing and the Epidemic of Alzheimer's Disease. New York, Thomas Dunne Books, 2004;p.36.
527 Waldman M, Lamb M. pp. 36, 42-48.
528 Dementia. World Health Organization. 2 Sep 2021. Retrieved: **https://www.who.int/news-room/factsheets/detail/dementia**. Accessed 2 Nov 2021.
529 Avramopoulos D. Genetics of Alzheimer's disease: recent advances. Genome Medicine. 2009;1(34): **https://doi.org/10.1186/gm34**.
530 Lerner A, Jeremia P, Matthias T. The World Incidence and Prevalence of Autoimmune Diseases is Increasing. Int J Celiac Disease
531 Osler W. On the visceral complications of the erythema excudativum multiforme. Am J Med Sci. 1895;110:629-646.
532 Osler W. On the visceral manifestations of the erythema group of skin diseases. Am J Med Sci. 1904;127:1-23.
533 Osler W. The visceral manifestations of the erythema group. Br J Dermatol. 1900;12:227-245.
534 Scofield RH, Oates JC. The place of William Osler in the description of systemic lupus erythematosus. Am J Med Sci. 2009;338(5):409-412.
535 Sequeira JH, Balean H. Lupus erythematosus: a clinical study of seventy-one cases. Br J Dermatol. 1902;14:367-379.
536 Libman E, Sacks B. A hitherto undescribed form of valvular and mural endocarditis. Trans Assoc Am Phys. 1923;38:46-61.
537 Tremaine MJ. Subacute Pick's disease (polyserositis) with polyarthritis and glomerulonephritis: a report of two fatal cases. N Engl J Med. 1934;211:754-759.
538 Christian HA. Long continued fever with inflammatory changes in serous and synovial membranes and eventual glomerulonephritis: clinical syndrome of unknown etiology. Med Clin North Am. 1935;18:1023-26.
539 Baehr G, Klemperer P, Schifrin A. A diffuse disease of the peripheral circulation (usually associated with lupus erythematosus and endocarditis). Trans Assoc Am Phys. 1935;50:139-156.
540 Hopkinson N. Epidemiology of systemic lupus erythematosus. Annals of Rheumatic Diseases. 1992;51:1292-1294.
541 Furst DE, Clarke AE, Fernandez AW, et al. Incidence and prevalence of adult systemic lupus erythematosus in a large US managed-care population. Lupus. 2013;22:99-105.
542 Lupus facts and statistics. Lupus Foundation of America. ND. Retrieved: **https://www.lupus.org/resources/lupus-facts-and-statistics**. Accessed 2 Jan 2022.
543 "About Autoimmunity." Autoimmune Association. ND. Retrieved: **https://autoimmune.org/resource-center/about-autoimmunity/**. Accessed 10 Dec 2022.
544 Kingwell E, Marriott JJ, Jetté N, et al. Incidence and prevalence of multiple sclerosis in Europe: a systematic review. BMC Neurology. 2013;13, 128. **https://doi.org/10.1186/1471-2377-13-128**.
545 Kister I, Bacon TE, Chamot E, et al. Natural History of Multiple Sclerosis Symptoms. Int J MS Care. 2013;15(3):146-156.
546 Murray, T. Jock. Multiple Sclerosis: The History of a Disease. New York, Demos Medical Publishing, 2005.
547 Murray, T. Jock. Multiple Sclerosis: The History of a Disease. New York, Demos Medical Publishing, 2005, p.4.
548 Koch-Henriksen N, Sorensen. Lancet Neurol. 2010;9:520-32.
549 World Health Organization (WHO). Atlas multiple sclerosis resources in the world 2008. 2008, Geneva: WHO Press.
550 Ng WK, Wong SH, Ng SC. Changing epidemiological trends in inflammatory bowel disease in Asia. Intest Res. 2016;14(2):111-119.
551 Snook J. Are the inflammatory bowel diseases autoim-

mune disorders? Gut. 1990;31(9):961-963.

552 Tjonneland A, Olsen K, Overvad K, et al. Linoleic acid, a dietary n-6 polyunsaturated fatty acid, and the aetiology of ulcerative colitis: a nested case-control study within a European prospective cohort study. Gut. 2009;58:1606-1611.

553 Dinse GE, Parks CG, Weinberg CR, et al. Increasing prevalence of antinuclear antibodies in the United States. Arthritis Rheumatol. 2020;72(6):1026-1035.

554 "Autoimmune Diseases." NIH, National Institute of Environmental Health Sciences. ND. Retrieved: **https://www.niehs.nih.gov/health/topics/conditions/autoimmune/index.cfm**. Accessed 5 Jan 2022.

555 Paray BA, Ableshr MF, Jan AT, Rather IA. Leaky Gut and Autoimmunity: An Intricate Balance in Individuals Health and the Diseased State. Int J Mol Sci. 2020;21(24):9770. **https://doi.org/10.3390/ijms21249770**.

556 Lin L, Zhang J. Role of intestinal microbiota and metabolites on gut homeostasis and human diseases. BMC Immunology. 2017;18, 2. **https://doi.org/10.1186/s12865-016-0187-3**.

557 Campos M. "Leaky gut: What is it, and what does it mean for you?" Harvard Health Publishing. 16 Nov 2021. Retrieved: **https://www.health.harvard.edu/blog/leaky-gut-what-is-it-and-what-does-it-mean-for-you-2017092212451**. Accessed 10 Jan 2022.

558 Aguayo-Patrón SV, Calderón de la Barca AM. Old Fashioned vs. Ultra-Processed-Based Current Diets: Possible Implication in the Increased Susceptibility to Type 1 Diabetes and Celiac Disease in Childhood. Foods. 2017;6(11):100; **https://doi.org/10.3390/foods6110100**.

559 Kaliannan K, Wang B, Li XY, et al. A host-microbiome interaction mediates the opposing effects of omega-6 and omega-3 fatty acids on metabolic endotoxemia. Scientific Reports. 2015;5:11276. DOI: 10.1038/srep11276.

560 Rohr MW, Narasimhulu CA, Rudeski-Rohr TA, Parthasarathy S. Negative Effects of a High-Fat Diet on Intestinal Permeability: A Review. Advances in Nutrition. 2020;11(1):77-91.

561 Rai P, Janardhan KS, Meacham J, et al. IRGM1 links mitochondrial quality control to autoimmunity. Nat Immunol. 2021;22(3):312-321.

562 Arnette R. Autoimmunity origins may lie in defective mitochondria. Environmental Factor. NIH, National Institutes of Environmental Health Sciences. March 2021. Retrieved: **https://factor.niehs.nih.gov/2021/3/papers/autoimmunity/index.htm**. Accessed 10 Jan 2022.

563 Manzel A, Muller DN, Hafler DA, et al. Role of "Western Diet" in Inflammatory Autoimmune Diseases. Curr Allerg Asthma Rep. 2014;14:404:1-8.

564 Mijac DD, Jankovic GLJ, Jorga J, Krstic MN. Nutritional status in patients with active inflammatory bowel diseases: prevalence of malnutrition and methods for routine nutritional assessment. Eur J Intern Med. 2010;21(4):315-9.

565 Prasad PS, Schwartz SD, Hubschman JP. Age-related macular degeneration: Current and novel therapies. Maturitas. 2010;66(1):46-50.

566 Jager RD, Mieler WF, Miller JW. Age-Related Macular Degeneration. N Engl J Med. 2008;358:2606-2617.

567 Leibowitz HM, Krueger DE, Maunder LR, et al. The Framingham Eye Study monograph: An ophthalmological and epidemiological study of cataract, glaucoma, diabetic retinopathy, macular degeneration, and visual acuity in a general population of 2631 adults, 1973-1975. Surv Ophthalmol. 1980;24(Suppl):335-610.

568 Wong WL, Su X, Li X, et al. Global prevalence of age-related macular degeneration and disease burden projection for 2020 and 2040: a systematic review and meta-analysis. Lancet Glob Health. 2014;2: e106-16.

569 Gehrs KM, Anderson DH, Johnson LV, Hageman GS. Age-related macular degeneration—emerging pathogenetic and therapeutic concepts. Annals of Medicine. 2006;38(7):450-471.

570 Swaroop A, Chew EY, Rickman CB, Abecasis GR. Unraveling a Multifactorial Late-Onset Disease: From Genetic Susceptibility to Disease Mechanisms for Age-Related Macular Degeneration. Annual Review of Genomics and Human Genetics. 2009;10:19-43.

571 Seddon JM, Cote J, Page WF, et al. The US Twin Study of Age-Related Macular Degeneration. Arch Ophthalmol. 2005;123:321-327.

572 Stix G. Traces of a distant past. Sci Am. 2008;299(1):56-63.

573 Ashe, A, Colot V, Oldroyd BP. How does epigenetics influence the course of evolution? Philosophical Transactions of the Royal Society B. 2021;376:20200111.

574. Hutchinson J, Tay W. Symmetrical central choroidal-retinal disease occurring in senile persons. R Lond Ophthalmic Rep. 1874;8:231-244.

575. de Jong PTVM. Elusive ageing macula disorder (AMD). Hist Ophthal Intern. 2015;1:139-152.

576. Fuchs, Ernest. Textbook of Ophthalmology. New York, D. Appleton and Company, 1892. P. 315.

577. Haab O. Atlas und Grundriss der Ophthalmoskopie und ophthalmoskopischen Diagnostik. Atlas and outline of ophthalmoscopy and ophthalmoscopic diagnosis. München, Lehmann; 1895.

578. Bird AC. Therapeutic targets in age-related macular disease. J Clin Invest. 2010;120(9):3033-3041.

579. Duke-Elder, W. Stewart. Recent Advances in Ophthalmology. Philadelphia, P. Blakiston's Son & Co., 1927.

580. May, Charles H. Manual of the Diseases of the Eye. Thirteenth Ed., Revised. New York: William Wood and Company; 1930: p. 188.

581. Verhoeff FH, Grossman HP. The pathogenesis of disciform degeneration of the Macula. Trans Am Ophthalmol Soc. 1937;35:262-94.

582. Duke-Elder WS. Textbook of Ophthalmology – Duke Elder, Vol. III, Diseases of the Inner Eye, St. Louis: The C.V. Mosby Company, 1940, p. 2372.

583. Kahn HA;, Leibowitz HM, Ganley JP, et al. The Framingham Eye Study II. Association of ophthalmic pathology with single variables previously measured in the Framingham Heart Study. Am J Epidemiol. 1977;106:33.

584. Kahn HA, Leibowitz HM, Ganley JP, et al. The Framingham Eye Study I. Outline and major prevalence findings. Am J Epidemiol. 1977;106(1):17-32.

585. Kini MM, Leibowitz HM, Colton T, et al. Prevalence of senile cataract, diabetic retinopathy, senile macular degeneration, and open angle glaucoma in the Framingham Eye Study. Am J Ophthalmol. 1978;85(1):28-34.

586. Evans J, Wormald R. Is the incidence of registrable age-related macular degeneration increasing? Br J Ophthalmol. 1996;80:9-14.

587. Smith W, Assink J, Klein R, et al. Risk factors for age-related macular degeneration: Pooled findings from three continents. Ophthalmol. 2001;108(4):697-704.

588. Moore DS, McCabe GP. Introduction to the Practice of Statistics. 1989. Original Source: Occupational Mortality: The Registrar General's Decennial Supplement for England and Wales, 1970-1972, Her Majesty's Stationary Office, London, 1978.

589. Peace LR. A Time Correlation Between Cigarette Smoking and Lung Cancer. Journal of the Royal Statistical Society. Series D (The Statistician). 1985;34(4):371-381.

590. Frost J. Introduction to Statistics. 2019, 97-103.

591. Knobbe, Chris A. Ancestral Dietary Strategy to Prevent and Treat Macular Degeneration. Springville, Utah, Vervante Corp, 2016.

592. Genetic and Rare Diseases Information Center. National Institutes of Health (NIH). ND. Retrieved: **https://rarediseases.info.nih.gov/diseases/pages/31/faqs-about-rare-diseases**. Accessed 2 Dec 2021.

593. Wakap SN, Lambert DM, Olry A, et al. Estimating cumulative point prevalence of rare diseases: analysis of the Orphanet database. Eur J Human Genetics. 2020;28:165-173.

594. "Life Expectancy." Wikipedia. ND. Retrieved: **https://en.wikipedia.org/wiki/Life_expectancy**. Accessed: 4 Jan 2022.

595. "Life Expectancy at Birth." World Health Organization (WHO). Retrieved: **https://www.who.int/whosis/whostat2006DefinitionsAndMetadata.pdf**. Accessed: 4 Jan 2022.

596. Robine JM, Allard M, Herrmann FR, Jeune B. The Real Facts Supporting Jeanne Calment as the Oldest Ever Human. The Journals of Gerontology. 2019; Series A, 74(Suppl 1):S13-S20.

597. Roser M, Ritchie H, Dadonaite B. "Child and Infant Mortality." Published online at OurWorldInData.org. Retrieved: **https://ourworldindata.org/child-mortality**. Accessed 5 Jan 2022.

598. "Child mortality rate (under five years old) in the United States, from 1800 to 2020." Statista. Statista 2022. Retrieved: **https://www.statista.com/statistics/1041693/united-states-all-time-child-mortality-rate/**. Accessed 10 Jan 2022.

599. Achievements in Public Health, 1900-1999: Healthier Mothers and Babies. CDC MMWR. 1 Oct 1999;48(38):849-858. Retrieved: **https://www.cdc.gov/mmwr/preview/mmwrhtml/mm4838a2.htm**. Accessed 2 Jan 2022.

600. Volk AA, Atkinson JA. Infant and child death in the

human environment of evolutionary adaptation. Evolution and Human Behavior. 2013;34(3):182-192.

601 Gurven M, Kaplan H. Longevity Among Hunter-Gatherers: A Cross-Cultural Examination. Population and Development Review. 29 May 2007. https://doi.org/10.1111/j.1728-4457.2007.00171.x.

602 Roser M, Ortiz-Ospina E, Ritchie H. "Life Expectancy." Published online at OurWorldInData.org. Retrieved: https://ourworldindata.org/life-expectancy#mortality-and-life-expectancy-by-age. Accessed: 10 Jan 2022.

603 Lambert T. A History of Life Expectancy in the UK. Local Histories. ND. Retrieved: https://localhistories.org/a-history-of-life-expectancy-in-the-uk/. Accessed 4 Jan 2022.

604 Rappaport SM, Genetic Factors Are Not the Major Causes of Chronic Disease. PLoS One. 2016;11(4): e0154387.

605 "Human Genome Project FAQ." NIH National Human Genome Research Institute. ND. Retrieved: https://www.genome.gov/human-genome-project/Completion-FAQ. Accessed 10 Jan 2022.

606 Cooke Bailey JN, Pericak-Vance MA, Haines JL. The Impact of the Human Genome Project on Complex Disease. Genes (Basel). 2014;5(3):518-535.

607 Wade, Nicholas. "A Decade Later, Genetic Map Yields Few New Cures." New York Times. 12 June, 2010. Retrieved: https://www.nytimes.com/2010/06/13/health/research/13genome.html. Accessed 10 Jan 2022.

608 Rechsteiner MC. The human genome project: misguided science policy. Trends Biochem Sci. 1991;16(12):455, 457, 459.

609 McCain J. The Future of Gene Therapy. Biotechnology Healthcare. 2005;2(3):52-54.

610 Naldini L. Gene therapy returns to centre stage. Nature. 2015;526(7573):351-360.

611 "How are genetic conditions treated or managed?" NIH National Library of Medicine. Medline Plus. ND. Retrieved: https://medlineplus.gov/genetics/understanding/consult/treatment/. Accessed 10 Jan 2022.

612 Fitzsimmons JS. A Handbook of Clinical Genetics. London, William Heinemann Medical Books Ltd, 1980.

613 Haggarty, P. Chapter 41, Epigenetics. In: Ross AC, Caballero B, Cousins RJ, Tucker KL, Ziegler TR. Modern Nutrition in Health and Disease, Eleventh Edition. Baltimore, Maryland, Lippincott Williams & Wilkins, 2014, pp. 534-539.

614 Mazzio EA, Soliman KFA. Basic concepts of epigenetics – impact of environmental signals on gene expression. Epigenetics. 2012;7(2):119-130.

615 Choi S-W, Friso S. Epigenetics: A New Bridge between Nutrition and Health. Adv Nutr. 2010;1(1):8-16.

616 Lieu EL, Nguyen T, Rhyne S, Kim J. Amino acids in cancer. Experimental & Molecular Medicine. 2020;52:15-30.

617 Crider KS, Yang TP, Berry RJ, Bailey LB. Folate and DNA Methylation: A Review of Molecular Mechanisms and the Evidence for Folate's Role. Adv Nutr. 2012;3(1):21-38.

618 Kuzawa CW, Sweet E. Epigenetics and the embodiment of race: developmental origins of US racial disparities in cardiovascular health. Am J Hum Biol. 2009;21:2-15.

619 Thaye ZM, Kuzawa CW. Biological memories of past environments: epigenetic pathways to health disparities. Epigenetics. 2011;6:798-803.

620 Lu MC, Kotelchuck M, Hogan V, et al. Closing the Black-White gap in birth outcomes: a life-course approach. Ethn Dis. 2010;20:62-76.

621 Dailey DE. Social Stressors and strengths as predictors of infant birth weight in low-income African American women. Nurs Res. 2009;58:340-347.

622 Brooks PE. Ethnographic evaluation of a research partnership between two African American communities and a university. Ethn Dis. 2010;20:21-29.

623 Rappaport SM. Genetic Factors Are Not the Major Causes of Chronic Diseases. PLoS One. 2016;11(4): e0154387.

624 Eaton SB, Konner M. Paleolithic Nutrition – A Consideration of Its Nature and Current Implications. NEJM. 1985;312(3):283-289.

625 Templeton AR. Has Human Evolution Stopped? Rambam Maimonides Med J. 2010;1(1): e0006.

626 Cochran G, Harpending H. The 10,000 Year Explosion: How Civilization Accelerated Human Evolution. New York, NY, Basic Books, 2009.

627 Institute of Medicine (US) Committee on Nutritional Status During Pregnancy and Lactation. Nutrition

During Pregnancy: Part I Weight Gain: Part II Nutrient Supplements. National Academies Press (US); 1990.

628 Salmeron J, Ascherio A, Rimm EB, et al. Dietary fiber, glycemic load, and risk of NIDDM in men. Diabetes Care. 1997;20:545-550.

629 Salmeron J, Manson JE, Stampfer MJ, et al. Dietary fiber, glycemic load, and risk of non-insulin dependent diabetes mellitus in women. JAMA. 1997;277:472-477.

630 Lundgren H, Bengtsson C, Blohme G, et al. Dietary habits and incidence of noninsulin-dependent diabetes mellitus in a population study of women in Gothenburg, Sweden. Am J Clin Nutr. 1989;49:708-712.

631 Colditz GA, Manson JE, Stampfer MJ, et al. Diet and risk of clinical diabetes in women. Am J Clin Nutr. 1992;55:1018-1023.

632 Sheard NF, Clark NG, Brand-Miller JC, et al. Dietary Carbohydrate (Amount and Type) in the Prevention and Management of Diabetes: A statement by the American Diabetes Association. Diabetes Care. 2004;27(9):2266-2271.

633 Hudgins LC, Hellerstein M, Seidman C, et al. Human fatty acid synthesis is stimulated by a eucaloric low fat, high carbohydrate diet. J Clin Invest. 1996;97:2081-91.

634 Hudgins LC, Seidman CE, Diakun J, Hirsch J. Human fatty acid synthesis is reduced after the substitution of dietary starch for sugar. Am J Clin Nutr. 1998;67:631-9.

635 Spector AA, Kim H-Y. Discovery of essential fatty acids. J Lipid Res. 2015;56(1):11-21. doi: 10.1194/jlr.R055095.

636 Burr GO, Burr MM. A new deficiency disease produced by the rigid exclusion of fat from the diet. J Biol Chem. 1929;82:345-367.

637 Burr GO, Burr MM. On the nature and role of the fatty acids essential in nutrition. J Biol Chem. 1930;86:587-621.

638 Bernhard K, Schoenheimer R. The inertia of highly unsaturated fatty acids in the animal, investigated with deuterium. J Biol Chem. 1940;133:707-712.

639 Schoenheimer R, Rittenberg D. The study of intermediary metabolism of animals with the aid of isotopes. Physiol Rev. 1940;20:218-248.

640 Sanders, Thomas AB. The Role of Fats in the Human Diet. In: Sanders, Thomas A.B. (ed). Functional Dietary Lipids – Food Formulation, Consumer Issues and Innovation for Health. Cambridge, U.K., Woodhead Publishing, 2016; Chapter 1, pp. 1-20.

641 Malcicka M, Visser B, Ellers J. An Evolutionary Perspective on Linoleic Acid Synthesis. Evol Biol. 2018;45:15-26.

642 Mead, James F, Fulco Armand J. The Unsaturated and Polyunsaturated Fatty Acids in Health and Disease. Springfield, Illinois, Charles C. Thomas, Publisher, 1976, pp. p. 107-114.

643 Hewavitharana GG, Perera DN, Navaratne SB, Wickramasinghe I. Extraction methods of fat from food samples and preparation of fatty acid methyl esters for gas chromatography: A review. Arabian Journ of Chemistry. 2020;13(8):6865-6875.

644 FAO/WHO. Fats and Oils in Human Nutrition Report of a Joint Expert Consultation. Food and Agriculture Organization of the United Nations and the World Health Organization. FAO Food Nutr Pap. 1994;57:1-147.

645 Hansen HS. The essential nature of linoleic acid in mammals. Trends in Biochemical Sciences. 1986;11(6):263-265.

646 Theophrast Paracelsus: works. Vol. 2, Darmstadt, 1965, pp. 508-513.

647 Gantenbein, Urs Leo. Chapter 1 – Poison and Its Dose: Paracelsus on Toxicology. In: Wexler, Philip. Toxicology in the Middle Ages and Renaissance: History of Toxicology and Environmental Health. Academic Press, 2017, pp.1-10.

648 Gardner JW. Death by water intoxication. Mil Med. 2002;167(5):432-4.

649 Jenkinson SG. Oxygen toxicity. New Horizons (Baltimore, MD). 1993;1(4):504-511.

650 Tinoco J. Dietary Requirements and Functions of α-Linolenic Acid in Animals. Prog Lipid Res. 1982;21:1-45.

651 Pudelkewicz C, Seufert J, Holman RT. Requirements of the Female Rat for Linoleic and Linolenic Acids. J Nutrition. 1968;94(2):138-46.

652 Tomaino RM, Parker JD, Larick DK. Analysis of Free Fatty Acids in Whey Products by Solid-Phase Microextraction. J Agric Food Chem. 2001;49(3):3993-3998.

653 Institute of Medicine. 2005. Dietary Reference Intakes

for Energy, Carbohydrate, Fiber, Fat, Fatty Acids, Cholesterol, Protein, and Amino Acids. Washington, DC: The National Academies Press. **https://doi.org/10.17226/10490**.

654 Ameer F, Scandiuzzi L, Hasnain S, et al. De novo lipogenesis in health and disease. Metabolism. 2014;63(7):895-902.

655 Keim NL, Levin RJ, Havel PJ. Carbohydrates. In: Ross AC, Caballero B, Cousins RJ, et al. Modern Nutrition in Health and Disease, Eleventh Edition. Baltimore, MD, Lippincott Williams & Wilkins, 2014, pp.48-49.

656 Collins JM, Neville MJ, Pinnick KE, et al. De novo lipogenesis in the differentiating human adipocyte can provide all fatty acids necessary for maturation. J Lipid Res. 2011;52(9):1683-92.

657 Hellerstein MK. Synthesis of Fat in Response to Alterations in Diet: Insights from New Stable Isotope Methodologies. Lipids. 1996;31 Suppl:S117-25.

658 Wu J HY, Lemaitre RN, Imamura F, et al. Fatty acids in the de novo lipogenesis pathway and risk of coronary heart disease: the Cardiovascular Health Study. Am J Clin Nutr. 2011;94(2):431-438.

659 Ibarguren M, López DJ, Escribá PV. The effect of natural and synthetic fatty acids on membrane structure, microdomain organization, cellular functions and human health. Biochim Biophys Acta. 2014;1838(6):1518-28.

660 Rao GA, Siler K, Larkin EC. Diet-induced alterations in the discoid shape and phospholipid fatty acid compositions of rat erythrocytes. Lipids. 1979;14(1):30-8.

661 Beynen AC, Hermus RJJ, Hautvast JGAJ. A mathematical relationship between the fatty acid composition of the diet and that of the adipose tissue in man. Amer J Clin Nutr. 1980;33:81-85.

662 Baylin A, Kabagambe EK, Siles X, Campos H. Adipose tissue biomarkers of fatty acid intake. Am J Clin Nutr. 2002;76:750-7.

663 Hirsch J, Farquhar JW, Ahrens EH, et al. Studies of Adipose Tissue in Man. A Microtechnic for Sampling and Analysis. Amer J Clin Nutr. 1960;8:499-511.

664 Beynen AC, Hermus RJJ, Hautvast JGAJ. A mathematical relationship between the fatty acid composition of the diet and that of the adipose tissue in man. Am J Clin Nutr. 1980;33(1):81-5.

665 Hodson L, Skaeff CM, Fielding BA. Fatty acid composition of adipose tissue and blood in humans and its use as a biomarker of dietary intake. Progress in Lipid Research. 2008;47(5):348-80.

666 Hawkins, M. Were warriors once low carb? Commentary on New Zealand Māori nutrition and anthropometrics over the last 150 years. J Prim Health Care. 2021;13(2):1-6.

667 Cook J, Wharton WJL. Captain Cook's Journal During His First Voyage Round the World. London, Elliot Stock, 1893.

668 Banks J, Beaglehole JC. The Endeavour journal of Joseph Banks, 1768-1771. Sydney: Trustees of the Public Library of New South Wales in association with Angus an Robertson; 1963.

669 Buck PH. Māori Diet. Med J Aust. 1927;5(Suppl):146-150.

670 Thomson, AS. Contribution to the Natural History of the New Zealand Race of Men: Being Observations on Their Stature, Weight, Size of Chest, and Physical Strength. Journal of the Statistical Society of London. 1854;17(1):27-33.

671 Price, Weston A. Nutrition and Physical Degeneration. Lemon Grove, CA: The Price-Pottenger Nutrition Foundation Inc; 1939, pp. 181-191.

672 Price, Weston A. Nutrition and Physical Degeneration. Lemon Grove, CA: The Price-Pottenger Nutrition Foundation Inc; 1939, p.188.

673 Coad J, Pedley K. Nutrition in New Zealand: Can the Past Offer Lessons for the Present and Guidance for the Future? Nutrients. 2020;12(11):3433.

674 Shorland FB, Czochanska Z, Prior IAM. Studies on Fatty Acid Composition of Adipose Tissue and Blood Lipids of Polynesians. Amer J Clin Nutr. 1969;22(5):594-605.

675 Sutherland WHF, Woodhouse SP, Heyworth MR. Physical Training and Adipose Tissue Fatty Acid Composition in Men. Metabolism – Clinical and Experimental. 1981;30(9):839-844.

676 Prior IAM, Harvey HPB, Neave MN, Davidson F. The Health of Two Groups of Cook Island Māoris. Medical Research Council of New Zealand and the Department of Health. Department of Health, Special Report Series, 1966;no. 26.

677 Pollock, Nancy J. These Roots Remain: Food Habits in Islands of the Central and Eastern Pacific Since Western Contact. The Institute for Polynesian Studies, University of Hawaii, 1992, pp 191-192.

678 Neel, JV. Diabetes mellitus: A "thrifty" genotype rendered detrimental by "progress." American J Human Genetics. 1962;14:354-362.

679 Baker P. Modernization and the biological fitness of Samoans. In Fleming and Prior. Migration, adaptation, and health in the South Pacific. 1981.

680 Prior, Ian. Nutritional problems in Pacific Islanders, New Zealand. Nutrition Society of New Zealand, Annual Proceedings, 1977.

681 Zimmet P. Blood pressure studies in two Pacific populations with varying degrees of modernization. New Zealand Medical J. 1980;657:249-252.

682 Ministry of Health. Excess Body Weight: New Zealand Health Survey. Wellington: Ministry of Health. 2015.

683 Ministry of Health. Tracking the Obesity Epidemic: New Zealand 1977-2003. Wellington: Ministry of Health, 2004.

684 Annual Data Explorer: New Zealand Health Survey 2016/17. Review: Ministry of Health, New Zealand Health System. Retrieved: http://www.health.govt.nz/nz-health-statistics/health-statistics-and-data-sets/obesity-statistics. Accessed 20 Jan 2022.

685 Diabetes. Ministry of Health, New Zealand Health System. ND. Retrieved: https://www.health.govt.nz/our-work/populations/Māori-health/tatau-kahukura-Māori-health-statistics/nga-mana-hauora-tutohu-health-status-indicators/diabetes. Accessed: 20 Jan 2022.

686 Kingsbury KJ, Crossley SPA, Morgan DM. The Fatty Acid Composition of Human Depot Fat. Biochem J. 1961;78:541.

687 Krut LH, Singer R. Steatopygia: The Fatty Acid Composition of Subcutaneous Adipose Tissue in the Hottentot. Am J Phys Anthropol. 1963;21(2):181-187.

688 Hegsted DM, Jack CW, Stare FJ. The Composition of Human Adipose Tissue from Several Parts of the World. Am J Clin Nutr. 1962;10:11-18.

689 Bakker N, Van't Veer P, Zock PL, the EURAMIC Study Group. Adipose Fatty Acids and Cancers of the Breast, Prostate and Colon: An Ecological Study. Int J Cancer. 1997;72:587-591.

690 Cottet V, Vaysse C, Scherrer M-L, et al. Fatty acid composition of adipose tissue and colorectal cancer: a case-control cancer: a case-control study. Am J Clin Nutr. 2015;101:192-201.

691 Kunesova M, Hlavaty P, Tvrzicka E, et al. Fatty acid composition of adipose tissue triglycerides after weight loss and weight maintenance: the DIOGENES study. Physiol Res. 2012;61:597-607.

692 Hellmuth C, Demmelmair H, Schmitt I, et al. Association between Plasma Nonesterified Fatty Acids Species and Adipose Tissue Fatty Acid Composition. PLoS ONE. 2013;8(10):e74927.

693 Mead, James F, Fulco Armand J. The Unsaturated and Polyunsaturated Fatty Acids in Health and Disease. Springfield, Illinois, Charles C. Thomas, Publisher, 1976, pp. 22-34, 52.

694 Bergqvist U, Holmberg J. 4th International Conference on Biochemistry. Problems of Lipids, HM Sinclair, Ed., 1958, p. 60.

695 Dickman, John Theodore. "The Nature of the Fatty Acids of Human Depot Fat." Dissertation, Ohio State University. 1960. Dissertation preserved at University Microfilms, Inc., Ann Arbor Michigan, Mic 60-4073. Retrieved: https://etd.ohiolink.edu/apexprod/rws_etd/send_file/send?accession=osu1486477735978598&disposition=inline. Accessed 4 March 2021.

696 Gertow K, Rosell M, Sjögren P, et al. Fatty acid handling protein expression in adipose tissue, fatty acid composition of adipose tissue and serum, and markers of insulin resistance. Eur J Clin Nutr. 2006;60:1406-1413.

697 Neovius M, Teixeira-Pinto A, Rasmussen F. Shift in the composition of obesity in young adult men in Sweden over a third of a century. Intern Journ of Obesity. 2008;32:832-836.

698 Neovius M, Jansen A, Rössner S. Prevalence of Obesity in Sweden. Obesity Reviews. 2006;7(1):1-3.

699 Lean M, Gruer L, Alberti G, Sattar N. ABC of obesity. Obesity—can we turn the tide? BMJ. 2006;333(7581):1261-4.

700 Moody, A. Health Survey for England 2019 – Overweight and obesity in adults and children. NHS Digital. Retrieved: https://files.digital.nhs.uk/9D/4195D5/HSE19-Overweight-obesity-rep.pdf. Accessed 4 Jan 2022.

701 Fat, Linda Ng. Health Survey for England – 2019 Adults. NHS Digital. Retrieved: https://files.digital.nhs.uk/23/6B5DEA/HSE19-Adult-health-rep.pdf. Accessed 20 Jan 2022.

702 "Facing the Facts: The Impact of Chronic Disease in the United Kingdom." World Health Organization. ND. Retrieved: **https://www.who.int/chp/chronic_disease_report/media/UK.pdf**. Accessed 25 Jan 2022.

703 Brand-Miller J, Barclay AW. Declining consumption of added sugars and sugar-sweetened beverages in Australia: a challenge for obesity prevention. Am J Clin Nutr. 2017;105:854-63.

704 Flood J. Archeology of the Dreamstime. Sydney, Collins, 1983.

705 O'Dea K. Diabetes in Australian Aborigines: impact of western diet and lifestyle. Journ Intern Med. 1992;232:103-117.

706 Price, Weston A. Nutrition and Physical Degeneration. Lemon Grove, CA: The Price-Pottenger Nutrition Foundation Inc; 1939, pp. 154-155.

707 Price, Weston A. Nutrition and Physical Degeneration. Lemon Grove, CA: The Price-Pottenger Nutrition Foundation Inc; 1939, p.162.

708 Price, Weston A. Nutrition and Physical Degeneration. Lemon Grove, CA: The Price-Pottenger Nutrition Foundation Inc; 1939, p.166.

709 Bussey C. Food security and traditional foods in remote Aboriginal communities: A review of the literature. Australian Indigenous Health Bulletin. 2013;13(2):April – June 2013.

710 Profile of Indigenous Australians. Australian Government, Australian Institute of Health and Welfare. 16 Sep 2021. Retrieved: **https://www.aihw.gov.au/reports/australias-welfare/profile-of-indigenous-australians**. Accessed 27 Jan 2022.

711 Barclay AW, Brand-Miller J. The Australian Paradox: A Substantial Decline in Sugars Intake over the Same Timeframe that Overweight and Obesity Have Increased. Nutrients. 2011;3:491-504.

712 Huse O, Hettiarachchi J, Gearon E, et al. Obesity in Australia. Obesity Research & Clinical Practice. 2018;12(1):29-39.

713 National Health Survey: First results. Australian Bureau of Statistics. 2017-18. Retrieved: **https://www.abs.gov.au/statistics/health/health-conditions-and-risks/national-health-survey-first-results/latest-release**. Accessed 24 Jan 2022.

714 Diabetes. Australian Government, Australian Government, Australian Institute of Health and Welfare. 23 Jul 2020. Retrieved: **https://www.aihw.gov.au/reports/australias-health/diabetes**.

715 Pereira Machado P, Martinez Steele E, Bertazzi Levey R, et al. Ultra-processed food consumption and obesity in the Australian adult population. Nutr Diabetes. 2020;10(1):39.

716 Brand-Miller JC, Barclay AW. Declining consumption of added sugars and sugar-sweetened beverages in Australia: a challenge for obesity prevention. Am J Clin Nutr. 2017;105:854-63.

717 "Diet compositions by macronutrient." OurWorldInData.org. Diet composition by macronutrient, Australia. Retrieved: **https://ourworldindata.org/diet-compositions#diet-compositions-by-macronutrient**. Accessed 26 Jan 2022.

718 National Institutes of Health (NIH), National Cancer Institute. "Identification of Top Food Sources of Various Dietary Components." Table 11. Food sources of linoleic acid (PFA 18:2), listed in descending order by percentages of their contribution to intake, based on data from the National Health and Nutrition Examination Survey 2005-2006. Epidemiology and Genomics Research Program website, Retrieved: **https://epi.grants.cancer.gov/diet/foodsources/top-food-sources-report-02212020.pdf#search=dietary%20sources%20of%20linoleic%20acid**. p. 42. Updated Nov 30, 2019: **https://epi.grants.cancer.gov/diet/foodsources**.

719 "Sweet potato diversity in Papua New Guinea." Global Education – Teacher Resources to Encourage a Global Perspective Across the Curriculum. Environment, Food Security, in Papua New Guinea. Retrieved: **https://globaleducation.edu.au/case-studies/sweet-potato-diversity-in-papua-new-guinea.html**. Accessed 30 Jan 2022.

720 Sinnett PF, Whyte HM. Epidemiological Studies In A Total Highland Population, Tukisenta, New Guinea – Cardiovascular Disease and Relevant Clinical Electrocardiographic, Radiological and Biochemical Findings. J Chron Dis. 1973;26:265-290.

721 Barnes R. Incidence of heart disease in a native hospital of Papua. Med J Aust. 1961;2:540-42.

722 Campbell CH, Arthur RK. A study of 2000 admissions to the medical ward of the Port Moresby General Hospital. Med J Aust. 1964;1:989-992.

723 Korner MH. A sample of heart disease in hospital patients in New Guinea. Med J Aust. 1964;2:368-370.

724 National Heart Foundation of Australia. Reports by Drs Hetzel PS (1962), Grice KG (1964), Studkey D (1966), and Galea EG (1968), Canberra.

725 Sinnett PF, Whyte HM. Epidemiological Studies in a Highland Population of New Guinea: Environment, Culture, and Health Status. Human Ecology. 1973;1(3):245-277.

726 Hipsley EH, Clements FW. Report of the New Guinea Nutrition Survey Expedition, 1947. Department of External Territories, Canberra.

727 Norgan NG, Ferro-LUZZI A, Durnin JVGA. The Energy and Nutrient Intake and the Energy Expenditure of 204 New Guinean Adults. Philosophical Transactions of the Royal Society of London. 1974;B. 268:309-348.

728 Beulens JW, Booth SL, van den Heuvel EGHM, et al. The role of menaquinones (vitamin K2) in human health. British Journ Nutrition. 2013;110(8):1357-1368.

729 West CE, Eilander A, Van Lieshout M. Consequences of revised estimates of carotenoid bioefficacy for the Dietary Control of Vitamin A Deficiency in Developing Countries. J Nutr. 2002;132:2920S-2926S.

730 Willett WC, Stampfer MJ, Underwood BA, et al. Vitamins A, E, and carotene: effects of supplementation on their plasma levels. Amer J Clin Nutr. 1983;38(4):559-566.

731 "Cardiovascular diseases." World Health Organization (WHO). 11 Jun 2021. Retrieved: **https://www.who.int/en/news-room/fact-sheets/detail/cardiovascular-diseases-(cvds)**. Accessed 31 Jan 2022.

732 Diehl, Hans. Reversing Coronary Heart Disease. In: Temple, Norman J., Burkitt, Denis P. Western Diseases: Their Dietary Prevention and Reversibility. Totowa, New Jersey, Humana Press, 1994, p.281.

733 Keys, Ancel. Diet and the Epidemiology of Coronary Heart Disease. JAMA. 1957;164(17):1912-1919.

734 DuBroff R, de Lorgeril M. Fat or fiction: the diet-heart hypothesis. BMJ Evidence-Based Medicine. 2021;26:3-7.

735 Steinberg D. In celebration of the 100th anniversary of the lipid hypothesis of atherosclerosis. J Lipid Res. 2013;54(11):2946-9.

736 Steinberg D. Hypercholesterolemia and Atherosclerosis in Humans: Causally Related? In: The Cholesterol Wars. Academic Press, 2007.

737 Ravnskov U. The fallacies of the lipid hypothesis. Scandinavian Cardiovascular Journal. 2008;42(4):236-239.

738 Ware WR. The mainstream hypothesis that LDL cholesterol drives atherosclerosis may have been falsified by non-invasive imaging of coronary artery plaque burden and progression. Medical Hypotheses. 2009;73(4):596-600.

739 Jakobsen MU, O'Reilly EJ, Heitmann BL, et al. Major types of dietary fat and risk of coronary heart disease: a pooled analysis of 11 cohort studies. Am J Clin Nutr. 2009;89:1425-1432.

740 Mente A, de Koning L, Shannon HS, et al. A systematic review of the evidence supporting a causal link between dietary factors and coronary heart disease. Arch Intern Med. 2009;169:659-669.

741 Skeaff CM, Miller J. Dietary fat and coronary heart disease: summary of evidence from prospective cohort and randomized controlled trials. Ann Nutr Metab. 2009;55:173-201.

742 Siri-Rarino PW, Sun Q, Hu FB, et al. Meta-analysis of prospective cohort studies evaluating the association of saturated fat with cardiovascular disease. Am J Clin Nutr. 2010. 2010;91:535-546.

743 Chowdury R, Warnakula S, Kunutsor S, et al. Association of dietary, circulating, and supplement fatty acids with coronary risk: a systematic review and meta-analysis. Ann Intern Med. 2014;160:398-406.

744 Farvid MS, Ding M, Pan A, et al. Dietary linoleic acid and risk of coronary heart disease: a systematic review and meta-analysis of prospective cohort studies. Circulation. 2014;130:1568-1578.

745 de Souza RJ, Mente A, Maroleanu A, et al. Intake of saturated and trans unsaturated fatty acids and risk of all cause mortality, cardiovascular disease, and type 2 diabetes: systematic review and meta-analysis of observational studies. BMJ. 2015;351:h3978.

746 Harcombe Z, Baker JS, DiNicolantonio JJ, et al. Evidence from randomized controlled trials does not support current dietary fat guidelines: a systematic review and meta-analysis. Open Heart. 2016;3:e000409.

747 Zhu Y, Bo Y, Liu Y. Dietary total fat, fatty acids intake, and risk of cardiovascular disease: a dose-response meta-analysis of cohort studies. Lipids Health Dis. 2019;18:91.

748 Sacks FM, Lichtenstein AH, Wu JHY, et al. Dietary fats and cardiovascular disease: a presidential advisory from the American Heart Association. Circulation.

2017;136:e1-e23.

749 Eckel RH, Jakicic JM, Ard JD. AHA/ACC guidelines on lifestyle management to reduce cardiovascular risk: a report of the American College of Cardiology/American Heart Association Task Force on practice guidelines. J Am Coll Cardiol. 2014;63:2960-2984.

750 "Cut Down on Saturated Fats." Dietary Guidelines for Americans 2015-2020, Eighth Edition. Retrieved: **https://health.gov/sites/default/files/2019-10/DGA_Cut-Down-On-Saturated-Fats.pdf**. Accessed 29 Jan 2022.

751 "Healthy diet." World Health Organization. 29 Apr 2020. Retrieved: **https://www.who.int/news-room/fact-sheets/detail/healthy-diet**. Accessed 29 Jan 2022.

752 Goldstein JL, Basu SK, Brown MS. Binding site on macrophages that mediates uptake and degradation of acetylated low density lipoprotein, producing massive cholesterol deposition. Proc Natl Acad Sci. USA. 1979;76(1):333-337.

753 Goldstein JL, Brown MS. The low-density lipoprotein pathway and its relation to atherosclerosis. Annu Rev Biochem. 1977;46:897-930.

754 "The Nobel Prize in Physiology or Medicine 1985." The Nobel Prize.

755 Witztum JL, Steinberg D. Role of Oxidized Low Density Lipoprotein in Atherogenesis. J Clin Invest. 1991;88(6):1785-1792.

756 Glass CK, Witztum JL. Daniel Steinberg, 1922-2015. Proc Natl Acad Sci. 2015;112(32):9791-9792.

757 Steinberg D, Witztum JL. Oxidized Low-Density Lipoprotein and Atherosclerosis. Arteriosclerosis, Thrombosis, and Vascular Biology. 2010;30(12):2311-2316.

758 Steinberg, Daniel. The Cholesterol Wars – The Skeptics vs the Preponderance of Evidence. 1st Edition. Amsterdam, Elsevier/Academic Press, 2007.

759 Reaven P, Parthasarathy S, Grasse BJ, Miller E, Steinberg D, Witztum JL. Effects of oleate-rich and linoleate-rich diets on the susceptibility of low density lipoprotein to oxidative modification in mildly hypercholesterolemic subjects. J Clin Invest. 1993;91(2):668-76.

760 Parthasarathy S, Litvinov D, Selvarajan K, et al. Lipid peroxidation and decomposition—conflicting roles in plaque vulnerability and stability. Biochim Biophys Acta. 2008;1781:221-31.

761 Jira W, Spitellar G, Carson W, et al. Strong increase in hydroxy fatty acids derived from linoleic acid in human low density lipoproteins of atherosclerotic patients. Chem Phys Lipids. 1998;91:1-11.

762 DiNicolantonio JJ, O'Keefe JH. Omega-6 vegetable oils as a driver of coronary heart disease: the oxidized linoleic acid hypothesis. Open Heart. 2018;5:e000898. Doi:10.1136/openhrt-2018-000898.

763 DiNicolantonio JJ. Good Fats versus Bad Fats: A Comparison of Fatty Acids in the Promotion of Insulin Resistance, Inflammation, and Obesity. Missouri Medicine. 2017;114(4):303-307.

764 McClelland RL, Chung H, Detrano R, et al. Distribution of Coronary Artery Calcium by Race, Gender, and Age. Circulation. 2005;113(1):30-37.

765 Holvoet P, Jenny NS, Schreiner PJ, Tracy RP, Jacobs DR. The relationship between oxidized LDL and other cardiovascular risk factors and subclinical CVD in different ethnic groups: the multi-ethnic study of atherosclerosis (MESA). Atherosclerosis. 2007;194:245-52.

766 Hecht HS. Coronary Artery Calcium Scanning – Past, Present, and Future. JACC Cardiovasc Imaging. 2015;8(5):579-596.

767 Schrauwen P, Westerterp KR. The role of high-fat diets and physical activity in the regulation of body weight. Brit J Nutr. 2000;84(4):417-427.

768 Dobrian AD, Davies MJ, Russell LP, Lauterio TJ. Development of Hypertension in a Rat Model of Diet-Induced Obesity. Hypertension. 2000;35(4):1009-1015.

769 Lai M, Chandrasekera PC, Barnard ND. You are what you eat, or are you? The challenges of translating high-fat-fed rodents to human obesity and diabetes. Nutrition & Diabetes. 2014;4:e135.

770 Keys A. Diet and the Epidemiology of Coronary Heart Disease. JAMA. 1957;164(17):1912-1919.

771 Duan Y, Zeng L, Zheng C, et al. Inflammatory Links Between High Fat Diets and Diseases. Front Immunol. 2018;9:2649.

772 Krogh, August and Krogh, Marie. A study of the diet and metabolism of Eskimos undertaken in 1908 on an expedition to Greenland. Vol 51, Issue 1 of Meddelelser om Grønland. Reitzel, 1913, pp. 1-45.

773 Lindeberg S, Berntorp E, Nilsson-Ehle P, et al. Age relations of cardiovascular risk factors in a traditional Melanesian society: the Kitava Study. Amer J Clin Nutr. 1997;66(4):845-852.

774 Ulijaszek SJ. Modernization and the diet of adults on Rarotonga, the Cook Islands. Ecology of Food and Nutrition. 2002;41(3):203-228.

775 Hawkes K, Hill K, O'Connell JF. Why Hunters Gather: Optimal foraging and the Aché of Paraguay. Journal of the American Ethnological Society. May 1982. https://doi.org/10.1525/ae.1982.9.2.02a00100.

776 Hilliard, Sam Bowers. Hog Meat and Hoecake – Food Supply in the Old South, 1840-1860. Athens and London, The University of Georgia Press. 1972.

777 Simopoulos AP. Omega-6 and omega-3 fatty acids: Endocannabinoids, genetics and obesity. EDP Sciences, 2020. Online: https://doi.org/10.1051/ocl/2019046.

778 Di Genova T, Guyda H. Infants and children consuming atypical diets: Vegetarianism and macrobiotics. Paediatr Child Health. 2007;12(3):185-188.

779 Gadsby, Patricia. The Inuit Paradox – How can people who gorge on fat and rarely see a vegetable be healthier than we are? Discover. 2004;25(10): Biology & Medicine.

780 Kaplan, Lawrence. "Inuit or Eskimo: Which name to use?" Alaska Native Language Center, University of Alaska Fairbanks. ND. Retrieved: https://www.uaf.edu/anlc/resources/inuit_or_eskimo.php. Accessed 24 Jan 2022.

781 Bjerregaard P, Mulvad G, Olsen J. Studying Health in Greenland: Obligations and Challenges. Int J Circumpolar Health. 2003;62(1):5-16.

782 Krogh, August and Krogh, Marie. A study of the diet and metabolism of Eskimos undertaken in 1908 on an expedition to Greenland. Vol 51, Issue 1 of Meddelelser om Grønland. Reitzel, 1913, pp. 1-45.

783 Villega R, Xiang Y-B, Elasy T, et al. Purine-rich foods, protein intake, and the prevalence of hyperuricemia: The Shanghai Men's Health Study. Nutr Metab Cardiovasc Dis. 2012;22(5):409-416.

784 Magdanz J, Wolfe RJ. The Production and Exchange of Seal Oil in Alaska. Special Publication No. SP1988-001. Alaska Department of Fish and Game. 1988. Retrieved: https://www.adfg.alaska.gov/specialpubs/SP2_SP1988-001.pdf. Accessed 10 Jan 2022.

785 Price, Weston A. Nutrition and Physical Degeneration. Lemon Grove, CA: The Price-Pottenger Nutrition Foundation Inc; 1939, p.55.

786 Bang HO, Dyerberg J. Lipid Metabolism and Ischemic Heart Disease in Greenland Eskimos. In: Draper HH (eds). Advances in Nutritional Research. Springer, Boston, MA. https://doi.org/10.1007/978-1-4757-4448-4_1.

787 Bang HO, Dyerberg J, Nielsen AB. Plasma lipid and lipoprotein pattern in Greenlandic West-coast Eskimos. Lancet. 1971;1:1143-1145.

788 Dyerberg J, Bang HO, Hjørne N. Fatty acid composition of the plasma lipids in Greenland Eskimos. Amer J Clin Nutr. 1975;28:958-966.

789 Bang HO, Dyerberg J, Sinclair HM. The composition of the Eskimo food in northwestern Greenland. Amer J Clin Nutr. 1980;33:2657-2661.

790 Dyerberg J, Bang HO. Eicosapentaenoic acid and Prevention of Thrombosis and Atherosclerosis? The Lancet. 1978;2(8081):117-9.

791 Bertelsen A. Grønlandsk medicinsk statistic og nosografi: Undersøgelser og erfaringer fra 30 aars grønlandsk laegevirksomhed. 'Greenland medical statistics and nosography. Studies and experience from 30 years of clinical work in Greenland. In Danish]. Vol 1: Grønlands befolkningsstatistik 1901-30. Meddelelser om Grønland 1935; 117(1). Vol. II: Sundhedsvilkaarene i Grønland. Meddelelser om Grønland 1937; 117(2). Vol. III: Det saedvanlige grønllandske sygdomsbillede. Meddelelser om Grønland 1940; 117(3). Vol. IV: Akutte infektionssygdomme I Grønland. Meddelelser om Grønland 1943;117(4).

792 Bang HO, Dyerberg J. Lipid Metabolism and Ischemic Heart Disease in Greenland Eskimos. In: Draper HH (eds). Advances in Nutritional Research. Springer, Boston, MA. https://doi.org/10.1007/978-1-4757-4448-4_1.

793 Lynge I, Vanggaard L. Bent Jørgen Harvald – in memoriam. Int J Circumpolar Health. 2006;65(5):382-384.

794 Harvald B. Third International Symposium on Circumpolar Health. ugeskrLaeg. 1974;136:2461-2462 (in Danish).

795 FAO (FAOSTAT), Denmark. Retrieved via Knoema.com: https://knoema.com/FAOFBS2017/food-balance-sheets. Accessed 22 Jan 2022.

796 Harris WS, Calder PC, Mozaffarian D, Serhan CN. Bang and Dyerberg's omega-3 discovery turns fifty. Nature Food. 2021;2:303-305. Published online: https://doi.org/10.1038/s43016-021-00289-7.

797 Fodor JG, Helis E, Yazdekhasti N, Vohnout B. "Fishing" for the Origins of the "Eskimos and Heart Disease" Story: Facts or Wishful Thinking? Can J Cardiol. 2014;30(8):P864-868.

798 DiNicolantonio JJ. Increase in the intake of refined carbohydrates and sugar may have led to the health decline of the Greenland Eskimos. Open Heart. 2016;3:e000444. Doi: 10.1136/openhrt-2016-000444.

799 Raitakari OT. Imaging of subclinical atherosclerosis in children and young adults. Annals of Med. 1999;31(sup1):33-40.

800 Bjerregaard P, Young TK, Hegele RA. Low incidence of cardiovascular disease among the Inuit—what is the evidence? Atherosclerosis. 2003;166(2):351-7.

801 Juel K, Sjøl A. Decline in Mortality From Heart Disease In Denmark: Some Methodological Problems. J Clin Epdemiol. 1995;48(4):467-472.

802 Baylin A, Kim MK, Donovan-Palmer A, et al. Fasting Whole Blood as a Biomarker of Essential Fatty Acid Intake in Epidemiologic Studies: Comparison with Adipose Tissue and Plasma. Am J Epidemiol. 2005;162:373-381.

803 Rosqvist F, Bjermo H, Kullberg J, et al. Fatty acid composition in serum cholesterol esters and phospholipids is linked to visceral and subcutaneous adipose tissue content in elderly individuals: a cross-sectional study. Lipids in Health and Disease. 2017;16:68.

804 Furtado JD, Beqari J, Campos H. Comparison of the Utility of Total Plasma Fatty Acids Versus those in Cholesteryl Ester, Phospholipid, and Triglyceride as Biomarkers of Fatty Acid Intake. Nutrients. 2019;11:2081; doi:10.3390/nu11092081.

805 Sowa F. Kalaalimernit: the Greenlandic taste for local foods in a globalized world. Polar Rec. 2015;51:290-300.

806 Pars T, Osler M, Bjerregaard P. Contemporary use of traditional and imported food among Greenland Inuit. Arctic. 2001;54:22-31.

807 Raghavan M, DeGiorgio M, Albrechtsen A, et al. The genetic prehistory of the New World Arctic. Science. 2014;345:1255832.

808 Senftleber NK, Overvad M, Dahl-Peteresen K, et al. Diet and physical activity in Greenland: genetic interactions and associations with obesity and diabetes. Appl Physiol Nutr Metab. 2021;46:849-855.

809 Koch A. Diabetes in Greenland – how to deliver diabetes care in a country with a geographically dispersed population. Int J Circumpolar Health. 2019;2019;78(sup 1), DOI:10.108/22423982.2019.16 68592

810 Sagild U, Littauer J, Jespersen CS, et al. Epidemiological studies in Greenland 1962-1964. Acta Med Scand. 2009;179(1):29-2.

811 Andersen S, Fleischer Rex K, Noahsen P, et al. Forty-Five Year Trends in Overweight and Obesity in an Indigenous Arctic Inuit Society in Transition and Spatiotemporal Trends. Am J Human Biology. 2014;26:511-517.

812 Greenland Obesity Prevalence. Global Obesity Observatory. Retrieved: **https://data.worldobesity.org/country/greenland-81/#data_prevalence**. Accessed 30 Jan 2022.

813 Bjerregaard P, Larsen CVL. Health Aspects of Colonization and the Post-Colonial Period in Greenland 1721-2014. Journal of Northern Studies. 2016;10(2):85-106.

814 Kjaergaard M, Andersen S. Holten M, et al. Low occurrence of ischemic heart disease among Inuit around 1963 suggested from ECG among 1851 East Greenland Inuit. Atherosclerosis. 2009;203:599-603.

815 Jørgensen ME, Bjerregaard P, Kjaergaard JJ, Borch-Johnsen K. High prevalence of markers of coronary heart disease among Greenland Inuit. Atherosclerosis. 2008;196:722-778.

816 Greenland. Imports and Exports. OEC. Animal and Vegetable Bi-Products. Retrieved: **https://oec.world/en/profile/country/grl**. Accessed 1 Feb 2022.

817 Bjorn-Mortensen K, Lynggaard F, Lynge Pedersen M. Incidence of Greenlandic stroke-survivors in Greenland: A 2-year cross-sectional study. Int J Circumpolar Health, 2013;72:22626.

818 He K, Song Y, Daviglus ML, et al. Fish Consumption and Incidence of Stroke – A Meta-Analysis of Cohort Studies. Stroke. 2004;35:1538-1542.

819 Wennberg M, Jansson J-H, Norberg M, et al. Fish consumption and risk of stroke: a second perspective case-control study from northern Sweden. Nutrition Journal. 2016;15:98.

820 Zhao W, Tang H, Yang X, et al. Fish Consumption and Stroke Risk: A Meta-Analysis of Prospective Cohort Studies. Journ Stroke Cerebrovasc Dis. 2019;28(3):604-611.

821 Donkor ES. Stroke in the 21st Century: A Snapshot of the Burden, Epidemiology, and Quality of Life. Stroke Research and Treatment. 2018. Article ID: 3238165.

https://doi.org/10.1155/2018/3238165.

822 Neises VM, Karpovich SA, Keogh MJ, et al. Regional, seasonal and age class blubber fatty acid signature analysis of harbor seals in Alaska from 1997 to 2010. Conservation Physiology. 2021;9(1):coab036, **https://doi.org/10.1093/conphys/coab036**.

823 Lockyer CH, McConnell C, Waters TD. The biochemical composition of fin whale blubber. Can J Zool. 1984;62(12):2553-2562.

824 Harris WS, Mozaffarian D, Rimm E, et al. Omega-6 fatty acids and risk for cardiovascular disease: a science advisory from the American Heart Association Nutrition Subcommittee of the Council on Nutrition, Physical Activity, and Metabolism; Council on Cardiovascular Nursing; and Council on Epidemiology and Prevention. Circulation. 2009;119(6):902-7.

825 "Saturated Fat." American Heart Association. Retrieved from: **https://www.heart.org/en/healthy-living/healthy-eating/eat-smart/fats/saturated-fats**. Accessed 6 Jun 2020.

826 De Looper M, Bhatia K. International health—how Australia compares. Australian Institute of Health and Welfare Canberra. AIHW cat. No. PHE 8. 1998.

827 Yam D, Eliraz A, Berry EM. Diet and disease—The Israeli paradox: Possible dangers of a high omega-6 polyunsaturated fatty acid diet. Israel Journal of Medical Sciences. 1996;32(11):1134-1143.

828 Kark JD, Kaufmann NA, Binka F, et al. Adipose tissue n-6 fatty acids and acute myocardial infarction in a population consuming a diet high in polyunsaturated fatty acids. Am J Clin Nutr. 2003;77:796-802.

829 Guggenheim K, Kaufmann NA. Nutritional health in a changing society – studies from Israel. World Rev Nutr Diet. Basel, Karger. 1976, vol 2, pp. 217-240.

830 FAO Food Balance Sheets: Israel. Retrieved: **https://knoema.com/FAOFBS2017/food-balance-sheets**. Accessed 31 Jan 2022.

831 "Diet compositions by macronutrient. OurWorldInData.org. Retrieved: **https://ourworldindata.org/diet-compositions**. Accessed: 2 Feb 2022.

832 Blondheim SH, Horne T, Davidovich R, et al. Unsaturated Fatty Acids in Adipose Tissue of Israeli Jews. Isr J Med Sci. 1976;12(7):658-61.

833 Seidelin KN. Fatty Acid Composition of Adipose Tissue In Humans. Implications for the Dietary Fat-Serum Cholesterol—CHD Issue. Pro Lipid Res. 1995;34(3):199-217.

834 Kark JD, Kaufmann NA, Binka F, et al. Adipose tissue n—6 fatty acids and acute myocardial infarction in a population consuming a diet high in polyunsaturated fatty acids. Am J Clin Nutr. 2003;77:796-802.

835 Kaluski D N, Berry EM. Prevalence of obesity in Israel. Obes Rev. 2005;6(2):115-6

836 "Results Summary, Prevalence of obesity among adults (ages 20-64)." Israel National Program for Quality Indicators in Community Healthcare." Years 2013-2019. Retrieved: **https://en.israelhealthindicators.org/blank-44**. Accessed 24 Jan 2022.

837 Health Information Services. Israel Ministry of Health. Retrieved: **http://www.health.gov.il/units/healthisrael/63.htm**, Accessed 1 April 2006.

838 Kalter-Leibovici O, Chetrit A, Lubin F, et al. Adult-onset diabetes among Arabs and Jews in Israel: a population-based study. Diabet Med. 2012;29(6):748-54.

839 De Looper M, Bhatia K. International health—how Australia compares. Australian Institute of Health and Welfare Canberra. AIHW cat. No. PHE 8. 1998.

840 Even, D. "Israel Leads West in Diabetes, Kidney Disease Deaths." Haaretz. 20 Jul 2011. Retrieved: **https://www.haaretz.com/1.5031222**. Accessed 4 Feb 2022.

841 Peritz E, Dreyfuss F, Halevi HS, Schmelz UO. Mortality of adult Jews in Israel 1950-1967. Jerusalem, Central Bureau of Statistics, 1973.

842 Dubnov G, Berry EM. Omega-6/omega-3 fatty acid ratio: the Israeli paradox. World Rev Nutr Diet. 2003;92:81-91.

843 Kark JD, Goldberger N, Fink R, et al. Myocardial infarction occurrence in Jerusalem: a Mediterranean anomaly. Atherosclerosis. 2005;178:129-138.

844 Goldberger N, Aburbeh M, Haklai Z. Leading causes of death in Israel. Ministry of Health, Health Information Division. Retrieved: **https://www.health.gov.il/PublicationsFiles/CausesOfDeaths2018_Summary.pdf**. Accessed 3 Feb 2022.

845 Dataset Records for Ministry of Health (Israel). 2008. **http://ghdx.healthdata.org/organizations/ministry-health-israel**. Review available: Robinson E, Ziv M, Keinan-Boker L. Cancer on the Global Stage: Incidence and Cancer-Related Mortality in Israel. The ASCO Post. 10 April 2016. Retrieved: **https://ascopost.com/issues/april-10-2016/cancer-on-the-global-stage-incidence-and-cancer-re-**

846. Barchana M, Lipshitz I, Rozen P. Trends in colorectal cancer incidence and mortality in the Israeli Jewish ethnic populations. Fam Cancer. 2004;3(3-4):207-14.

847. Rudd KE, Charlotte-Johnson S, Agesa KM, et al. Global, regional, and national sepsis incidence and mortality, 1990-2017: analysis for the Global Burden of Disease Study. The Lancet. 395(10219):P200-211.

848. "Standard of living in Israel." Wikipedia.org. Accessed 4 Feb 2022.

849. Samad N, Dutta S, Sodunke TE, et al. Fat-Soluble Vitamins and the Current Global Pandemic of COVID-19: Evidence-Based Efficacy from Literature Review. J Inflamm Res. 2021;14:2091-2110.

850. "Food and nutrition tips during self-quarantine. World Health Organization. ND. Retrieved: **https://www.euro.who.int/en/health-topics/health-emergencies/coronavirus-covid-19/publications-and-technical-guidance/food-and-nutrition-tips-during-self-quarantine**. Accessed 4 Feb 2022.

851. "Introduction: Magnitude, causes and consequences of micronutrient malnutrition." FAO.org. Retrieved: **https://www.fao.org/3/x0245e/x0245e01.htm**. Accessed: 4 Feb 2022.

852. Hennig B, Watkins BA. Linoleic acid and linolenic acid: Effect on permeability properties of cultured endothelial cell monolayers. Am J Clin Nutr. 1989;49:301-305.

853. Pisani DF, Amri EZ, Ailhaud G. Disequilibrium of polyunsaturated fatty acids status and its dual effect in modulating adipose tissue development and functions. OCL 2015;22:D405.

854. Vähäheikkilä M, Peltomaa T, Róg T, et al. How cardiolipin peroxidation alters the properties of the inner mitochondrial membrane. Chemistry and Physics of Lipids. 2018;214:15-23.

855. Ghosh S, Kewalramani G, Yuen G, et al. Induction of mitochondrial nitrative damage and cardiac dysfunction by chronic provision of dietary ω-6 polyunsaturated fatty acids. Free Radical Biology & Medicine. 2006;41:1413-1424.

856. Araya J, Rodrigo R, Videla LA, et al. Increase in long-chain polyunsaturated fatty acid n-6/n-3 ratio in relation to hepatic steatosis in patient with non-alcoholic fatty liver disease. Clinical Science. 2004;106:635-643.

857. Kopp W. How Western Diet and Lifestyle Drive the Pandemic of Obesity and Civilization Diseases. Diabetes Metab Syndr Obes. 2019;12:2221-2236.

858. Phillips CM, Goumidi L, Bertrais S, et al. Leptin receptor polymorphisms interact with polyunsaturated fatty acids to augment risk of insulin resistance and metabolic syndrome in adults. J Nutr. 2010;140:238-244.

859. Cheng L, Yu Y, Zhang Q, et al. Arachidonic acid impairs hypothalamic leptin signaling and hepatic energy homeostasis in ice. Mol Cell Endocrinol. 2015;5(412):12-18.

860. Simopoulos AP. Evolutionary aspects of diet and essential fatty acids. In: Hamazaki R, Okuyama H, (Eds). Fatty Acids and Lipids—New Findings. Basel, Switzerland, Karger, 2001;Vol 88, pp.18-27.

861. James MJ, Gibson RA, Cleland LG. Dietary polyunsaturated fatty acids and inflammatory mediator production. Am J Clin Nutr. 2000;71:343S-348S.

862. Alvheim AR, Torstensen BE, Lin YH, et al. Dietary linoleic acid elevates the endocannabinoids 2-AG and anandamide and promotes weight gain in mice fed a low fat diet. Lipids. 2014;49:59-69.

863. Banni S, Di Marzo V. Effect of dietary fat on endocannabinoids and related mediators: consequences on energy homeostasis, inflammation and mood. Mol Nutr Food Res. 2010;54:82-92.

864. Matias I, Di Marzo V. Endocannabinoids and the control of energy balance. Trends Enocrinol Metab. 2007;18:27-37.

865. Tracy RP. Emerging relationships of inflammation, cardiovascular disease and chronic diseases of aging. International Journal of Obesity. 2003;27:S29-S34.

866. Kauppinen A, Paterno JJ, Blasiak J, et al. Inflammation and its role in age-related macular degeneration. Cell Mol Life Sci. 2016;73:1765-1786.

867. Campbell A, Solaimani P. Oxidative and Inflammatory Pathways in Age-Related Chronic Disease Processes. In: Bondy S, Campbell A (eds). Inflammation, Aging, and Oxidative Stress. Oxidative Stress in Applied Basic Research and Clinical Practice. Springer, Cham. **https://doi.org/10.1007/978-3-319-33486-8_6**. 2016; pp 95-106.

868. Zhong S, Li L, Shen X. An update on lipid oxidation and inflammation in cardiovascular diseases. Free Rad-

ical Biology and Medicine. 2019;144(20):266-278.

869 Rael LT, Thomas GW, Craun ML, et al. Lipid Peroxidation and the Thiobarbituric Acid Assay: Standardization of the Assay When Using Saturated and Unsaturated Fatty Acids. J Biochem Mol Biol. 2004;37(6):749-52.

870 Ayala A, Muñoz, Argüelles. Lipid Peroxidation: Production, Metabolism, and Signaling Mechanisms of Malondialdehyde and 4-Hydroxy-2-Nonenal. Oxid Med Cell Longev. 2014;2014: 360438. Doi: 10.1155/2014/360438.

871 Lobo V, Patil A, Phatak A, Chandra, N. Free radicals, antioxidants and functional foods: Impact on human health. Pharmacognosy Review. 2010;4(8):118-126.

872 Frankel EN. Volatile lipid oxidation products. Prog Lipid Res. 1983;22:1-33.

873 Kerr BJ, Kellner TA, Shurson GC. Characteristics of lipids and their feeding value in swine diets. Journ Animal Sci Biotechnol. 2014;6:30. Doi: 10.1186/s40104-015-0028-x.

874 Zhou JF, Yan XF, Guo FZ, et al. Effects of cigarette smoking and smoking cessation on plasma constituents and enzyme activities related to oxidative stress. Biomedical and Environmental Sciences. 2000;13(1):44-55.

875 Lane N. Oxygen: The Molecule that Made the World. Oxford University Press; 2002.

876 Sender R, Fuchs S, Milo R. Revised Estimates for the Number of Human and Bacteria Cells in the Body. PLoS Biology. 2016;14(8):e1002533. **https://doi.org/10.137/journal.pbio.1002533.**

877 Pryor WA, Houk KN, Foote CS, et al. Free radical biology and medicine: it's a gas, man! Amer J Physiol – Regulatory, Integrative and Comparative Physiology. 2006;191:3:R491-R511.

878 Inagi R, Miyata T. Oxidative protein damage with carbohydrates and lipids in uremia: 'Carbonyl stress.' Blood Purif. 1999;17(2-3):95-8.

879 Spiteller G. Is Lipid Peroxidation of Polyunsaturated Acids the Only Source of Free Radicals that Induce Aging and Age-Related Diseases? Rejuvenation Research. 2010;13(1):91-103.

880 Ratcliffe N, Wieczorek T, Drabinska N, et al. A mechanistic study and review of volatile products from peroxidation of unsaturated fatty acids: an aid to understanding the origins of volatile organic compounds from the human body. Journal of Breath Research. 2020;14(3):034001.

881 Esterbauer H, Cheesman KH, Dianzani MU. Separation and characterization of the aldehydic products of lipid peroxidation stimulated by ADP-Fe2+ in rat liver microsomes. Biochemical Journal. 1982;208(1):129-140.

882 Innes JK, Calder PC. Omega-6 fatty acids and inflammation. Prostaglandins Leukot Essent Fatty Acids. 2018;132:41-48.

883 Toborek M, Lee YW, Garrido R, et al. Unsaturated fatty acids selectively induce an inflammatory environment in human endothelial cells. Am J Clin Nutr. 2002;75(1):119-25.

884 Bagga D, Wang L, Farias-Eisner R, et al. Differential effects of prostaglandin derived from omega-6 and omega-3 polyunsaturated fatty acids on COX-2 expression and IL-6 secretion. Proc Natl Acad Sci USA. 2003;100(4):1751-56.

885 Schmitz G, Ecker J. The opposing effects of n-3 and n-6 fatty acids. Prog Lipid Res. 2008;47(2):147-55.

886 Nagy L, Tontonoz P, Alvarez JGA, et al. Oxidized LDL Regulates Macrophage Gene Expression through Ligand Activation of PPAR⊠. Cell. 1998;93(2):229-240.

887 Poirier B, Michel O, Bazin R, et al. Conjugated dienes: a critical trait of lipoprotein oxidizability in renal fibrosis. Nephrol Dialysis Transplant. 2001;16(8):1598-1606.

888 Esterbauer H, Gebicki J, Puhl H, Jürgens G. The role of lipid peroxidation and antioxidants in oxidative modification of LDL. Free Radical Biol Med. 1992;13:341-390.

889 Schneider C, Tallman KA, Porter NA, Brash AR. Two distinct pathways of formation of 4-hydroxynonenal. Mechanisms of nonenzymatic transformation of the 9- and 13-hydroperoxides of linoleic acid to 4-hydroxyalkenals. J Biol Chem. 2001;276:20831-20838.

890 Stevens JF, Maier CS. Acrolein. Mol Nutr Food Res. 2008;52(1):7-25.

891 Ebrahem Q, Renganathan K, Sears J, et al. Carboxyethylpyrrole oxidative protein modifications stimulate neovascularization: Implications for age-related macular degeneration. PNAS. 2006;103(42):13480-13484.

892 Weber D, Milkovic L, Bennett SJ, et al. Measurement of HNE-protein adducts in human plasma and serum by ELISA—Comparison of two primary antibodies.

Redox Biology. 2013;1(1):226-233.

893 Claxson AWD, Hawkes GE, Richardson DP, et al. Generation of lipid peroxidation products in culinary oils and fats during episodes of thermal stressing: a high field ^{1}H NMR study. FEBS Lett. 1994;355(1):81-90.

894 Halvorsen BL, Blomhoff R. Determination of lipid oxidation products in vegetable oils and marine omega-3 supplements. Food & Nutrition Research. 2011;55(1):5792.

895 "Consumption of vegetable oils worldwide from 2013/14 to 2021/2022, by oil type. Statista. Retrieved: **https://www.statista.com/statistics/263937/vegetable-oils-global-consumption/**. Accessed 14 Feb 2022.

896 Roth DE, Abrams SA, Aloia J. Global prevalence and disease burden of vitamin D deficiency: a roadmap for action in low- and middle-income countries. Ann N Y Acad Sci. 2018;1430(1):44-79.

897 Stone NJ. Fish consumption, Fish Oil, Lipids, and Coronary Heart Disease. Circulation. 1996;94(9):2337-2340.

898 Jayedi A, Shab-Bidar S. Fish Consumption and the Risk of Chronic Disease: An Umbrella Review of Meta-Analyses of Prospective Cohort Studies. Advances in Nutrition. 2020;11(5):1123-1133.

899 Varlet V, Prost C, Serot T. Volatile aldehydes in smoked fish: Analysis methods, occurrence and mechanisms of formation. Food Chemistry. 2007;105:1536-1556.

900 Health Canada. Canadian Nutrient File (CNF) – Search by food. 29 Dec 2021. Retrieved: **https://food-nutrition.canada.ca/cnf-fce/index-eng.jsp**. Accessed 5 May 2022.

901 Claxson AWD, Hawkes GE, Richardson DP, et al. Generation of lipid peroxidation products in culinary oils and fats during episodes of thermal stressing: a high field ^{1}H NMR study. FEBS Letters. 1994;355:81-90.

902 Grootveld M, Atherton MD, Sheerin AN, et al. In Vivo Absorption, Metabolism, and Urinary Excretion of α, β-Unsaturated Aldehydes in Experimental Animals. Relevance to the development of cardiovascular diseases by the dietary ingestion of thermally stressed polyunsaturated-rich culinary oils. J Clin Invest. 1998;101(6):1210-8.

903 Grootveld M, Silwood CJL, Addis P, Claxson A. Health Effects of Oxidized Heated Oils. Foodservice Research International. 2001;13:41-55.

904 Grootveld M, Ruiz-Rodado V, Silwood CJL. Detection, monitoring and deleterious health effects of lipid oxidation products generated in culinary oils during thermal stressing episodes. Inform. Am Oil Chem Soc. 2014;25(10):614-24.

905 Grootveld M, Percival BC, Grootveld KL. Chronic non-communicable disease risks presented by lipid oxidation products in fried foods. Hepatobil Surg Nutr. 2018;7(4):305-12.

906 Moumtaz S, Percival BC, Parmar D, Grootveld KL, Jansson P, Grootveld M. Toxic aldehyde generation in and food uptake from culinary oils during frying practices: peroxidative resistance of a monounsaturated-rich algae oil. Scientific Reports. 2019;9:4125. **https://doi.org/10.1038/s41598-019-3967-1**.

907 Grootveld M, Percival BC, Leenders J, Wilson PB. Potential Adverse Public Health Effects Afforded by the Ingestion of Dietary Lipid Oxidation Product Toxins: Significance of Fried Food Sources. Nutrients. 2020;12:974. Doi:10.3390/nu12040974.

908 Mendick, R. "Cooking with vegetable oil releases toxic cancer-causing chemicals, say experts." The Telegraph. 7 Nov 2015. Retrieved: **https://www.telegraph.co.uk**. Accessed: 29 Jan 2022.

909 Vistoli G, De Maddis D, Cipak A, et al. Advanced glycoxidation and lipoxidation end products (AGEs and ALEs): an overview of their mechanisms of formation. Free Radical Research. 2013;47:sup1:3-27. DOI:10.3109/10715762.2013.815348.

910 Pamplona R. Advanced lipoxidation end-products. Chemico-Biological Interactions. 2011;192(1-2):14-20.

911 Moldogazieva NT, Mokhosoev IM, Mel'nikova TI, et al. Oxidative Stress and Advanced Lipoxidation and Glycation End Products (ALEs and AGEs) in Aging and Age-Related Diseases. Oxidative Medicine and Cellular Longevity. 2019;Article ID 3085756. **https://doi.org/10.1155/2019/3085756**.

912 Aldini G, Vistoli G, Stefek M, et al. Molecular strategies to prevent, inhibit, and degrade advanced glycoxidation and advanced lipoxidation and products. Free Radical Research. 2013;47,Suppl 1:93-137.

913 Anderson EJ, Taylor DA. Stressing the heart of the matter: re-thinking the mechanisms underlying therapeutic effects of n-3 polyunsaturated fatty acids. F1000 Medicine Reports. 2012;4:13, doi: 10.3410/M4-13.

914 Ayala A, Muñoz MF, Argüelles S. Lipid Peroxidation Products in Human Health and Disease 2014. Oxidative Medicine and Cellular Longevity.

2014;2014:360438. Doi: 10.1155/2014/360438.

915 Bolea G, Philouze C, Dubois M, et al. Digestive n-6 Lipid Oxidation, a Key Trigger of Vascular Dysfunction and Atherosclerosis in the Western Diet: Protective Effects of Apple Polyphenols. Molecular Nutrition Food Research. 2021;65(6):e2000487.

916 Rosenfeld ME, Palinski W, Yla-Herttuala S, et al. Distribution of oxidation specific lipid-protein adducts and apolipoprotein b in atherosclerosis lesions of varying severity from WHHL rabbits. Arteriosclerosis. 1990;10(3):336-349.

917 Palinksi W, Yla-Herttuala S, Rosenfeld ME, et al. Antisera and monoclonal antibodies specific for epitopes generated during oxidative modification of low density lipoprotein. Arteriosclerosis. 1990;10(3):325-335.

918 Yoritaka A, Hattori N, Uchida K, et al. Immunohistochemical detection of 4-hydroxynonenal protein adducts in Parkinson's disease. Proc Natl Acad Sci, USA. 1996;93(7):2696-2701.

919 Shibata N, Nagai R, Uchida K, et al. Morphological evidence for lipid peroxidation and protein glycoxidation in spinal cords from sporadic amyotrophic lateral sclerosis patients. Brain Res. 2001;917(1):97-104.

920 Okamoto K, Toyokuni S, Uchida K, et al. Formation of 8-hydroxy-2'-deoxyguanosine and 4-hydroxy-2-nonenal-modified proteins in human renal-cell carcinoma. Int J Cancer. 1994;58(6):825-859.

921 Mattson MP. Roles of the lipid peroxidation product 4-hydroxynonenal in obesity, the metabolic syndrome, and associated vascular and neurodegenerative disorders. Exp Gerontol. 2009;44(10):625-33.

922 Ethen CM, Reilly C, Feng X, et al. Age-related macular degeneration and retinal protein modification by 4-hydroxy-2-nonenal. Invest Ophthalmol Vis Sci. 2007;48(8):3469-79.

923 Soulage CO, Pelletier CC, Florens N, et al. Two Toxic Lipid Aldehydes, 4-hydroxy-2-hexanal (4-HHE) and 4-hydroxy-2-nonenal (4-HNE), Accumulate in Patients with Chronic Kidney Disease. Toxins (Basel). 2020;12(9):567. Doi: 10.3390/toxins12090567.

924 Rahman I, van Schadewijk AAM, Crowther ANL, et al. 4-Hydroxy-2-Nonenal, a Specific Lipid Peroxidation Product, Is Elevated in Lungs of Patients with Chronic Obstructive Pulmonary Disease. Amer J Resp Crit Care Med. 2002;166(4):490-5. Doi: 10.1164/rccm.2110101.

925 Romano A, Serviddio G, Calcagnini S, et al. Linking lipid peroxidation and neuropsychiatric disorders: focus on 4-hydroxy-2-nonenal. Free Radical Biology and Medicine. 2017;111:281-293.

926 Yamashima T. The Scourge of Vegetable Oil—Destroyer of Nations. Journal of Alzheimer's Disease & Parkinsonism. 2018;8(4):446.

927 Ma L, Liu G, Liu X. Amounts of malondialdehyde do not accurately represent the real oxidative level of all vegetable oils: a kinetic study of malondialdehyde formation. Int Journ Food Sci Technol. 2019;54:412-423.

928 Gorelik S, Ligumsky M, Kohen R, Kanner J. The stomach as a "bioreactor": when red meat meets red wine. Journ Agricult Food Chem. 2008;56:5002-5007.

929 Ma L, Liu G. Simultaneous analysis of Malondialdehyde, 4-Hydroxy-2-hexanal, and 4-Hydroxy-2-nonenal in vegetable oil by reversed-phase high-performance liquid chromatography. Journ Agricult Food Chem. 2017;65:11320-11328.

930 Voulgaridoiu GP, Anestopoulos I, Franco R, et al. DNA damage induce by endogenous aldehydes: Current state of knowledge. Mutation Research/Fundamental and Molecular Mechanisms of Mutagenesis. 2011;711:13-27.

931 Douny C, Tihon A, Bayonnet P, et al. Validation of the analytical procedure for the determination of malondialdehyde and three other aldehydes in vegetable oil using liquid chromatography coupled to tandem mass spectrometry (LC-MS/MS) and applications to linseed oil. Food Analytical Methods. 2015;8:1425-1435.

932 Reaven PD, Witztum JL. Oxidized Low Density Lipoproteins In Atherogenesis: Role of Dietary Modification. Annu Rev Nutr. 1996;16:51-71.

933 Papastergiadis A, Fatouh A, Jacxsens L, et al. Exposure assessment of Malondialdehyde, 4-Hydroxy-2-€-Nonenal and 4-Hydroxy-2-€-Hexanal through specific foods available in Belgium. Food and Chemical Toxicology. 2014;73:51-58.

934 Long AC, Kaiser JL, Katz GE. Lipids in infant formulas: Current and future innovations. Lipid Technology. 2013;25(6): DOI: 10.1002/lite.201300279.

935 Cesa S. Malondialdehyde contents in infant milk formulas. Journ Agricult Food Chem. 2004;52:2119-2122.

936 Papastergiadis A, Fatouh A, Jacxsens L, et al. Exposure assessment of Malondialdehyde, 4-Hydroxy-2-(E)-

Nonenal and 4-Hydroxy-2-(E)-Hexanal through specific foods available in Belgium. Food and Chemical Toxicology. 2014;73:51-58.

937 Singh Z, Karthigesu IP, Singh P, Kaur R. Use of Malondialdehyde as a Biomarker for Assessing Oxidative Stress in Different Disease Pathologies: a Review. Iranian Journal Public Health. 2014;43(Suppl No 3):7-16.

938 Prázný M, Škrha J, Hilgertová J. Plasma malondialdehyde and Obesity: Is there a Relationship? Clin Chem Lab Med 1999;37(11/12):1129-1130.

939 "Toxicological Review of Acrolein." Environmental Protection Agency (EPA). CAS No. 107-02-8. May 2003. Retrieved: **https://cfpub.epa.gov/ncea/iris/iris_documents/documents/toxreviews/0364tr.pdf**. Accessed 2 Jan 2022.

940 Moghe A, Ghare S, Lamoreau B, et al. Molecular Mechanisms of Acrolein Toxicity: Relevance to Human Disease. Toxicological Sciences. 2015;143(2):242-255.

941 Stevens JF, Maier CS. Acrolein: Sources, metabolism, and biomolecular interactions relevant to human health and disease. Mol Nutr Food Res. 2008;52(1):7-25.

942 "McDonald's Large French Fries Nutrition Facts." Fast Food Nutrition. ND. Retrieved: **https://fastfoodnutrition.org/mcdonalds/french-fries/large**. Accessed 4 Feb 2022.

943 Gomes DR, Meek ME. Concise International Chemical Assessment Document 43 ACROLEIN. Geneva: World Health Organization, 2002.

944 "Acceptable daily intakes for agricultural and veterinary chemicals." Australian Government, Australian Pesticides and Veterinary Medical Authority. Edition 4/2021, current as of 31 December 2021. Retrieved: **https://apvma.gov.au/node/26596#Alpha%20list%20of%20chemicals**. Accessed 12 Feb 2022.

945 Roemer E. Stabbert R, Rustemeier K, et al. Chemical composition, cytotoxicity and mutagenicity of smoke from US commercial and reference cigarettes smoked under two sets of machine smoking conditions. Toxicology. 2004;195:31-52.

946 Feng Z, Hu W, Hu Y, Tang M-s. Acrolein is a major cigarette-related lung cancer agent: Preferential binding at p53 mutational hotspots and inhibition of DNA repair Proc Natl Acad Sci USA. 2006;103(42):15404-9.

947 Metayer C, Wang Z, Kleinerman RA, et al. Cooking oil fumes and risk of lung cancer in women in rural Gansu, China. Lung Cancer. 2002;35:111-117.

948 Henning RJ, Johnson GT, Coyle JP, Harbison RD. Acrolein Can Cause Cardiovascular Disease: A Review. Cardiovasc Toxicol. 2017;17(3):227-236.

949 Jiang C, Jiang L, Li Q, et al. Acrolein induces NLRP3 inflammasome-mediated pyroptosis and suppresses migration via ROS-dependent autophagy in vascular endothelial cells. Toxicology. 2018;410:26-40.

950 Huang Y-J Jin M-H, Pi R-B, et al. Acrolein induces Alzheimer's disease-like pathologies in vitro and in vivo. Toxicol Lett. 2013;217(3):184-191.

951 Hong J-H, Lee PAH, Lu Y-C, et al. Acrolein contributes to urothelial carcinomas in patients with chronic kidney disease. Urol Oncol. 2020;38(5):465-475.

952 Liu J-H, Wang T-W, Lin Y-Y, et al. Acrolein is involved in ischemic stroke-induced neurotoxicity through spermidine/spermine-N1-acetyltransferase activation. Exp Neurol. 2020;323:113066.

953 Jia L, Liu Z, Sun L, et al. Acrolein, a toxicant in cigarette smoke, causes oxidative damage and mitochondrial dysfunction in RPE cells: protection by (R)-alpha-lipoic acid. Invest Ophthalmol Vis Sci. 2007;48(1):339-48.

954 Salomon RG, Hong L, Hollyfield JG. The Discovery of Carboxyethylpyrroles (CEPs): Critical Insights into AMD, Autism, Cancer, and Wound Healing from Basic Research on the Chemistry of Oxidized Phospholipids. Chem Res Toxicol. 2011;24(11):1803-1816.

955 Gu X, Meer SG, Miyagi M et al. Carboxyethylpyrrole protein adducts and autoantibodies, biomarkers for age-related macular degeneration. J Biol Chem. 2003;278:42027-42035.

956 Gu J, Paeur GJ, Yue X, et al. Assessing susceptibility to age-related macular degeneration with proteomic and genomic biomarkers. Mol Cell Proteomics. 2009;8:1338-1349.

957 Bressler SB, Maguire MG, Bressler NM, Fine SL. Relationship of drusen and abnormalities of the retinal pigment epithelium to the prognosis of neovascular macular degeneration. The Macular Photocoagulation Study Group. Arch Ophthalmol. 1990;108:1442-1447.

958 Siddiq A, Ambreen G, Hussain K, Baig SG. Oxidative stress and lipid per-oxidation with repeatedly heated mix vegetable oils in different doses in comparison with single time heated vegetable oils. Pak J Pharm Sci.

2019;32(5):2099-2105.

959 Alberts B, Johnson A, Lewis J, et al. Molecular Biology of the Cell. 4th Edition. New York: Garland Science; 2002. How Cells Obtain Energy from Food. Available from: **https://www.ncbi.nlm.nih.gov/books/NBK26882**.

960 Mulkidjanian AY, Shalaeva DN, Lyamzaev KG, Chernyak BV. Does Oxidation of Mitochondrial Cardiolipin Trigger a Chain of Apoptotic Reactions? Biochemistry (Moscow). 2018;83(10):1263-1278.

961 Dudek J. Role of Cardiolipin in Mitochondrial Signaling Pathways. Front Cell Dev Biol. 5:90. doi: 10.3389/fcell.2017.0090.

962 Haines TH, Dencher NA. Cardiolipin: A proton trap for oxidative phosphorylation. FEBS Lett. 2002;528:35-39.

963 Lee H-J, Mayette J, Rapoport SI, Bazinet RP. Selective remodeling of cardiolipin fatty acids in the aged rat heart. Lipids in Health and Disease. 2006;5:2. Doi:10.1186/1476-511X-5-2.

964 Dyer JR, Greenwood CE. Dietary Essential Fatty Acids Change the Fatty Acid Profile of Rat Neural Mitochondria Over Time. J Nutr. 1991;121(10):1548-53.

965 McGee CD, Lieberman P, Greenwood CE. Dietary Fatty Acid Composition Induces Comparable Changes in Cardiolipin Fatty Acid Profile of Heart and Brain Mitochondria. Lipids. 1996;31(6):611-616.

966 Rieger B, Krajčová, Duwe P, Busch KB. ALCAT1 Overexpression Affects Supercomplex Formation and Increases ROS in Respiring Mitochondria.

967 Allingham MJ, Mettu PS, Cousins SW. Phase 1 Clinical Trial of Elamipretide in Intermediate Age-Related Macular Degeneration and High-Risk Drusen: ReCLAIM High-Risk Drusen Study. Ophthalmology Science. 2022;2(1):100095.

968 Birk AV, Chao WM, Bracken C, et al. Targeting Mitochondrial Cardiolipin and the Cytochrome C/Cardiolipin Complex to Promote Electron Transport and Optimize Mitochondrial ATP Synthesis. Br J Pharmacol. 2014;171(8):2017-2028.

969 Szeto HH. First-in class cardiolipin-protective compound as a therapeutic agent to restore mitochondrial bioenergetics. Br J Pharmacol. 2014;171(8):2029-2050.

970 Apostolova N, Victor VM. Molecular strategies for targeting antioxidants to mitochondria: therapeutic implications. Antioxidants & Redox Signaling. 2015;22(8):686-729.

971 Murphy MP. How Mitochondria Produce Reactive Oxygen Species. The Biochemical Journal. 2009;417(1):1-13.

972 Paradies G, Paradies V, Ruggiero FM. Oxidative Stress, Cardiolipin and Mitochondrial Dysfunction in Nonalcoholic fatty liver disease. World Journal of Gastroenterology. 2014;20(39):14205-14218.

973 Li J, Romestang C, Han X, et al. Cardiolipin Remodeling by ALCAT1 Links Oxidative Stress and Mitochondrial Dysfunction to Obesity. Cell Metabolism. 2010;12:154-165.

974 Houstis N, Rosen ED, Lander ES. Reactive oxygen species have a causal role in multiple forms of insulin resistance. Nature. 2006;440:944-948.

975 Meigs JB, Larson MG, Fox CS, et al. Association of oxidative stress, insulin resistance, and diabetes risk phenotypes

976 Pérez-Carreras M, Del Hoyo P, Martin MA, et al. Defective hepatic mitochondrial respiratory chain in patients with nonalcoholic steatohepatitis. Hepatology. 2003;38:999-1007.

977 Gasanoff ES, Yaguzhinsky LS, Garab G. Cardiolipin, Non-Bilayer Structures and Mitochondrial Bioenergetics: Relevance to Cardiovascular Diseases. Cells. 2021;10,1721. **https://doi.org/10.3390/cells10071721**.

978 Modica-Napolitano JS, Singh KK. Mitochondrial dysfunction in cancer. Mitochondrion. 2004;4(5-6):755-762.

979 Falabella M, Vernon HJ, Hanna MG, et al. Cardiolipin, Mitochondria, and Neurological Disease. Trends in Endocrinology & Metabolism. 2021;32(4):224-237.

980 Nashine S, Potential Therapeutic Candidates for Age-Related Macular Degeneration (AMD). Cells. 2021;10:2483. **https://doi.org/10.3390/cells10092483**.

981 Filler K, Lyon D, Bennett J, et al. Association of mitochondrial dysfunction and fatigue: A review of the literature. BBA Clin. 2014;1:12-23.

982 Diaz-Vegas A, Sanchez-Aguilera P, Krycer JR, et al. Is Mitochondrial Dysfunction a Common Root of Noncommunicable Chronic Disease? Endocrine Reviews. 2020;41(3):1-27.

983 Wallace DC. Mitochondrial diseases in man and mouse. Science. 1999;183:1482-1488.

984 Schwarz K, Siddiqi N, Sing S, Neil CJ, et al. The breath-

ing heart – mitochondrial respiratory chain dysfunction in cardiac disease. Int J Cardiol. 2014;171:134-143. Doi: 10.1016/j.ijcard.2013.12.014.

985 Monteiro-Cardoxo VF, Oliveira MM, Melo T, et al. Cardiolipin Profile Changes are Associated to the Early Synaptic Mitochondrial Dysfunction in Alzheimer's Disease. Journ Alzheimer's Disease. 2015;43(4):1375-1392.

986 Masterjohn C. Vitamin D toxicity redefined: Vitamin K and the molecular mechanism. Medical Hypotheses. 2007;68:1026-1034.

987 Masterjohn C. On the Trail of the Elusive X-Factor: A Sixty-Two-Year-Old Mystery Finally Solved. The Weston A. Price Foundation. 14 Feb 2008. Retrieved: https://www.westonaprice.org/health-topics/abcs-of-nutrition/on-the-trail-of-the-elusive-x-factor-a-sixty-two-year-old-mystery-finally-solved/. Accessed 20 Feb 2022.

988 Kennedy BK, Berger SL, Brunet A, et al. Geroscience: Linking Aging to Chronic Disease. Cell. 2014;159(4):709-713.

989 Neufeld HN Goldbourt U. Coronary heart disease: genetic aspects. Circulation. 1983;1983;67(5):943-954.

990 Chiu KC, Permutt MA. Genetic factors in the pathogenesis of NIDDM. In: Pickup JC, Williams G (eds). Textbook of Diabetes. Oxford: Blackwell Science, 1997, Ch.18, pp.1-16.

991 Dowling JE, Wald G. Vitamin A Deficiency and Night Blindness. Proc Natl Acad Sci USA. 1958;44:648-661.

992 Guy, RA. The History of Cod Liver Oil As A Remedy. Am J Dis Child. 1923;26(2):112-116.

993 Guy, "The History of Cod Liver Oil as a Remedy" (n. 15), 112. Thomas Percival's quote is taken from Theophilus Thompson, "Clinical Lectures on Diseases of the Chest: Lecture V: Cod-Liver Oil," London Lancet. 1851;2:343.

994 Thompson T. Effects of cod-liver oil on the blood. Med Chron Montreal Monthly J Med Surg. 1855.2:111.

995 Nozeran A. De l'héméralopie des pays chauds. Thèse no. 61. Montpellar: Gras, 1865.

996 McArdle TE. Cod-liver oil—a food and a medicine. J Pract Med. 1896;6:279-282.

997 Grad R. Cod and the Consumptive: A Brief History of Cod-Liver Oil in the Treatment of Pulmonary Tuberculosis. Pharmacy in History. 2004;46(3):106-120.

998 Bloch CE. Klinische Untersuchungen uber Dystrophie und Xeropthamic bei jungen Kindern. Jahrb Kinderheilk. 1919;89:305-341.

999 Wolf G. A history of vitamin A and retinoids. FASEB J. 1996;10:1102-1107.

1000 Blegvad O. Xerophthalmia, Keratomalacia and Xerosis Conjunctivae. Amer Journ Ophthalmol. 1924;7(2):89-117.

1001 Sommer A, West KP. Vitamin A deficiency: health, survival and vision. New York, Oxford University Press, 1995.

1002 Green HN, Pindar D, Davis G, Mellanby E. Diet as a prophylactic agent against puerperal sepsis. BMJ. 1931;2:595-8.

1003 Clausen SW. Nutriton and infection. JAMA. 1935;104:793-8.

1004 Renewed interest in vitamin A. Lancet. 1931;217:708.

1005 Green HN, Mellanby E. Vitamin A as an anti-infective agent. London, Publisher not identified, 1928. Available: https://wellcomecollection.org/works/at9ms6tg.

1006 Semba RD, Bloem MW. The anemia of vitamin A deficiency: epidemiology and pathogenesis. European J Clin Nutr. 2002;56:271-281.

1007 Olsen JA. Vitamin A, Retinoids and Carotenoids. In: Modern Nutrition in Health and Disease, 8th ed. Shils ME, Olson JA, Shike M, eds. Lea & Febiger, Philadelphia, PA, 1994; 287-307.

1008 Underwood BA. Methods for Assessment of Vitamin A Status. Journal of Nutrition. 1990;120(suppl 11):1459-1463.

1009 Wald G, Heghers H, Arminio J. An Experiment in Human Dietary Night-Blindness. Am J Physiol. 1938;123:732.

1010 Hecht S, Mandelbaum J. The Relation Between Vitamin A and Dark Adaptation. JAMA. 1939;112(19):1910-1916.

1011 Dow DJ, Steven DM. An Investigation of Simple Methods For Diagnosing Vitamin A Deficiency By Measurements of Dark Adaptation. J Physiol. 1941;100:256-262.

1012 Owsley C, McGwin G, Jackson GR. Effect of Short-Term, High-Dose Retinol on Dark Adaptation in Aging and Early Age-Related Maculopathy. Invest Ophthalmol Vis Sci. 2006;47(4):1310-1318.

1013 Mellanby E (Study Compiled by E.M Hume and H.A. Krebs). Vitamin A Requirement of Human Adults – An Experimental Study of Vitamin A Deprivation In Man. Medical Research Council Special Report Series

No. 264. London. 1949.

1014 West CE, Eilander A, Van Lieshout M. Consequences of revised estimates of carotenoid bioefficacy for the Dietary Control of Vitamin A Deficiency in Developing Countries. J Nutr. 2002;132:2920S-2926S.

1015 Sauberlich HE, Hodges RE, Kolder WH, et al. Vitamin A Metabolism and Requirements in the Human Studied with the Use of Labeled Retinol. Vitamins & Hormones. 1975;32:251-275.

1016 Vitamin A – Fact Sheet for Health Professionals. National Institutes of Health (NIH), Office of Dietary Supplements. 14 Feb 2020. Retrieved: **https://ods.od.nih.gov/factsheets/VitaminA-HealthProfessional/#:~:text=According%20to%20an%20analysis%20of,women%20(580%20mcg%20RAE)**.

1017 Shah AK, Dhalla NS. Effectiveness of Some Vitamins in the Prevention of Cardiovascular Disease: A Narrative Review. Front Physiol. 08 Oct 2021. **https://doi.org/10.3389/fphys.2021.729255**.

1018 Ong DE, Chytil F. Vitamin A and Cancer. Vitamins & Hormones. 1983;40:105-144.

1019 Sommer, Alfred. Vitamin A Deficiency – Health, Survival, and Vision. Oxford, Oxford University Press, 1996.

1020 Timoneda J, Rodríguez-Fernández L, Zaragozá R, et al. Vitamin A Deficiency and the Lung. Nutrients. 2018;10:1132; doi:10.3390/nu10091132.

1021 Tanoury ZA, Piskunov A, Rochette-Egly C. Vitamin A and retinoid signaling: genomic and nongenomic effects. Thematic Review Series: Fat Soluble Vitamins: Vitamin A. J Lipid Res. 2013;54:1761-1775.

1022 Hammerling U. Retinol as electron carrier in redox signaling, a new frontier in vitamin A research. Hepatobiliary Surg Nutr. 2016;5(1);15-28.

1023 Passmore R, Hollingsworth DF, Robertson J. Prescription for a better British diet. Br Med J. 1979;1:527-531.

1024 Conlan R, Sherman E. Unraveling the Enigma of Vitamin D. National Academy of Sciences, Beyond Discovery – The Path From Research to Human Benefit. Oct 2000. Retrieved: **http://www.nasonline.org/publications/beyond-discovery/vitamin-d.pdf**. Accessed 22 Feb 2022.

1025 DeLuca HF. History of the discovery of vitamin D and its active metabolites. BoneKEy Reports. 2014;Reports 3, Article number:479.

1026 Mellanby E. An experimental investigation on rickets. Lancet. 1919;1:407-412.

1027 McCollum EV, Simmonds N, Becker JE, Shipley PG. An experimental demonstration of the existence of a vitamin which promotes calcium deposition. J Biol Chem. 1922;53:293-298.

1028 Huldschinsky K. Heilung von rachitis durch künstlich hohen-sonne. Deut MedWochenscher. 1919;45:712-713. Orthopad Chir. 1920;39:426 as described in Bills CE. In: Sebrell Jr WH, Harris RS (eds). The Vitamins. Vol II. Academic Press: New York, 1954, p.162.

1029 Chick H, Palzell EJ, Hume EM. Studies of rickets in Vienna 1919-1922. Medical Research Council, Special Report: 1923, No. 77.

1030 Nicolaysen R. Studies upon the mode of action of vitamin D. III. The influence of vitamin D on the absorption of calcium and phosphorus in the rat. Biochem J. 1937;31:122-129.

1031 Nicolaysen R, Eeg-Larsen N, Malm QJ. Physiology of calcium metabolism. Physiol Rev. 1953;33:424-444.

1032 Patrick RP, Ames BN. Vitamin D and the omega-3 fatty acids control serotonin synthesis and action, part 2: relevance for ADHD, bipolar disorder, schizophrenia, and impulsive behavior. FASEB J. 2015;29(6):2207-22.

1033 Hossein-nezhad A, Holick MF. Vitamin D for Health: A Global Perspective. Mayo Clin Proc. 2013;88(7):720-755.

1034 Holick MF, Binkley NC, Bischoff-Ferrari H, et al. Endocrine Society. Evaluation, treatment, and prevention of vitamin D deficiency: an Endocrine Society clinical practice guideline. J Clin Endocrinol Metab. 2011;96:1911-30.

1035 Ginde AA, Liu MC, Camargo CA Jr. Demographic differences and trends of vitamin D insufficiency in the US population, 1988-2004. Arch Intern Med. 2009;169:626-632.

1036 Bailey RL, Fulgoni VL 3rd, Keast DR, Dwyer JT. Examination of vitamin intakes among US adults by dietary supplement use. J Acad Nutr Dietetics. 2012;112:657-663.

1037 Mansback JM, Ginde AA, Camargo CA Jr. Serum 25-hydroxyvitamin D levels among US children aged 1 to 11 years: do children need more vitamin D? Pediatrics. 2009;124:1404-1410.

1038 Holick MF, Chen TC. Vitamin D deficiency: a worldwide problem with health consequences. Am J Clin Nutr. 2008;87(suppl):1080S-6s.

1039 Naeem Z. Vitamin D Deficiency- An Ignored Epidemic. Int J Health Sci (Qassim). 2010;4(1):V-VI.

1040 Schmid A, Walther B. Natural Vitamin D Content in Animal Products. Adv Nutr. 2013;4(4):453-462.

1041 American Academy of Dermatology. "Sunscreen FAQS." ND. Retrieved: **https://www.aad.org/public/everyday-care/sun-protection**. Accessed 22 Feb 2022.

1042 Wolpowitz D, Gilchrest BA. The vitamin D questions: how much do you need and how should you get it? J Am Acad Dermatol. 2006;54:301-17.

1043 Matsuoka LY, Ide L, Wortsman J, et al. Sunscreens suppress cutaneous vitamin D3 synthesis. J Clin Endocrinol Metab. 1987;64:1165-8.

1044 Chowdury R, Kunutsor S, Vitezova A, et al. Vitamin D and risk of cause specific death: Systematic review and meta-analysis of observational cohort and randomized intervention studies. BMJ. 2014;348:g1903.

1045 Lindqvist, PG, Epstein E, Nielsen K, et al. Avoidance of sun exposure as a risk factor for major causes of death: A competing risk analysis of the melanoma in Southern Sweden cohort. J Int Med. 2016;280(4):375-387.

1046 Reichrath J. The challenge resulting from positive and negative effects of sunlight: How much solar UV exposure is appropriate to balance between risks of vitamin D deficiency and skin cancer? Progress in Biophysics and Molecular Biology. 2006;92:9-16.

1047 Sorenson MB, Grant WB. Embrace the Sun. U.S.A. ISBN: 978-0-692-07600-2, p.XVII.

1048 Sorenson MB, Grant WB. Embrace the Sun. U.S.A. ISBN: 978-0-692-07600-2, pp.4-5.

1049 Sorenson MB, Grant WB. Embrace the Sun. U.S.A. ISBN: 978-0-692-07600-2, p.8.

1050 Sorenson MB, Grant WB. Embrace the Sun. U.S.A. ISBN: 978-0-692-07600-2, pp.9-10.

1051 Mawson AR. Role of Fat-Soluble Vitamins A and D in the Pathogenesis of Influenza: A New Perspective. ISRN Infectious Diseases. Volume 2013, Article ID 246737.

1052 Barolet D, Christiaens F, Hamblin MR. Infrared and skin: Friend or foe. Journal of Photochemistry and Photobiology, B: Biology. 2016;155:78-85.

1053 Tan DX, Manchester LC, Liu X, Rosales-Corral SA, Acuna-Castroviejo D, Reiter RJ. J Pineal Res. 2013;54(2):127-38.

1054 Aulinas A. Physiology of the Pineal Gland and Melatonin. Endotext [Internet]. National Library of Medicine. 10 Dec. 2019. Retrieved: **https://www.ncbi.nlm.nih.gov/books/NBK550972/**. Accessed 19 Apr 2022.

1055 Reiter RJ, Ma Q, Sharma R. Melatonin in Mitochondria: Mitigating Clear and Present Dangers. Physiology. 2020;35:86-95.

1056 Suofu Y, Jean-Alphonse FG, Friedlander RM. Dual role of mitochondria in producing melatonin and driving GPCR signaling to block cytochrome c release. PNAS. 2017;114(38):E7997-E8006.

1057 He C, Wang J, Zhang Z, et al. Mitochondria Synthesize Melatonin to Ameliorate Its Function and Improve Mice Oocyte's Quality under in Vitro Conditions. Int J Mol Sci. 2016;17(6):E939.

1058 Wang L, Feng C, Zheng X, et al. Plant mitochondria synthesize melatonin and enhance the tolerance of plants to drought stress. J Pineal Res. 2017;63(3):E12429.

1059 Odinokov D, Hamblin MR. Aging of lymphoid organs: Can photobiomodulation reverse age-associated thymic involution via stimulation of extrapineal melatonin synthesis and bone marrow stem cells? Journ Biophotonics. 2018;11(8):e201700282.

1060 Zimmerman S, Reiter RJ. Melatonin and the Optics of the Human Body. Melatonin Research. 2019;2(1):138-160.

1061 Martin M, Macías M, Escames G, et al. Melatonin but not vitamins C and E maintains glutathione homeostasis in t-butyl hydroperoxide-induced mitochondrial oxidative stress. FASEB J. 2000;14:1677-79.

1062 Acuña-Castroviejo D, López LC, Escames G, et al. Melatonin-mitochondria interplay in health and disease. Curr Top Med Chem. 2011;11:221-240.

1063 Jou MJ, Peng TI, Reiter RJ, et al. Visualization of the antioxidative effects of melatonin at the mitochondrial level during oxidative stress-induced apoptosis of rat brain astrocytes. J Pineal Res. 2004;37:55-70.

1064 White, Ellen G. The Health Reformer, May 1, 1871. HL 230.2.

1065 Price, Weston A. Nutrition and Physical Degeneration. Self-Published, 1945.

1066 Price, Weston A. Nutrition and Physical Degeneration. Lemon Grove, CA: The Price-Pottenger Nutrition Foundation Inc; 1939, pp.241-243.

1067 McKee RW, Binkley SB, MacCorquodale SA, et al. The Isolation of Vitamins K1 and K2. Journal Am Chem Soc. 1939;61(5):1295-1295.

1068 Vermeer C, Hamulyak K. Vitamin K: lessons from the

past. J Thromb Haemost. 2004;2(12):2115-7.
1069 Beulens JWJ, Booth SL, van den Heuvel EGHM, et al. The role of menaquinones (vitamin K2) in human health. Brit J Nutr. 2013;110:1357-1368.
1070 Billeter M, Martius C. Über die Umwandlung von Phyllochinon (Vitamin K1) in Vitamin K2(20) im Tierkörper. Biochem Z. 1960;333:430-439.
1071 Thijssen HHW, Drittij-Reijnders MJ. Vitamin K distribution in rat tissues: dietary phylloquinone is a source of tissue menaquinone-4. Br J Nutr. 1994;72:415-425.
1072 Ronden JE, Thijssen HHW, Vermeer C. Tissue distribution of K-vitamins under different nutritional regimens in the rat. Biochim Biophys Acta. 1998;1379:16-22.
1073 Cranenberg ECM, Schurgers LJ, Vermeer C. Vitamin K: The coagulation vitamin that became omnipotent. Thromb Haemost. 2007;98(01):120-125.
1074 Akbulut AC, Pavlic A, Petsophonsakul P, et al. Vitamin K2 Needs an RDI Separate from Vitamin K1. Nutrients. 2020;12:1852.
1075 Schurgers LJ, Vermeer C. Determination of phylloquinones and menaquinones in food. Haemostasis. 2000;30:298-307.
1076 Schurgers LJ, Teunissen KJF, Hamulyák K, et al. Vitamin K-containing dietary supplements: comparison of synthetic Vitamin K1 and natto-derived menaquinone-7. Blood. 2007;109:3279-3283.
1077 Vermeer C, Raes J, van't Hoofd C, et al. Menaquinone content of cheese. Nutrients. 2018;10:446.
1078 Sato T, Schurgers LJ, Uenishi K. Comparison of menaquinone-4 and menaquinone-7 bioavailability in healthy women. Nutr J. 2012;11:93.
1079 Oliva A, Ragione FD, Fratta M, et al. Effect of retinoic acid on osteocalcin gene expression in human osteoblasts. Biochem Biophys Res Commun. 1993;191(3):908-914.
1080 Koshihara Y, Hoshi K. Vitamin K2 enhances osteocalcin accumulation in the extracellular matrix of human osteoblasts in vitro. J Bone Miner Res. 1997;12(3):431-8.
1081 Berkner KL, Runge W. The physiology of vitamin K nutriture and vitamin K-dependent protein function in atherosclerosis. J Thromb Haemost. 2004;2(12):2118-32.
1082 Flore R, Ponziani FR, Di Rienzo TA, et al. Something more to say about calcium homeostasis: the role of vitamin K2 in vascular calcification and osteoporosis. European Review for Medical and Pharmacological Sciences. 2013;17:2433-2440.
1083 Greenland P, Bonow RO, Brundage BH, et al. ACCF/AHA clinical expert consensus document on coronary artery calcium scoring by computed tomography in global cardiovascular risk assessment and in evaluation of patients with chest pain: a report of the American College of Cardiology Foundation Clinical Expert Consensus Task Force (ACCF/AHA Writing Committee to Update the 2000 Expert Consensus Document on Electron Beam Computed Tomography) developed in collaboration with the Society of Atherosclerosis Imaging and Prevention and the Society of Cardiovascular Computed Tomography. J Am Coll Cardiol. 2007;49:378-402.
1084 Okuyama H, Langsjoen PH, Ohara N, et al. Medicines and Vegetable Oils as Hidden Causes of Cardiovascular Disease and Diabetes. Pharmacology. 2016;98:134-170.
1085 Institute of Medicine 2001. Dietary Reference Intakes for Vitamin A, Vitamin K, Arsenic, Boron, Chromium, Copper, Iodine, iron, Manganese, Molybdenum, Nickel, Silicon, Vanadium, and Zinc. Washington, DC: The National Academies Press. **https://doi.org/10.17226/10026**.
1086 National Institutes of Health Office of Dietary Supplements. Vitamin K – Fact Sheet for Health Professionals. Updated 29 March 2021. Retrieved: **https://ods.od.nih.gov/factsheets/VitaminK-HealthProfessional/?print=1#en3**. Accessed 24 Feb 2022.
1087 Wright NC, Looker AC, Saag KG, et al. The Recent Prevalence of Osteoporosis and Low Bone Mass in the United States Based on Bone Mineral Density at the Femoral Neck or Lumbar Spine. J Bone Miner Res. 2014;29(11):2520-2526.
1088 Rippe JM, Angelopoulos TJ. Relationship between Added Sugars Consumption and Chronic Disease Risk Factors: Current Understanding. Nutrients. 2016;8,697; doi: 10.3390/nu8110697.
1089 Lustig RH, Schmidt LA, Brindis CD. The toxic truth about sugar. Nature. 2012;482:27-29.
1090 Sievenpiper JL. Sickeningly Sweet: Does Sugar Cause Chronic Disease? No. Canadian Journal of Diabetes. 2016;40:287-295.
1091 Yudkin, John. Pure, White and Deadly. The New Facts About the Sugar You Eat as a Cause of Heart Disease, Diabetes, and Other Killers. Davis-Poynter Limited.

SBN 0706700562, ISBN13:9780706700565.

1092 Taubes, Gary. "What if It's All Been a Big Fat Lie?" The New York Times Magazine. 7 July 2002. Retrieved: https://www.nytimes.com/2002/07/07/magazine/what-if-it-s-all-been-a-big-fat-lie.html. Accessed 4 Feb 2022.

1093 Lustig, Robert H. "Sugar: The Bitter Truth." A University of California Television lecture. 27 July 2009. Retrieved: https://www.uctv.tv/shows/sugar-the-bitter-truth-16717. Accessed 4 Feb 2022.

1094 Lustig, Robert H. FAT Chance – Beating the Odds Against Sugar, Processed Food, Obesity, and Disease. New York, NY, Penguin Group, 2012.

1095 World Health Organization. "Why excess sugar is bad for you – limit sugar for healthier life." WHO. Retrieved: https://cdn.who.int/media/docs/default-source/searo/myanmar/factsheet-sugar.pdf?sfvrsn=d0cdcffa_4#:~:text=WHO%20recommends%20adults%20and%20children,approx%205%20g%20of%20sugar. Accessed 20 Feb 2022.

1096 Aragno M, Mastrocola R. Dietary Sugars and Endogenous Formation of Advanced Glycation Endproducts: Emerging Mechanisms of Disease. Nutrients. 2017;9(4),385. https://doi.org/10.3390/nu9040385.

1097 Livesey G, Taylor R. Fructose consumption and consequences for glycation, plasma triacylglycerol, and body weight: Meta-analyses and meta-regression models of intervention studies. Am J Clin Nutr. 2008;88:1419-1437.

1098 Rahbar S. The discovery of glycated hemoglobin: a major event in the study of nonenzymatic chemistry in biological systems. Ann N Y Acad Sci. 2005;1043:9-19.

1099 Cibičková L, Karásek D, Langová K, et al. Correlation of Lipid Parameters and Markers of Insulin Resistance: Does Smoking Make a Difference? Physiol Res. 2014;63(Suppl. 3):S387-S393.

1100 Haire-Hoshu D, Glasgow RE, Tibbs TL. Smoking and Diabetes. American Diabetes Association. 2004;27:S74-5. DOI:10.2337/diacare.27.2007.S74.

1101 Pan DA, Storlien LH. Dietary Lipid Profile Is a Determinant of Tissue Phospholipid Fatty Acid Composition and Rate of Weight Gain in Rats. J Nutr. 1993;123(3):512-9.

1102 Deol P, Evans JR, Dhahbi J, et al. Soybean Oil Is More Obesogenic and Diabetogenic than Coconut Oil and Fructose in Mouse: Potential Role for the Liver. PLoS One. 2015;10(7): e0132672. Doi: 10.1371/journal.pone.0132672.

1103 Khitan Z, Kim DH. Fructose: A Key Factor in the Development of Metabolic Syndrome and Hypertension. Journal of Nutrition and Metabolism. 2013;Article ID: 682673. https://doi.org/10.1155/2013/682673.

1104 Midtbo LK, Ibrahim MM, Myrmel LS, et al. Intake of farmed Atlantic salmon fed soybean oil increases insulin resistance and hepatic lipid accumulation in mice. PLoS One. 2013; 3: e53094. Doi: 10.1371/journal.pone.0053094 PMID: 23301026.

1105 Alvheim AR, Torstensen BE, Lin YH, et al. Dietary linoleic acid elevates endogenous 2-arachidonoylglycerol and anandamide in Atlantic salmon (Salmo salar L.) and mice, and induces weight gain and inflammation in mice. Br J Nutr. 2013;109:1508-1517.

1106 Alvheim AR, Malde MK, Osei-Hyiaman D, et al. Dietary linoleic acid elevates endogenous 2-AG and anandamide and induces obesity. Obesity. 2012;20:1984-1994.

1107 Poonamjot Deol. Fahrmann J, Yang J, et al. Omega-6 and omega-3 oxylipins are implicated in soybean oil-induced obesity in mice. Scientific Reports. 2017;7:12488. DOI:10.1038/s41598-017-12624-9.

1108 Ambreen G, Siddiq A, Hussain K. Association of long-term consumption of repeatedly heated mix vegetable oils in different doses and hepatic toxicity through fat accumulation. Lipids in Health and Disease. 2020;19:69. https://doi.org/10.1186/s12944-020-01256-0.

1109 Ghosh S, Kewalramani G, Yuen G, et al. Induction of mitochondrial nitrative damage and cardiac dysfunction by chronic provision of dietary omega-6 polyunsaturated fatty acids. Free Radic Biol Med. 2006;41(9):1413-24.

1110 Hipkiss AR, Worthington VC, Himsworth DTJ, Herwig W. Protective effects of carnosine against protein modification mediated by malondialdehyde and hypochlorite. Biochimica et Biophysica Acta. 1998;1380:46-54.

1111 Aldini G, Carini M, Beretta, et al. Carnosine is a quencher of 4-hydroxy-nonenal: through what mechanism of reaction? Biochim and Biophysical Res Communications. 2002;198(5):699-706.

1112 Aldini G, Facino RM, Beretta G, Carini M. Carnosine and related dipeptides as quenchers of reactive carbonyl species: From structural studies to therapeutic perspectives. BioFactors. 2005;24:77-87.

1113 Burcham PC, Kaminskas LM, Tan D, Pyke SM. Carbonyl-Scavenging Drugs & Protection Against Carbonyl Stress – Associated Cell Injury. Mini-Reviews Med Chem. 2008;8:319-30.

1114 Ghodsi R, Kheirouri S. Carnosine and advanced glycation end products: a systematic review. Amino Acids. 2018;50:177-1186.

1115 Rashid I, van Reyk DM. Davies MJ. Carnosine and its constituents inhibit glycation of low-density lipoproteins that promotes foam cell formation in vitro. FEBS Letters. 2007;581(5):1067-1070.

1116 Boldyrev AA, Aldini G, Derave W. Physiology and pathophysiology of carnosine. Physiol Rev. 2013;93:1803-1845.

1117 Hipkiss A.R. "Chapter 3: Carnosine and Its Possible Roles in Nutrition and Health." Advances in Food and Nutrition Research. 2009;Vol 57. ISSN: 1043-4526, DOI: 10.1016/S1043-4526(09)57003-9.

1118 Harris RC, Jones G, Hill CH, et al. The carnosine content of vastus lateralis in vegetarians and omnivores. FASEB J. 2007;21:76.

1119 Artioli GG, Gualano B, Smith A, et al. Role of Beta-alanine Supplementation on Muscle Carnosine and Exercise Performance. Med Sci Sports Exerc. 2010;42(6):1162-73.

1120 di Pierro F, Bertuccioli A, Bressnan A, Rapacioli G. Carnosine-based supplement. Nutra foods. 2011;10(2):1-5.

1121 O'Toole TE, Li X, Riggs DW, et al. Urinary Levels of the Acrolein Conjugates of Carnosine Are Associated with Cardiovascular Disease Risk. Int J Mol Sci. 2021;22,1383. **https://doi.org/10.3390/ijms22031383**.

1122 Kondo N. What Has Made Japan Healthy? Harvard School of Public Health, Takemi Program 30th Anniversary Symposium, Tokyo, 2013. Retrieved: **https://www.ncbi.nlm.nih.gov/pmc/articles/PMC4130084/pdf/jmaj-57-24.pdf**. Accessed 27 Feb 2022.

1123 Willcox BJ, Willcox DC, Todoriki H, et al. Caloric Restriction, the Traditional Okinawan Diet, and Healthy Aging. The Diet of the World's Longest-Lived People and Its Potential Impact on Morbidity and Lifespan. Ann N.Y. Acad Sci. 2007;1114:434-455.

1124 World History Encyclopedia. "Food & Agriculture in Ancient Japan." 20 Jun 2017. Retrieved: **https://www.worldhistory.org/article/1082/food--agriculture-in-ancient-japan/**. Accessed 27 Feb 2022.

1125 Ishigi, Naomichi. The History and Culture of Japanese Food. Kegan Paul, London, New York, 2001, p.17.

1126 Ishigi, Naomichi. The History and Culture of Japanese Food. Kegan Paul, London, New York, 2001, pp. 20-21.

1127 MayaIncaAztec.com. "Food in Ancient Japan." ND **https://www.mayaincaaztec.com/medievel-japan/food-in-ancient-japan**. Accessed 27 Feb 2022.

1128 Smil V, Kobayashi K. Japan's Dietary Transition and its Impacts (Cambridge, MA: The MIT Press, 2012, p. 49.

1129 Sho H. History and characteristics of Okinawan longevity food. Asia Pacific J Clin Nutr. 2001;10:159-164.

1130 Japan-Guide.com. "Post War History (since 1945). Japan-Guide. ND. Retrieved: **https://www.japan-guide.com/e/e2124.html**. Accessed 26 Feb 2022.

1131 Office of The Historian. "Occupation and Reconstruction of Japan, 1945-52." Department of State, United States of America. Retrieved: **https://history.state.gov/milestones/1945-1952/japan-reconstruction**. Accessed 27 Feb 2022.

1132 Tetsuji, Okazaki. . "Lessons from the Japanese Miracle: Building the Foundations for a New Growth Paradigm. Nippon.com. ND. Retrieved: https://www.nippon.com. Accessed: 27 Feb 2022.

1133 Popkin BM. Nutritional Patterns and Transitions. Population and Development Review. 1993;19(1):138-157.

1134 Facts and Details. "Restaurants and Fast Food In Japan: Michelin Stars, McDonald's, Bento Boxes and Plastic Food. ND. Retrieved: **https://factsanddetails.com/japan/cat19/sub123/item648.html#chapter-15**. Accessed 27 Feb 2022.

1135 Adachi H, Hino A. Trends in Nutritional Intake and Serum Cholesterol Levels over 40 Years in Tanushimaru, Japanese Men. Journ Epidemiol. 2005;15(3):85-89.

1136 Willcox DC, Scapagnini G, Willcox BJ. Healthy aging diets other than the Mediterranean: A focus on the Okinawan diet. Mechanisms of Ageing and Development. 2014;136-137:148-162.

1137 Sugano M, Hirahara F. Polyunsaturated fatty acids in the food chain in Japan. Am J Clin Nutr. 2007;71(Suppl):189S-196S.

1138 Yoshiike N, Kaneda F, Takimoto H. Epidemiology of obesity and public health strategies for its control in Japan. Asia Pacific J Clin Nutr. 2002;11(Suppl):S727-S731.

1139 Nishi N. Monitoring Obesity Trends in Health Japan 21. J Nutr Si Vitaminol. 2015;61:S17-S19.

1140 Kuzuya T. Prevalence of diabetes mellitus in Japan compiled from literature. Diabetes Research and Clinical Practice. 1994;24 Suppl:S15-S21.

1141 Nanri A, Shimazu T, Takachi R. Dietary patterns and type 2 diabetes in Japanese men and women: the Japan Public Health Center-based Prospective Study. Eur J Clin Nutr. 2013;67:18-24.

1142 Saika K, Sobue T. Epidemiology of Breast Cancer in Japan and the US. JMAJ. 2009;52(1):39-44.

1143 Ichikawa H. The visual functions and aging, Rinsho Ganka. Jpn J Clin Ophthalmol. 1981;35:9-26.

1144 Hoshino M, Mizuno K, Ichikawa H. Aging alterations of retina and choroid of Japanese: light microscopic study of macular region of 176 eyes. Jpn J Ophthalmol. 1984;28(1):89-102.

1145 Yasuda M, Kiyohara Y, Hata Y, at al. Nine-year incidence and risk factors for age-related macular degeneration in a defined Japanese population: the Hisayama study. Ophthalmology. 2009;116(11):2135-40.

1146 Nakata I, Yamashiro K, Nakanishi H, et al. Prevalence and characteristics of age-related macular degeneration in the Japanese population: the Nagahama study. Am J Ophthalmol. 2013;156(5):1002-1009.

1147 Tanaka H, Shimabukuro T, Shimabukuro M. High Prevalence of Metabolic Syndrome among Men in Okinawa. Journal of Atherosclerosis and Thrombosis. 2005;12:284-288.

1148 Todoriki H, Willcox DC, Willcox BJ. The Effects of Post-War Dietary Change on Longevity and Health in Okinawa. The Okinawa Journal of American Studies. 2004;1:52-61.

1149 NCD Risk Factor Collaboration (NCD-RisC). Trends in adult body-mass index in 200 countries from 1975 to 2014: a pooled analysis of 1698 population-based measurement studies with 19.2 million participants. The Lancet. 2016;387(10026):P1377-1396.

1150 Drexler M. "Obesity – Can we stop the epidemic?" Harvard Public Health. Spring 2017. Retrieved: https://www.case.org/system/files/media/file/Obesity-Can%20we%20stop%20the%20epidemic-PDF.pdf. Accessed 4 Feb 2022.

1151 Knoema. "Energy from vegetable oils." Original data: FAOSTAT (FAO). Available: https://www.knoema.com/atlas.

1152 Knoema. Vegetable Oils, Aggregate data, all countries. https://www.fao.org/faostat/en/#home. Original data: FAO.org (FAOSTAT).

1153 Harvard Health Publishing. "No need to avoid healthy omega-6 fats." Harvard Health Publishing – Harvard Medical School. 20 Aug 2019. Retrieved: https://www.health.harvard.edu/newsletter_article/no-need-to-avoid-healthy-omega-6-fats#:~:text=Omega%2D6%20fats%20from%20vegetable,of%20something%2C%20or%20the%20end. Accessed: 4 Feb 2022.

1154 IHME. "The Lancet: Latest global disease estimates reveal perfect storm of rising chronic diseases and public health failures fueling COVID-19 pandemic. 15 Oct 2020. Retrieved: https://www.healthdata.org. Accessed 27 Feb 2022.

1155 NCD Risk Factor Collaboration (NCD-RisC). Trends in adult body mass index in 200 countries from 1975 to 2014: a pooled analysis of 1698 population-based measurement studies with 19.2 million participants. Lancet. 2016;387:1377-96.

1156 Nuttall FQ. Body Mass Index. Nutr Today. 2015;50(3):117-128.

1157 Liu B, Du Y, Wu Y, et al. Trends in obesity and adiposity measures by race or ethnicity among adults in the United States 2011-18: population based study. BMJ. 2021;372: n365.

1158 NCD Risk Factor Collaboration (NCD-RisC). Worldwide trends in diabetes since 1980: a pooled analysis of 751 population-based studies with 4.4 million participants. The Lancet. 2016;387:1513-30.

1159 FAO Statistics Division 2010, Food Balance Sheets, Food and Agriculture Organization of the United Nations, Rome, Italy, viewed 17th March, 2011, <http://faostat.fao.org/

1160 Carbohydrates in Human Nutrition. FAO Food and Nutrition Paper – 66, Consultation Rome, 14-18 Apr, 1997 http://www.fao.org/3/W8079E/w8079e0g.htm

1161 FAO Statistics Division 2010, Food Balance Sheets, Food and Agriculture Organization of the United Nations, Rome, Italy, viewed 17th March, 2011, <http://faostat.fao.org/

1162 Donnelly JF, Winston-Salem NC, Flowers CE, et al. Parental, fetal, and environmental factors in perinatal mortality. Am Journ Obst Gyn. 1957;74(6):1245-

1256.

1163 Refsum H. Folate, vitamin B12 and homocysteine in relation to birth defects and pregnancy outcome. British Journal of Nutrition. 2001;85(Suppl 2):S109-S113.

1164 Li Z, Shen J, Wu WKK, et al. Vitamin A Deficiency Induces Congenital Spinal Deformities in Rats. PLoS One. 2012;7(10):e46565. Doi: 10.1371/journal.pone.0046565.

1165 Hollis BW, Wagner CL. New insights into the vitamin D requirements during pregnancy. Bone Res. 2017;5:17030. https://doi.org/10.1038/boneres.2017.30.

1166 Brines J, Billeaud C. Breast-Feeding from an Evolutionary Perspective. Healthcare. 2021;9:1458.

1167 Stevens EE, Patrick TE, Pickler R. A History of Infant Feeding. The Journal of Perinatal Education. 2009;18(2):32-39.

1168 Long AC, Kaiser JL, Katz GE. Lipids in infant formulas: Current and future innovations. Lipid Technology. 2013;25(6):127-129.

1169 Lönnerdal B. Breast milk: a truly functional food. Nutrition. 2000;16(7/8:509-511.

1170 Walker A. Breast Milk as the Gold Standard for Protective Nutrients. Journ Pediatr. 2010;156(2):S3-S7.

1171 Andreas NJ, Kampmann B, Mehring Le-Doare K. Human breast milk: A review on its composition and bioactivity. Early Human Development. 2015;91(11):629-635.

1172 Bravi F, Wiens F, Decarli A, et al. Impact of maternal nutrition on breast-milk composition: a systematic review. Am J Clin Nutr. 2016;104(3):646-662.

1173 Taha AY. Linoleic acid – good or bad for the brain? NPJ Science of Food. 2020;4:1; https://doi.org/10.1038/s41538-019-0061-9.

1174 Putnam JC, Carlson SE, DeVoe PW, Barness LA. The effect of variations in dietary fatty acids on the fatty acid composition of erythrocyte phosphatidylcholine and phosphatidylethanolamine in human infants. Am J Clin Nutr. 1982;36:106-114.

1175 Jenness R. The composition of human milk. SSemin. Perinatol. 1979;3:225-239.

1176 Bernard JY, Armand M, Garcia C, et al. The association between linoleic acid levels in colostrum and child cognition at 2 and 3 y in the EDEN cohort. Pediatric Research. 2015;77:829-835.

1177 Bernard JY, Armand M, Peyre H, et al. Breastfeeding, Polyunsaturated Fatty Acid Levels in Colostrum and Child Intelligence Quotient at Age 5-6 Years. Journ Pediatr. 2017;183:43-50.e3.

1178 Cooperstock MS, Steffen E, Yolken R, Onderdonk A. Clostridium difficile in Normal Infants and Sudden Infant Death Syndrome: An Association with Infant Formula Feeding. Pediatrics. 1982;70(1):91-95.

1179 Boyd CA, Quigley MA, Brocklehurst P. Donor breast milk versus infant formula for preterm infants: systematic review and meta-analysis. Archives of Disease in Childhood – Fetal and Neonatal Edition. 2007;92:F169-F175.

1180 Stettler N, Stallings VA, Troxel AB, et al. Weight Gain in the First Week of Life and Overweight in Adulthood. Circulation. 2005;111:1897-1903.

1181 Dewey KG. Nutrition, growth, and complementary feeding of the breastfed infant. Pediatr Clin North Am. 2001;48:87-104.

1182 Baker JL, Michaelsen KF, Rasmussen KM, Sorensen TI. Maternal prepregnant body mass index, duration of breastfeeding, and timing of complementary food introduction are associated with infant weight gain. Am J Clin Nutr. 2004;80:1579-1588.

1183 von Kries R, Koletzko B, Sauerwald T, et al. Breast feeding and obesity: cross sectional study. BMJ. 1999;319:147-150.

1184 Gillman MW, Rifas-Shiman SL, Camargo CA Jr, et al. Risk of overweight among adolescents who were breastfed as infants. JAMA. 2001;285:2461-2467.

1185 Fujita K, Kakuya F, Ito S. Vitamin K1 and K2 status and faecal flora in breast fed and formula fed 1-month-old infants. Eur J Pediatr. 1993;152:852-855.

1186 Widdowson EM, Dauncey MJ, Gairdner DM, et al. Body fat of British and Dutch Infants. Br Med J. 1975;1(5959):653-5.

1187 Statista. "Sales of the leading baby formula (powder) brands of the United States in 2016." Statista.com. Retrieved: http://www.statista.com. Accessed 28 Feb 2022.

1188 Abbott. "Similac Advance." ND. Retrieved: https://www.similac.com/products/baby-formula/advance-powder/20-6oz.html. Accessed 1 Mar 2022.

1189 Ailhaud G. n-6 Fatty acids and adipogenesis. Scand J Food Nutr. 2006;50(52):17-20.

1190 Massiera F, Guesnet P, Ailhaud G. The Crucial Role of Dietary n-6 Polyunsaturated Fatty Acids in Excessive

Adipose Tissue Development: Relationship to Childhood Obesity. In: Lucas A, Sampson HA (eds): Primary Prevention by Nutrition Intervention in Infancy and Childhood. Nestlè Nutr Workshop Scr Pediatr Program, vol 57, pp 235-245, Nestec Ltd., Vevey/S. Karger AG, Basel, 2006.

1191 Moon RJ, Harvey NC, Robinson SM, et al. Maternal plasma polyunsaturated fatty acid status in late pregnancy is associated with offspring body composition in childhood. J Clin Endocrinol Metab. 2013;98(1):299-307.

1192 MacLennan M, Ma D. Role of dietary fatty acids in mammary gland development and breast cancer. Breast Cancer Res. 2010;12(5):211.

1193 Brown RA. Bioactive Oxidized Products of Omega-6 and Omega-3, Excess Oxidative Stress, Oxidized Dietary Intake and Antioxidant Nutrient Deficiencies, in the Context of a Modern Diet. Omega-3 Fatty Acids, 2016;349-383. Doi:10.1007/978-3-319-40458-5_28.

1194 "Most Popular Countries and Cities for Vegans in 2020 (Jan-2021 Update." ChefsPencil. 5 Jan 2021. Retrieved: **https://www.chefspencil.com/most-popular-countries-and-cities-for-vegans-in-2020-jan-2021-update/**. Accessed 11 Feb 2022.

1195 O'Leary F, Samman S. Vitamin B12 in Health and Disease. Nutrients. 2010;2:299-316.

1196 McCollum, E.V. The Newer Knowledge of Nutrition – The Use of Food For the Preservation of Vitality and Health. New York, The MacMillan Company, 1918, pp.150-151.

1197 Price, WA. Studies of Relationships Between Nutritional Deficiencies and (a) Facial and Dental Arch Deformities and (b) Loss of Immunity to Dental Caries Among South Sea Islanders and Florida Indians. Dental Cosmos. 1935;77(11):1033-45.

1198 Price, Weston A. Nutrition and Physical Degeneration. Lemon Grove, CA: The Price-Pottenger Nutrition Foundation Inc; 1939, p.250.

1199 Watanabe F. Vitamin B12 Sources and Bioavailability. Experimental Biology and Medicine. 2007;232(10):1266-1274.

1200 Herrmann W, Schorr H, Obeid R, Geisel J. Vitamin B-12 status, particularly holotranscobalamin II and methylmalonic acid concentrations, and hyperhomocysteinemia in vegetarians. Am J Clin Nutr. 2003;78:131-6.

1201 Antony AC. Vegetarianism and vitamin B-12 (cobalamin) deficiency. Am J Clin Nutr. 2003;78(1):3-6.

1202 Wood MM, Elwood PC. Symptoms of Iron Deficiency Anaemia – A Community Survey. Brit J Prev Soc Med. 1966;20:117-121.

1203 Soppi E. Iron Deficiency Without Anemia – Common, Important, Neglected. Clinical Case Reports and Reviews. 2019. Doi: 10.1576/CCRR.1000456.

1204 Richter M, Boeing H, Grünewald-Funk, et al. Vegan Diet – Position of the German Nutrition Society (DGE). The German Nutrition Society (DGE). Ernahrungs Umschau. 2016;63(04):92-102. Erratum in: 63(05): M262. DOI: 10.4455/eu.2016.021.

1205 Gordon, Ali. "Vegan diet 'could have severe consequences,' professor warns. BBC News. 5 Jan 2019. Retrieved: **https://www.bbc.com/news/uk-northern-ireland-46616637**. Accessed 2 Feb 2022.

1206 "7 Dangerous Side Effects of Vegan Diet." Times of India. Retrieved: **https://timesofindia.indiatimes.com/life-style/food-news/7-dangerous-side-effects-of-vegan-diet/photostory/77717097.cms**. Accessed 2 Feb 2022.

1207 Hauner H. [Vegetarian/vegan diet – reasonable or dangerous?]. MMW Fortschr Med. 2015;157(10:41-3.

1208 López-Moreno M, Garcé-Rimón, Miguel M. Antinutrients: Lectins, goitrogens, phytates and oxalates, friends or foe? Journ Functional Foods. 2022;8(:104938.

1209 Di Genova T, Guyda H. Infants and children consuming atypical diets: Vegetarianism and macrobiotics. Paediatr Child Health. 2007;12(3):185-188.

1210 Roschitz B, Plecko B, Huemer M, Biebl A, et al. Nutritional infantile vitamin B12 deficiency: Pathobiochemical considerations in seven patients. Arch Dis Child Fetal Neonatal Ed. 2005;90:F281-2.

1211 Second Opinions. Vegan Child Abuse. Retrieved: **http://www.second-opinion.co.uk/child_abuse.html**.

1212 Grinberg E. Vegan parents on trial for baby's death, allegedly from malnutrition. Retrieved: **http://news.findlaw.com/court_tv/s/20051018/18oct2005172836.html**.

1213 Farberov S. "US vegan parents who eat only raw fruit and vegetables are charged with MURDER for the starvation death of their 18-month-old son who was found weighing only 17lbs." DailyMail.com. 19 Dec 2019. Retrieved: **https://www.dailymail.co.uk/news/article-7810073/Vegan-parents-charged-murder-baby-sons-starvation-death.html**. Accessed 10 Feb 2022.

1214 Dupri, A. "Vegan Parents on Trial, Charged with Neglect, After Baby's Death." KissRichmond.com. ND. Retrieved: https://kissrichmond.com/1646962/vegan-parents-on-trial-charged-with-neglect-after-babys-death/. Accessed 10 Feb 2022.

1215 Brook B, Graham B. "Parents sentenced over neglect of child on vegan-only diet." News.com.au. 22 Aug 2019. Retrieved: https://www.news.com.au/national/nsw-act/crime/parents-sentenced-over-neglect-of-child-on-veganonly-diet/news-story/68bedf9fd-1b86a2e04864c27349233d2. Accessed 10 Feb 2022.

1216 Price, Weston A. Nutrition and Physical Degeneration. Lemon Grove, CA: The Price-Pottenger Nutrition Foundation Inc; 1939, p.265.

1217 Price, Weston A. Nutrition and Physical Degeneration. Lemon Grove, CA: The Price-Pottenger Nutrition Foundation Inc; 1939, p.264.

1218 Bazzano LA, Hu T, Reynolds K, et al. Effects of Low-Carbohydrate and Low-Fat Diets. Ann Intern Med. 2014;161(5):309-18.

1219 Chawla S, Silva FT, Medeiros SA, et al. The Effect of Low-Fat and Low-Carbohydrate Diets on Weight Loss and Lipid Levels: A Systematic Review and Meta-Analysis. Nutrients. 2020;12(12):3774.

1220 Dyson P. Low Carbohydrate Diets and Type 2 Diabetes: What is the Latest Evidence? Diabetes Therapy. 2015;6:411-424.

1221 Naude CE, Schoonees A, Senekal M, et al. Low Carbohydrate versus Isoenergetic Balanced Diets for Reducing Weight and Cardiovascular Risk: A Systematic Review and Meta-Analysis. PLOS ONE. 2014;9:e100652.

1222 NIH National Cancer Institute. "Identification of Top Food Sources of Various Dietary Components." Epidemiology and Genomics Research Program website, updated Nov 30, 2019, https://epi.grants.cancer.gov/diet/foodsources. Retrieved: https://epi.grants.cancer.gov/diet/foodsources/top-food-sources-report-02212020.pdf. Accessed 2 Mar 2022.

1223 Teicholz, Nina. The Big FAT Surprise – Why Butter, Meat, and Cheese Belong in a Healthy Diet. New York, Simon & Schuster. 2014.

1224 Teicholz, Nina. Via personal email, on 2 Mar 2022.

1225 Centers for Disease Control and Prevention (CDC). "What Are the Risk Factors for Lung Cancer?" CDC. ND. Retrieved: https://www.cdc.gov/cancer/lung/basic_info/risk_factors.htm#:~:text=Tobacco%20smoke%20is%20a%20toxic,people%20who%20do%20not%20smoke. Accessed: 4 April 2022.

1226 Centers for Disease Control and Prevention. "Smoking & Tobacco Use – Health Effects." ND. Retrieved: https://www.cdc.gov/tobacco/basic_information/health_effects/index.htm#:~:text=Smoking%20causes%20cancer%2C%20heart%20disease,immune%20system%2C%20including%20rheumatoid%20arthritis. Accessed 4 Apr 2022.

1227 Hayes, A. Wallace. Principles and Methods of Toxicology, Fifth Edition. Boca Raton, FL, CRC Press, Taylor & Francis Group, 2008.

1228 Rose G. Incubation period of coronary heart disease. BMJ. 1982;284:1600-1601.

1229 Phillipe P. Sartwell's incubation period model revisited in the light of dynamic modeling. J Clin Epidemiol. 1994;47(4):419-433.

1230 Armenian HK, Lilienfeld AM. The Distribution of Incubation Periods of Neoplastic Diseases. Amer J Epidemiol. 1974;99(2):92-100.

1231 Horner RD. Age at Onset of Alzheimer's Disease: Clue to the Relative Importance of Etiologic Factors? Am J Epidemiol. 1987;126(3):409-414.

1232 Hall KD, Chen KY, Guo J, et al. Energy expenditure and body composition changes after an isocaloric ketogenic diet in overweight and obese men. Am J Clin Nutr. 2016;104(2):324-333.

1233 Hall KD, Bemis T, Brychta R, et al. Calorie for Calorie, Dietary Fat Restriction Results in More Body Fat Loss than Carbohydrate Restriction in People with Obesity. Cell Metabollsm. 2015;22(3):P427-436.

1234 Vahter M. Health Effects of Early Life Exposure to Arsenic. Basic and Clinical Pharmacology & Toxicology. 2008;102(2):204-211.

1235 Jomova K, Jenisova Z, Feszterova M, et al. Arsenic: toxicity, oxidative stress and human disease. J Applied Toxicol. 2011;31(2):95-107.

1236 Hossain K, Himeno S, Islam MS, et al. Chronic arsenic exposure, endothelial dysfunction and risk of cardiovascular diseases. In: Zhu, Guo, Bhattacharya, Ahmad, Bundschuh, Naidu (eds). Environmental Arsenic in a Changing World. 2018. ISBN: 978-1-138-48609-6.

1237 Cheng T-J, Chuu J-J, Chang C-Y, et al. Atherosclerosis induced by arsenic in drinking water in rats through altering lipid metabolism. Toxicology and Applied

Pharmacology. 2011;256(2):146-153.
1238 Hughes MF. Arsenic toxicity and potential mechanisms of action. Toxicology Letters. 2002;133:1-16.
1239 Farkhondeh T, Samarghandian S, Azimi-Nezhad M. The role of arsenic in obesity and diabetes. J Cell Physiol. 2019;234:12516-12529.
1240 Spratlen MJ, Grau-Perez M, Best LG, et al. The Association of Arsenic Exposure and Arsenic Metabolism With the Metabolic Syndrome and its Individual Components: Prospective Evidence From the Strong Heart Family Study. Am J Epidemiol. 2018;187(8):1598-1612.
1241 Giakoumis EG. Analysis of 22 vegetable oils' physico-chemical properties and fatty acid composition on a statistical basis, and correlation with the degree of unsaturation. Renewable Energy. 2018, doi: 10.1016/J.renene.2018.03.057.
1242 Orsavova J, Misurcova L, Ambrozova JV, et al. Fatty Acids Composition of Vegetable Oils and Its Contribution to Dietary Energy Intake and Dependence of Cardiovascular Mortality on Dietary Intake of Fatty Acids. Int J Mol Sci. 2015;16(6):12871-12890.
1243 Dyer JM, Stymne S, Green AG, Carlsson AS. High-value oils from plants. The Plan Journal. 2008;54:640-655.
1244 Bonaccio M, Di Castelnuovo A, Bonanni A, et al. Adherence to a Mediterranean diet is associated with a better health-related quality of life: a possible role of high dietary antioxidant content. BMJ Open. 2013;e003003. Doi: 10.1136/bmjopen-2013-003003.
1245 Boateng L, Ansong R, Owusu W, Steiner-Asiedu M. Coconut oil and palm oil's role in nutrition, health and national development: A review. Ghana Medical Journal. 2016;50(3):
1246 Ramadan MF. Fruit Oils: Chemistry and Functionality. Switzerland, Springer, Cham, 2019.
1247 Hernandez M L, Sicardo MD, Balaj A, Martinez-Rivas JM. The Oleic/Linoleic Acid Ratio in Olive (Olea europaea L.) Fruit Mesocarp Is Mainly Controlled by OeFAD2-2 and OeFAD2-5 Genes Together With the Different Specificity of Extraplastidial Acytransferase Enzymes. Front Plant Sci 2021;12:653997. Doi: 10.3389/fpls.2021.653997.
1248 Tan CX. Virgin avocado oil: An emerging source of functional fruit oil. Journ Functional Foods. 2019;54:381-392.
1249 Mailer RJ, Gafner S. Adulteration of Olive (Olea europaea) Oil. Botanical Adulterants Prevention Bulletin. Austin, TX: ABC-AHP-NCNPR Botanical Adulterants Prevention Program: 2020.
1250 **FoodFraud.org**
1251 Whitaker, Bill. "Agromafia." 60 Minutes, CBS News. Retrieved: **https://www.cbsnews.com/news/60-minutes-agromafia-food-fraud/**. Accessed 2 Mar 2022.
1252 Rodriguez C. The Olive Oil Scam: If 80% Is Fake, Why Do You Keep Buying It? Forbes. Retrieved: **https://www.forbes.com/sites/ceciliarodriguez/2016/02/10/the-olive-oil-scam-if-80-is-fake-why-do-you-keep-buying-it/?sh=7d4782cc639d**. Accessed 2 Mar 2022.
1253 Kosma I, Badeka A, Vatavali K, et al. Differentiation of Greek extra virgin olive oils according to cultivar based on volatile compound analysis and fatty acid composition. Eur J Lpid Sci Technol. 2016;118:849-861.
1254 Stefanoudaki E, Kotsifaki F, Koutsaftakis A. Classification of Virgin Olive Oils of the Two Major Cretan Cultivars Based on Their Fatty Acid Composition. JAOCS. 1999;76(5):623-626.
1255 Sheorey SD, Sengupta R, Hinge MA. Heart Healthy Nuts. Int J Curr Pharm Rev Res. 2011;2(3):145-160.
1256 Mayo Clinic Staff. "Nuts and your heart: Eating nuts for heart health." Mayo Clinic. ND. Retrieved: **https://www.mayoclinic.org/diseases-conditions/heart-disease/in-depth/nuts/art-20046635#:~:text=The%20American%20Heart%20Association%20recommends,of%20a%20heart%2Dhealthy%20diet**. Accessed: 2 Mar 2022.
1257 Vecka M, Staňková B, Kutová S. Comprehensive sterol and fatty acid analysis in nineteen nuts, seeds, and kernel. SN Applied Sciences. 2019;1,Article no: 1531.
1258 Green America. "Dean Foods." ND. Retrieved: **https://www.greenamerica.org/dean-foods#:~:text=Cows%20living%20on%20industrialized%20farms,to%20feeding%20livestock%20and%20poultry**. Accessed: 3 Mar 2022.
1259 Van Eenennaam AL. GMOs in animal agriculture: time to consider both costs and benefits in regulatory evaluations. J Animal Sci Biotechnol. 2013;4(1):37.
1260 Nürnberg K, Wegner J, Ender K. Factors influencing fat composition in muscle and adipose tissue of farm animals. Livestock Production Science. 1998;56:145-156.
1261 Maia MRG, Chaudhary LC, Bestwick CS, et al. Toxicity of unsaturated fatty acids to the biohydrogenating ruminal bacterium, Butyrivibrio fibrisolvens. BMC Microbiol. 2010;10:52.
1262 Daley CA, Abbott A, Doyle PS, et al. A review of

fatty acid profiles and antioxidant content in grass-fed and grain-fed beef. Nutrition Journal. 2010;9, Article number: 10.

1263 Cuhra M. Review of GMO safety assessment studies: glyphosate residues in Roundup Ready crops is an ignored issue. Environmental Sciences Europe. 2015;27, Article number: 20.

1264 Smith, Jeffrey M. Seeds of Deception: Exposing Industry and Government Lies About the Safety of the Genetically Engineered Foods You're Eating. Yes! Books, 2003.

1265 USDA FoodData Central. Chicken, broiler or fryers, breast, skinless, boneless, meat only, cooked, braised. **https://fdc.nal.usda.gov/fdc-app.html#/food-details/331960/nutrients**.

1266 Data courtesy of Karl Holovach, Frog Eye Vineyard, Medallion Labs Independent Analysis, 3 Mar 2021.

1267 Holovach, Karl. Frog Eye Vineyard. Knoxville, Maryland. Laboratory testing performed independently: Medallion Labs, Minneapolis, MN, 8 Jan 2021.

1268 De Marchi M, Costa A, Pozza M, et al. Detailed characterization of plant-based burgers. Scientific Reports. 2021;11, Article number: 2049.

1269 Angel Acres Farms egg data. Testing completed independently at The Fenton Lab, Michigan State University.

1270 Lutter CK, Iannotti LL, Stewart CP. The potential of a simple egg to improve maternal and child nutrition. Maternal and Child Nutrition. 2018;14(53):e12678.

1271 Washington State Department of Health. "Farmed Salmon vs. Wild Salmon. Washington State Department of Health. ND. Retrieved: **https://doh.wa.gov/community-and-environment/food/fish/farmed-salmon**. Accessed 3 Mar 2022.

1272 Carbonara F, dos Santos HMC, Montanher PF, et al. Distinguishing wild and farm-raised freshwater fish through fatty acid composition: Application of statistical tools. Eur J Lipid Sci Technol. 2014;30 May. **https://doi.org/10.1002/ejlt.201300339**.

1273 Jensen I-J. Eilertsen K-E, Otnaes CHA, et al. An Update on the Content of Fatty Acids, Dioxins, PCBs and Heavy Metals in Farmed, Escaped and Wild Atlantic Salmon (Salmo salr L.) in Norway. Foods. 2020;9:1901; doi:10.339/foods9121901.

1274 Burger J, Stern AH, Gochfeld M. Mercury in Commercial Fish: Optimizing Individual Choices to Reduce Risk. Environmental Health Perspectives. 2005;113(3). **https://doi.org/10.1289/ehp.7315**.

1275 EPA, United States Environmental Protection Agency. EPA-FDA Fish Advice: Technical Information. ND. Retrieved: **https://www.epa.gov/fish-tech/epa-fda-fish-advice-technical-information**. Accessed 3 Mar 2022.

1276 Muñoz A, Costa M. Nutritionally Mediated Oxidative Stress and Inflammation. Oxidative Medicine and Cellular Longevity. 2013; Article ID: 610950. **http://dx.doi.org/10.1155/2013/610950**.

1277 Jaarin K, Mustafa MR, Leong X-F. The effects of heated vegetable oils on blood pressure in rats. Clinics. 2011;66(12):2125-2132.

1278 Ng C-Y, Leong X-F, Masbah N, et al. Heated vegetable oils and cardiovascular disease risk factors. Vascular Pharmacology. 2014;61(1):1-9.

1279 Kaur N, Chugh V, Gupta AK. Essential fatty acids as functional components of foods- a review. Journ Food Sci Technol. 2014;51:2289-2303.

1280 Cisse V, Yemiscioglu F. Cacao Butter and Alternative Production. Cukurova J Agric Food Sci. 2019;34(1):37-50.

1281 Schroder KEE. Effects of fruit consumption on body mass index and weight loss in a sample of overweight and obese dieters enrolled in a weight-loss intervention trial. Nutrition. 2010;26(7-8):727-734.

1282 Conceição de Oliveira M, Sichieri R, Mozzer RV. A low-energy dense diet adding fruit reduces weight and energy intake in women. Appetite. 2008;51(2):291-295.

1283 Whigham LD, Valentine AR, Johnson LK, et al. Increased vegetable and fruit consumption during weight loss effort correlates with increased weight and fat loss. Nutrition and Diabetes. 2012, 2, e48.

1284 van der Windt DAWM, Jellema P, Mulder CJ. Diagnostic Testing for Celiac Disease Among Patients With Abdominal Symptoms. JAMA. 2010;303(17):1738-1746.

1285 U.S. Food & Drug Administration (FDA). GMO Crops, Animal Food, and Beyond. ND. Retrieved: **https://www.fda.gov/food/agricultural-biotechnology/gmo-crops-animal-food-and-beyond**. Accessed 4 Mar 2022.

1286 Seneff, Stephanie. Toxic Legacy – Howe the Weedkiller Glyphosate Is Destroying Our Health and the Environment. White River Junction, VT, Chelsea Green Publishing, 2021.

1287 American Academy of Environmental Medicine (AAEM). "Genetically Modified Foods." ND. Retrieved: **https://www.aaemonline.org/genetical-**

1288 Greenhill C. Benefits of time-restricted feeding. Nature Reviews Endocrinology. 2018;14:626.

1289 Boyd P, O'Connor SG, Heckman-Stoddard BM, Sauter ER. Time-Restricted Feeding Studies and Possible Human Benefit. JNCI Cancer Spectrum. 2022;6(3):pkac032.

1290 Cienfuegos S, McStay M, Gabel K, Varady KA. Time restricted eating for the prevention of type 2 diabetes. Journ Physiol. August 2021, **https://doi.org/10.1113/JP281101**.

1291 Gabel K, Cienfuegos S, Kalam F, et al. Time-Restricted Eating to Improve Cardiovascular Health. Current Atherosclerosis Reports. 2021:23, Article number: 22.

1292 Christensen RAG, Kirkham AA. Time-Restricted Eating: A Novel and Simple Dietary Intervention for Primary and Secondary Prevention of Breast Cancer and Cardiovascular Disease. Nutrients. 2021;13(10), 3476; **https://doi.org/10.3390/nu13103476**.

1293 Currenti W, Godos J, Castellano S, et al. Time restricted feeding and mental health: a review of possible mechanisms on affective and cognitive disorders. Int J Food Sci Nutr. 2020;72(6), **https://doi.org/10.1080/09637486.2020.1866504**.

1294 Long H, Panda S. Time-restricted feeding and circadian autophagy for long life. Nature Reviews Endocrinology. 2022;18:5-6.

1295 Al-Hadramy MS, Zawawi TH, Abdelwahab SM. Altered cortisol levels in relation to Ramadan. Eur J Clin Nutr. 1988;42(4):359-362.

1296 Sliman AF. Effect of fasting on some blood hormones in healthy Muslim males. Mu'tah J Res Stud. 1993;8:91-109.

1297 Bahammam A. Effect of fasting during Ramadan on sleep architecture, daytime sleepiness and sleep pattern. Sleep Biol Rhythms. 2004;2(2):135-143.

1298 Röjdmark S, Wetterberg L. Short-term fasting inhibits the nocturnal melatonin secretion in healthy man. Clin Endocrinol. 1989;30(4):451-457.

1299 Almeneessier AS, BaHammam AS. How does diurnal intermittent fasting impact sleep, daytime sleepiness, and markers of the biological clock? Current insights. Nature and Science of Sleep. 2018;10:439-452.

1300 Raza SA, Ishtiaq O, Unnikrishnan AG, et al. Thyroid diseases and Ramadan. Indian J Endocr Metab. 2012;16(4):522-524.

1301 Ikhsan M, Siregar MFG, Muharam R. The relationship between Ramadan fasting with menstrual cycle pattern changes in teenagers. Middle East Fertility Society Journal. 2017;22(1):43-47.

1302 Harsh C. "What Does it Really Mean to Eat Like a Pig?" World Animal Protection. 10 Jun 2021. Retrieved: **https://www.worldanimalprotection.us/**. Accessed 4 Mar 2022.

1303 Manusevich A. What Do Chickens Eat in a Day? World Animal Protection. 16 Dec 2021. Retrieved: **https://www.worldanimalprotection.us/blogs/what-do-chickens-eat-day**. Accessed 4 Mar 2022.

1304 Colombo SM, Mazal X. Investigation of the nutritional composition of different types of salmon available to Canadian consumers. Journal of Agriculture and Food Research. 2020;2:100056.

1305 Zheng T, Jia R, Cao L, et al. Effects of chronic glyphosate exposure on antioxidant status, metabolism and immune response in tilapia (GIFT, Oreochromis niloticus). Comp Biochem Physiol C Toxicol Pharmacol. 2021;239:108878.

1306 Price, Weston A. Nutrition and Physical Degeneration. Lemon Grove, CA: The Price-Pottenger Nutrition Foundation Inc; 1939, p.241.

1307 Sözen T, Özisik L, Basaran NC. An overview and management of osteoporosis. Eur J Rheumatol. 2017;4(1):46-56.

1308 Christakos S, Dhawan P, Porta A, et al. Vitamin D and Intestinal Calcium Absorption. Mol Cell Endocrinol. 2011;347(1-2):25-29.

1309 Fallon S, Enig MG. Cod Liver Oil Basics and Recommendations. 9 Feb 2009. Retrieved: **https://www.westonaprice.org/health-topics/cod-liver-oil/cod-liver-oil-basics-and-recommendations/**. Accessed 3 Mar 2022.

1310 Mora JC, Valencia WM. Exercise and Older Adults. Clin Geriatr Med. 2018;34(1):145-162.

1311 Karlsen T, Aamot I-L, Haykowsky M, Tognmo Ø. High Intensity Interval Training for Maximizing Health Outcomes. Progress in Cardiovascular Disease. 2017;60(1):67-77.

1312 Shillon RJS, Hasni S. Pathogenesis and Management of Sarcopenia. Clin Geriatr Med. 2017;33(1):17-26.

1313 Mesinovic J, Zengin A, De Courten B, et al. Sarcopenia and type 2 diabetes mellitus: a bidirectional relationship. Diabetes Metab Syndr Obes. 2019;12:1057-72.

1314 Sinclair AJ, Abdelhafiz AH, Rodriguez-Manas L. Frailty and sarcopenia—newly emerging and high impact complications of diabetes. J Diabetes Complications. 2017;31:1465-73.

1315 Lee JH, Yoon JS, Lee HW, et al. Risk factors affecting amputation in diabetic foot. Yeungnam Univ J Med. 2020;37:314-320.

1316 Kang SH, Do JY, Kim JC. The relationship between disability and clinical outcomes in maintainence dialysis patients. Yeungnam Univ J Med. 2020;38:127-35.

1317 Wu Z-J, Wang Z-Y, Gao H-E, et al. Impact of high-intensity interval training on cardiorespiratory fitness, body composition, physical fitness, and metabolic paramaters in older adults: A meta-analysis of randomized controlled trials. Experimental Gerentology. 2021;150:111345. Doi: 10.1016/j.exger.2021.111345.

ABOUT THE AUTHORS

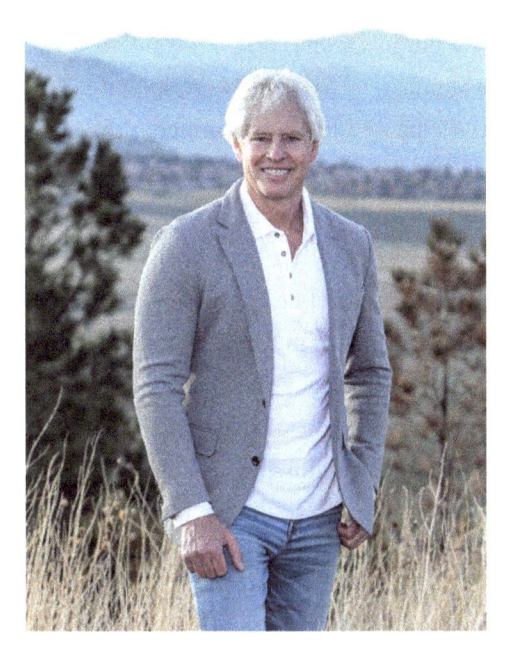

Chris A. Knobbe, MD

Chris A. Knobbe, MD, is a physician, ophthalmologist, nutrition researcher, published scientist, speaker, and Associate Clinical Professor Emeritus, formerly of the University of Texas Southwestern Medical Center, Dallas, Texas. Dr. Knobbe, a Weston A. Price acolyte since 2013, is known primarily for his research, papers, and presentations regarding the devastating effects of seed oils ('vegetable oils'). Knobbe is also known for his revolutionary hypothesis, research, and published science connecting Westernized diets and seed oils to the potentially blinding eye disease, age-related macular degeneration (AMD). Dr. Knobbe's research is deeply invested in seed oils ('vegetable oils') and their unequaled contributions to Westernized diseases, including heart disease, hypertension, stroke, cancers, type 2 diabetes, metabolic syndrome, obesity, and other chronic diseases. Dr. Knobbe and colleagues have a published paper regarding his hypothesis and supportive research regarding AMD in the journal *Medical Hypotheses*. Knobbe is the author of the book *Ancestral Dietary Strategy to Prevent and Treat Macular Degeneration*, available via online book retailers everywhere. Knobbe is a frequent speaker and lecturer to medical and lay audiences all across the U.S. and is now reaching international audiences via both online and in-person conferences.

Dr. Knobbe has been a frequent presenter for the Ancestral Health Symposium, the Weston A. Price Foundation, and the Macular Degeneration Association. He has presented to colleague physicians, researchers, ophthalmologists, optometrists, and vision scientists at these conferences as well as the Public Health Collaboration UK (University of Bristol, England), Metabolix (Tel Aviv, Israel), ALLDocs Annual Convention, Low Carb Denver, the Christian Ophthalmology Society, and the Eye Care Center of Northern Colorado. He has also been the featured guest on numerous podcasts and articles, including reviews and podcasts by Epoch Health, Dr. Joe Mercola, Dr. Eric Berg, Dr. Paul Saladino, Dr. Shawn Baker, and numerous others. In 2020, Dr. Knobbe was appointed the prestigious position of Honorary Board of Directors member for the Ocular Wellness & Nutrition Society (OWNS), where he also delivered the "keynote address" at their annual convention. Knobbe also recently gave the keynote address for the semi-annual convention of the American Academy for

Oral & Systemic Health (AAOSH), as well as the keynote address for the "Collaboration Cures" annual convention, which is the combined meeting of AAOSH and the American Academy of Physiological Medicine and Dentistry (AAPMD).

Dr. Knobbe is the proud father of daughter, Kyla, who has brought him more joy and blessings in life than anything else.

Dr. Knobbe has been certified by the American Board of Ophthalmology since 1997. He is the Founder and Director of both the Ancestral Health Foundation and Cure AMD Foundation, both IRS-qualified 501(c)(3) organizations. Dr. Knobbe accepts no book royalties or compensation for his research or roles in directing either organization.

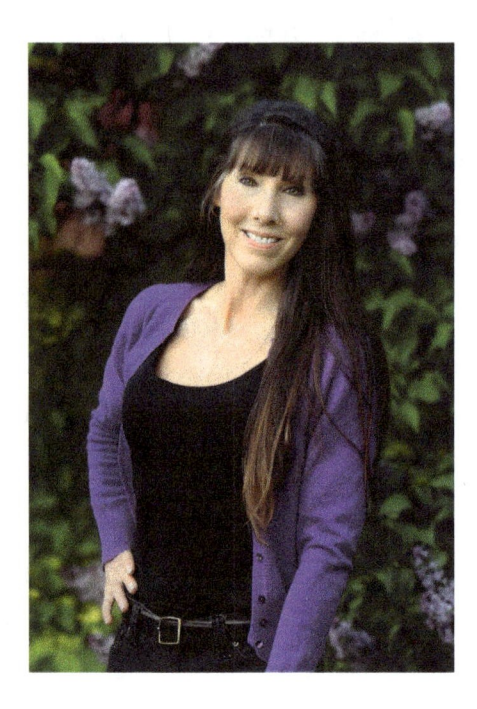

Suzanne Alexander, M.Ed.

Suzanne is a multi-award-winning educator with 30 years of experience in the classroom and an accomplished health and nutrition researcher with more than 40 years of research to her credit. She received her bachelor's and master's degrees in education from the State University of New York at Cortland. Additionally, Suzanne attended the Hartt School of Music at the University of Hartford in Connecticut with a major in Opera.

Suzanne was Miss New York State 1981 and Top Ten Finalist and Talent winner at the 1982 Miss America Pageant, where she never thought she'd find herself competing. Ironically, Suzanne was far more comfortable helping her father raise wild raccoons, skunks, foxes, squirrels, rats, and dogs, climbing trees, and running barefoot in nature while joyfully singing throughout each day. With this, she observed and studied how wild animals thrived, eating their species-specific diets and living in their natural habitats. Thus, she began implementing this knowledge into her own life to heal the health issues that plagued her since early childhood.

As family, friends, and colleagues know her, "Suz" studied health and nutrition for many decades and simultaneously educated her clients about healing their chronic illnesses utilizing an ancestral diet. She is now using her vast knowledge and experiences to work alongside Dr. Knobbe as a health and nutrition researcher and educator.

Suz is the Executive Director of Public Relations and Philanthropy at the Ancestral Health Foundation and Cure AMD Foundation. You can reach her via the foundations' website contact pages and social media on Facebook and Instagram.

Suzanne believes her greatest accomplishments and blessings are giving birth to and raising her two beautiful daughters, Alexandra and Roxana, and being a grandmother to her precious granddaughter, Claire.

Suz considers God as the author of her life. He is the center of all that she is and does!

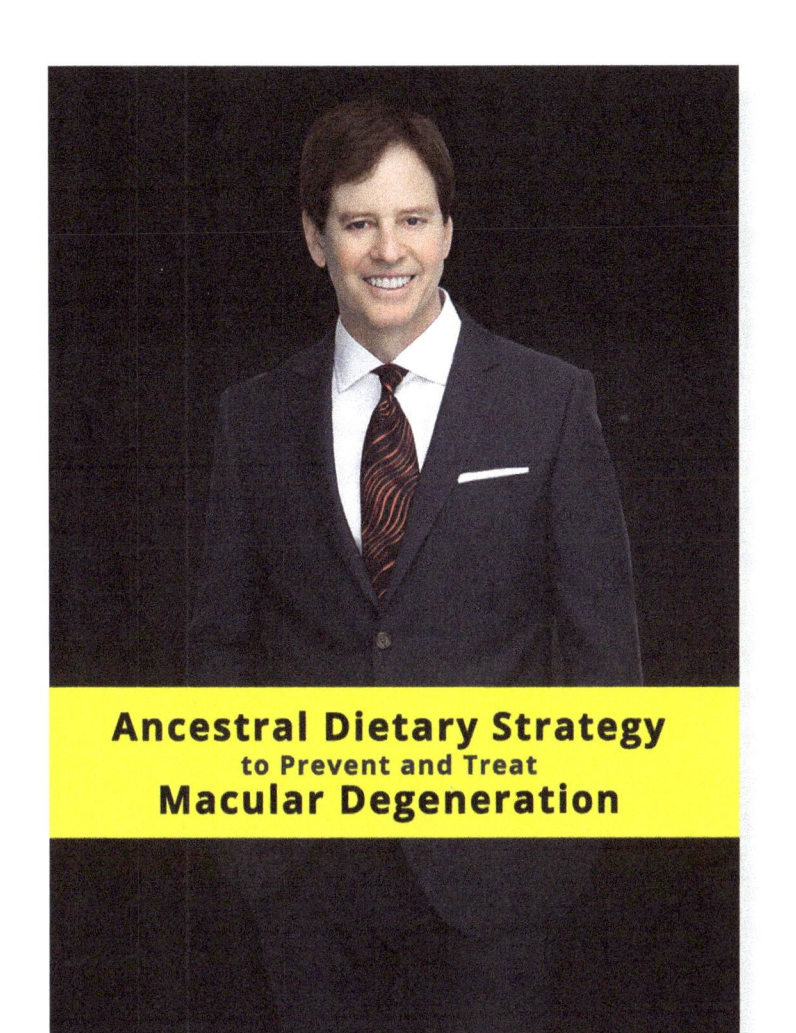

Ancestral Dietary Strategy
to Prevent and Treat
Macular Degeneration

CHRIS A. KNOBBE, M.D.
OPHTHALMOLOGIST & ASSOCIATE CLINICAL PROFESSOR EMERITUS
FOUNDER & PRESIDENT – CURE AMD FOUNDATION™

Seed Oil Free
Is the Key to
Being Disease Free

ANCESTRAL HEALTH FOUNDATION

Cure AMD Foundation

© C. Knobbe, 2022. Ancestral Health Foundation

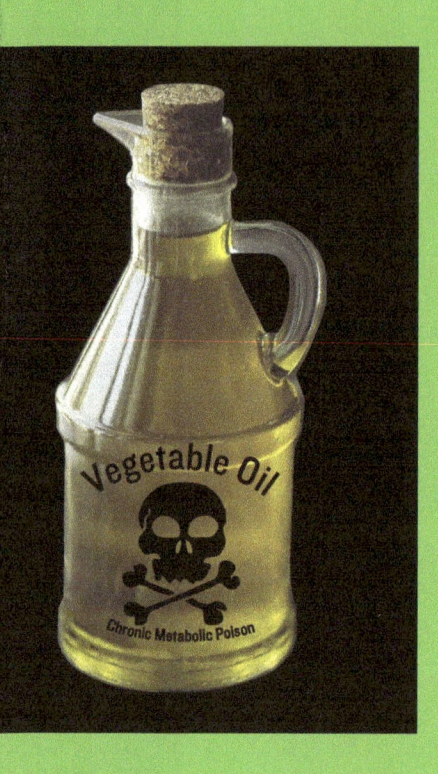

Vegetable Oil — Chronic Metabolic Poison

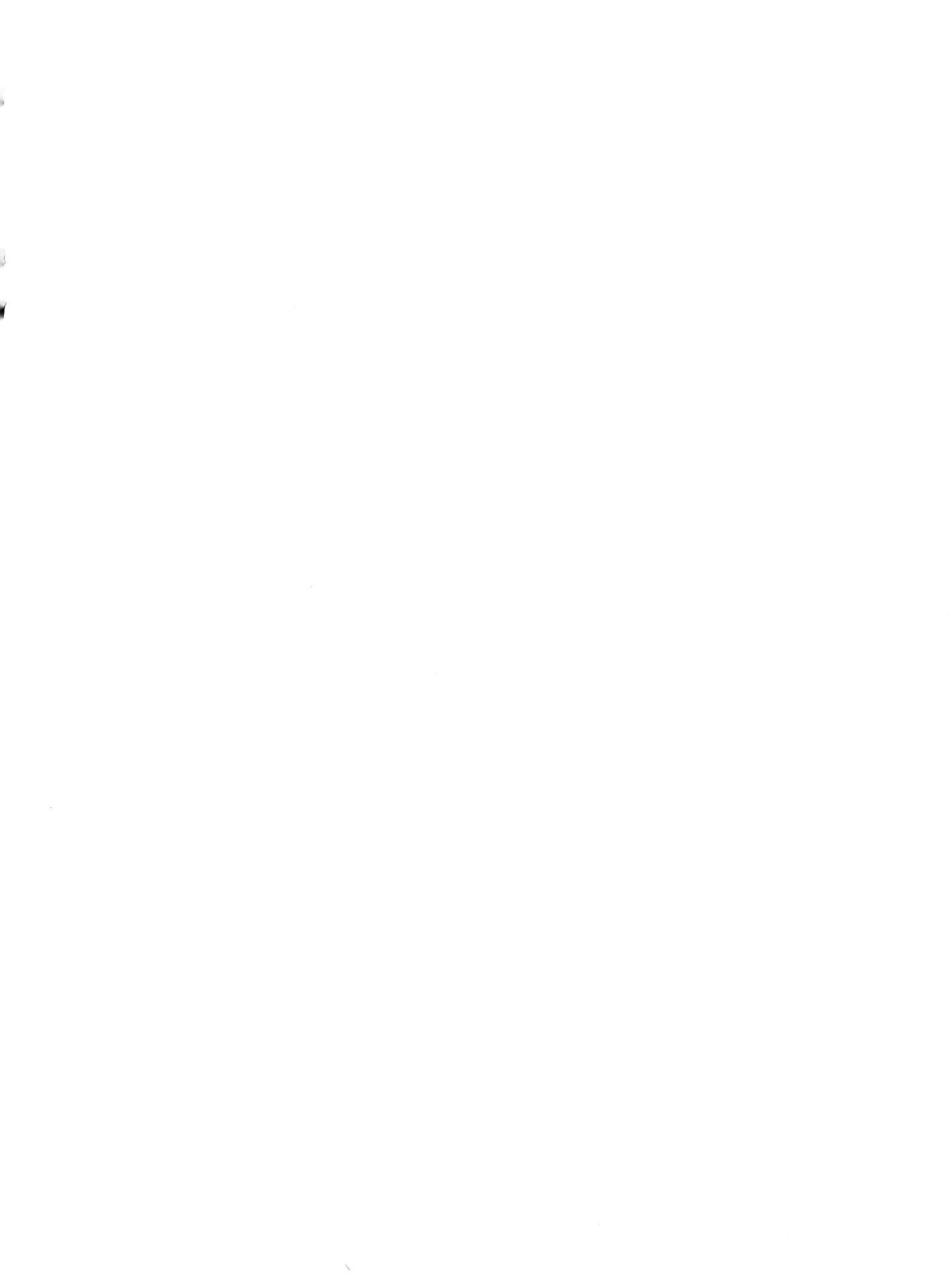

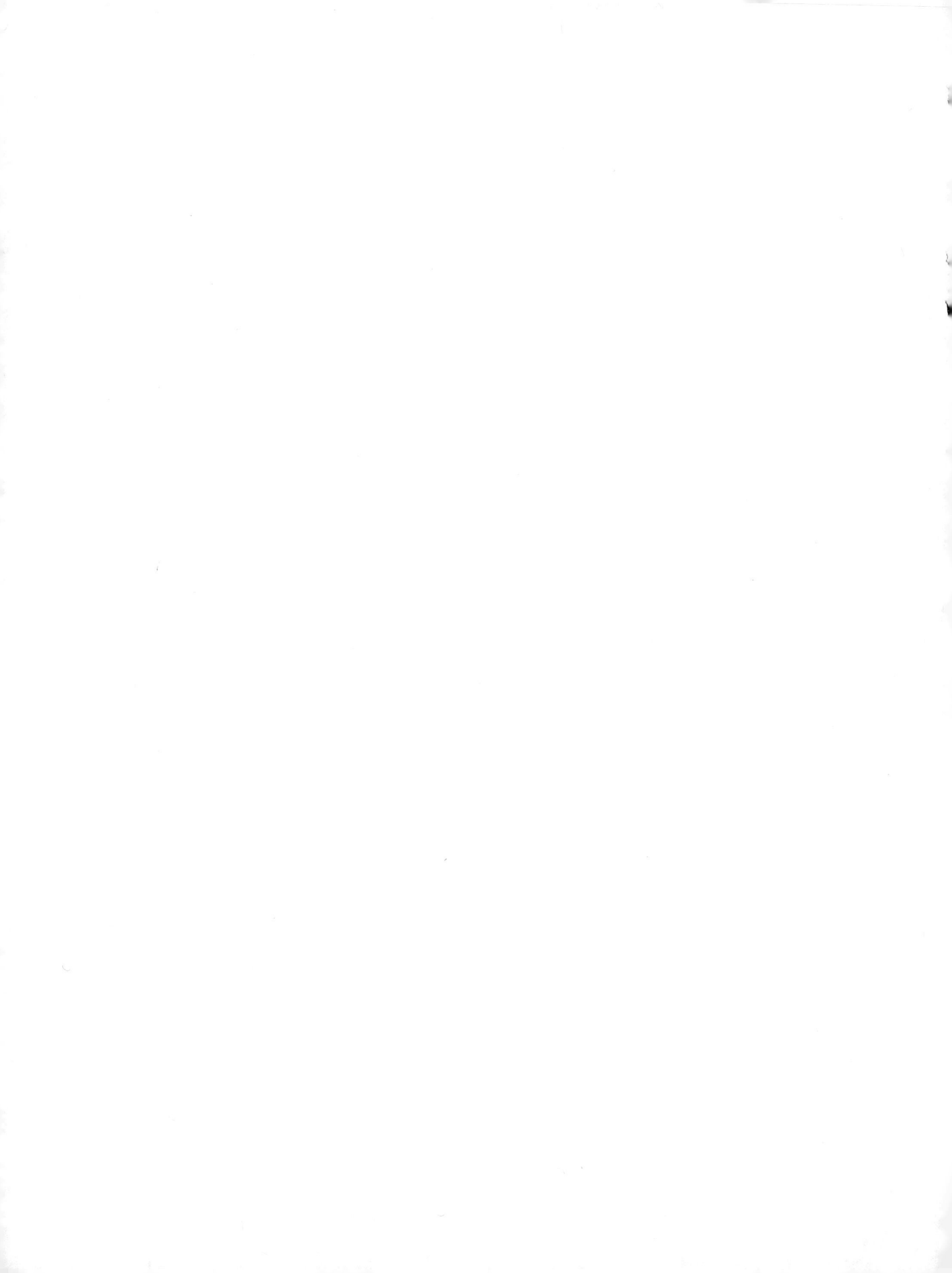

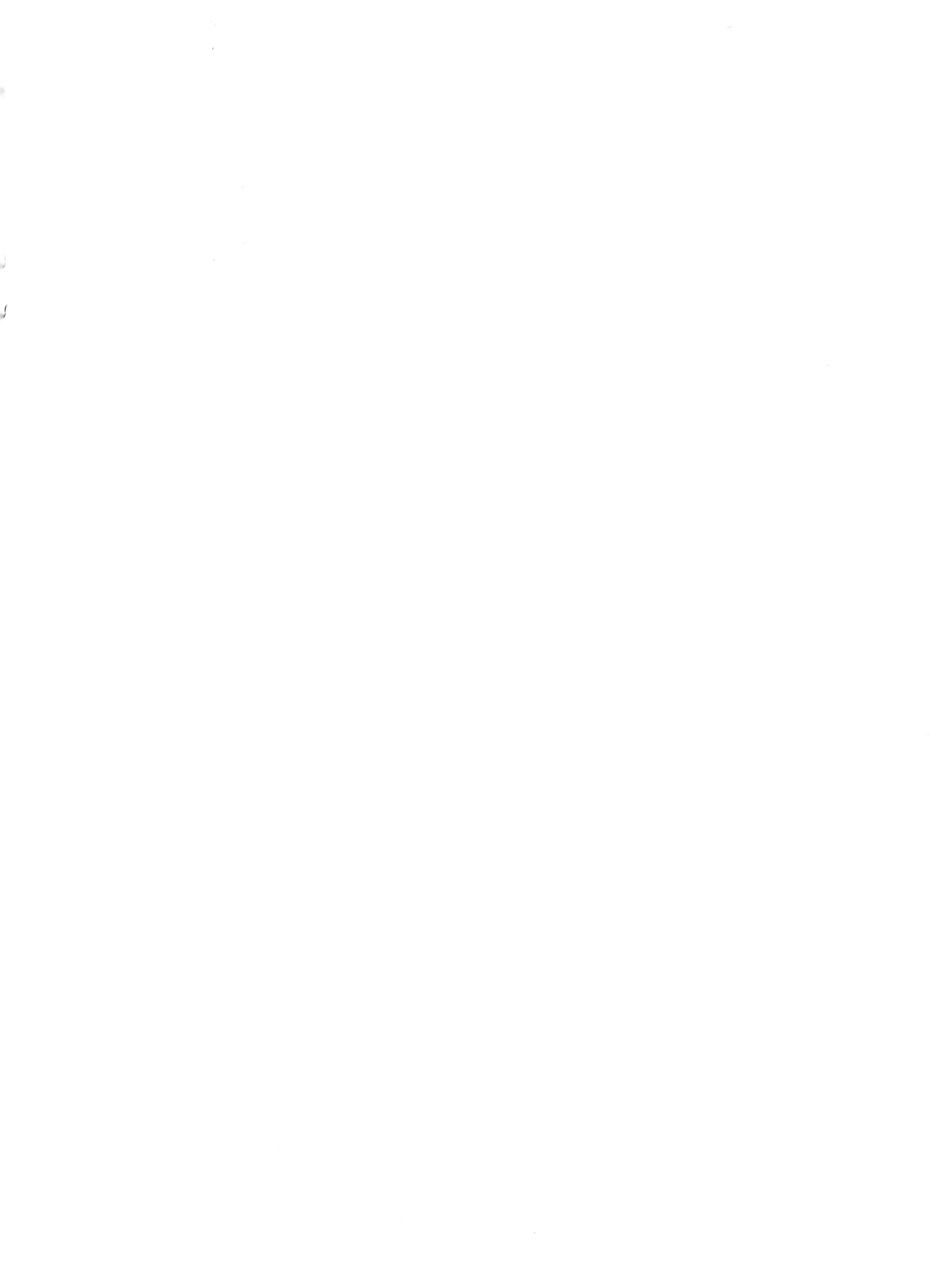